Biomedical Advances
in Aging

GWUMC Department of Biochemistry
Annual Spring Symposia

Series Editors:
Allan L. Goldstein, Ajit Kumar, and J. Martyn Bailey
The George Washington University Medical Center

BIOLOGY OF CELLULAR TRANSDUCING SIGNALS
Edited by Jack Y. Vanderhoek

BIOMEDICAL ADVANCES IN AGING
Edited by Allan L. Goldstein

CARDIOVASCULAR DISEASE
Molecular and Cellular Mechanisms, Prevention, and Treatment
Edited by Linda L. Gallo

CELL CALCIUM METABOLISM
Physiology, Biochemistry, Pharmacology, and Clinical Implications
Edited by Gary Fiskum

DIETARY FIBER IN HEALTH AND DISEASE
Edited by George V. Vahouny and David Kritchevsky

EUKARYOTIC GENE EXPRESSION
Edited by Ajit Kumar

NEURAL AND ENDOCRINE PEPTIDES AND RECEPTORS
Edited by Terry W. Moody

PROSTAGLANDINS, LEUKOTRIENES, AND LIPOXINS
Biochemistry, Mechanism of Action, and Clinical Applications
Edited by J. Martyn Bailey

THYMIC HORMONES AND LYMPHOKINES
Basic Chemistry and Clinical Applications
Edited by Allan L. Goldstein

Biomedical Advances in Aging

Edited by
Allan L. Goldstein
The George Washington University Medical Center
Washington, D.C.

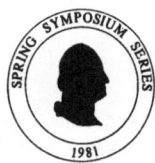

Plenum Press • New York and London

Library of Congress Cataloging-in-Publication Data

Biomedical advances in aging / edited by Allan L. Goldstein.
        p.   cm. -- (GWUMC Department of Biochemistry annual spring
symposia)
    Based on the VIII Annual International Spring Symposium on Health
Sciences, held at the George Washington University School of
Medicine in Washington, D.C. in 1988.
    Includes bibliographical references.
    ISBN-13: 978-1-4612-7844-3   e-ISBN-13: 978-1-4613-0513-2
    DOI: 10.1007/978-1-4613-0513-2

    1. Aging--Molecular aspects--Congresses. 2. Aging--Physiolical
aspects--Congresses. 3. Aged--Diseases--Congresses.   I. Goldstein,
Allan L. II. International Spring Symposium on Health Sciences (8th
: 1988 : George Washington University School of Medicine)
III. Series.
    [DNLM: 1. Aging--congresses.   WT 104 B6158 1988]
QP86.B527 1990
618.97'07--dc20
DNLM/DLC
for Library of Congress   89-72140
                                                              CIP

© 1990 Plenum Press, New York
Softcover reprint of the hardcover 1st edition 1990

A Division of Plenum Publishing Corporation
233 Spring Street, New York, N.Y. 10013

Preface

The VIIIth Annual International Spring Symposium on Health Sciences held at the George Washington University School of Medicine in Washington, D.C., attracted over three hundred fifty scientists from twenty-five countries. The leading scientific experts in the field reported on recent biomedical advances in aging. They provided an up-to-date account of the molecular, genetic, nutritional, and immunological mechanisms associated with the aging process and approaches to intervention and treatment of the major disorders associated with the aging process, including Alzheimer's disease.

A unique aspect of this meeting was a concurrent one-day hearing of the U.S. Senate Sub-Committee on Aging, organized by the Alliance for Aging Research. The theme for the hearing was "Advances in Aging Research." Seven scientists attending our aging symposium were asked to testify. They were Drs. Carl Cotman (University of California–Irvine), Trudy Bush (Johns Hopkins University), Takashi Makinodan (University of California–Los Angeles), William Ershler (University of Wisconsin–Madison), Gino Doria (ENEA, Rome), Mr. Dan Perry (Director of the Alliance for Aging Research), and myself.

At the symposium the Abraham White Distinguished Scientific Award was presented to the Nobel laureate Dr. D. Carleton Gajdusek and his colleague Dr. C. Joseph Gibbs, Jr., who were honored for their pioneering research and scientific contributions in the field of virology. These distinguished scientists were also the first recipients of the Lifetime Science and Humanitarian medal of the Institute for Advanced Studies in Immunology and Aging. Also honored at the meeting was Representative Claude Pepper, who received the annual Public Service award, and who was the recipient of the Lifetime Public Service and Humanitarian award from the Institute for Advanced Studies in Immunology and Aging. Representative Pepper was honored for his creative leadership and outstanding achievements over the past fifty years in the United States Senate and in the House of Representatives, and for his longtime commitment to support for biomedical research and improving the health and welfare of older Americans.

This volume, which contains 56 chapters, provides new information dealing with molecular and immunological mechanisms, intervention and clinical approaches to treatment of diseases associated with aging, and with the aging process itself. The volume is divided into six major sections. Part I deals with the molecular biology, virology, and genetics of Alzheimer's disease. This section includes contributions by leading virologists and geneticists who discuss the role of viruses in neurodegenerative diseases and molecular, biochemical, and immunological aspects of Alzheimer's disease and senile dementia. The second section of the book deals with metabolic, membrane, and cellular markers and models for aging. The section contains a number of interesting hypotheses developed to provide insights into the aging process. The third section of the volume deals with the latest advances in nutritional, dietary, and immune factors in the pathogenesis of aging, and includes outstanding chapters on "nutritional requirements in aging" by David Kritchevsky, and the "effects of caloric restriction and longevity" by Richard Weindruch. The fourth section of the volume deals with studies on the characterization of the key immunological components and mechanisms of immune regulation in the aging process. These reports suggest that the thymus plays a vital role in the functioning of T cells and in the aging of the immune system. Part 5 of the volume deals with the brain, neuroendocrine circuits, pathology, and plasticity. In this section we learn from Drs. Robert Terry, Marian Diamond, Donald Ingram, and other specialists on changes in the neuronal populations in the brain that occur with the aging process, and on the apparent resiliency of the aging brain, along with the potential for modeling age-related memory dysfunctions.

The last section of the volume, which is primarily clinical research, deals with immunological, endocrine, and pharmacological approaches to the treatment of diseases of aging. In these chapters, Drs. Ershler, Shen, and their colleagues present data documenting the ability to enhance immune function in normal elderly people using administration of thymosin and other immune modulators. These studies show very clearly that there is a resiliency to the decaying immune system with age that can be enhanced by immunological intervention. Drs. Miller, LaRosa, and Muesing present exciting new data regarding the potential role of estrogen in altering lipid and lipoprotein changes in postmenopausal women and in lowering the incidence of cardiovascular disease in this high-risk population. Finally, Dr. Charles Hennekens provides an update on the potential role of aspirin in lowering the risks of cardiovascular disease in the Physicians' Health Study.

What is emerging in the clinical arena is a clear recognition that it is possible to intervene in the aging process as regards improving the health of elderly individuals through hormonal, immunological, and pharmacological intervention. Whether these studies will translate into prolongevity itself has not yet been established. This volume should be of interest not only to the basic scientist interested in understanding the most recent advances in the biochemical, immunological, and genetic components of aging, but also to clinicians, gerontologists, and geriatricians involved in providing better health care for the elderly. The volume also provides many insights into the future directions of aging research.

Allan L. Goldstein

Washington, D.C.

Contents

PART V—THE BRAIN, NEUROENDOCRINE CIRCUITS, PATHOLOGY, AND PLASTICITY

Molecular Biology, Virology, and Genetics of Alzheimer's Disease

I

Brain Amyloidoses

Precursor Proteins and the Amyloids of Transmissible and Nontransmissible Dementias: Scrapie–Kuru–CJD Viruses as Infectious Polypeptides or Amyloid-Enhancing Factors

D. CARLETON GAJDUSEK and C. JOSEPH GIBBS, JR.

1. INTRODUCTION

Kuru and the transmissible virus dementias are in a group of virus-induced slow infections that we have described as *subacute spongiform virus encephalopathies* because of the strikingly similar histopathological lesions they induce. Scrapie, mink encephalopathy, the chronic wasting disease with spongiform encephalopathy of captive mule deer and of captive elk, and bovine spongiform encephalopathy all appear, from their histopathology, pathogenesis, and the similarities of their infectious agents, to belong to the same group (Gajdusek and Gibbs, 1975; Gajdusek *et al.*, 1965, 1966; Hope *et al.*, 1988; Masters *et al.*, 1981a,b; Wilesmith *et al.*, 1988; Williams and Young, 1980, 1982; Williams *et al.*, 1982). The basic neurocytological lesions in all these diseases are a progressive vacuolation in the dendritic and axonal processes and cell bodies of neurons and, to a lesser extent, in astrocytes and oligodendrocytes; an extensive astroglial hypertrophy and proliferation; and spongiform change or status spongiosis of gray matter and extensive neuronal loss (Beck *et al.*, 1975, 1982; Klatzo *et al.*, 1959).

These atypical infections differ from other diseases of the human brain subsequently demonstrated to be slow virus infections in that they do not evoke a virus-associated inflammatory response in the brain (i.e., no perivascular cuffing or invasion of the brain parenchyma with leukocytes); they usually show no pleocytosis or marked rise in protein in the cerebrospinal fluid (CSF) throughout the course of infection (Gajdusek, 1985b; Gajdusek and Zigas, 1957, 1959; Traub *et al.*, 1977). Furthermore, they show no evidence of an immune response to the causative virus, and there are no recognizable virions in sections of the brain

D. CARLETON GAJDUSEK and C. JOSEPH GIBBS, JR. • Laboratory of Central Nervous System Studies, National Institute of Neurological Disorders and Stroke, National Institutes of Health, Bethesda, Maryland 20892.

visualized by electron microscopy, whereas in other virus encephalopathies virions have been readily observed. Instead, they show ultrastructural alteration in the plasma membrane lining the vacuoles (Beck *et al.*, 1982), piled-up neurofilament in some swollen nerve cells (Beck *et al.*, 1975, 1982; Klatzo *et al.*, 1959; Lampert *et al.*, 1971), and strange arrays of regularly arrayed tubules that look like particles in cross section in postsynaptic processes (Baringer *et al.*, 1979, 1981; David-Ferreira *et al.*, 1968; Field and Narang, 1972; Field *et al.*, 1969; Lamar *et al.*, 1974; Narang, 1973, 1974a,b; Narang *et al.*, 1972, 1980; Vernon *et al.*, 1970; ZuRhein and Varakis, 1976).

The pursuit of the transmissibility and viral etiology of kuru (Gajdusek and Zigas, 1957, 1959; Gajdusek *et al.*, 1966; Klatzo *et al.*, 1959) and the presenile dementia of the Creutz-feldt–Jakob disease (CJD) type (Gajdusek, 1977; Gajdusek and Gibbs, 1975; Gibbs *et al.*, 1968) has led to the definition of the unconventional viruses as a new group of microbes. Because of their very atypical physical, chemical, and biological properties, this new definition has stimulated a worldwide quest to elucidate their structures and resolve the many paradoxes they present to the basic tenets of microbiology and to solve the enormous clinical and epidemiological problems these viruses pose. The unanticipated ramifications of the discovery of these slow infections and the peculiar properties of the unconventional viruses, which have even challenged the central dogma of modern molecular biology, have led to a series of discoveries, each of which has wide implications for microbiological and neurobiological research (Braig and Diringer, 1985; Diringer *et al.*, 1983; Gajdusek, 1977, 1984, 1985a,b,c; Gajdusek and Gibbs, 1975; Masters *et al.*, 1981a,b, 1985a,b; Multhaup *et al.*, 1985; Oesch *et al.*, 1985; Prusiner, 1982, 1984; Prusiner *et al.*, 1983, 1984; Robertson *et al.*, 1985; Rohwer, 1984a,b,c, 1985; Rohwer and Gajdusek, 1980; Rohwer *et al.*, 1979). We now believe these viruses are infectious proteins autonucleating and autopatterning a configurational change in a host precursor protein to an infectious form (see Fig. 1).

2. INTERFERENCE WITH AXONAL TRANSPORT LEADS TO AMYLOID FORMATION FROM A HOST PRECURSOR PROTEIN IN TRANSMISSIBLE AND NONTRANSMISSIBLE DEMENTIAS

The cytoskeleton of all cells contains three ultrastructurally distinct elements made of fibrous macromolecules: microtubules 24 nm in diameter, intermediate filaments 10 nm in diameter, and microfilaments ~5 nm in diameter and composed of polymerized actin.

Neurofilaments, also called neuronal intermediate filaments, are antigenically distinct from the intermediate filaments of other cells. They extend from the cell body down the whole length of the axon; they are composed of three proteins of 200, 150, and 68 kilodaltons (kDa), respectively. Our work on the etiology of kuru (Gajdusek, 1977, 1984, 1985a,b,c; Gajdusek and Gibbs, 1975; Gajdusek and Zigas, 1957, 1959; Gajdusek *et al.*, 1965, 1966; Klatzo *et al.*, 1959) and on the cause of amyotrophic lateral sclerosis and parkinsonism dementia (ALS/PD) with the early appearance of neurofibrillary tangles (NFT) (Anderson *et al.*, 1979; Chen, 1981) in the populations in high-incidence foci in the Western Pacific (Gajdusek, 1988; Gajdusek and Salazar, 1982; Garruto *et al.*, 1982, 1984, 1986; Perl *et al.*, 1982) has pointedly emphasized the pooling and stagnation of this molecular complex in chromatolytic neurons (Gajdusek, 1984, 1985a,b,c; Hirano and Inoue, 1980; Hirano *et al.*, 1984a,b).

Interference with axonal transport is responsible for such stagnation or pooling of

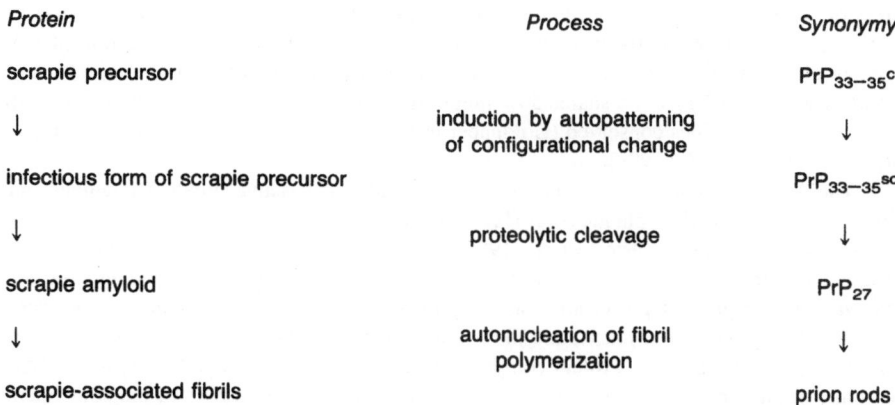

Protein	Process	Synonymy
scrapie precursor		$PrP_{33-35}{}^c$
↓	induction by autopatterning of configurational change	↓
infectious form of scrapie precursor		$PrP_{33-35}{}^{sc}$
↓	proteolytic cleavage	↓
scrapie amyloid		PrP_{27}
↓	autonucleation of fibril polymerization	↓
scrapie-associated fibrils		prion rods

FIGURE 1. *De novo* generation of infectious scrapie proteins from scrapie precursor.

cytoskeletal elements and for the subsequent degradation to amyloid fibrils of the sequestered or trapped proteins to form paired helical filaments (PHF) in the NFT and the straight filaments of neuritic plaques that characterize Alzheimer's disease (AD) (Autilio-Gambetti *et al.*, 1983; Gambetti *et al.*, 1983; Bizzi *et al.*, 1983; Dahl and Bignami, 1985; Gambetti *et al.*, 1983a,b; Hirano and Inoue, 1980; Hirano *et al.*, 1984a,b; Inoue and Hirano, 1979; Klatzo *et al.*, 1965; Rasool and Selkoe, 1985; Selkoe *et al.*, 1986; Sotelo *et al.*, 1980b; Terry and Pena, 1965). Furthermore, it now appears that amyloid deposits in the nervous system, particularly the amyloid plaques of Alzheimer's disease and those of Down's syndrome, Pick's disease, and the normal aging and the perivascular accumulations of amyloid in the central nervous system (CNS) and in the vascular walls extending out into the meninges are derived from a precursor protein (amyloid β-protein or A4) trapped in these cytoskeletal accumulations, while the paired helical filaments of NFT may represent yet further intracellular degradation of the same precursor protein in the stagnated cytoskeletal elements (Glenner and Wong, 1984a,b; Guiroy *et al.*, 1987; Kidd *et al.*, 1985; Masters *et al.*, 1985a,b; Schubert *et al.*, 1988). We earlier presumed that the precursor for these brain amyloid fibrils is the 200-kDa component of the protein triad from which 10-nm neurofilaments are formed or microtubule-associated proteins τ (MAP-τ) (Anderton *et al.*, 1982; Gajdusek, 1984, 1985a). However, Goldgaber *et al.* (1987a,b) isolated, sequenced, and characterized complementary DNA (cDNA) clones coding for this precursor protein from the adult human brain cDNA library. This gene was localized on chromosome 21 in man. Kang *et al.* (1987) also isolated and sequenced the cDNA coding for the same protein from the fetal human brain cDNA library; Tanzi *et al.* (1987) and Robakis *et al.* (1987) later isolated the same gene. Down's syndrome patients carry three copies of this gene and overexpress this precursor and thus express NFT, amyloid plaque cores (APC), and congophilic angiopathy (CA) 50 years earlier than do normal subjects (Delabar *et al.*, 1987), but we cannot reconfirm that AD patients carry three copies of the gene as we first reported (Delabar *et al.*, 1987). However, since virtually every human brain shows NFT, APC, or CA by 100 years of age, no abnormal gene is needed for the production of this amyloid.

The normal amyloid precursor β-protein gene is overexpressed in brains of Alzheimer's disease patients (Higgins *et al.*, 1988; Schmerchle *et al.*, 1988; Cohen *et al.*, 1988). It also encodes several different messenger RNA (mRNA) that are identical except for the expression of a 168-basepair (bp)-long exon, or an added 225-bp-long exon immediately following, at position 289 (between the G and TT of a GTT valine codon) of the full mRNA without either of these inserts. This alternative splicing results in a 57- or a 76-amino acid insert. The 168-bp-long exon shares 50% homology to Kunitz-type protease inhibitors, with all six cysteine residues conserved (Goldgaber et al., 1988; Kitaguchi et al., 1988; Ponte et al., 1988; Tanzi et al., 1988).

The 4.1 kDa subunit polypeptide (42 amino acids) of vascular amyloid (Glenner and Wong, 1984a,b), amyloid plaque cores (Masters et al., 1985b), as well as the PHF from NFT of Alzheimer's disease (Masters et al., 1985a) all have the same amino acid sequence with progressively more N-terminal heterogeneity (Masters et al., 1985a,b). This finding indicates that vascular amyloid deposits are least degraded from the host precursor protein, core amyloid of amyloid plaques next, and the amyloid polypeptide of PHF most degraded from this same precursor protein. Protein components of microtubules (α- and β-tubulin or MAP proteins) might well be copolymerized or passively caught in the masses of amyloid fibers which appear in perivascular deposits or in neuritic or amyloid plaques and NFT. It appears that the β-protein precursor of amyloid, the gene for which we have identified on chromosome 21 in humans, is an excreted or membrane-anchored protein caught in this mass of collapsed pooled cytoskeletal elements (Schubert et al., 1988).

Hirano and co-workers demonstrated ultrastructurally minute masses of amyloid fibers and of regular paracrystalline arrays of particles or tubules within packed masses of piled up NF in spheroids that have formed from such swollen perikaryons or axonal swellings in motor neurons of the spinal cord in amyotrophic lateral sclerosis (Inoue and Hirano, 1979; Hirano and Inoue, 1980; Hirano et al., 1984a,b). Kirschner et al. (1986) pointed out that the α-helical structure of the 200-kDa component of neurofilaments does not lend itself to degeneration to the β-pleated sheet structure common to all brain amyloids and that perhaps MAP-τ is the more likely precursor. It too is accumulated in pooled masses of neurofilaments (Grundke-Iqbal et al., 1986; Kosik et al., 1986; Wood et al., 1986). Copolymerization or firm associations of the amyloid β-protein fibrils with a β-pleated peptide derived from MAP-τ appears to be likely (Gajdusek, 1988b; Guiroy and Gajdusek, 1988). However, we do not yet know the normal function of the precursor protein for aging brain amyloid polypeptide formation.

Thus, interference with axonal transport of neurofilament may be a basic mechanism of pathogenesis that leads to (1) pooling of the cytoskeletal elements, associated proteins, and matrix proteins in the perikaryon or axonal cylinders and lysis of the neuron as in ALS and other motor neuron diseases; (2) amyloid and neuritic plaque formation, from degradation in AD and many other CNS degenerations of a precursor β-protein, which is a transmembrane protein anchored to the external membrane surface or excreted; and (3) neurofibrillary tangle formation with the same precursor protein further modified to form paired helical filaments probably copolymerized or otherwise associated with numerous proteins of the cytoskeleton. We know that the precursor β-protein is synthesized in neurons and probably in microglial and oligodendroglial and some cerebrovascular endothethial cells as well (Bahmanyar et al., 1987; Fukatsu et al., 1984a,b; Goldgaber et al., 1987a,b; Schmechle et al., 1988). It is released into the extracellular space by all these cells and has a very high turnover rate.

3. TWO FORMS OF AMYLOID IN CEREBRAL PLAQUES

The larger more regular amyloid plaques of kuru, of CJD and its Gerstmann–Sträussler variant, and of scrapie are thus composed of a scrapie amyloid protein (PrP_{27-30}), a configurationally changed and proteolytically cleaved product of a normal host-specified scrapie precursor protein (PrP$_{35-37}$c) (Fig. 1). The cDNA for this precursor protein has been sequenced (Oesch *et al.*, 1985) and much of the oligonucleotide sequence confirmed by amino acid sequencing of parts of the isolated precursor (Multhaup *et al.*, 1985). The gene for this precursor protein of the amyloid of the transmissible dementias is located on chromosome 20 in man, on 2 in mouse.

Prusiner calls this scrapie-modified host-specified scrapie amyloid protein his "prion" protein (PrP$_{27-30}$) (Bendheim *et al.*, 1984; Bolton *et al.*, 1985; Multhaup *et al.*, 1985; Oesch *et al.*, 1985; Prusiner, 1982, 1984; Prusiner *et al.*, 1983, 1984; Rohwer, 1984c). In CJD, the amyloid in plaque cores carries the same immunologic specificity as those of kuru and scrapie (Bendheim *et al.*, 1984; Bockman *et al.*, 1985; Braig and Diringer, 1985; Brown *et al.*, 1986a; Manuelidis, 1985; Manuelidis *et al.*, 1985) and very closely the same amino acid sequence as does the purified scrapie amyloid protein (27–30 kDa) of scrapie-associated fibrils (SAF) from hamsters or mice. The microheterogeneity of the CJD plaque polypeptide is the result of cleavage from different regions of the same host precursor protein.

In sharp contrast, the amyloid of AD and Down's syndrome and normal aging brain is composed of a self-aggregating 4.1-kDa amyloid polypeptide subunit of 42 amino acids (β-protein or A4 protein) (Glenner and Wong, 1984a; Masters *et al.*, 1985a,b; Wong *et al.*, 1985). The cDNA clones coding for this amyloid subunit have been isolated and characterized by D. Goldgaber and M. Lerman and their co-workers (1987a,b) and by Kang *et al.* (1987), Robakis *et al.* (1987), and Tanzi *et al.* (1987). This aging brain amyloid precursor protein yields a 42 amino acid nonglycosylated polypeptide monomer very different from the glycosylated 27–30 kDa monomer of kuru–CJD–scrapie amyloid. It is specified by a gene on chromosome 21 in man, on 16 in mouse.

Thus there are two forms of brain amyloid: that of the transmissible dementias caused by infectious polypeptides (unconventional viruses) and that of Alzheimer's disease, aged Down's syndrome, Guamanian ALS/PD, and normal aging. The respective precursors are specified by different genes located in man on chromosomes 20 and 21, respectively (in mouse on chromosomes 2 and 16, respectively). Whether these amyloids are formed from a neuronal, microglial, or serum-borne precursor has been the problem. It now appears that the amyloid in NFT is formed from neuronal synthesized precursor; extracellular amyloid of plaques and congophilic angiopathy may be of microglial and vascular endothelial origin (Fukatsu, 1984a,b; Higgins *et al.*, 1988).

The intramolecular mechanism of configurational changes that occur to produce the regularly oriented β-pleated sheet configuration of amyloid proteins from the precursor is unknown. The known sequences of the amyloid in perivascular deposits (Glenner and Wong, 1984a,b; Wong *et al.*, 1985), plaque cores (Masters *et al.*, 1985b), and PHF of neurofibrillary tangles (Masters *et al.*, 1985a; Guiroy *et al.*, 1987), which are all alike, do not correspond with the amino acid sequence of the amyloid protein of SAF (Bondheim *et al.*, 1985; Bolton *et al.*, 1985; Multhaup *et al.*, 1985; Oesch *et al.*, 1985; Prusiner *et al.*, 1984). Furthermore, neither precursor shows any homology with the sequences for the major components of the cytoskeleton: the three proteins components of neurofilaments, α- or β-tubulin, or MAP II or MAP-τ or actin (Geisler *et al.*, 1985; Lewis and Cowan, 1985). Thus, we are dealing with two different precursor proteins and two different amyloid polypeptides, or small proteins, derived from them in the transmissible and the nontransmissible dementias, respectively. The two host-specified precursor proteins are transmembrane proteins protruding from the cell surface of normal cells. The normal function of the scrapie precursor protein is completely unknown. The aging brain amyloid precursor of β/A4 protein subunit of aging and Alzheimer's disease has recently been found to be protease nexin-II, a protease inhibitor that forms inhibitory complexes with epidermal growth factor-binding protein and the γ subunit of nerve growth factor (Van Nostrand *et al.*, 1989).

In the course of scrapie infection, the scrapie precursor protein undergoes a configurational change in secondary structure to an infectious form without change in amino acid sequence. This configurational change renders it protease-resistant and insoluble. It can still be cleaved at only one site to form the scrapie amyloid protein, which is easily polymerized into fibrils (SAF) (see Fig. 1).

4. SCRAPIE-ASSOCIATED FIBRILS

In density-gradient preparations of scrapie-affected brain suspensions, Merz and Somerville demonstrated amyloid-like two-stranded fibers—each fiber composed of two protofibrils—that increase in quantity with virus titer (Merz *et al.*, 1981, 1984a,b). We have found these structures in the brain of CJD patients and in the brain of primates with experimental CJD and kuru, but not in normal control brains or brains of patients with other neurodegenerative diseases (Brown *et al.*, 1985; Gajdusek, 1985c; Merz *et al.*, 1984a,b). It was early postulated that these structures may represent the scrapie or CJD or kuru infectious agent (Gajdusek, 1985b; Merz *et al.*, 1981, 1984a,b; Prusiner, 1984; Prusiner *et al.*, 1983). It now appears that this monomeric scrapie amyloid subunit is infectious (Ceroni et al., 1989; Safar *et al.*, 1989a,b,c). Such structures bring to mind the filamentous plant viruses and filamentous phage fd, which are of about the same diameters. No nucleic acid has been demonstrated in purified preparations of SAF proteins. SAF are still more intriguing, as they are the central core of cigar-like tubulofilamentous structures in scrapie and CJD brains (Narang *et al.*, 1987) but are obscured by an outer coat of proteinaceous material and an inner coat of host single-stranded DNA (Narang *et al.*, 1988).

These scrapie-associated fibrils (SAF), which are composed of infectious monomers, are distinguishable ultrastructurally from the paired helical filaments (PHF) of neurofibrillary tangles and the fibrils of brain amyloid (Merz *et al.*, 1981, 1984a,b). However, their similarity is misleading because they do not share antigenicity with the PHF of NFT or with the amyloid fibrils in the amyloid plaques of aging, Alzheimer's disease, and Down's syndrome. Thus, some antisera, both polyclonal and monoclonal, to the PHF of Alzheimer's disease NFT cross-react with the purified subunit protein of amyloid from plaque cores of senile plaques (Autilio-Gambetti *et al.*, 1983; Gambetti *et al.*, 1983a,b; Rasool and Selkoe, 1985; Selkoe *et al.*, 1985). However, most antisera to amyloid plaque cores do not react with NFT. Neither of these antisera reacts, however, with the SAF of scrapie (Kingsbury *et al.*, 1985; Manuelidis, 1985).

Antibodies to scrapie amyloid protein of SAF cross-react strongly on Western blots with the subunit protein of SAF from CJD- (Bendheim *et al.*, 1985; Brown *et al.*, 1985) and kuru- (Brown *et al.*, 1986a) affected brains. However, such SAF-specific sera do not react with neurofilaments nor with PHF or plaque core amyloid from Alzheimer's disease (Bendheim *et al.*, 1985; C. J. Gibbs, Jr., and D. C. Gajdusek, unpublished data).

5. VIRUSES PROVOKING NO IMMUNE RESPONSE AND EVIDENCING NO NONHOST ANTIGEN

The CJD–kuru–scrapie-like slow viruses first invade the reticuloendothelial cells and particularly low-density lymphocytes in the spleen. Yet, they provoke no antibody response that can be demonstrated using as antigen live virus preparation of high infectious titers (Gajdusek, 1985a,b; Gajdusek and Gibbs, 1975; Kasper et al., 1981; McFarlin et al., 1971). With the inability to demonstrate any antiviral antibody response or any immune response directed against nonhost viral components or capable of neutralizing the virus activity, these unconventional viruses become unique in their immunological behavior in microbiology. Natural and experimental infection with these viruses elicits no antibody response in the host, nor does immunosuppression with whole-body radiation, cortisone, antileukocytic serum, or cytotoxic drugs alter the incubation period, progress, or pattern of disease, or duration of illness to death. Finally, in vivo and in vitro study of both B-cell and T-cell function demonstrated no abnormality early or late in the course of illness and no in vitro sensitization of the cells taken from diseased animals to high-titer preparations of these viruses (Gajdusek, 1977, 1985b,c; Gajdusek and Gibbs, 1975). Since high-titer infective material in both crude suspension and highly purified also fails to elicit an immunological response against nonhost components, even when used with adjuvants, this becomes the first group of microbes in which such immunological inertness has been demonstrated which has evoked the speculation that the replication of these viruses does not involve production of a virus-specified nonhost antigen (Gajdusek, 1977; Prusiner, 1982). Instead, their protein component must be specified by host genes and therefore be recognized as self.

The scrapie amyloid protein obtained from highly purified preparations of SAF (prion protein PrP_{27-30}) is the subunit of the SAF, which are a fibrillary aggregation of such subunits. It aggregates into dimer, tetramer, octomer, and hexadecamer polymers, as does the different 4.1-kDa subunit polypeptide of amyloid of Alzheimer's disease and aging brain (Braig and Diringer, 1985; Masters et al., 1985b; Multhaup et al., 1985). Antibody to same scrapie amyloid protein has been made in rabbits; such polyclonal antibody reacts well with SAF by an enzyme-linked immunosorbent assay (ELISA) (Brown et al., 1985), Western blotting technique (Brown et al., 1985, 1986a; Manuelidis et al., 1985), and gold bead decoration immunoelectron microscopy (Manuelidis et al., 1985). Such antibodies to the scrapie SAF cross-react well with the SAF of kuru and of CJD and the Gerstmann–Sträussler form of CJD (Bendheim et al., 1985; Brown et al., 1985; Manuelidis et al., 1985) and already provide a quick means of diagnosis of these diseases (Brown et al., 1986a). These antisera to SAF cross-react with the amyloid plaques of kuru, CJD, and scrapie, but they do not cross-react with the amyloid plaques of Alzheimer's disease or the aging brain (Brown et al., 1985; Gibbs, C. J., Jr., and Gajdusek, D. C., unpublished data; Kitramoto et al., 1986). Such antibody possesses low level neutralizing activity against purified infectious form of the scrapie precursor protein (Safar et al., 1989).

6. ENORMOUS RESISTANCE TO PHYSICAL AND CHEMICAL INACTIVATION

The demonstration of the resistance of the unconventional viruses to high concentrations of formaldehyde or glutaraldehyde, psoralens, and most other antiviral and antiseptic substances (Brown et al., 1982a, 1986b, 1989) and to ultraviolet (UV) and ionizing radiation, ultrasonication, and heat, as well as the further demonstration of iatrogenic transmission through implanted surgical electrodes, contaminated surgical instruments, corneal transplantation, injections of human growth hormone derived from pituitary glands obtained from cadavers (Brown et al., 1985), and dura mater obtained from cadavers and "sterilized" by ionizing radiation, and possibly through dentistry, have led to the necessity of changing autopsy room and operating theater techniques throughout the world as well as the precautions used in handling older and demented patients. Many of the gentle organic disinfectants, including detergents and the quaternary ammonium salts, often used for disinfection and even hydrogen peroxide, formaldehyde, ether, chloroform, iodine, phenol, and acetone, are inadequate for sterilization of the unconventional viruses, as is the use of the ethylene oxide sterilizer. More recently, it has been shown that formaldehyde-fixed brain tissue is much more resistant to inactivation by autoclaving than is unfixed fresh scrapie-infected brain (Taylor and McConnell, 1988, Brown *et al.*, 1989). This demands revision of previously acceptable procedures for decontamination and disinfection (Brown *et al.*, 1982a,b, 1984, 1986b, 1989).

These unconventional viruses are also resistant, even when partially purified, to all nucleases, to β-propiolactone, ethylenediaminetetraacetic acid (EDTA), and sodium deoxycholate. They are moderately sensitive to most membrane-disrupting agents in high concentration such as phenol (60%), chloroform, ether, urea (6M), periodate (0.01 M), 2-chloroethanol, alcoholic iodine, acetone, chloroform–butanol, hypochlorite, and alkalai, to chaotropic ions such as thiocyanate and guanadinium and trichloroacetate, and to proteinase K and trypsin when partially purified (Prusiner, 1982), but these only inactivated 99–99.9% of the infectious particles leaving behind highly resistant infectivity (Rohwer, 1984b). Sodium hydroxide (1.0 N) and hypochlorite (5%), however, quickly inactivate more than 10^5 ID_{50} of the virus (Brown *et al.*, 1984). They have a UV inactivation action spectrum with a sixfold increased sensitivity at 237 nm over that at 254 nm or 280 nm, and 50-fold increased sensitivity at 220 nm (Gibbs *et al.*, 1977; Haig *et al.*, 1969; Latarjet, 1979; Latarjet *et al.*, 1970). Moreover, they show remarkable resistance to ionizing radiation that would indicate a target size, if such a naive calculation is applicable to a highly aggregated "semisolid" array of associated proteins, of under 100 kDa (Gibbs *et al.*, 1977; Latarjet, 1979; Latarjet *et al.*, 1970; Rohwer and Gajdusek, 1980).

Many investigators have seen regular arrays of particles that appear to be tubular structures seen in cross section, in postsynaptic terminals of neurons in experimental animals infected with CJD, kuru, and scrapie (Baringer *et al.*, 1979, 1981; David-Ferreira *et al.*, 1968; Field and Narang, 1972; Field *et al.*, 1969; Lamar *et al.*, 1974; Narang, 1973, 1974a,b; Narang *et al.*, 1972, 1980; Vernon *et al.*, 1970; ZuRhein and Varakis, 1976). Structures more typical of virions are not recognized on electron microscopic study of infected cells *in vivo* or *in vitro*, nor are they recognized in highly infectious preparations of virus concentrated by density-gradient banding in the zonal rotor.

These atypical properties have led to speculation that the infectious agents lack a nucleic acid and that they may be a self-replicating protein (perhaps by derepressing or causing misreading of cellular DNA bearing information for their own synthesis), even a self-replicating membrane fragment that serves as a template for laying down abnormal plasma membrane, including itself (Bendheim *et al.*, 1985; Bolton *et al.*, 1982, 1984, 1985; Gajdusek, 1984, 1985a,b,c; Oesch *et al.*, 1985; Prusiner, 1982, 1984; Prusiner *et al.*, 1983, 1984). We have often suggested that they are replicating polypeptides, autonucleating and autopatterning a configurational change in the secondary structure of the host precursor protein, autocatalytically to an infectious form (Gajdusek, 1977, 1984, 1985a,b,c, 1989). More recently, we suggested that the fibril amyloid-enhancing factors offer a good model for scrapie replication (Gajdusek, 1988; Guiroy and Gajdusek, 1988).

Analogies with defective or "contaminated" seed crystals or simple nucleating molecules specifying the crystallization of their own distinct crystal structure come to mind, as do mineral nucleation of protein crystallization (McPherson and Shlichta, 1988). The presence of mineral deposits in neurons in the form of hydroxyapatites often containing aluminum (Bizzi *et al.*, 1984; Nikaido *et al.*, 1972; Perl and Brody, 1980), silicon (Austin *et al.*, 1973, 1978; Iler, 1985; Nikaido *et al.*, 1972), and other atoms as the antecedents to NFT formation with the amyloid protein of PHF has been shown in the high-incidence foci of ALS/PD, and associated early appearance of NFT in the Western Pacific (Gajdusek and Salazar, 1982; Garruto *et al.*, 1982, 1984; Perl *et al.*, 1982). More recently, Masters *et al.* (1985a) and Candy *et al.* (1986) found silicon and aluminum deposits in the center of amyloid plaque cores in Alzheimer's disease. The aluminum silicate, perhaps in the form of montmorillo-nites, are in the center of amyloid plaque cores. Candy *et al.* (1986) have therefore suggested that, because of this location, they are the initiating elements of the amyloid deposition. We wonder whether a nucleus of a cation-binding mineral lattice may initiate the change to amyloid configuration of some keratinoid type host protein (Gajdusek, 1989; Iler, 1985; Rees and Cragg, 1983; Weiss, 1981).

7. MENDELIAN SINGLE-GENE AUTOSOMAL-DOMINANT INHERITANCE DETERMINES EXPRESSION IN FAMILIAL CJD

Creutzfeldt–Jakob disease became the first human infectious disease in which a single gene was demonstrated to control susceptibility and occurrence of the disease. The CJD virus is isolated from the brain of such familial cases. The autosomal-dominant behavior of the disease in such families, including the appearance of the disease in 50% of siblings who survive to the age at which the disease usually appears, has evoked the possibility of virus etiology in other familial dementias. The presence of CJD patients in the families of well-known familial Alzheimer's disease and the familial occurrence of the spinocerebellar ataxic form of CJD—Gerstmann–Sträussler syndrome—which is also transmissible, have led to renewed interest in familial dementias of all types (Masters *et al.*, 1981a,b; Traub *et al.*, 1977).

Four different mutations have now been found in families with CJD: three cause single amino acid replacements and one causes a large (c.144 bp) insertion near the N-terminus (position 53). Five different families with the GSS form of CJD have the same mutation, changing a proline in position 102 to a leucine; one CJD family has a mutation changing a glutamine in position 200 to lysine; and several other CJD patients have a mutation changing a methionine in position 129 to a valine. We now believe that most sporadic CJD cases result from spontaneous conversion of the host precursor protein to the infectious CJD virus from a change in secondary structure of the precursor. This spontaneous *de novo* creation of a virus occurs as a rare event, at a rate of 1 per million population per annum (the world-wide incidence of CJD). However, in familial cases where one of the four mutations is present, the likelihood of this conformational change to occur spontaneously increases a million-fold. Thus, the disease appears to be an autosomal dominant trait.

8. AUTOIMMUNE ANTIBODY TO 10-NM NEUROFILAMENT IN SSVE PATIENTS

The demonstration by Sotelo and co-workers of a very specific autoimmune antibody directed against 10-nm neurofilaments and no other component of the CNS in more than 60% of the patients with kuru and CJD as a phenomenon appearing late in the disease was the first demonstration of an immune phenomenon in the subacute spongiform virus encephalopathies (SSVE) and an exciting new avenue of approach for the study of the transmissible dementias (Aoki *et al.*, 1982; Bahmanyar *et al.*, 1983, 1984; Sotelo *et al.*, 1980a,b). This autoimmune antibody behaves like many other autoimmune antibodies, such as the rheumatoid factor and the anti-DNA antibody in lupus and the antithyroglobulin antibody in Hashimoto's thyroiditis, in that it is often present in normal subjects and is more often present in subjects closely related to the patients. Although found in more than one half of patients with transmissible virus dementia, it was not detected in 40% of patients with classic CJD. It does develop in other gray matter diseases, including Alzheimer's and Parkinson's diseases, but at far lower incidence than in CJD (Bahmanyar *et al.*, 1983; Sotelo *et al.*, 1980a). Furthermore, it was not detected in patients with other immune diseases such as disseminated lupus erythematosus and chronic rheumatoid arthritis (Bahmanyar *et al.*, 1983). We have demonstrated that on Western blots separating the three proteins comprising the 10-nm neurofilament triad of 200 kDa, 150 kDa, and 68 kDa, most positive sera have antibodies directed against the 200-kDa protein with some cross-reaction with the 150-kDa protein, some sera react better with the 150-kDa protein, and rare sera only with the 68-kDa protein, thought to be an internal component of the neurofilament (Bahmanyar *et al.*, 1984; Toh *et al.*, 1985a,b). Sheep with scrapie, however, often react best with a 62-kDa neurofilament-associated protein (Toh *et al.*, 1985b). Some investigators noted a higher incidence of these specific antibodies in normal subjects than we have found (Stefansson *et al.*, 1985). Nonetheless, the same problem is posed: Why are there antibodies to the neurofilament proteins and not to other CNS antigens?

9. UNCONVENTIONAL VIRUSES: SUBVIRAL PATHOGENS, DEVOID OF A NUCLEIC ACID OR A NONHOST PROTEIN

The scrapie virus has been partially purified by density-gradient sedimentation in the presence of specific detergents. Scrapie virus has been more than 1000-fold purified relative to other quantifiable proteins in the original brain suspension (Bolton *et al.*, 1982, 1984; Diringer *et al.*, 1983; Manuelidis and Manuelidis, 1983; Multhaup *et al.*, 1985; Prusiner *et al.*, 1984; Rohwer and Gajdusek, 1980; Rohwer *et al.*, 1979). In such preparations, the virus is susceptible to high concentrations of proteinase K and trypsin digestion, but it is not inactivated by any nuclease (Prusiner, 1982). Sedimented, washed, and resuspended virus has been banded into peaks of high infectivity with the use of cesium chloride, sucrose, and metrizamide density gradients in the ultracentrifuge. Attempts to demonstrate a nonhost nucleic acid in scrapie virus preparations using DNA homology and transfection and nuclease inactivation have been unsuccessful (Borras and Gibbs, 1985; Borras *et al.*, 1982; Hunter *et al.*, 1976). No significant quantities of nucleic acid are present in purified preparations of 27- to 30-kDa SAF associated-protein (PrP_{27-30}), (Diringer *et al.*, 1983; Manuelidis, 1985; Multhaup *et al.*, 1985; Oesch *et al.*, 1985). R. G. Rowher (personal communication) has shown that there is no nonhost DNA by subtracting total normal host brain DNA from scrapie-infected brain DNA using polymerase chain reaction.

The atypical action spectrum for inactivation of scrapie virus by UV implies the absence of DNA or RNA, but should not be taken as absolute proof thereof (Gibbs *et al.*, 1977; Haig *et al.*, 1969; Latarjet, 1979; Latarjet *et al.*, 1970). UV resistance also depends greatly on small RNA size, as has been shown by the high resistance of the purified, very small, tobacco ring spot satellite virus RNA (~80 kDa). However, virus resistance to temperatures above 270°C rules out any nucleic acid as an essential component (Brown et al., 1990).

Moreover, the unconventional viruses possess numerous properties in which they resemble classic viruses (Gajdusek, 1977, 1985b; Rohwer, 1984a,b, 1985; Rohwer and Gajdusek, 1980); some of these properties suggest far more complex genetic interaction between virus and host than one might expect for genomes with a molecular mass of only 10^5 kDa. Rohwer (1985) showed that the scrapie virus replicates in hamster brain at a constant rate, with no eclipse phase, and with a doubling time of 5.2 days. Examination of the kinetics of its inactivation and the demonstrated association or aggregation of scrapie virus particles into polymers or clusters that can be disrupted by ultrasonication have cast doubt on the calculation of its small size from ionizing radiation inactivation data and inferences about its structure from resistance to chemical inactivating agents. Thus, aggregates necessitate "multiple hits" for inactivation, whereas free virus is killed by a single event (Rohwer, 1985).

In plant virology we have been forced to modify our concepts of a virus to include subviral pathogens such as the newly described viroids causing 11 natural plant diseases—potato spindle tuber disease, chrysanthemum stunt disease, citrus exocortis disease, Cadang-Cadang disease of coconut palms, cherry chloratic mottle, cucumber pale fruit disease, hop stunt disease, avocado sunblotch disease, tomato bunchy top disease, tomato "planta macho" disease, and burdock stunt disease—and the virusoids of four natural plant diseases (velvet tobacco mottle virus, solanum nodiflorum mottle virus, lucerne transient streak virus, subterranean clover mottle virus) to which we may turn for analogy (Diener and Hadidi, 1977; Sänger, 1982). All the viroids are small circular RNA containing no structural protein or membrane, and all been fully sequenced and their fine structures determined. They have only partial base pairing as the circle collapses on itself. They contain only 246–574 ribonucleotides and replicate by a "rolling circle" copying of their RNA sequences in many sequential rotations to produce an oligomeric copy, which is then cut into monomers or sometimes dimers. No protein is synthesized from their genetic information, and only the replication machinery of the cell is used. These subviral pathogens have caused us to give much thought to possible similarities to the unconventional viruses. However, we and others have shown that the unconventional viruses differ markedly from the plant viroids on many counts (Diener and Hadidi, 1977; Gajdusek, 1985b,c; Prusiner, 1982; Sänger, 1982); in fact, many of their properties are diametrically opposite those of the viroids. Thus, the intellectually stimulating analogies of the unconventional viruses to viroids and virusoids prove spurious, yet these subviral pathogens of plants have served to alert us to the possibility of extreme departure from conventional virus structures.

Recent work on amyloid-enhancing factors, particularly fibril amyloid-enhancing factor (Niewold et al., 1987), strongly suggests that an autocatalytic nucleating process directing fibril growth according to its own specified fibril structure appears to give us the most challenging model for scrapie replication (Gajdusek, 1988; Guiroy and Gajdusek, 1988). It is now clear that the scrapie infectious monomer causes the progressive slow modification of the normal scrapie precursor protein to an infectious form (Ceroni et al., 1989; Safar et al., 1989a,b,c). This infectious form represents a configurational change in the whole length of molecule which slowly renders it protease resistant and capable of polymerizing into insoluble amyloid fibrils. Differential solubility permits the separation of the infectious monomer ($PrP_{35-37}sc$) from the normal noninfectious precursor ($PrP_{35-37}c$) with the same amino acid sequence (Safar et al., 1989a,b,c). It still can be cleaved at one peptide bond which produces the still-infectious scrapie amyloid protein of 27–30 kDa size (PrP_{27-30}). Spontaneous poly-merization of this scrapie amyloid protein results in SAF and further crystallization or aggregation produces scrapie–kuru–CJD amyloid plaques (Fig. 1).

10. CONCLUDING HYPOTHESIS: A REPLICATING POLYPEPTIDE AND A FANTASY OF A "VIRUS" FROM THE INORGANIC WORLD

We are at an exciting moment in the study of the unconventional viruses. The monomer of the scrapie-altered form of the normal scrapie precursor protein ($PrP_{35-37}sc$) and its cleavage product, the scrapie amyloid protein (PrP_{27}) are the infectious agent directing its own synthesis by autonucleation and autopatterning of configurational change in the normal host precursor protein. Polymerization or fibril crystallization of this infectious scrapie amyloid monomer (PrP_{27}) forms the SAF and scrapie–kuru–CJD plaques. Only protein crystallographers can fully resolve for us the details of the process of configurational change by which a normal host protein is changed to the infectious self-inducing, insoluble, protease-resistant amyloid-like infectious viruses. It might also involve an autoinduction of altered posttranslational processing such as change in crosslinkage, glycosylation (Bolton et al., 1985; Manuelidis et al., 1985; Multhaup et al., 1985), phosphorylation (Sternberger et al., 1985), or the induction of an alternatively spliced form of the precursor protein.

This paradigm assumes the de novo creation of the infectious protein (or scrapie–kuru–CJD virus). In familial cases of CJD (or its GSS variant) this occurrence becomes one million-fold more likely, as the result of any one of four different mutations three of which cause a one-amino-acid change in the precursor. Thus we would not expect these de novo generated viruses of CJD in familial cases to "breed true," but rather to replicate infectious progeny in an inoculated host which carried the normal host amino acid sequence, and did not carry the mutation. Similarly, we would expect the infectious viruses of kuru, CJD, and scrapie all to have the same amino acid sequence in a given host: that of the precursor protein gene of goat, squirrel monkey, or spider monkey, or other hosts in which they replicated. This will soon be tested.

Recently Brown et al. (1990) confirmed complete resistance of scrapie infectivity to autoclaving at 137°C once the virus protein is crosslinked by formaldehyde; in dry lyophilized form much infectivity resists 270°C and some even 360°C dry oven heat for one hour. A mineral or mineral–protein complex would be the replicating agent we seek for such heat resistance. We must allow for the possibility that such a mineral–amyloid complex might serve as a nucleating agent and template for conversion of normal host precursor protein to the infectious form. For aging brain amyloid, hydroxyapatite–aluminum silicate inorganic nidi have been found in NFT and in the center of amyloid plaque in AD. Thus these mineral nidi are candidates for the initiation or nucleation of amyloidogenesis and the degenerative amyloidoses of brain. In scrapie–kuru–CJD slow virus infections, a microfibril or oligomer of the scrapie amyloid protein may be its own nucleating agent and crystallization template for epitaxial crystal growth. In AD, Pick's disease, and Down's syndrome, a 4.1 kDa polypeptide or its polymers complexed as an amyloid protein to a calcium–aluminum–silicate apparently can cause such nucleation and trigger self-aggregation to the mineral amyloid aggregates or paracrystalline arrays we see in NFT (Garruto et al., 1984; Perl et al., 1982) and the amyloid plaque cores (Austin, 1978; Candy *et al.*, 1985; Masters *et al.*, 1985a; Nikaido *et al.*, 1972). Only in the nondividing neuron does this slow degenerative process eventually kill the cell.

Thus, our atypical slow "virus" may simply be similar to a crystal template directing its own crystallization or crystal lattice from a source of presynthesized host precursor proteins, and an inorganic cation receptor nucleus. If the recently reported (Brown *et al.*, 1990) resistance to such temperatures as 360°C are confirmed, we would be forced to assume that a mineral complex carries the crystallographically necessary pattern for nucleation of the conformational change of the precursor to the infectious form. If so, inorganic polymer chemistry and crystallography may provide better insights than the normal paradigms of modern molecular biology (Connors, 1985; Iler, 1985; McPherson and Schlichta, 1988; Wise, 1981).

The authors would prefer to call the infectious agent of scrapie a *virus*, even if it proves to be as romantically exotic as a polypeptide directing an autocatalytically patterned degradation of a stagnated, pooled host-specific protein to an infectious amyloid. The potent abstract concept of a virus as a self-specifying transmissible entity requiring the machinery of the host for its replication does not specify any specific structure. Mathematicians playing with computers have not hesitated to use the term *virus* for the *virus infections* of computer memories they have produced (Dewdney, 1985a,b). Dewdney (1984), with his Core Wars program, initiated computer virology. The fact that their software viruses contain no nucleic acid, and that nucleic acids are in no way involved in the pathology that these viral diseases produce, has not prevented computer scientists from appropriately calling them viruses (Denning, 1988).

REFERENCES

Anderson, F. H., Richardson, E. P., Jr., Okazaki, H., and Brody, J. A., 1979, Neurofibrillary degeneration on Guam. Frequency in Chamorros and non-Chamorros with no known neurological disease, Brain 102:65–77.

Anderton, B. H., Breinburg, D., Downes, M. J., Green, P. J., Tomlinson, B. E., Ulrich, J., Wood, J. N., and Kahn, J., 1982, Monoclonal antibodies show that neurofibrillary tangles and neurofilaments share antigenic determinants, *Nature (Lond.)* 298: 84–86.

Aoki, T., Gibbs, C. J., Jr., Sotelo, J., and Gajdusek, D. C., 1982, Heterogenic autoantibody against neurofilament protein in the sera of the animals with experimental kuru and Creutzfeldt–Jakob disease and natural scrapie infection, *Infection Immun.* 38:316–324.

Austin, J. H., Rinehart, R., Williamson, J., Burcar, P., Russ, K., Nikaido, T., and Lafrance, M., 1973, Studies in ageing of the brain. III. Silicon levels in postmortem tissues and body fluids, *Prog. Brain Res.* 40:485–495.

Austin, J. H., 1978, Silicon levels in human tissues, in: *Biochemistry of Silicon and Related Problems* (G. Bendz and I. Lindqvist, eds.), Plenum, New York, pp. 255–268.

Autilio-Gambetti, L., Gambetti, P, and Crane, R. C., 1983, Paired helical filaments: Relatedness to neurofilaments shown by silver staining and reactivity with monoclonal antibodies, in: *Biological Aspects of Alzheimer's Disease* (R. Katzman, ed.), Banbury Report 15, Cold Spring Harbor Laboratory, Cold Spring Harbor, New York, pp. 117–124.

Bahmanyar, S., Moreau-Dubois, M. C., Brown, P., and Gajdusek, D. C., 1983, Serum antineurofilament antibodies in patients with neurological and non-neurological disorders and healthy controls using rat spinal cord, *J. Neuroimmunol.* 5:191–196.

Bahmanyar, S., Liem, R. K. H., Griffin, J. W., and Gajdusek, D. C., 1984, Characterization of antineurofilament autoantibodies in Creutzfeldt–Jakob disease, *J. Neuropathol. Exp. Neurol.* **43**:369–375.

Bahmanyar, S., Higgins, G. A., Goldgaber, D., Lewis, D. A., Morrison, J. H., Wilson, M. C., Shankar, S. K., and Gajdusek, D. C., 1987, Localization of amyloid β-protein messenger RNA in brains from Alzheimer's disease patients, *Science* **237**:77–80.

Baringer, J. R., Wong, J., Klassen, T., and Prusiner, S. B., 1979, Further observations of the neuropathology of experimental scrapie in mouse and hamster, in: *Slow Transmissible Diseases of the Nervous System*, Vol. 2. (S. B. Prusiner and W. J. Halow, eds.), Academic, New York, pp. 111–121.

Baringer, J. R., Prusiner, S. B., and Wong, J. S., 1981, Scrapie-associated particles in postsynaptic processes. Further ultrastructural studies, *Neuropathol. Exp. Neurol.* **40**:281–288.

Beck, E., Bak, I. J., Christ, J. F., Gajdusek, D. C., Gibbs, C. J., Jr., and Hassler, R., 1975, Experimental kuru in the spider monkey. Histopathological and ultrastructural studies of the brain during early stages of incubation, *Brain* **98**:595–612.

Beck, E., Daniel, P. M., Davey, A. J., Gajdusek, D. C., and Gibbs, C. J., Jr., 1982, The pathogenesis of spongiform encephalopathies: An ultrastructural study, *Brain* **105**:755–786.

Bendheim, P. E., Barry, R. A., DeArmond, S. J., Stites, D. P., and Prusiner, S. B., 1984, Antibodies to a scrapie-prion protein, *Nature (Lond.)* **310**:418–421.

Bendheim, P. E., Bockman, J. O., McKinley, M. P., Kingsbury, D. T., and Prusiner, S. B., 1985, Scrapie and Creutzfeldt–Jakob disease prion proteins share physical properties and antigenic determinants, *Proc. Natl. Acad. Sci. USA* **82**: (February), 997–1001.

Bizzi, A., Crane, R. C., and Autilio-Gambetti, L., and Gambetti, P., 1984, Aluminum effect on slow axonal transport: A novel impairment of neurofilament transport, *J. Neurosci.* **4**:722–731.

Bockman, J. M., Kingsbury, D. T., McKinley, M. P., Bendheim, P. E., and Prusiner, S. B., 1985, Creutzfeldt–Jakob disease prion proteins in human brains, *N. Engl. J. Med.* **312**:73–78.

Bolton, D. C., McKinley, M. P., and Prusiner, S. B., 1982, Identification of a protein that purifies with the scrapie prion, *Science* **218**:1309–1311.

Bolton, D. C., McKinley, M. P., and Prusiner, S. B., 1984, Molecular characteristics of the major scrapie prion protein, *Biochemistry* **23**:5898–5905.

Bolton, D. C., Meyer, R. K., and Prusiner, S. B., 1985, Scrapie PrP 27–30 is a sialoglycoprotein, *J. Virol.* **53**:596–606.

Borras, M. T., and Gibbs, C. J., Jr., 1986, Molecular hybridization studies with scrapie brain nucleic acids. I. Search for specific DNA sequences, *Arch. Virol.* **88**:67–78.

Borras, M. T., Kingsbury, D. T., Gajdusek, D. C., and Gibbs, C. J., Jr., 1982, Inability to transmit scrapie by transfection of mouse embryo cells *in vitro*, *J. Gen. Virol.* **58**:263–271.

Borras, M. T., Merendino, J. J., and Gibbs, C. J., Jr., 1986, Molecular hybridization studies with scrapie brain nucleic acids. II. Differential expression in scrapie hamster brains, *Arch. Virol.* **88**:79–90.

Braig, H. R., and Diringer, H., 1985, Scrapie: Concept of a virus induced amyloidosis of the brain, *Eur. J. Mol. Biol.* **4**:2309–2311.

Brown, P., Gibbs, C. J., Jr., Amyx, H. L., Kingsbury, D. T., Rohwer, R. G., Sulima, M. P., and Gajdusek, D. C., 1982a, Chemical disinfection of Creutzfeldt–Jakob disease virus, *N. Engl. J. Med.* **306**:1279–1282.

Brown, P., Rohwer, R. G., Green, E. M., and Gajdusek, D. C., 1982b, Effect of chemicals, heat and histopathological processing on high infectivity hamster-adapted scrapie virus, *J. Infect. Dis.* **145**:683–687.

Brown, P., Rohwer, R. G., and Gajdusek, D. C., 1984, Sodium hydroxide decontamination of Creutzfeldt–Jakob disease virus, *N. Engl. J. Med.* **310**:727.

Brown, P., Gajdusek, D. C., Gibbs, C. J., Jr., and Asher, D. M., 1985, Potential epidemic of Creutzfeldt–Jakob disease from human growth hormone therapy, *N. Engl. J. Med.* **313**:728–731.

Brown, P., Coker-Vann, M., Pomeroy, B. S., Asher, D. M., Gibbs, C. J., Jr., and Gajdusek, D. C., 1986a, Diagnosis of Creutzfeldt–Jakob disease by Western blot identification of marker protein in human brain tissue, *N. Engl. J. Med.* **314**:547–551.

Brown, P., Rohwer, R. G., and Gajdusek, D. C., 1986b, Newer data on the inactivation of scrapie virus or Creutzfeldt–Jakob disease virus in brain tissue, *J. Infect. Dis.* **153:**1145–1148.

Brown, P., Wolf, A., Liberski, P. P., and Gajdusek, D. C., 1990, Resistance of scrapie infectivity to steam autoclaving after formaldehyde fixation and limited survival above 360°C: practical and theoretical implications, *Journ. Infec. Dis.* (in press).

Candy, J. M., Oakley, A. E., Klinowski, J., Carpenter, T. A., Perry, R. H., Atack J. R., Perry, E. K., Blessed, G., Fairbairn, A., and Edwardson, J. A., 1986, Aluminosilicates contribute to senile plaque formation in Alzheimer's disease, *Lancet* **1:**354–356.

Ceroni, M., Piccardo, P., Safar, J., Gajdusek, D. C., and Gibbs, C. J. Jr., 1989, Scrapie infectivity and scrapie amyloid protein are distributed in the same pH range in Agarose iselectric focusing (in press).

Chen, L., 1981, Neurofibrillary change on Guam, *Arch. Neurol.* **38:**16–18.

Cohen, M. L., Golde, T. E., Usiak, M. F., Younkin, L. H., and Younkin, S. G., 1988, In situ hybridization of nucleus basalis neurons shows increased β-amyloid mRNA in Alzheimer's disease, *Proc. Natl. Acad. Sci. USA* **85:**1227–1231.

Connors, L. H., 1985, *In vitro* formation of amyloid fibrils, *Biochem. Biophys. Res. Commun.* **131:**1063–1068.

Dahl, D., and Bignami, A., 1985, Two different populations of neurofibrillary tangles in Alzheimer's dementias revealed by neurofilament immunoreactivity and Congo Red staining, in: Molecular Mechanisms of Pathogenesis of Central Nervous System Disorders (A. Bignami, L. Bolis, and D. C. Gajdusek, eds.), *Discussions in Neuroscience,* Vol. 3:80–82.

David-Ferreira, J. F., David-Ferreira, K. L., Gibbs, C. J., Jr., and Morris, J. A., 1968, Scrapie in mice: Ultrastructural observations in the cerebral cortex, *Proc. Soc. Exp. Biol. Med.* **127:**313–320.

Delabar, J-M., Goldgaber, D., Lamour, Y., Nicole, A., Huret, J-L., DeGrouchy, J., Brown, P., Gajdusek, D. C., and Sinet, P-M., 1987, β-Amyloid gene duplication in Alzheimer's disease and karyotypically normal Down syndrome, *Science* **235:**1390–1392.

Denning, P. J., 1988, The science of computing. Computer viruses, *Am. Sci.* **76:**236–238.

Dewdney, A. K., 1984, Computer recreations: In the game called Core Wars hostile program's engage in a battle of bits, *Sci. Am.* **250:**14,18–20,22.

Dewdney, A. K., 1985a, Computer recreations: A core war bestiary of viruses, worms and other threats to computer memories, *Sci. Am.* **252:**14,19–23.

Dewdney, A. K., 1985b, Analog gadgets that solve a diversity of problems and array of questions, *Sci. Am.* **252:**18,22,24,25,28,29.

Diener, T., and Hadidi, A., 1977, Viroids, in: *Comprehensive Virology,* Vol. 11 (H. Fraenkel-Conrat and R. R. Wagner, eds.), pp. 285–337, Plenum, New York.

Diringer, H., Gelderblom, H., Hilmert, H., Özel, M., Edelbluth, C., and Kimberlin, R. H., 1983, Scrapie infectivity, fibrils, and low molecular weight protein, *Nature (Lond.)* **306:** 476–478.

Field, E. J., and Narang, H. K., 1972, An electron microscopic study of natural scrapie in the rat: Further observations on "inclusion bodies" and virus-like particles, *J. Neurol. Sci.* **17:**347–364.

Field, E. J., Mathews, J. D., and Raine, C. S., 1969, Electron microscopic observations on the cerebellar cortex in kuru, *J. Neurol. Sci.* **8:**209–224.

Fukatsu, R., Gibbs, C. J., Jr., Amyx, H. L., and Gajdusek, D. C., 1984a, Amyloid plaque formation along the needle track in experimental murine scrapie, *J. Neuropathol. Exp. Neurol.* **43:**313.

Fukatsu, R., Gibbs, C. J., Jr., and Gajdusek, D. C., 1984b, Cerebral amyloid plaques in experimental murine scrapie, in: *Proceedings of the Workshop on Slow Transmissible Diseases* (J. Tateishi, ed.), Research Committee on Slow Virus Infections, Japanese Ministry of Health, August 31, Tokyo, pp. 71–84.

Gajdusek, D. C., 1977, Unconventional viruses and the origin and disappearance of kuru, *Science* **197:** 943–960.

Gajdusek, D. C., 1984, Interference with axonal transport of neurofilament: The underlying mechanism of pathogenesis in Alzheimer's disease, amyotrophic lateral sclerosis and many other degenerations of the CNS, The Merrimon Lecture, School of Medicine, University of North Carolina, Chapel Hill.

Gajdusek, D. C., 1985a, Hypothesis: Interference with axonal transport of neurofilament as a common pathogmatic mechanism in certain diseases of the central nervous system, *N. Engl. J. Med.* **312:**711–719.

Gajdusek, D. C., 1989b, Unconventional viruses causing subacute spongiform encephalopathies, in: *Virology* (B. N. Fields *et al.*, eds.), 2nd edition, Raven, New York.

Gajdusek, D. C., 1985c, Subacute spongiform virus encephalopathies caused by unconventional viruses, in: *Subviral Pathogens of Plants and Animals: Viroids and Prions* (K. Maramorosch, ed.), Academic, Orlando, Florida, pp. 483–544.

Gajdusek, D. C., 1989a, Cycad toxicity not the cause of high incidence amyotrophic lateral sclerosis/Parkinsonism–dementia on Guam, Kii Peninsula of Japan or in West New Guinea, in: *Amyotrophic Lateral Sclerosis: concepts in Pathogenesis and Etiology* (A. J. Hudson, ed.), University of Toronto Press, Toronto.

Gajdusek, D. C., 1988b, Etiology versus pathogenesis: The causes of post-translational modifications of host specified brain proteins to amyloid configuration, in: *Abstracts of the génétique et maladie d'Alzheimer*, 174–176, Foundation IPSEN pour la Recherche Thérapeutique, Paris.

Gajdusek, D. C., and Gibbs, C. J., Jr., 1975, Slow virus infections of the nervous system and the laboratories of slow, latent and temperate virus infections, in: *The Nervous System* (D. B. Tower, ed.), Vol. 2: *The Clinical Neurosciences* (T. N. Chase, ed.), Raven Press, New York, pp. 113–135.

Gajdusek, D. C., and Salazar, A., 1982, Amyotrophic lateral sclerosis and parkinsonian syndromes in high incidence among Anga and Jakai peoples of West New Guinea, *Neurology (NY)* **32:**107–126.

Gajdusek, D. C., and Zigas, V., 1957, Degenerative disease of the central nervous system in New Guinea. The endemic occurrence of "kuru" in the native population, *N. Engl. J. Med.* **257:**974–978.

Gajdusek, D. C., and Zigas, V., 1959, Kuru: Clinical, pathological and epidemiological study of an acute progressive degenerative disease of the central nervous system among natives of the Eastern Highlands of New Guinea, *Am. J. Med.* **26:** 442–469.

Gajdusek, D. C., Gibbs, C. J., Jr., and Alpers, M. (eds.), 1965, *Slow, Latent and Temperate Virus Infections*, NINCDB Monograph No. 2, National Institutes of Health, PHS Publication No. 1378, U.S. Government Printing Office, Washington, D. C.

Gajdusek, D. C., Gibbs, C. J., Jr., and Alpers, M., 1966, Experimental transmission of a kuru-like syndrome in chimpanzees, *Nature (Lond.)* **209:**794–796.

Gambetti, P., Autilio-Gambetti, L., Perry, G., Shecket, G., and Crane, R. C., 1983a, Antibodies to neurofibrillary tangles of Alzheimer's disease raised from human and animal neurofilament fractions, *Lab. Invest.* **49:**430–435.

Gambetti, P., Shecket, G., Ghetti, B., Hirano, A. and Dahl, D., 1983b, Neurofibrillary changes in human brain. An immunocytochemical study with a neurofilament antiserum, *J. Neuropathol. Exp. Neurol.* **42:**69–79.

Garruto, R. M., Yanagihara, R., Arion, D. M., Daum, C. A., and Gajdusek, D. C., 1982, *Bibliography of Amyotrophic Lateral Sclerosis and Parkinsonism–Dementia of Guam*, National Institutes of Health, Bethesda, U.S. Government Printing Office, Washington, D.C.

Garruto, R. M., Fukatsu, R., Yanagihara, R., Gajdusek, D. C., Hook, G., and Fiori, C. E., 1984, Imaging of calcium and aluminum in neurofibrillary tangle-bearing neurons in parkinsonism–dementia of Guam, *Proc. Natl. Acad. Sci. USA* **81:**875–879.

Garruto, R. M., Swyt, C., Yanagihara, R., Fiori, C. E., and Gajdusek, D. C., 1986, Intraneuronal colocalization of silicon with calcium and aluminum in amyotrophic lateral sclerosis and parkinsonism with dementia of Guam, *N. Engl. J. Med.* **315:**711–712.

Geisler, N., Plassmann, U., and Weber, K., 1985, The complete amino acid sequence of the major mammalian neurofilament protein (NF-L), *Fed. Eur. Biol. Soc.* **182:**475–478.

Gibbs, C. J., Jr., Gajdusek, D. C. and Latarjet, R., 1977, Unusual resistance to UV and ionizing radiation of the viruses of kuru, Creutzfeldt–Jakob disease, and scrapie (unconventional viruses), *Proc. Natl. Acad. Sci. USA* **75:**6268–6270.

Gibbs, C. J., Jr., Gajdusek, D. C., Asher, D. M., Alpers, M. P., Beck, E., Daniel, P. M., and Matthews, W. B., 1968, Creutzfeldt–Jakob disease (subacute spongiform encephalopathy): Transmission to the chimpanzee, *Science* **161**:388–389.

Glenner, G. G., and Won, C. W., 1984a, Alzheimer's disease: Report of the purification and characterization of a novel cerebrovascular amyloid protein, *Biochem. Biophys. Res. Commun.* **120**:885–890.

Glenner, G. G., and Wong, C. W., 1984b, Alzheimer's disease and Down's syndrome: Sharing of a unique cerebrovascular fibril protein, *Biochem. Biophys. Res. Commun.* **122**:1131–1135.

Goldfarb, L. G., Brown, P., Goldgaber, D., Asher, D. M., Rubenstein, R., Brown, W. T., Kascsak, R. J., and Gajdusek, D. C., 1989, Creutzfeldt–Jakob disease and kuru patients lack a mutation consistently found in Gerstmann–Sträussler–Scheinker syndrome, *Experimental Neurology* (in press).

Goldgaber, D., Goldfarb, L. G., Brown, P., Asher, D. M., Brown, W. T., Lin, S., Teener, J. W., Feinstone, S. M., Rubenstein R., Kascsak, R. J., Boellard, J. W., and Gajdusek, D. C., 1989, Mutations in familial Creutzfeldt–Jakob disease and Gerstmann–Sträussler's syndrome, *Experimental Neurology* **106**:515–528.

Goldgaber, D., Lerman, M., McBride, W., Saffiotti, U., and Gajdusek, D. C., 1987a, Isolation, characterization and chromosomal localization of cDNA clones coding for the precursor protein of amyloid of brain in Alzheimer disease, Down's syndrome, and aging, in: (S. H. Corkin and J. H. Growden, eds.) *Advances in Basic Research Therapies.* Proceedings of the Fourth Meeting of the International Study Group on the Pharmacology of Memory Disorders Associated with Aging, Zurich, Switzerland, January 16–18, 1987, Center for Brain Science and Metabolism Charitable Trust, Cambridge, Massachusetts, 1987, pp. 209–217.

Goldgaber, D., Lerman, M., McBride, W., Saffiotti, U., and Gajdusek, D. C., 1987b, Characterization and chromosomal localization of cDNA encoding brain amyloid of Alzheimer's disease, *Science* **235**:877–880.

Goldgaber, D., Teener, J. W., and Gajdusek, D. C., 1988, Alternative cDNA clones of amyloid β-protein precursor gene encode proteinase inhibitor, *Disc. Neurosci.* **5**:40.

Gorevic, P., Goni, F., Pons-Estel, B., Alvarez, F., Peress, R., and Frangiohe, B. (1990), Isolation and partial characterization of neurofibrillary tangles and amyloid plaque cores in Alzheimer's disease. Immunological studies, *J. Neuropathol. Exp. Neurol.* (in press).

Grundke-Iqbal, I., Iqbal, K., Tung, Y.-C., Quinlan, M., Wiesniewski, H., and Binder, L. I., 1986, Abnormal phosphorylation of the microtubule-associated protein t (tau) in Alzheimer cytoskeletal pathology, *Proc. Natl. Acad. Sci. USA* **83**:4913–4917.

Guiroy, D. C., and Gajdusek, D. C., 1988, Fibril-derived amyloid enhancing factors as nucleating agents in Alzheimer's disease and transmissible virus dementias, *Disc. Neurosci.* **5**:69–73.

Guiroy, D. C., Miyazaki, M., Multhaup, G., Fischer, P., Garruto, R. M., Beyreuther, K., Masters, C., Simms, G., Gibbs, C. J., Jr., and Gajdusek, D.C., 1987, Amyloid of neurofibrillary tangles of Guamanian parkinsonism–dementia and Alzheimer's disease share identical amino acid sequence, *Proc. Natl. Acad. Sci.* **84**:2073–2077.

Haig, D. C., Clarke, M. C., Blum, E., and Alper, T., 1969, Further studies on the inactivation of the scrapie agent by ultraviolet light, *J. Gen. Virol.* **5**:455–457.

Higgins, G. A., Lewis, D. A. Bahmanyar, S., Goldgaber, D., Gajdusek, D. C., Young, W. G., Morrison, J. H., and Wilson, M. C., 1988, Differential regulation of amyloid β-protein mRNA expression with hippocampal neuronal subpopulations in Alzheimer disease, *Proc. Natl. Acad. Sci. USA* **85**:1297–1301.

Hirano, A., and Inoue, K., 1980, [Early pathological changes in amyotrophic lateral sclerosis. Electron microscopic study of chromatolysis, spheroids, and Bunina bodies], *Neurol. Med. (Tokyo)* **13**:148–160.

Hirano, A., Donnenfeld, H., Sasaki, S., and Nakano, I., 1984a, Fine structural observations of neurofilamentous changes in amyotrophic lateral sclerosis, *J. Neuropathol. Exp. Neurol.* **43**:461–470.

Hirano, A., Nakano, I., Kurland, L. T., Mulder, D. W., Holley, P. W., and Saccomanno, G., 1984*b*, Fine structural study of neurofibrillary changes in a family with amyotrophic lateral sclerosis, *J. Neuropathol. Exp. Neurol.* **43:** 471–480.

Hope, J., Reekie, L. J. D., Hunter, N., Multhaup, G., Beyreuther, K., White, H., Scott, A. C., Stack, M. J., Dawson, M., and Wells, G. A. H., 1988, Fibrils from brains of cows with new cattle disease contain scrapie-associated protein, *Nature* **336:**390–392.

Hsiao, K., Baker, H. F., Crow, T. J., Poulter, N., Owen, F., Terwilliger, J. D., Westaway, D., Ott, J., and Prusiner, S. B., 1989, Linkage of a prion protein missense variant to Gerstmann–Strässler syndrome, *Nature* **338:**342–345.

Hsiao, K., Doh-ura, K., Kitamoto, T., Tateishi, J., and Prusiner, S. B., 1989, A prion protein amino acid substitution in ataxic Gerstmann–Strässler syndrome, *Ann. Neurol.* (Abstr.) **26:**137.

Hunter, G. D., Collis, S. C., Millson, G. C., and Kimberlin, R. H., 1976, Search for scrapie-specific RNA and attempts to detect an infectious DNA or RNA, *J. Gen. Virol.* **32:**157–162.

Iler, R. K., 1985, Hydrogen-bond complexes of silicon with organic compounds, in: *Biochemistry of Silicon and Related Problems* (G. Bendz and I. Lindqvist, ed.), Plenum, New York, pp. 53–76.

Inoue, K., and Hirano, A., 1979, [Early pathological changes in amyotrophic lateral sclerosis. Autopsy findings of a case of ten months duration], *Neurol. Med. (Tokyo)* **11:**448–455.

Kang, J., Lemaire, H-G., Unterbeck, A., Slabaum, J. M., Masters, C. L., Grzeschik, K-H., Multhaup, G., Beyreuther, K., Muller-Hill, B., 1987, The precursor of Alzheimer's disease amyloid A4 protein resembles a cell-surface receptor, *Nature (Lond.)* **1:**733–736.

Kasper, K. C., Bowman, K., Stites, D. P., and Prusiner, S. B., 1981, Toward development of assays for scrapie-specific antibodies, in: *Hamster Immune Responses in Infectious and Oncogenic Diseases* (J. W. Streilein, D. A. Hart, J. Stein-Sterilein, W. R. Duncan, and R. E. Billingham, eds.), Plenum, New York, pp. 401–413.

Kidd, M., Allsop, D., and Landon, M., 1985, Senile plaque amyloid, paired helical filaments and cerebrovascular amyloid in Alzheimer's disease are all deposits of the same protein, *Lancet* **1:**278.

Kingsbury, D. T., Prusiner, S. B., Bockman, J. M., McKinley, M. P., and Barry, R. A., 1985, Reply to the Editor: Laura Manuelidis: Creutzfeldt–Jakob disease prion proteins in human brains, *N. Engl. J. Med.* **312:**1644–1645.

Kirschner, D. A., Abraham, C., and Selkoe, D. J., 1986, X-ray diffraction from intraneuronal paired helical filaments and extraneuronal amyloid fibers in Alzheimer disease indicates cross β-conformation, *Proc. Natl. Acad. Sci. USA* **83:**503–507.

Kitaguchi, N., Takahashi, Y., Tokushima, Y., Shiojiri, S., and Ito, H., 1988, Novel precursor of Alzheimer's disease amyloid protein shows protease inhibitory activity, *Nature (Lond.)* **331:**530–532.

Kitramoto, T., Tateishi, J., Tashima, T., Takeshita, I., Barry, R. A., DeArmond, S. J., and Prusiner, S. B., 1986, Amyloid plaques in Creutzfeldt–Jakob disease stain with prion protein antibodies, *Ann. Neurol.* **20:**204–208.

Klatzo, I., Gajdusek, D. C., and Zigas, V., 1959, Pathology of kuru, *Lab. Invest.* **8:**799–847.

Klatzo, I., Wisniewski, H., and Streicher, E. J., 1965, Experimental production of neurofibrillary degeneration. 1. Light microscopic observations, *J. Neuropathol. Exp. Neurol.* **24:**187–199.

Kosik, K. S., Joachim, C. L., and Selkoe, D. J., 1986, Microtubule-associated protein tau (τ) is a major antigenic component of paired helical filaments in Alzheimer disease, *Proc. Natl. Acad. Sci. USA* **83:**4044–4048.

Lamar, C. H., Gustafson, D. P., Krashnovich, M., and Hinsman, E. J., 1974, Ultrastructural studies of spleens, brains and brain cell cultures of mice with scrapie, *Vet. Pathol.* **11:**13–19.

Lampert, P. W., Gajdusek, D. C., and Gibbs, C. J., Jr., 1971, Experimental spongiform encephalopathy (Creutzfeldt–Jakob disease) in chimpanzees. Electron microscopic studies, Presented at a meeting of the American Association of Pathologists and Bacteriologists, St. Louis, March 7, 1970, *J. Neuropathol. Exp. Neurol.* **30:**20–32.

Latarjet, R., 1979, Inactivation of the agents of scrapie, Creutzfeldt–Jakob disease and kuru by radiation, in: *Slow Transmissible Diseases of the Nervous System*, Vol. 2 (S. B. Prusiner and W. J. Hadlow, eds.), pp. 387–407, Academic, New York.

Latarjet, R., Muel, B., Haig, D. A., Clarke, M. C. and Alper, T., 1970, Inactivation of the scrapie agent by near-monochromatic ultraviolet light, *Nature (Lond.)* **227:**1341–1343.

Lewis, S. A., and Cowan, N. J., 1985, Genetics, evolution, and expression of the 68,000-molecular-weight neurofilament protein: Isolation of a cloned cDNA probe, *J. Cell Biol.* **100:**843–850.

Manuelidis, L., 1985, Creutzfeldt–Jakob disease prion proteins in human brains (Letter to the editor), *N. Engl. J. Med.* **312:**1643–1644.

Manuelidis, L., and Manuelidis, E. E., 1983, Fractionation and infectivity studies in Creutzfeldt–Jakob disease, in: *Biological Aspects of Alzheimer's Disease*, Banbury Report No. 15 (R. Katzman, ed.), Cold Spring Harbor Laboratory, Cold Spring Harbor, New York, pp. 399–412.

Manuelidis, L., Valley, S., and Manuelidis, E. E., 1985, Specific proteins associated with Creutzfeldt–Jakob disease and scrapie share antigenic and carbohydrate determinants, *Proc. Natl. Acad. Sci. USA* **82:**4263–4267.

Masters, C. L., Gajdusek, D. C., and Gibbs, C. J., Jr., 1981*a*, The familial occurrence of Creutzfeldt–Jakob disease and Alzheimer's disease, *Brain* **104:**535–558.

Masters, C. L., Gajdusek, D. C., and Gibbs, C. J., Jr., 1981*b*, Creutzfeldt–Jakob disease virus isolations from the Gerstmann–Sträussler syndrome, with an analysis of the various forms of amyloid plaque deposition in the virus-induced spongiform encephalopathies, *Brain* **104:**559–588.

Masters, C. L., Multhaup, G., Simms, G., Pottgiesser, J., Martins, R. N., and Beyreuther, K., 1985*a*, Neuronal origin of a cerebral amyloid: Neurofibrillary tangles of Alzheimer's disease contain the same protein as the amyloid of plaque cores and blood vessels, *Eur. J. Mol. Biol.* **4:**2757–2763.

Masters, C. L., Simms, G., Weinman, N. A., Multhaup, G., McDonald, B. L., and Beyreuther, K., 1985*b*, Amyloid plaque core protein in Alzheimer's disease and Down's syndrome, *Proc. Natl. Acad. Sci. USA* **82:**4245–4249.

McFarlin, D. E., Rott, M. C., Simpson, L., and Nehlson, S., 1971, Scrapie in immunologically deficient mice, *Nature (Lond.)* **233:**336.

McPherson, A., and Schlichta, P., 1988, Heterogeneous and epitaxial nucleation of protein crystals on mineral surfaces, *Science* **239:**385–387.

Merz, P. A., Somerville, R. A., Wisniewski, H. M., and Iqbal, K., 1981, Abnormal fibrils from scrapie-infected brain, *Acta Neuropathol. (Berl.)* **54:**63–74.

Merz, P. A., Rohwer, R. G., Kascsak, R., Wisniewski, H. M., Somerville, R. A., Gibbs, C. J., Jr., and Gajdusek, D. C., 1984a, Identification of a disease-specific particle in scrapie-like slow virus diseases, *Science* **225:**437–440.

Merz, P. A., Somerville, R. A., Wisniewski, H. M., Manuelidis, L., and Manuelidis, E. E., 1984b, Scrapie associated fibrils in Creutzfeldt–Jakob disease, *Nature (Lond.)* **306:**474–476.

Merz, P. A., Wisniewski, H. M., Rubenstein, R., and Kascsak, R. J., 1986, Immunological studies on paired helical filaments and amyloid of Alzheimer's disease, *Disc. Neurosci.* **3:**58–68.

Multhaup, G., Diringer, H., Hilmert, H., Prinz, H., Heukeshoven, J., and Beyreuther, K., 1985, The protein component of scrapie-associated fibrils is a glycosylated low-molecular-weight protein, *Eur. J. Mol. Biol.* **4:**1495–1501.

Narang, H. K., 1973, Virus-like particles in natural scrapie of the sheep, *Res. Vet. Sci.* **14:**108–110.

Narang, H. K., 1974a, An electron microscopic study of natural scrapie sheep brain: Further observations on virus-like particles and paramyxovirus-like tubules, *Acta Neuropathol. (Berl.)* **28:**317–329.

Narang, H. K., 1974b, An electron microscopic study of the scrapie mouse and rat: Further observations on virus-like particles with ruthenium red and lanthanum nitrate as a possible trace and negative stain, *Neurobiology* **4:**349–363.

Narang, H. K., Shenton, B. K., Giorgi, P. P., and Field, E. J., 1972, Scrapie agent and neuron, *Nature (Lond.)* **240:**105–107.

Narang, H. K., Chandler, R. L., and Anger, H. S. 1980, Further observations on particulate structures in scrapie affected brain, *Neuropathol. Appl. Neurobiol.* **6**:23–28.

Narang, H. K., Asher, D. M., and Gajdusek, D. C., 1987, Tubulofilaments in negatively stained scrapie-infected brains: Relationship to scrapie-associated fibrils, *Proc. Natl. Acad. Sci. USA* **84**:7730–7734.

Narang, H. K., Asher, D. M., and Gajdusek, D. C., 1988, Evidence that DNA is present in abnormal tubulofilamentous structures found in scrapie, *Proc. Natl. Acad. Sci. USA* **85**:3575–3579.

Niewold, Th. A., Hol, P. R., van Andel, A. C. J., Lutz, E. T. G., and Gruys, E., 1987, Enhancement of amyloid induction by amyloid fibril fragments in hamsters, *Lab. Invest.* **56**:544–549.

Nikaido, T., Austin, J., Truch, L., and Reinhart, R., 1972, Studies in ageing of the brain. II. Microchemical analyses of the nervous system in Alzheimer patients, *Arch. Neurol.* **27**:549–554.

Oesch, B., Westaway, D., Wälchli, M., McKinley, M. P., Kent, S. B. H., Aebersold, R., Barry, R. A., Tempst, P., Teplow, D. B., Hood, L. E., Prusiner, S. B., and Weissmann, C., 1985, A cellular gene encodes scrapie PrP 27–30 protein, *Cell* **40**:735–746.

Owen, F., Poulter, M., Lofthouse, R., Collinge, J., Crow, T. J., Rishy, D., Baker, H. F., Ridley, R. M., Hsiao, K., and Prusiner, S. B., 1989, Insertion in prion protein gene in familial Creutzfeldt–Jakob disease, *Lancet* **1**:51–52.

Perl, D. P., and Brody, A. R., 1980, Alzheimer's disease: X-ray spectrometric evidence of aluminum accumulation in neurofibrillary tangle-bearing neurons, *Science* **208**:297–299.

Perl, D. P., Gajdusek, D. C., Garruto, R. M., Yanagihara, R. T., and Gibbs, C. J., Jr., 1982, Intraneuronal aluminum accumulation in amyotrophic lateral sclerosis and parkinsonism–dementia of Guam, *Science* **217**:1053–1055.

Piccardo, P., Safar, J., Ceroni, M., Gajdusek, D. C., and Gibbs, C. J., Jr., 1990, Immunohistochemical localization of scrapie amyloid protein in spongiform encephalopathies and normal brain tissue (in press).

Ponte, P., Gonzalez-DeWhitt, P., Schilling, J., Miller, J., Hsu, D., Greenberg, B., Davis, K. Wallace, W., Lieberburg, I., Fuller, F., and Cordell, B., 1988, A new A4 amyloid mRNA contains a domain homologous to serine proteinase inhibitors, *Nature (Lond.)* **331**:525–527.

Prusiner, S. B., 1982, Novel proteinaceous infectious particles cause scrapie, *Science* **216**:136–144.

Prusiner, S. B., 1984, Some speculations about prions, amyloid and Alzheimer's disease, *N. Engl. J. Med.* **310**:661–663.

Prusiner, S. B., McKinley, M. P., Bowman, K. A., Bolton, D. C., Benheim, P. D., Groth, D. F., and Glenner, G. G., 1983, Scrapie prions aggregate to form amyloid-like birefringent rods, *Cell* **35**:349–358.

Prusiner, S. B., Groth, D. F., Bolton, D. C., Kent, S. B., and Hood, L. E., 1984, Purification and structural studies of a major scrapie prion protein, *Cell* **38**:127–134.

Rasool, C. G., and Selkoe, D. J., 1985, Sharing of specific antigens by degenerating neurons in Pick's disease and Alzheimer's disease, *N. Engl. J. Med.* **312**:700–705.

Rees, S., and Cragg, B., 1983, Is silica involved in neuritic (senile) plaque formation?, *Acta Neuropathol.* **59**:31–40.

Robakis, N. K., Wisnieski, H. M., Jenkins, E. C., Devine-Gage, E. A., Housck, G. E., Xiu-Lan Yao, Ramakrishna, N., Wolfe, G., Silverman, W. P., and Brown, W. T., 1987, Chromosome 21q21 sublocalization of gene encoding β-amyloid peptide in cerebral vessels and neuritic (senile) plaques of people with Alzheimer disease and Down syndrome, *Lancet* **1**:384.

Robertson, H. D., Branch, A. D., and Dahlberg, J. E., 1985, Focusing on the nature of the scrapie agent, *Cell* **40**:725–727.

Rohwer, R. G., 1984a, Scrapie shows a virus-like sensitivity to heat inactivation, *Science* **223**:600–602.

Rohwer, R. G., 1984b, Scrapie: Virus-like size and virus-like susceptibility to inactivation of the infectious agent, *Nature (Lond.)* **308**:658–662.

Rohwer, R. G., 1984c, Scrapie-associated fibrils (Letter to the editor), *Lancet* **2**:36.

Rohwer, R. G., 1990, Growth kinetics of hamster scrapie strain 263K: Sources of slowness in a slow virus infection, *Virology*, Raven Press, New York.

Rohwer, R. G., and Gajdusek, D. C., 1980, Scrapie—virus or viroid: The case for a virus, in: *Search for the Cause of Multiple Sclerosis and Other Chronic Diseases of the Central Nervous System,* Proceedings of the First International Symposium of the Hertie Foundation, Frankfurt am Main, September, 1979 (A. Boese, ed.), Verlag Chemie, Weinheim, pp. 333–355.

Rohwer, R. G., Brown, P. W., and Gajdusek, D. C., 1979, The case of sedimentation to equilibrium as a step in the purification of the scrapie agent, in: *Slow Transmissible Diseases of the Nervous System* (S. B. Prusiner and W. J. Hadlow, eds.), Academic, New York, pp. 465–478.

Safar, J., Ceroni, M., Piccardo, P., Gajdusek, D. C., and Gibbs, C. J., Jr., 1989, Scrapie precursor proteins: Antigenic relationship between species and immunocytochemical localization in normal, scrapie and Creutzfeldt–Jakob disease brains, (in press).

Safar, J., Ceroni, M., Piccardo, P., Liberski, P. P., Miyazaki, M., Gajdusek, D. C., and Gibbs, C. J., Jr., 1989, Subcellular distribution and physicochemical properties of scrapie precursor protein and relationship with scrapie infectivity, (in press).

Safar, J., Wang, W., Paogett, M. P., Ceroni, M., Piccardo, P., Zopf, D., Gibbs, C. J., Jr., and Gajdusek, D. C., 1989, Molecular mass, biochemical composition and physicochemical behavior of the infectious form of the scrapie precursor protein monomer, (in press).

Sänger, H. L., 1982, Biology, structure, functions, and possible origins of plant viroids, in: *Nucleic Acids and Proteins in Plants,* Vol. II. Encyclopaedia of Plant Pathology, New Series, 14B, Springer-Verlag, Berlin. pp. 368–454.

Schmechel, D. E., Goldgaber, D., Burkhart, D. S., Gilbert, J. R., Gajdusek, D. C., and Roses, A. D., 1988, Cellular localization of amyloid-beta-protein messenger RNA in postmortem brain in Alzheimer's disease patients, *Int. J. Alzheimer's Dis. Rel. Dis.* 2:96–111.

Schubert, D., Schroeder, R., LaCorbiere, M., Saiton, T., and Cole, G., 1988, Amyloid β-protein precursor is possibly a heparin sulfater proteoglycan core protein, *Science* 241:223–226.

Selkoe, D. J., Abraham, C. R., Podlinsky, M. D., and Duffy, L. K., 1986, Isolation of low molecular weight proteins from amyloid plaque fibers in Alzheimer's disease, *J. Neurochem.* 146:1820–1834.

Sotelo, J., Gibbs, C. J., Jr., and Gajdusek, D. C., 1980a, Autoantibodies against axonal neurofilaments in patients with kuru and Creutzfeldt–Jakob disease, *Science* 210:190–193.

Sotelo, J., Gibbs, C. J., Jr., Gajdusek, D. C., Toh, B. H., and Wurth, M., 1980b, Method for preparing cultures of central neurons: Cytochemical and immunochemical studies, *Proc. Natl. Acad. Sci. USA* 77:653–657.

Stefansson, K., Marton, L. S., Dieperink, M. E., Molnar, G. K., Schlaepfer, W. W., and Helgason, C. M., 1985, Circulating autoantibodies to the 200,000-dalton protein of neurofilaments in the serum of healthy individuals, *Science* 228:1117–1119.

Sternberger, N. H., Sternberger, L. A., and Ulrich, J., 1985, Aberrant neurofilament phosphorylation in Alzheimer's disease, *Proc. Natl. Acad. Sci. USA* 82:4274–4276.

Tanzi, R. E., Gusella, J. F., Watkins, P. C., Bruas, G. A. P., St. George-Hyslop, P., VanKeuren, M. L., Patterson, D., Pagan, S., Kuruit, D. M., and Neve, R. L., 1987, Amyloid β-protein gene: cDNA, mRNA distribution, and genetic linkage near the Alzheimer locus, *Science* 235:880–884.

Tanzi, R. E., McClatchey, A. I., Lamperti, E. D., Villa-Komaroff, L., Gusella, J. F., and Neve, R. L., 1988, Protease inhibitor domain encoded by an amyloid protein precursor mRNA associated with Alzheimer's disease, *Nature (Lond.)* 331:528–530.

Taylor, D. M., and McConnell, I., 1988, Autoclaving does not decontaminate formal-fixed scrapie tissues, *Lancet* 1:1463–1464.

Terry, R. D., and Pena, C. J., 1965, Experimental production of neurofibrillary degeneration. 2. Electron microscopy, phosphatase histochemistry and electron probe analysis, *Neuropathol. Exp. Neurol.* 24:200–210.

Toh, B. H., Gibbs, C. J., Jr., Gajdusek, D. C., Goudsmit, J., and Dahl, D., 1985a, The 200- and 150-kDa neurofilament proteins react with IgG autoantibodies from patients with kuru, Creutzfeldt–Jakob disease and other neurologic diseases, *Proc. Natl. Acad. Sci. USA* 82:3485–3489.

Toh, B. H., Gibbs, C. J., Jr., Gajdusek, D. C., Tuthill, D. D., and Dahl, D., 1985b, The 200- and 150-kDA neurofilament proteins react with IgG autoantibodies from chimpanzees with kuru,

Creutzfeldt–Jakob disease and 62-kDa neurofilament-associated protein reacts with sera from sheep with natural scrapie, *Proc. Natl. Acad. Sci. USA* **82**:3894–3896.

Traub, R., Gajdusek, D. C., and Gibbs, C. J., Jr., 1977, Transmissible virus dementias. The relation of transmissible spongiform encephalopathy to Creutzfeldt–Jakob disease, in: *Aging and Dementia* (M. Kinsbourne and L. Smith, eds.), pp. 91–146, Spectrum, Flushing, New York.

Troncoso, J. C., Hoffman, P. N., Griffin, J. W., Hess-Kozlow, K. M., and Price, D. L., 1985, Aluminum intoxication: A disorder of neurofilament transport in motor neurons, *Brain Res.* **342**:172–175.

Van Nostrand, W. E., Wagner, S. L., Suzuki, M., Choi, B. H., Farrow, J. S., Geddes, J. W., Cotman, C. W., Cunningham, D. D., 1989, Protease nexin-II, a potent antichymotrypsin, shows identity to amyloid β-protein precurser, *Nature* **341**:546–549.

Vernon, M. L., Horta-Barbosa, L., Fuccillo, D. A., Sever, J. L., Barringer, J. R., and Burnbaum, G., 1970, Virus-like particles and nuclear protein type filaments in brain tissue from two patients with Creutzfeldt–Jakob disease, *Lancet* **1**:964–967.

Weiss, A., 1981, Replication and evolution of inorganic systems, *Angew. Chem. Int. Ed. Engl.* **20**:850–860.

Westaway, D., Goodman, P. A., Mirenda, C. A., McKinley, P., Carlson, G. A., and Prusiner, S. B., 1987, Distinct prion proteins in short and long scrapie incubation period mice, *Cell* **51**:651–662.

Wilesmith, J. W., Wells, G. A. H., Cranwell, M. P., and Ryan, J. B. M., 1988, Bovine spongiform encephalopathy: Epidemiological studies, *Vet. Record* **123**:638–644.

Williams, E. S., and Young, S., 1980, Chronic wasting disease of captive mule deer: A spongiform encephalopathy, *J. Wildl. Dis.* **16**:89–98.

Williams, E. S., and Young, S., 1982, Spongiform encephalopathy of Rocky Mountain elk, *J. Wildl. Dis.* **18**:465–471.

Williams, E. S., Young, S., and Marsh, R. F., 1982, Preliminary evidence of the transmissibility of chronic wasting disease of mule deer, in: *Proceedings of the Wildlife Disease Associate Annual Conference, August 19, 1982, Madison, Wisconsin* (abst. 22).

Wong, C. W., Quaranta, V., and Glenner, G. G., 1985, Neuritic plaques and cerebral vascular amyloid in Alzheimer disease are antigenically related, *Proc. Natl. Acad. Sci. USA* **82**: 8729–9732.

Wood, J. G., Mirra, S. S., and Binder, L. I., 1986, Neurofibrillary tangles of Alzheimer disease share antigenic determinants with the axonal microtubule-associates protein tau (t), *Proc. Natl. Acad. Sci. USA* **83**:4040–4043.

ZuRhein, G. M., and Varakis, J., 1976, Subacute spongiform encephalopathy, in: *Slow Virus Diseases of Animal and Man* (R. H. Kimberlin, ed.), North-Holland, Amsterdam, pp. 359–380.

2

Prions Causing Neurodegenerative Diseases

Immunoaffinity Purification and Neutralization of Scrapie Infectivity

RUTH GABIZON, MICHAEL P. McKINLEY,
DARLENE GROTH, and STANLEY B. PRUSINER

1. INTRODUCTION

Amyloid deposits in Alzheimer's disease (AD) are an invariant feature of the disease. Amyloid deposition has been found primarily within neurofibrillary tangles (NFT), plaques, and cerebral vasculature. These structures are defined as amyloid primarily on the basis of their binding of Congo red and the green-gold birefringence they exhibit under polarized light. Whether any or all of these amyloid deposits in AD are etiologic remains to be established.

Scrapie is a degenerative neurological disease of sheep and goats that can be transmitted to laboratory rodents. Much evidence argues that the infectious agent is not a virus, but rather an unprecedented particle, termed *prion* (Prusiner, 1982). Whether prions contain only protein or possess a second molecule such as a nucleic acid is unknown.

In the prion disorders of humans and animals, amyloid deposits appear to be composed largely of an abnormal isoform of the prion protein (PrP). This abnormal PrP molecule is also a component of the infectious prion particle that causes these neurodegenerative diseases (Prusiner, 1987). In humans, prions cause Creutzfeldt–Jakob disease (CJD), kuru, and Gerstmann–Sträussler syndrome (GSS).

The only macromolecule in preparations highly enriched for prion infectivity identified to date is a protein of 33–35 kDa, designated the scrapie isoform of the prion protein (PrPSc) (Prusiner, 1987). Removal of the N-terminal 67 amino acids of hamster PrPSc by limited proteinase K digestion yields a prion protein (PrP) of 27–30 kDa designated PrP 27–30

RUTH GABIZON, MICHAEL P. McKINLEY, and DARLENE GROTH • Department of Neurology, University of California–San Francisco, San Francisco, California 94143-0518.   STANLEY B. PRUSINER • Departments of Neurology and Biochemistry and Biophysics, University of California–San Francisco, San Francisco, California 94143-0518.

(Basler et al., 1986). Many lines of evidence support the idea that PrPSc is a component of the infectious particle:

1. PrPSc and the scrapie agent copurify in fractions prepared by detergent extraction, differential centrifugation, limited proteinase K digestion, and sucrose-gradient sedimentation (Prusiner et al., 1982a, 1983; Bolton et al., 1982; Diringer et al., 1983).
2. The PrP 27–30 concentration is proportional to the prion titer (McKinley et al., 1983).
3. Procedures that denature, hydrolyze, or selectively modify PrP 27–30 also diminish the prion titer (Bolton et al., 1984). The unusual kinetics of PrP 27–30 proteolysis have been shown to correlate with the diminution of the scrapie-agent titer (McKinley et al., 1983).
4. The PrP gene (Prn-p) in mice is linked to a gene controlling scrapie incubation times (Prn-i) (Diringer et al., 1983; Carlson et al., 1986). The pre-eminent role of PrP in the pathogenesis of scrapie has been made more compelling by the discovery of a correlation between PrP amino acid sequence and scrapie incubation times (Westaway et al., 1987).
5. PrP 27–30 and scrapie infectivity copartition into many different forms: membranes, rods, spheres, detergent–lipid–protein complexes (DLPC), and liposomes (Gabizon et al., 1987).
6. Scrapie and Creutzfeldt–Jakob disease (CJD) isoforms of the prion protein have been identified only in the tissues of animals and humans with transmissible neurodegenerative diseases, and not in murine systemic amyloidosis, AD, anoxic encephalopathy, or non-neurologic disorders (Bockman et al., 1985; Brown et al., 1986; Roberts et al., 1986; Bockman et al., 1987).
7. Cultured murine neuroblastoma cells have been infected with both scrapie and CJD prions. Clones of the scrapie-infected cells were found to produce PrPSc, whereas clones showing no infectivity lacked PrPSc (Butler et al., 1988).

Although the evidence is considerable that PrPSc is an integral component of the prion, some investigators continue to believe that PrPSc is a pathological product of infection that copurifies with the scrapie agent (Braig and Diringer, 1985; Manuelidis et al., 1987; Clawson, 1988).

For several years, the only highly purified preparations of scrapie prions were in the form of rod-shaped amyloid polymers (Prusiner et al., 1982a, 1983; Diringer et al., 1983). Recently, we developed a protocol to disperse these rod-shaped polymers into DLPC and liposomes with full retention of infectivity (Gabizon et al., 1987). This protocol was subsequently adapted for DLPC formation directly from brain microsomes, which avoids the aggregation of PrPSc (Gabizon et al., 1988). Before the development of protocols for obtaining infectious prion DLPC and liposomes, many studies were not possible because purified preparations that retained infectivity were composed of the insoluble prion amyloid rods.

We reasoned that PrP monoclonal antibody (mAb) affinity chromatography would copurify solubilized PrPSc and prion infectivity if PrPSc is a component of the infectious scrapie particle. On the other hand, this procedure should separate PrPSc from infectivity if the two are unrelated. Upon testing this hypothesis, we found that PrPSc and prion infectivity copurify, implying that the molecular properties of PrPSc and the infectious particles must be extremely similar. This copurification is all the more significant, since it has now been achieved by two completely independent methods based on different biophysical principles (Prusiner et al., 1982a, 1983). As reported here, fractions eluted from the immunoaffinity column at alkaline pH contained one protein, PrPSc, and high titers of scrapie infectivity. We also demonstrate that rabbit polyclonal PrP 27–30 antisera can neutralize scrapie infectivity. These results, coupled with earlier observations summarized above, provide strong support favoring our contention that PrPSc is a component of the infectious scrapie particle.

2. EXPERIMENTAL PROCEDURES

2.1. Materials

Na cholate, Na dodecyl sarcosinate (Sarkosyl), Tris buffer, Na deoxycholate, and Nonidet P-40, were obtained from Sigma (St. Louis, Missouri). Protein A–Sepharose CL-4B was purchased from Pharmacia (Piscataway, New Jersey), dimethylpimelimidate from Pierce Chemical (Rockford, Illinois), sodium dodecyl sulfate (SDS) from BDH (London), phosphatidylcholine (PC) from Avanti (Birmingham, Alabama), and proteinase K from Beckman (Palo Alto, California).

2.2. Scrapie Prion Propagation and Bioassay

Hamster scrapie prions (Marsh and Kimberlin, 1975) were passaged five times in golden hamsters (LVG/LAK) purchased from Charles River Laboratories, Lakeview Colony. Propagation of prions was performed in golden hamsters inoculated intracerebrally with $\sim 10^7$ ID_{50} units of scrapie agent and sacrificed 70 days later. Bioassays for scrapie infectivity were performed in hamsters by incubation time measurements (Prusiner et al., 1982b).

2.3. Analytical Procedures

Protein was measured using the bicinchoninic acid (BCA) (Pierce Chemical, Rockford, Illinois) dye method with crystalline bovine serum albumin (BSA) as standard (Bradford, 1976). Samples with low protein concentrations were precipitated by chloroform–methanol (1 : 2) before measurement with BCA. Radioiodination of PrP 27–30 was accomplished using [^{125}I]-Bolton–Hunter reagent purchased from Amersham (Arlington Heights, Illinois) (1 mCi, 2000 Ci/mmole) (Bolton and Hunter, 1973). Sodium dodecyl sulfate–polyacrylamide gel electrophoresis (SDS–PAGE) was performed according to the method of Laemmli (1970). Western blots (Towbin et al., 1979) and silver staining of gels (Heukeshoven and Dernick, 1985) were performed as described previously with 0.01% SDS in the electrotransfer buffer (Butler et al., 1988). Concentration of PrP was estimated visually by comparing the volume of a given fraction required for detection on Western blot as well as the intensity of staining with that of standards.

2.4. Preparation of Immunoaffinity Resin

PrP mAb 13A5 was purified by a protein A–Sepharose CL-4B column in the presence of 0.5 M NaCl with a pH of 8.5; ~ 10 mg of antibody was obtained from 1 liter of hybridoma medium (Barry and Prusiner, 1986). The PrP mAb (10 mg) were crosslinked to protein A–Sepharose CL-4B (4 ml) using 20 mM dimethylpimelimidate dihydrochloride (Schneider et al., 1982), washed with phosphate-buffered saline, and stored at 4°C in a suspension containing 0.02% sodium azide. Alternatively, the IgG fraction from a polyclonal rabbit PrP

27–30 antiserum (RO17) (Butler et al., 1988) or a polyclonal rabbit human immunodeficiency virus (HIV)-GP120 synthetic peptide antiserum was crosslinked to protein A–Sepharose CL-4B. This PrP 27–30 antiserum was raised against the prion rods, which had been denatured in 0.5% SDS and boiled for 5 min. The synthetic peptide antiserum was raised against amino acids 465–480 of the HIV-GP120 (CFRPGGGDMRDNWRSEL) and was kindly provided by Dr. Tom Krowka.

2.5. Purification of Brain Microsomes

Scrapie-infected hamster brains were homogenized with a Polytron for 10 sec in 320 mM sucrose to produce a 10% (w/v) homogenate. All procedures were performed at 4°C unless otherwise stated. After centrifugation at 5000g for 10 min, the pellet was discarded and the supernatant centrifuged for 1 hr at 100,000g. The resulting pellet was resuspended in a minimal volume of a buffer containing 10 mM Tris–HCl (pH 7.4), 150 mM NaCl, and then subjected to osmotic shock by a 100-fold dilution into 10 mM Tris–HCl (pH 7.4), 2 mM phenylmethylsulfonylfluoride. After 20 min, the suspension was centrifuged for 1 hr at 100,000g and the osmotic shock step repeated. The purified microsomal membranes were resuspended at a concentration of 5 mg/ml protein and either used immediately or stored at −70°C.

2.6. Preparation of DLPC

We added 10 ml of microsomes purified from scrapie-infected brains to a glass test tube containing 100 mg of dry PC, vortexed before the addition of Sarkosyl to a final concentration of 2% (w/v) (Gabizon et al., 1987, 1988). The mixture was then sonicated for 10 min in a cylindrical bath sonicator and centrifuged at 100,000g for 1 hr. The supernatant fraction contained DLPC, which were used for further purification.

2.7. Immunoaffinity Chromatography

The DLPC fraction was incubated overnight at 4°C with PrP mAb Protein A–Sepharose beads on a rocking platform oscillating 30 times per min. The DLPC bound to resin was transferred to a column (2.5 × 15 cm) and washed with the following buffers: (1) 0.05 M NaCl, 0.05 M Tris–HCl (pH 8.2), 1% (w/v) Sarkosyl, 2 mg/ml PC (4 vol); (2) the same buffer with 0.5% (v/v) Nonidet P-40 instead of Sarkosyl (3 vol); and (3) 0.15 M NaCl, 0.5% (w/v) Na deoxycholate, 1 mg/ml PC (3 vol). PrP was then eluted by a discontinuous gradient of alkali pH: (1) 10 ml of 0.05 M triethylamine (pH 9.5) + 0.5% Na deoxycholate + 1 mg/ml PC; (2) the same solution titrated to pH 10.0; and (3) the same solution at pH 11.2. After elution, the samples were immediately titrated to neutrality with 2-N-(morpholino) ethane sulfonic acid (MES) buffer.

2.8. Immunoprecipitation and Neutralization

Iodine-125-labeled PrP 27–30 in purified prion rods was prepared using the Bolton–Hunter reagent (Bolton and Hunter, 1973), methanol-precipitated and solubilized into DLPC by the addition of 2% cholate and 5 mg/ml PC. The protein concentration was 5 µg/ml. The DLPC was then incubated with an IgG fraction of PrP antiserum or PrP mAb in a 1.5-ml Eppendorf tube and rocked overnight at 4°C. Protein A–Sepharose beads were added to the PrP antibody–DLPC mixture and incubated for 1 hr before centifugation in a microfuge for

10 min. The protein adsorbed by the beads was carefully separated from the supernatant fluid and the [125I] in each fraction measured in a Beckman gamma counter.

For the neutralization experiments, nonradioactive [[127I]-PrP 27–30 was solubilized into DLPC and incubated with the relevant antibody, as described above. After an overnight incubation, the samples were either directly inoculated into hamsters after dilution with inoculation buffer or incubated with protein A–Sepharose before fractionation and inoculation. In most of the experiments, the protein concentration of PrP 27–30 was 5 µg/ml, the lipid concentration 3 mg/ml, and the concentration of the antiserum IgG fraction 10 mg/ml.

3. RESULTS

A microsomal membrane fraction was prepared from scrapie-infected brains containing 50% of the scrapie infectivity and 50% of the PrP. The microsomes were solubilized by a combination of Sarkosyl (2% w/v) and PC (10 mg/ml). The DLPC formed by this procedure were subjected to ultracentrifugation and the supernatant applied to a PrP mAb affinity matrix. MAb raised against PrP 27–30 were crosslinked to protein A–Sepharose in an effort to minimize the leakage of the antibodies. After an overnight incubation at 4°C, the immunoaffinity matrix was washed with buffers containing increasing concentrations of salt and different detergent as well as 2% (w/v) PC. The PC was included to prevent aggregation of PrP^{Sc} while bound to the matrix and during elution.

The elution of PrP from the matrix was accomplished with increasing concentrations of alkali. The pH value of the eluate was increased progressively from 9.5 to 11.2. At pH 9.5, the first detectable PrP was eluted. Acid was also examined, but it was not efficient in eluting the prion protein. Because alkali is known to inactivate scrapie infectivity (Prusiner *et al.*, 1981), samples were titrated immediately after elution to pH 7.

Selected fractions of the immunoaffinity purification procedure were analyzed by SDS–PAGE. Most of the unbound PrP was eluted in the void volume; that not all of the PrP molecules are bound to the matrix may result from some PrP molecules possessing a configuration that is unfavorable for binding. No PrP was detected in subsequent washes prior to increasing the pH of the eluate buffer to 9.5, as judged by Western blotting (Fig. 1). Approximately 9% of the PrP was recovered in the alkaline eluate, representing ~20% of the PrP in the microsome fraction. An equal amount of PrP was found in the flowthrough fraction. At least 20% of the unaccounted for PrP remained bound to the column and was eluted by additional washes with the pH 11.2 buffer. The extent of PrP purification was approximately 5700-fold, and the purity of the PrP as judged by SDS–PAGE with silver staining was excellent. Similar results were obtained when the IgG fraction of a polyclonal rabbit PrP 27–30 antiserum was coupled to protein A–Sepharose and used in place of the PrP mAb columns.

Aliquots eluted from the immunoaffinity column at alkaline pH were examined by electron microscopy after negative staining with uranyl formate. Amorphous vesicles, but no prion rods, were seen (data not shown).

Some of the prion proteins in purified fractions are probably the cellular isoform of the prion protein (PrP^C) since all our PrP mAbs to date bind to both PrP isoforms. In order to estimate the amount of PrP^{Sc} in the purified fractions, we digested the fractions with proteinase K, which catalyzes the hydrolysis of PrP^C and the conversion of PrP^{Sc} to PrP 27–30. Most of the purified PrP^{Sc} is converted to PrP 27–30, as evidenced by the intensity of

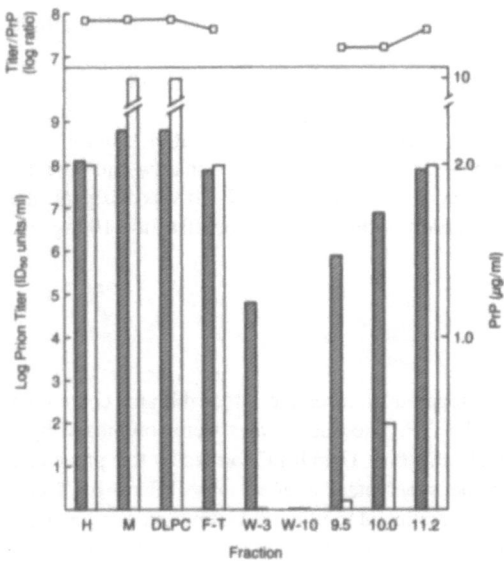

FIGURE 1. Immunoaffinity purification of PrPSc. Microsomes isolated from 15 scrapie-infected hamster brains were solubilized by a combination of Sarkosyl and PC. The resulting DLPC were incubated with PrP mAb (13A5) resin overnight at 4°C. The resin was then loaded into a column and washed sequentially with the following buffers: (1) 50 mM Tris–HCl (pH 8.2), 0.5 M NaCl, 1% (w/v) Sarkosyl, 2 mg/ml PC (4 washes); (2) 50 mM Tris–HCl, 0.5M NaCl, 1% (v/v) Nonidet P-40, 2 mg/ml PC (3 washes); (3) 0.15 M NaCl, 0.5% (w/v) Na deoxycholate, 1 mg/ml PC (3 washes). Each wash was equivalent to one column volume of 15 ml. The PrPSc bound to the resin was eluted by addition of alkali. Aliquots of selected fractions were analyzed by bioassays for scrapie infectivity and SDS–PAGE Western blotting for PrP. (Top) Log ratio of infectivity titer to PrP concentration for fractions listed on the horizontal axis. H, homogenate; M, microsomes; DLPC, detergent–lipid–protein complexes; F-T, flowthrough; W-3, wash 3; W-10, wash 10; 9.5, pH 9.5 eluate; 10.0, pH 10.0 eluate; 11.2, pH 11.2 eluate. (Bottom) Log titer (hatched bars) and the PrP concentration (open bars) for each fraction. Titer units are logarithmic, while PrP units are arithmetic.

immunostaining as well as silver staining on SDS–PAGE. From these digestions, we conclude that most of the PrP in our purified fractions is PrPSc.

Aliquots of fractions from the PrP immunoaffinity column were inoculated into hamsters for bioassay of scrapie prion titer. Those fractions that contain PrPSc also contain scrapie infectivity, while those fractions with no detectable PrPSc contain either low levels of scrapie prions or none (Fig. 1). Moreover, the amount of PrPSc recovered from the column was a function of the eluate pH and was roughly proportional to the prion titer. Although the specific infectivity (ID_{50} units/mg protein) increased by 4000-fold during purification, the ID_{50} units per μg PrP remained constant. We recovered ~4% of the total infectivity in the pH 11.2 eluate, corresponding to ~10% of infectivity found in the microsome fraction. An additional ~10% of the microsome infectivity was found in the flowthrough fraction. How much of the unaccounted infectivity remains bound to column and how much is inactivated during alkali elution remains to be determined. The imprecision of the animal bioassay (Prusiner *et al.*, 1982b) for scrapie infectivity complicates attempts to determine accurately the degree of purification and the recovery for a particular step. Even though the prion titers given in Fig. 1 represent the means from three separate experiments, it may be more prudent to claim a 10^3- to 10^4-fold purification of scrapie infectivity than the ~4000-fold, as described above.

In order to establish the specificity of our immunoaffinity purification protocol, we constructed an immunoaffinity matrix using an unrelated antibody raised against a synthetic peptide of GP120 of HIV. The results of the chromatography are depicted in Fig. 2. No PrPSc was eluted from the column regardless of the buffer pH, establishing that the binding of the PrP^{Sc} to the column was not nonspecific. Aliquots of the fractions from this experiment were bioassayed in hamsters. Prion infectivity was recovered only in the flowthrough; none was found in fractions eluted with alkali. Comparing the recoveries of prion infectivity eluted by alkali for the two columns reveals an impressive difference of ~10^8 (Figs. 1 and 2).

Concurrent with the development of an immunoaffinity purification protocol, we examined the immunoprecipitation of purified PrP 27–30 rods dispersed into DLPC. Polyclonal rabbit PrP 27–30 antiserum (RO18) precipitated ~50% of the radioiodinated PrP 27–30 in DLPC in the presence of protein A–Sepharose. Preimmune serum precipitated 1–2% of the PrP 27–30. The monoclonal PrP antibody (13A5) was unable to precipitate a significant portion of the PrP 27–30 in the presence of protein A–Sepharose; presumably, this was due to the relatively poor binding of murine IgG molecules to protein A. The efficacy of PrP mAb immunoprecipitation was substantially increased by using rabbit antiserum (RO21) raised against the PrP mAb (13A5) as second antibody to facilitate the binding to protein A–Sepharose. With all the PrP antibodies tested, it was necessary to use high concentrations in order to obtain maximal immunoprecipitation of [^{125}I]-PrP 27–30 in DLPC.

The immunoprecipitated fractions were also assessed for scrapie infectivity. The prion titers of samples treated with rabbit PrP 27–30 antiserum were reduced by a factor of 100, while exposure to preimmune serum did not alter the titer. In contrast to the polyclonal rabbit PrP antiserum, PrP mAb as well as polyclonal rabbit antiserum raised against the PrP mAb failed to neutralize scrapie infectivity associated with the DLPC.

In order to extend our finding that PrP 27–30 antiserum can neutralize scrapie infectivity, we incubated PrP 27–30 DLPC with increasing concentrations of antiserum. Preimmune serum failed to alter prion titer while immune serum caused a progressive decrease in

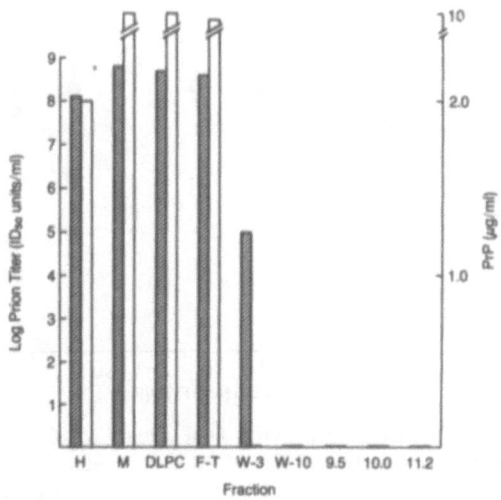

FIGURE 2. Immunoaffinity chromatography of PrP^{Sc} with a heterologous antibody. An immunoaffinity resin constructed by crosslinking the IgG fraction from a polyclonal rabbit HIV-GP120 synthetic peptide antiserum was coupled to protein A–Sepharose CL-4B. Microsomes isolated from 15 scrapie-infected hamster brains were solubilized by a combination of Sarkosyl and PC. The resulting DLPC were incubated with constant mixing using rocking platform overnight at 4°C in the presence of the immunoaffinity resin. The resin was then loaded into a column and washed sequentially with the three buffers described in Fig. 1. Log titer (hatched bars) and PrP concentration (open bars) are depicted for each fraction listed on the horizontal axis. Fractions are defined in Fig. 1.

titer (Fig. 3). A correlation between the ratio of PrP antiserum to PrP 27–30 and diminishing infectivity was found.

4. DISCUSSION

The immunoaffinity purification and neutralization studies reported here provide the first direct immunological and chromatographic demonstrations of a link between PrPSc and prion infectivity. Before developing techniques for the dispersion of PrPSc or PrP 27–30 into DLPC and liposomes (Gabizon et al., 1987, 1988), the experimental protocols described above could not have been performed, since they depend on the functional solubilization of scrapie prions. Our results combined with other immunologic, biochemical, and genetic data make it difficult to contend that PrPSc is not a component of the infectious particle but rather a pathological product of scrapie infection.

Investigators from many laboratories have confirmed the presence of PrPSc in brains infected with the scrapie or CJD agent (Braig and Diringer, 1985; Bockman et al., 1985, 1987; Brown et al., 1986; Roberts et al., 1986; Manuelidis et al., 1987). The amino acid sequence of PrP has also been confirmed (Oesch et al., 1985; Chesebro et al., 1985; Robakis et al., 1986; Basler et al., 1986), and there is agreement that PrP is glycosylated (Bolton et al., 1985; Manuelidis et al., 1985), but some investigators continue to suggest that PrP 27–30 may not be a component of the scrapie agent (Chesebro et al., 1985; Braig and Diringer, 1985; Manuelidis et al., 1987; Clawson, 1988). One argument focuses on the loss of CJD infectivity after binding to a lectin column (Manuelidis et al., 1987). However, the CJD preparations were composed of insoluble aggregates of PrP that were not amenable to chromatographic fractionation. Indeed, no studies to date have reported fractions with high levels of scrapie infectivity containing less than one PrP 27–30 molecule per infectious unit.

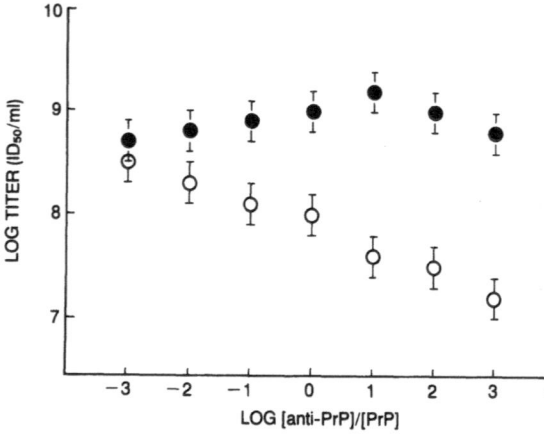

FIGURE 3. Neutralization of scrapie prion infectivity with polyclonal PrP 27–30 antiserum. DLPC were formed from purified prion rods containing 5 μg/ml PrP 27–30 by dispersion in a mixture of 2% cholate and 5 mg/ml PC. The 10-mg/ml IgG fraction of rabbit preimmune serum (–●–) or antiserum (R018) (–○–) raised against SDS–PAGE-purified PrP 27–30 was mixed with DLPC and incubated in an Eppendorf tube on a rocking platform at 4°C overnight. α-PrP and DLPC as well as diluent when necessary were added to each sample to obtain a final volume of 100 μl. Seven samples contained the following volumes in μl of α-PrP and DLPC, respectively: (1) 0.05, 50; (2) 0.5, 50; (3) 5, 50; (4) 50, 50; (5) 50, 5; (6) 50, 0.5; and (7) 50, 0.05. The samples were then inoculated into hamsters for bioassay. Samples were not frozen at any time after the DLPC were formed. Scrapie prion titer is plotted as a function of the ratio of the volume of PrP 27–30 antiserum to the volume of DLPC containing PrP 27–30.

Attempts to neutralize scrapie infectivity in fractions containing prion amyloid rods were unsuccessful (Barry and Prusiner, 1987). Only after the rods were dispersed into DLPC was a reduction of scrapie infectivity found with PrP antibodies (Fig. 3). Presumably, the DLPC expose epitopes, allowing neutralizing antibodies to bind; these same epitopes in rods may be buried and inaccessible to antibodies. Neutralization of viruses by antibodies has been widely studied and is thought to be a complex process that can occur through a variety of different pathways (Dimmock, 1987). Antibodies have also been used to assign a biological activity to a specific protein using neutralization or immunoprecipitation procedures (Allard and Lienhard, 1985; Barzilai et al., 1987; Targoff and Reichlin, 1987). The precise mechanism by which antibodies raised against SDS-PAGE-purified PrP 27-30 cause a reduction in scrapie infectivity remains to be established.

In part, the need for high concentrations of PrP antiserum to demonstrate neutralization may be due to the high particle-to-infectivity ratio. We estimate that the ratio of PrP^{Sc} molecules per ID_{50} unit in our immunoaffinity-purified fractions is $\sim 10^5$. This particle-to-infectivity ratio is similar to that previously reported for the prion amyloid rods, where it ranges from 10^4 to 10^6 (Prusiner et al., 1982a, 1983).

For many years, investigators searched for a detergent that would solubilize scrapie prion infectivity (Millson and Manning, 1979; Prusiner et al., 1980). Attempts at purification as well as characterization of the scrapie agent were plagued by the smearing of scrapie infectivity across centrifugation gradients, electrophoretic fractions, and chromatography profiles (Siakotos et al., 1976; Prusiner et al., 1978). Even fractionation of scrapie infectivity by precipitation or differential centrifugation was not efficient. Once PrP 27-30 was identified, the search shifted to detergents which could solubilize this protein without denaturing it. While no such detergent was found, combinations of detergents and phospholipids have been identified which are capable of functional solubilization (Gabizon et al., 1987, 1988). The utility of solubilizing PrP^{Sc} or PrP 27-30 under nondenaturing conditions that permit retention of scrapie infectivity is underscored by the immunoaffinity purification protocol reported here (see Fig. 1). The necessity of solubilization is emphasized by the control experiments using an unrelated antibody in which no detectable PrP or prion infectivity was detected in the alkaline eluate (see Fig. 2).

Because no effective protocols were available for complete solubilization, many earlier studies on the scrapie agent yielded confusing results. Agarose gel electrophoresis (Prusiner et al., 1980), SEC-HPLC (Prusiner, 1982) and sedimentation analyses (Prusiner et al., 1977, 1978; Malone et al., 1978) indicated that a portion of the infectious scrapie particles were small as well as demonstrating larger aggregates. The SEC studies suggested that the scrapie prion might have a monomeric molecular weight of 50,000 (Prusiner, 1982), in good agreement with ionizing radiation studies of homogenates, purified prion rods, and liposomes, giving a target size of 55,000 daltons (Alper et al., 1966; Bellinger-Kawahara et al., 1988). Of note, the apparent molecular weight of proteins based on SEC elution profiles can be inaccurate as a result of hydrophobic interactions between the protein and column matrix (Prusiner, 1982; Nozaki et al., 1976; Diringer and Kimberlin, 1983).

The experimental results of the complementary immunologic approaches reported here combined with results of biochemical and genetic studies mount a convincing argument for PrP^{Sc} being a major component of the infectious scrapie prion. This is an important feature distinguishing prions from viruses, since PrP is encoded by a host gene and not by a nucleic acid within the prion particle. Our results argue neither for nor against a second molecule within the prion, such as a small nucleic acid; however, all attempts to demonstrate a scrapie-specific polynucleotide have proved unsuccessful, to date. The development of an immunoaffinity purification protocol and procedures for chromatography will undoubtedly facilitate structural studies of prions as well as experiments focusing on how prions multiply.

The most compelling genetic evidence for a central role of PrP in the pathogenesis of scrapie comes from molecular cloning showing that inbred mice with short scrapie-incubation times (New Zealand white mice) and long scrapie incubation times (I/Ln mice) have distinct prion proteins (Westaway et al., 1987). A comparison of the PrP sequences of New Zealand white mice and I/Ln mice shows that the amino acid at codon 108 is changed from leucine to phenylalanine and that the amino acid at codon 189 is changed from threonine to valine. Although codon 189 is conserved in humans, hamsters, and most mice, codon 108 is not. All mice with short and intermediate scrapie incubation times that have been examined have been found to possess a leucine at codon 108 and a threonine at codon 189; all three inbred strains of mice known to have long incubation times have variant amino acids at these two codons. The correlation between scrapie incubation times and PrP sequence emphasizes the pivotal role of PrPSc in the pathogenesis of scrapie.

The cellular origin of prion proteins and the slow amplification mechanisms that account for the replication of prions make these unique macromolecules interesting candidates to explore with respect to many diseases that occur later in life. More important, the study of prion diseases has emphasized the need to learn how normal cellular proteins are converted into abnormal isoforms that polymerize into insoluble filaments (Prusiner, 1984). Although Alzheimer's disease has not been transmitted to laboratory animals (Gajdusek, 1977; Goudsmit et al., 1980), abnormal protein polymers do accumulate in Alzheimer's disease as amyloids; whether these polymers have a role in the pathogenesis of these disorders or accumulate only as pathological products remains to be determined (Prusiner, 1984).

5. SUMMARY

Prions are novel infectious pathogens causing scrapie of sheep and goats as well as Creutzfeldt–Jakob disease of humans. Biochemical and genetic studies contend that the scrapie isoform of the prion protein (PrPSc) is a major component of the prion. Limited proteinase K digestion of PrPSc produced PrP 27–30. After dispersion of brain microsomes isolated from scrapie-infected hamsters into detergent–lipid–protein complexes (DLPC), copurification of PrPSc and scrapie infectivity was obtained with PrP 27–30 monoclonal antibody affinity columns. PrPSc was enriched ~5700-fold with respect to total brain protein, while scrapie prion infectivity was enriched ~4000-fold. The ratio of prion titer to PrPSc remained constant throughout purification. Heterologous monoclonal antibody columns failed to bind either PrPSc or scrapie infectivity. Polyclonal rabbit PrP antiserum raised against SDS–PAGE-purified PrP 27–30 reduced scrapie infectivity dispersed into DLPC by a factor of 100. These results represent the first direct immunologic and chromatographic demonstrations of a relationship between PrPSc and prion infectivity as well as providing additional support for the contention that PrPSc is a major component of the infectious scrapie particle. Since PrPSc is a host-encoded protein, this is an important feature distinguishing prions from viruses.

ACKNOWLEDGMENTS. This work was supported by research grants AG02132 and NS14069 from the National Institutes of Health, by grant NS22786 from the Senator Jacob Javits Center of Excellence in Neuroscience, and by a grant from the American Health Assistance

Foundation, as well as by gifts from Sherman Fairchild Foundation and RJR–Nabisco, Inc. Portions of this manuscript are adapted from a paper entitled "Immunoaffinity Purification and Neutralization of Scrapie Prion Infectivity" published in *Proc. Natl. Acad. Sci. USA* (85:6617–6621), 1988. The authors thank Ms. Marion Vincent for excellent technical assistance, Dr. Eric Turk for helpful discussions, Dr. Ronald Barry and Dr. Dan Serban for production of PrP antibodies, and L. Gallagher for document production assistance. R. G. was supported by a Chaim Weizmann Postdoctoral Fellowship for Scientific Research.

REFERENCES

Allard, W. J., and Lienhard, G. E., 1985, Monoclonal antibodies to the glucose transporter from human erythrocytes, *J. Biol. Chem.* **260**:8668–8675.

Alper, T., Haig D. A., and Clarke, M. C., 1966, The exceptionally small size of the scrapie agent, *Biochem. Biophys. Res. Commun.* **22**:278–284.

Barry, R. A., and Prusiner, S. B., 1986, Monoclonal antibodies to the cellular and scrapie prion protein, *J. Infect. Dis.* **154**:518–521.

Barry, R. A., and Prusiner, S. B., 1987, Immunology of prions, in: *Prions—Novel Infectious Pathogens Causing Scrapie and Creutzfeldt–Jakob Disease* (S. B. Prusiner and M. P. McKinley, eds.), Academic, Orlando, Florida, pp. 239–275.

Barzilai, A., Spanier, R., and Rahamimoff, H., 1987, Immunological identification of the synaptic plasma membrane Na^+–Ca^{2+} exchanger, *J. Biol. Chem.* **262**:10315–10320.

Basler, K., Oesch, B., Scott, M., Westaway, D., Wälchli, M., Groth, D. F., McKinley, M. P., Prusiner, S. B., and Weissmann, C., 1986, Scrapie and cellular PrP isoforms are encoded by the same chromosomal gene, *Cell* **46**:417–428.

Bellinger-Kawahara, C. G., Kempner, E., Groth, D., Gabizon, R., and Prusiner, S. B., 1988, Scrapie prion liposomes and rods exhibit target sizes of 55,000 Da, *Virology* **164**:537–541.

Bockman, J. M., Kingsbury, D. T., McKinley, M. P., Bendheim, P. E., and Prusiner, S. B., 1985, Creutzfeldt–Jakob disease prion proteins in human brains, *N. Engl. J. Med.* **312**:73–78.

Bockman, J. M., Prusiner, S. B., Tateishi, J., and Kingsbury, D. T., 1987, Immunoblotting of Creutzfeldt–Jakob disease prion proteins: Host species-specific epitopes, *Ann. Neurol.* **21**:589–595.

Bolton, A. E., and Hunter, W. M., 1973, The labeling of proteins to high specific radioactivities by conjugation to a 125-I containing acylating agent, *Biochem. J.* **133**:529–539.

Bolton, D. C., McKinley, M. P., and Prusiner, S. B., 1982, Identification of a protein that purifies with the scrapie prion, *Science* **218**:1309–1311.

Bolton, D. C., McKinley, M. P., and Prusiner, S. B., 1984, Molecular characteristics of the major scrapie prion protein, *Biochemistry* **23**:5898–5905.

Bolton, D. C., Meyer, R. K., and Prusiner, S. B., 1985, Scrapie PrP 27–30 is a sialoglycoprotein, *J. Virol.* **53**:596–606.

Bradford, M. M., 1976, A rapid and sensitive method for the quantitation of microgram quantities of protein utilizing the principle of protein–dye binding, *Anal. Biochem.* **72**:248–254.

Braig, H., and Diringer, H., 1985, Scrapie: Concept of a virus-induced amyloidosis of the brain, *EMBO J.* **4**:2309–2312.

Brown, P., Coker-Vann, M., Pomeroy, K., Franko, M., Asher, D. M., Gibbs, C. J., Jr., and Gajdusek, D. C., 1986, Diagnosis of Creutzfeldt–Jakob disease by Western blot identification of marker protein in human brain tissue, *N. Engl. J. Med.* **314**:547–551.

Butler, D. A., Scott, M. R. D., Bockman, J. M., Borchelt, D. R., Taraboulos, A., Hsiao, K. K., Kingsbury, D. T., and Prusiner, S. B., 1988, Scrapie-infected murine neuroblastoma cells produce protease-resistant prion proteins, *J. Virol.* **62**:537–541.

Carlson, G. A., Kingsbury, D. T., Goodman, P., Coleman, S., Marshall, S. T., DeArmond, S. J.,

Westaway, D., and Prusiner, S. B., 1986, Linkage of prion protein and scrapie incubation time genes, *Cell* **46**:503–511.

Chesebro, B., Race, R., Wehrly, K., Nishio, J., Bloom, M., Lechner, D., Bergstrom, S., Robbins, K., Mayer, L., Keith, J. M., Garon, C., and Haase, A., 1985, Identification of scrapie prion protein-specific mRNA in scrapie-infected and uninfected brain, *Nature (Lond.)* **315**:331–333.

Clawson, G. A., 1988, Antiheretical speculations on the "prion" protein and scrapie, *Perspect. Biol. Med.* **31**:212–223.

Dimmock, N. J., 1987, Multiple mechanisms of neutralization of animal viruses, *Trends Biochem. Sci.* **12**:70–75.

Diringer, H., Gelderblom, H., Hilmert, H., Ozel, M., Edelbluth, C., and Kimberlin, R. H., 1983, Scrapie infectivity, fibrils and low molecular weight protein, *Nature (Lond.)* **306**:476–478.

Diringer, H., and Kimberlin, R. H., 1983, Infectious scrapie agent is apparently not as small as recent claims suggest, *Biosci. Rep.* **3**:563–568.

Gabizon, R., McKinley, M. P., and Prusiner, S. B., 1987, Purified prion proteins and scrapie infectivity copartition into liposomes, *Proc. Natl. Acad. Sci. USA* **84**:4017–4021.

Gabizon, R., McKinley, M. P., Groth, D. F., Kenaga, L., and Prusiner, S. B., 1988, Properties of scrapie prion liposomes, *J. Biol. Chem.* **263**:4950–4955.

Gajdusek, D. C., 1977, Unconventional viruses and the origin and disappearance of kuru, *Science* **197**:943–960.

Goudsmit, J., Morrow, C. H., Asher D. M., Yanagihara, R. T., Masters, C. L., Gibbs, C. J., Jr., and Gajdusek, D. C., 1980, Evidence for and against the transmissibility of Alzheimer's disease, *Neurology (NY)* **30**:945–950.

Heukeshoven, S., and Dernick, R., 1985, Simplified method for silver staining of proteins in poly-acrylamide gels and the mechanism of silver staining, *Electrophoresis* **6**:103–112.

Laemmli, U. K., 1970, Cleavage of structural proteins during the assembly of the head of bacteriophage T-4, *Nature (Lond.)* **227**:680–685.

Malone, T. G., Marsh, R. F., Hanson, R. P., and Semancik, J. S., 1978, Membrane-free scrapie activity, *J. Virol.* **25**:933–935.

Manuelidis, L., Sklaviadis, T., and Manuelidis, E. E., 1987, Evidence suggesting that PrP is not the infectious agent in Creutzfeldt–Jakob disease, *EMBO J.* **6**:341–347.

Manuelidis, L., Valley, S., and Manuelidis, E. E., 1985, Specific proteins associated with Creutzfeldt–Jakob disease and scrapie share antigenic and carbohydrate determinants, *Proc. Natl. Acad. Sci. USA* **82**:4263–4267.

Marsh, R. F., and Kimberlin, R. H., 1975, Comparison of scrapie and transmissible mink encephalopathy in hamsters. II. Clinical signs, pathology and pathogenesis, *J. Infect. Dis.* **131**:104–110.

McKinley, M. P., Bolton, D. C., and Prusiner, S. B., 1983, A protease-resistant protein is a structural component of the scrapie prion, *Cell* **35**:57–62.

Millson, G. C., and Manning, E. J., 1979, The effect of selected detergents on scrapie infectivity, in: *Slow Transmissible Diseases of the Nervous System*, Vol. 2, (S. B. Prusiner and W. J. Hadlow, eds.), Academic, New York, pp. 409–424.

Nozaki, Y., Schechter, M., Reynolds, J. A., and Tanford, C., 1976, Use of gel chromatography for the determination of the Stokes radii of proteins in the presence and absence of detergents: a reexamination, *Biochemistry* **15**:3884–3890.

Oesch, B., Westaway, D., Wälchli, M., McKinley, M. P., Kent, S. B., Aebersold, R., Barry, R. A., Tempst, P., Teplow, D. B., Hood, L. E., Prusiner, S. B., and Weissmann, C., 1985, A cellular gene encodes scrapie PrP 27–30 protein, *Cell* **40**:735–746.

Prusiner, S. B., 1982, Novel proteinaceous infectious particles cause scrapie, *Science* **216**:136–144.

Prusiner, S. B., 1984, Some speculations about prions, amyloid, and Alzheimer's disease, *N. Engl. J. Med.* **310**:661–663.

Prusiner, S. B., 1987, Prions and neurodegenerative diseases, *N. Engl. J. Med.* **317**:1571–1581.

Prusiner, S. B., Bolton, D. C., Groth, D. F., Bowman, K. A., Cochran, S. P., and McKinley, M. P., 1982a, Further purification and characterization of scrapie prions, *Biochemistry* **21**:6942–6950.

Prusiner, S. B., Cochran, S. P., Groth, D. F., Downey, D. E., Bowman, K. A., and Martinez, H. M., 1982b, Measurement of the scrapie agent using an incubation time interval assay, *Ann. Neurol.* **11**:353–358.

Prusiner, S. B., Groth, D. F., Bildstein, C., Masiarz, F. R., McKinley, M. P., and Cochran, S. P., 1980, Electrophoretic properties of the scrapie agent in agarose gels, *Proc. Natl. Acad. Sci. USA* **77**:2984–2988.

Prusiner, S. B., Groth, D. F., Cochran, S. P., Masiarz, F. R., McKinley, M. P., and Martinez, H. M., 1980, Molecular properties, partial purification, and assay by incubation period measurements of the hamster scrapie agent, *Biochemistry* **19**:4883–4891.

Prusiner, S. B., Groth, D. F., McKinley, M. P., Cochran, S. P., Bowman, K. A., and Kasper, K. C., 1981, Thiocyanate and hydroxyl ions inactivate the scrapie agent, *Proc. Natl. Acad. Sci. USA* **78**:4606–4610.

Prusiner, S. B., Hadlow, W. J., Eklund, C. M., and Race, R. E., 1977, Sedimentation properties of the scrapie agent, *Proc. Natl. Acad. Sci. USA* **74**:4656–4660.

Prusiner, S. B., Hadlow, W. J., Garfin, D. E., Cochran, S. P., Baringer, J. R., Race, R. E., and Eklund, C. M., 1978, Partial purification and evidence for multiple molecular forms of the scrapie agent, *Biochemistry* **17**:4993–4997.

Prusiner, S. B., McKinley, M. P., Bowman, K. A., Bolton, D. C., Bendheim, P., E., Groth, D. F., and Glenner, G. G., 1983, Scrapie prions aggregate to form amyloid-like birefringent rods, *Cell* **35**:349–358.

Robakis, N. K., Sawh, P. R., Wolfe, G. C., Rubenstein, R., Carp, R. I., and Innis, M. A., 1986, Isolation of a cDNA clone encoding the leader peptide of prion protein and expression of the homologous gene in various tissues, *Proc. Natl. Acad. Sci. USA* **83**:6377–6381.

Roberts, G. W., Lofthouse, R., Brown, R., Crow, T. J., Barry, R. A., and Prusiner, S. B., 1986, Prion protein immunoreactivity in human transmissible dementias, *N. Engl. J. Med.* **315**:1231–1233.

Schneider, C., Newman, R. A., Sutherland, D. R., Asser, U., and Greaves, M. F., 1982, A one-step purification of membrane proteins using a high efficiency immunomatrix, *J. Biol. Chem.* **257**:10766–10769.

Siakotos, A. N., Gajdusek, D. C., Gibbs, C. J., Jr., Traub, R. D., and Bucana, C., 1976, Partial purification of the scrapie agent from mouse brain by pressure disruption and zonal centrifugation in sucrose-sodium chloride gradients, *Virology* **70**:230–237.

Targoff, I. N., and Reichlin, M., 1987, Measurement of antibody to Jo-1 by ELISA and comparison to enzyme inhibitory activity, *J. Immunol.* **138**:2874–2882.

Towbin, H., Staehelin, T., and Gordon, J., 1979, Electrophoretic transfer of proteins from poly-acrylamide gels to nitrocellulose sheets: procedure and some applications, *Proc. Natl. Acad. Sci. USA* **76**:4350–4354.

Westaway, D., Goodman, P. A., Mirenda, C. A., McKinley, M. P., Carlson, G. A., and Prusiner, S. B., 1987, Distinct prion proteins in short and long scrapie incubation period mice, *Cell* **51**:651–662.

3

The Molecular Genetics of Alzheimer's Disease

J. A. HARDY, M. J. OWEN, A. M. GOATE, L. A. JAMES,
A. R. HAYNES, R. WILLIAMSON, P. ROQUES,
M. N. ROSSOR, and M. J. MULLAN

1. INTRODUCTION

In 1932, a case of apparent hereditary Alzheimer's disease was reported (Schottky, 1932); reports of similar families subsequently appeared in the literature (Lowenburg and Waggoner, 1934; Essen-Moller, 1946; Wheelan, 1959; Gillespie, 1938), but such cases were considered very rare. Since then, epidemiological studies suggest that familial Alzheimer's disease may be frequent (Sjögren *et al.*, 1952; Heston and Mastri, 1977; Heston *et al.*, 1981; Heyman *et al.*, 1983), and a number of extensive pedigrees with autosomal-dominant, histologically confirmed Alzheimer's disease have been reported (e.g., Nee *et al.*, 1983). The major problem with discerning a hereditary factor in Alzheimer's disease from prevalence data is the late age of onset. Studies such as those by Heyman and co-workers (1983) and by Breitner and colleagues (e.g., Mohs *et al.*, 1987) have suggested that a large proportion of cases might have a genetic basis.

Despite the uncertainty about the proportion of Alzheimer's disease that is genetic in origin, it is clear that the few, large, early-onset pedigrees in which Alzheimer's disease shows autosomal-dominant inheritance offer an opportunity to investigate the pathogenesis of the disease in more detail. In such pedigrees, the technique of linkage analysis offers a route to chromosomal localization, isolation, and finally, characterization of the defective gene and its product.

Linkage analysis relies on the fact that alleles of DNA sequences close together on a chromosome will be co-inherited more often than the 50% predicted for unlinked markers. The closer they are together, the more frequently alleles will co-segregate. Molecular genet-

J. A. HARDY, M. J. OWEN, A. M. GOATE, L. A. JAMES, A. R. HAYNES, and R. WILLIAMSON • Department of Biochemistry and Molecular Genetics, St. Mary's Hospital Medical School, London W2 1PG, England. P. ROQUES, M. N. ROSSOR, and M. J. MULLAN • Department of Neurology, St. Mary's Hospital Medical School, London W2 1PG, England.

ics permits the segregation of such sequence alleles, restriction fragment length polymorphisms RFLP), to be followed through families. Since the chromosomal positions of a large number of RFLP are now known, the inheritance of these can be followed through families to see whether any of the loci are close (i.e., genetically linked) to the disease locus.

2. CHROMOSOME 21 AND ALZHEIMER'S DISEASE

The observation that infants with Down's syndrome who survive into midlife develop histopathological features similar to those found in Alzheimer's disease suggested that abnormalities of the expression of a gene or set of genes on chromosome 21 can lead to the development of the disease. This finding implied that linkage analysis using probes to loci on this chromosome might be a fruitful strategy. This has recently been proved to be so, and linkage of two polymorphic loci (D21S1/S11 and D21S16) to a locus causing early-onset Alzheimer's disease has been reported. Since these loci are on the proximal segment of the long arm of chromosome 21 (21q1-2) (St. George-Hyslop *et al.*, 1987a), it follows that a familial Alzheimer's disease locus must also be in this region.

This localization of the Alzheimer gene was surprising for two reasons. First, although people had predicted that the Alzheimer gene might be on chromosome 21, they had thought that it would be at the end of the long arm, since individuals with just this segment triplicated (by translocation) develop phenotypic Down's syndrome. For this reason, the distal third of the long arm is termed the *pathological segment*. Second, at the same time that the Alzheimer's gene was localized, the amyloid precursor gene (a protein component of the senile plaques and cerebrovascular amyloid) was cloned and localized to the same chromosomal region (Kang *et al.*, 1987; Goldgaber *et al.*, 1987; Tanzi *et al.*, 1987b). A4-amyloid was an excellent candidate for the Alzheimer gene; its localization to the correct chromosomal region naturally prompted speculation that the genetic locus leading to Alzheimer's disease may be at or within the A4-amyloid gene. Expectations were further raised when it was reported that the A4-amyloid gene was duplicated in sporadic Alzheimer's disease (Delabar *et al.*, 1987). This suggested a unitary hypothesis for Alzheimer's disease with four tenets:

1. A4-amyloid deposition is central to the etiology of Alzheimer's disease.
2. Down's syndrome cases develop Alzheimer's disease because they have three copies of the A4-amyloid gene.
3. Sporadic Alzheimer's disease develops in people who have duplicated their A4-amyloid gene, i.e., they too have three copies.
4. Familial Alzheimer's disease is caused by overexpression or by expression of an abnormal variant of the A4-amyloid gene.

The attraction of this hypothesis is that tenets (3) and (4) are testable. Unfortunately, they do not stand up to experimental scrutiny. Further genetic analysis of families with Alzheimer's disease, using polymorphic markers of the A4-amyloid gene, clearly showed that there were recombinants between the two loci in several families. This strongly suggests the two loci are distinct (Van Broeckhoven *et al.*, 1987; Tanzi *et al.*, 1987c) and that the A4-amyloid gene is telomeric of the S1/S11 locus. Furthermore, other groups have not been able to replicate the observation of duplication of the amyloid gene locus in other affected individuals (Van Broeckhoven *et al.*, 1987; St. George Hyslop *et al.*, 1987b; Tanzi *et al.*, 1987a; Podlisny *et al.*, 1987).

3. HETEROGENEITY AND ALZHEIMER'S DISEASE

The identification of a genetic linkage of Alzheimer's disease to the loci S1/S11 and S16 should, in principle, make it a relatively straightforward task to determine whether other families, multiply affected by Alzheimer's disease, share the same disease locus. Clearly, linkage analysis of a number of new families should confirm the linkage between the chromosome 21 probes and the disease if there is only one disease locus. A multicenter collaboration has been established to determine the generality of the linkage to the chromosome 21 probes. So far, approximately 40 families have been analyzed (L. Farrer, unpublished data), with mean ages of onset ranging from 30 to 80 years of age. The null hypothesis being tested in this collaboration is that all familial cases of Alzheimer's disease are caused by the locus close to the probes D21S1/D21S11. The results analyzed so far are consistent with this hypothesis. In other words, there is at present no significant evidence for nonallelic genetic heterogeneity in the families tested, which included both young and old age of onset of the disease.

The localization of a familial Alzheimer's disease gene to the proximal end of the long arm of chromosome 21 is only the start of the endeavor to isolate the gene itself. Work in several laboratories is being directed toward determining precisely the position of the Alzheimer's disease gene on the linkage map of chromosome 21. The most complete linkage map of this chromosome is that of Watkins and co-workers, which gives a tentative probe order on chromosome 21 around the Alzheimer's disease locus (HGM9). However, the map does not include the other probe that has been linked to the Alzheimer's disease locus, S16. Van Broeckhoven (unpublished data, 1988) reported that S13 and S16 are physically close, and we have confirmed her data that these share common fragments by pulsed-field gel electrophoresis, as do S1 and S11.

These physical and genetic mapping data permit both determination of the position of S16 with respect to other probes and orientation of the genetic map with the Alzheimer's disease locus on it. The latest genetic analysis carried out by Farrer (unpublished data) suggests that the Alzheimer's disease locus is centromeric to all the probes on the genetic map of chromosome 21.

ACKNOWLEDGMENTS. We would like to thank Dr. P. Watkins, Dr. L. Farrer, Dr. P. St. George Hyslop, and Dr. C. Van Broeckhoven for access to data before publication, and Research into Ageing and the Medical Research Council for financial support.

REFERENCES

Delabar, J. M., Goldgaber, D., Lamour, Y., Nicole, A., Huret, J. L., de Grouchy, J., Brown, P., Gajdusek, D. C., and Sinet, P. M., 1987, Beta amyloid gene duplication in Alzheimer's disease and karyotypically normal Down syndrome, *Science* **235:**1390–1392.

Essen-Moller, E., 1946, A family with Alzheimer's disease, *Acta Psychiatr. Neurol. (Scand.)* **21:**233–244.

Gillespie, R. D., 1938, Discussion on the mental and physical symptoms of the presenile dementias, *Proc. R. Soc. Med.* **26:**1080–1084.

Goldgaber, D., Lerman, M. I., McBride, O. W., Saffiotti, U., and Gajdusek, D. C., 1987, Characterisation and chromosomal localisation of a cDNA encoding brain amyloid of Alzheimer's Disease, *Science* **235:**877–880.

Heston, L. L., and Mastri, A. R., 1977, The genetics of Alzheimer's disease. Associations with hematologic malignancy and Down's syndrome, Arch. Genet. Psychiatry 34:976–981.

Heston, L. L., Mastri, A. R., Anderson, V. E., and White, J., 1981, Dementia of the Alzheimer type. Clinical genetics, natural history and associated conditions, Arch. Gen. Psychiatry 38:1085–1090.

Heyman, A., Wilkinson, W. E., and Hurwitz, B. J., 1983, Alzheimer's disease: Genetic aspects and associate clinical disorders, Ann. Neurol. 14:507–515.

Kang, J., Lemaire, H-G., Unterbeck, A., Salbaum, J. M., Masters, C. L., Crzeschik, K-H., Multhaup, G., Beyreuther, K., and Muller-Hill, B., 1987, The precursor of Alzheimer's disease amyloid A4 protein resembles a cell-surface receptor, Nature (Lond.) 325:733–736.

Lowenberg, K., and Waggoner, R. W., 1934, Familial organic psychosis (Alzheimer's type), Arch. Neurol. Psychiatry 31:737–754.

Mohs, R. C., Breitner, J. C., Silverman, J. M., and Davis, K. L., 1987, Alzheimer's disease: morbid risk among first degree relatives approaches 50% by 90 years of age, Arch. Gen. Psychiatry 44:405–407.

Nee, L. E., Polinsky, R. J., Eldridge, R., Weingartner, H., and Smallberg, S., 1983, A family with histologically confirmed Alzheimer's Disease, Arch. Neurol. 40:203–208.

Podlisny, M. B., Lee, G., and Selkoe, D. J., 1987, Gene dosage of the amyloid beta precursor protein in Alzheimer's disease, Science 238:669–671.

Schottky, J., 1932, Uber prasenile Verblodungen, Ges. Neurol. Psych. 142:1–54.

Sjögren, T., Sjögren, J., and Lindgren, G. H., 1952, Morbus Alzheimer and Morbus Pick, Acta Psychiatr. Scand. 82(suppl.):9–63.

St. George-Hyslop, P., Tanzi, R. E., Polinsky, R. J., Haines, J. L., Nee, L., Watkins, P. C., Myers, R. H., Feldman, R. G., Pollen, D., Drachman, D., Growdon, J., Bruni, A., Foncin, J. F., Salmon, D., Frommelt, P., Amaducci, L., Sorbi, S., Piacentini, S., Stewart, G. D., Hobbs, W. J., Conneally, P. M., and Gusella, J. F., 1987a, The genetic defect causing familial Alzheimer's disease maps on chromosome 21, Science 235:885–889.

St. George Hyslop, P. H., Tanzi, R. E., Polinsky, R. J., Neve, R. E., Pollen, D., Drachman, D., Growdon, J., Cupples, L. A., Nee, L., Myers, R. H., O'Sullivan, D., Watkins, P. C., Amos, J. A., Deutsch, C. K., Bodfish, J. W., Kinsbourne, M., Feldman, R. G., Bruni, A., Amaducci, L., Foncin, J. F., and Gusella, J. F., 1987b, Absence of duplication of chromosome 21 genes in familial and sporadic Alzheimer's disease, Science 238:664–666.

Tanzi, R. E., Bird, E. D., Latt, S. A., and Neve, R. L., 1987a, The amyloid beta protein gene is not duplicated in brains from patients with Alzheimer's disease, Science 238:666–669.

Tanzi, R. E., Gusella, J. F., Watkins, P. C., Bruns, G. A. P., St. George-Hyslop, P., van Keuren, M. L., Patterson, D., Pagan, S., Kurnitt, D. M., and Neve, R. L., 1987b, Amyloid beta protein gene: cDNA, mRNA distribution and genetic linkage near the Alzheimer locus, Science 235:880–884.

Tanzi, R. E., St. George-Hyslop, P. H., Haines, J., Polinsky, R. J., Nee, L., Foncin, J. F., Neve, R. L., McClatchey, A. I., Conneally, P. M., and Gusella, J. F., 1987c, The genetic defect in familial Alzheimer's disease is not tightly linked to the amyloid beta-protein gene, Nature (Lond.) 329:156–157.

Van Broeckhoven, C., Genthe, A. M., Vandenberghe, A., Horsthemke, B., Backhovens, H., Raeymaekers, P., Van Hul, W., Wehnert, A., Gheuens, J., Cras, P., Bruyland, M., Martin, J., Salbaum, M., Multhaup, G., Masters, C. L., Beyreuther, K., Gurling, H. M. D., Mullan, M. J., Holland, A., Barton, A., Irving, A., Williamson, R., Richards, S-J., and Hardy, J. A., 1987, Failure of familial Alzheimer's disease to segregate with the A4-amyloid gene in several European families, Nature (Lond.) 329:153–155.

Wheelan, L., 1959, Familial Alzheimer's disease, Ann. Hum. Genet. 23:300–310.

4

A Developmental Genetic Approach to the Analysis of Aging Processes

THOMAS E. JOHNSON

1. INTRODUCTION

The biological processes collectively called *aging* are being dissected in our laboratory using classic genetic analyses akin to those used in the dissection of other fundamental biological processes, e.g., development or metabolism (Botstein and Mauer, 1982). Many pitfalls are inherent in the genetic analysis of components of fitness; many result from effects of inbreeding (Lints, 1978; Rose, 1984). These inbreeding effects have been avoided by the use of the small free-living nematode *Caenorhabditis elegans*. The hermaphroditic life-style of this animal facilitates the analysis of life span and senescence by permitting the direct isolation and genetic analysis of long-lived mutants and recombinant inbred (RI) lines without complications resulting from inbreeding problems (Johnson and Wood, 1982; T. E. Johnson, submitted for publication). Both approaches to obtaining long-lived genotypes have been used effectively in the analysis of the aging processes of *C. elegans* and the reader will find a brief summary of results below.

2. RECOMBINANT INBRED LINES

A series of RI lines have been derived from the progeny resulting from the mating of two wild-type strains followed by subsequent inbreeding (Johnson, 1986; Foltz and Johnson, submitted for publication) (Fig. 1). A few of these RI lines have life expectancies and maximum life spans significantly longer than those of wild-type strains (Fig. 2).

These long-lived lines were themselves derived from parents that had very similar life spans (Johnson and Wood, 1982). This can be explained by the existence of alternate allelic forms of genes at many loci that differ between the two parents. Estimates of the minimum number of these loci that differ in the two parents yield values of three to six and it is likely

THOMAS E. JOHNSON • Department of Molecular Biology and Biochemistry, University of California–Irvine, Irvine, California 92717.   *Present address:* Institute for Behavioral Genetics, University of Colorado, Boulder, Colorado 80309.

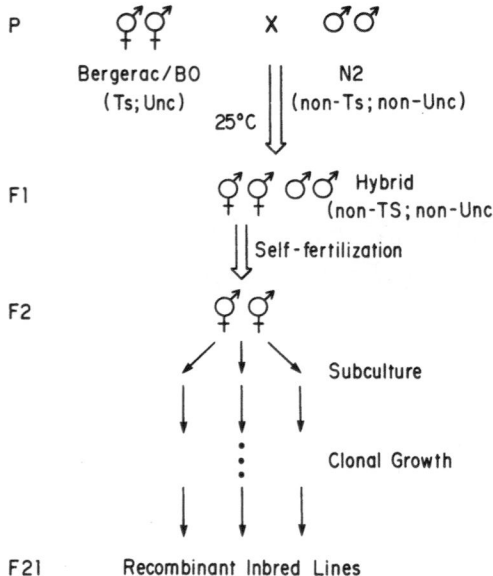

FIGURE 1. Scheme for constructing recombinant inbred lines in *Caenorhabditis elegans*. Two common laboratory wild types, N2 (Bristol) and Bergerac BO, were crossed. F1 cross-progeny were distinguished from self-progeny of the parental Bergerac hermaphrodites by the non-ts, non-unc phenotypes of the F1. Individual fourth larval stage F1 hermaphrodites were isolated to individual small petri plates containing NGM and preseeded with *Escherichia coli* OP50. Subsequent generations were produced by self-fertilization. Fourth larval stage hermaphrodites were transferred to a fresh NGM plates at each generation. This inbreeding procedure was continued for a total of 21 generations.

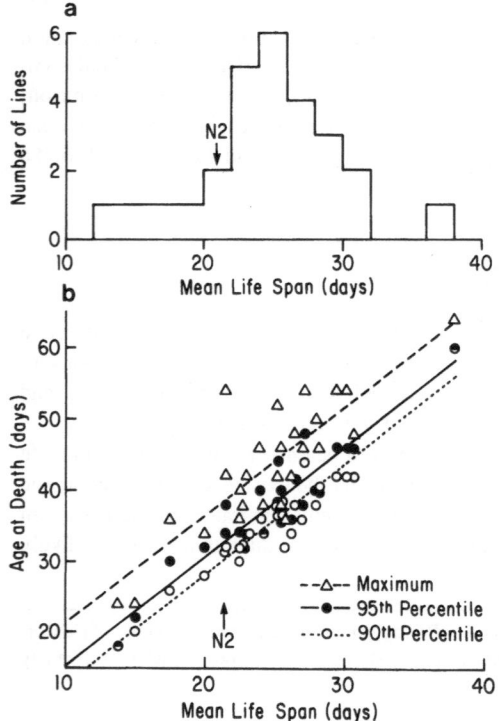

FIGURE 2. Life spans of hermaphrodites from recombinant inbred lines. (a) Mean life spans of 27 RI lines. A synchronous population of hermaphrodites was generated by permitting egg deposition by young adult hermaphrodite parents for 6 hr. Data are the average of two survival experiments, each containing 50 nematodes. Data were collected and analyzed as described earlier. The entire experiment involved the assay of 2950 nematodes; 2206 died of natural causes. (b) Regression of mean life span (same nematodes described in a) on either maximum life span, the 95th percentile of life span, or the 90th percentile of life span. Mean life span is highly correlated ($p \ll 0.001$) with maximum life span ($r = 0.83$), the 95th percentile of life span ($r = 0.93$), and the 90th percentile of life span ($r = 0.96$). (From Johnson, 1987.)

from the limitations inherent in these estimates that there are many more genes affecting length of life (Johnson, 1986; Foltz and Johnson, submitted for publication).

3. MUTANTS

A more powerful approach to the genetic dissection of the aging processes is the isolation of long-lived mutants (Klass, 1983). One such mutant has been identified and

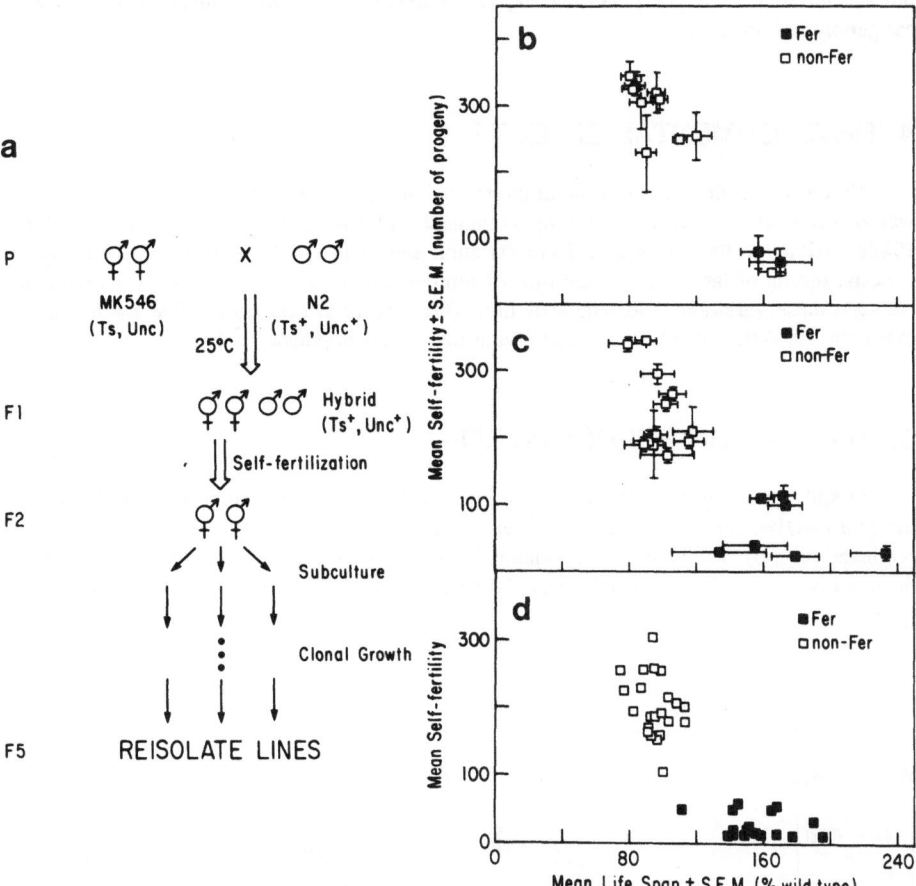

FIGURE 3. (a) Method for constructing homozygous populations from crosses between N2 and MK546. (b,c) Life expectancy at 20° of reisolates from the cross of MK546 [age-1(hx546) fer-15(b26ts) II; unc-31(z1) IV] to N2 is plotted relative to hermaphrodite self-fertility. (b) F5 reisolates from experiment 1. (c) F5 reisolates from experiment 2. (d) Life expectancy at 25° of F10 reisolates from crosses of MK542 [age-1(hx542) fer-15(b26ts) II; unc-31(z2) IV] Fer (o) and non-Fer (o) stocks are indicated; because of the large number of points, standard errors are not shown in Fig. 3d but ranged from 5% to 15% of the mean life span, while self-fertility is the average of three to five hermaphrodites whose progeny were counted collectively rather than individually. (From Friedman and Johnson, 1988.)

studied in some detail (Friedman and Johnson, 1988a,b). Mutants in a gene called *age-1* are responsible for a 70% increase in life expectancy and a 110% increase in maximum life span (Friedman and Johnson, 1988a). The *age-1* mutation also results in a fivefold decrease in the number of progeny produced (Friedman and Johnson, 1988a). Both long life and reduced fertility remain together in crosses (Fig. 3) and both are genetically closely linked to another mutant gene *fer-15* that is responsible for a temperature-sensitive (ts) sperm defect and was already present in the original strains in which *age-1* was isolated to facilitate mutant isolation (Klass, 1983). The strategy used to map *age-1* illustrates a further advantage of the self-fertilizing hermaphroditic life-style of this nematode in facilitating the mapping of long-life mutants through the production of homozygous mapping strains containing animals of identical genotype (Fig. 3a).

4. DEVELOPMENTAL EFFECTS

No change in the timing of larval molts, age of fertility (Fig. 4), or the rate of growth was detected in an analysis of the *age-1* mutant and wild type (Friedman and Johnson, 1988a). Although there was significant variation among the RI lines in length of embryogenesis, timing of larval molts, and time of reproduction (Fig. 5), there was no correlation between these variations and length of life. Thus, the processes responsible for life-span extension are different from those specifying rate of development.

5. EFFECTS ON REPRODUCTION

Despite the fact that *age-1* shows a fivefold reduction in progeny production, the length of the reproductive period is unaffected after normalizing to the number of progeny actually produced (Fig. 6). The RI lines vary among themselves in timing of fecundity (Fig. 5) and in the number of offspring produced at any given age. This variation was not correlated with life span.

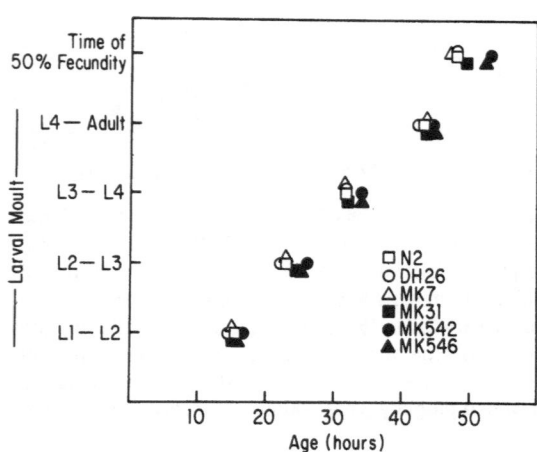

FIGURE 4. Time of intermolt lethargus and time of reproductive maturity for N2, DH26, MK7, MK31, MK542, and MK546. Points represent the time of minimal proportion of animals displaying pharyngeal pumping and the time at which 50% of hermaphrodites carried visible eggs. Two of the three synchronous cultures were slightly asynchronous at the L3–L4 larval molt. (From Friedman and Johnson, 1988.)

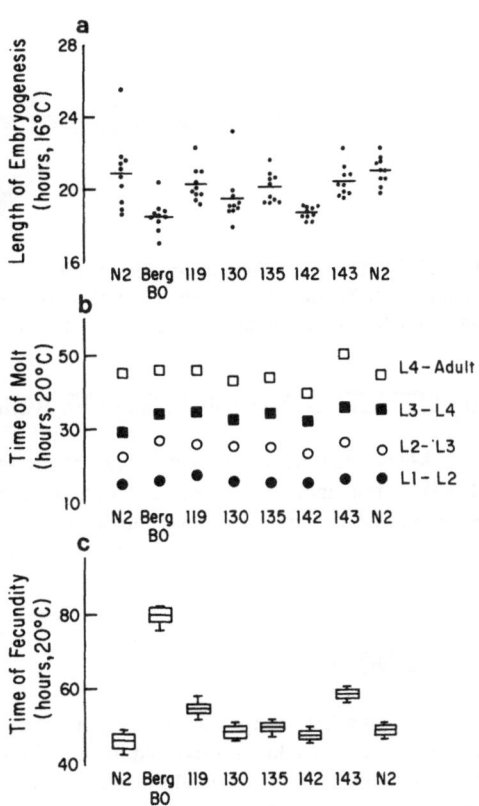

FIGURE 5. Duration of development. (a) Length of embryonic development was determined by measuring the period from the two-cell stage to hatching at 16°. Ten two-cell stage eggs were dissected out of fecund hermaphrodites of the appropriate genotype and followed until hatch; 16° was chosen for convenience of assay. Horizontal lines represent the means. (b) Times of larval molts. The time of molting was determined by monitoring pharyngeal lethargus using a Nikon Microphot equipped with DIC optics. Fifty worms from a larger population were assayed, approximately hourly, throughout the period of larval development. The time point at which fewest worms were pumping was taken as the midpoint for each molt and is recorded here. (c) The time of 50% fecundity was determined by assays of 50 worms of each genotype as in Fig. 5b. Shown here are Tukey Box Plots illustrating 10th, 25th, 50th, 75th, and 90th percentiles of fecundity. (From Johnson, 1987.)

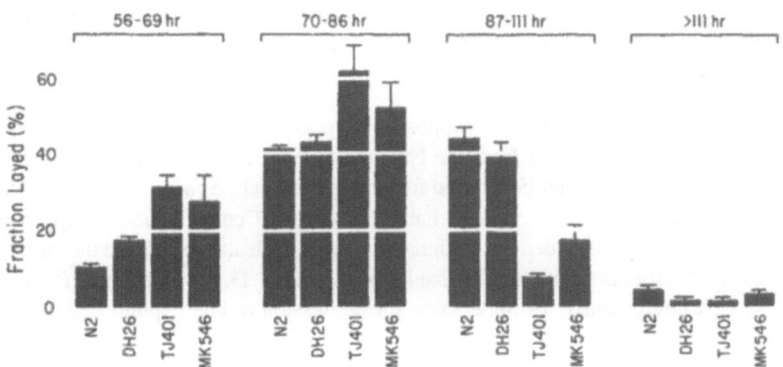

FIGURE 6. Relative age-specific fertilities of wild-type and *age-1* strains. Relative fertility (fraction of total progeny produced) was obtained from measurements on progeny produced during four consecutive periods of the fertile portion of adult life, 56 hr after hatch to sterility. Total hermaphrodite self-fertilities (mean ±SEM) were as follows: N2: 302.6 ± 7.3 (N = 10); DH26: 317.4 ± 14.9 (N = 7); TJ401: 71.9 ± 3.9 (N = 9); MK546: 30.9 ± 3.8 (N = 10). (From Friedman and Johnson, 1988.)

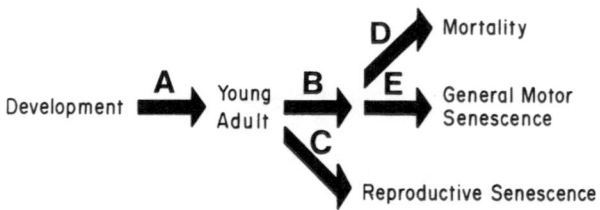

FIGURE 7. Diagram describing the order of dependency of events in senescence of *Caenorhabditis elegans*. Arrows indicate independent genetic specification and do not necessarily imply causal relationships. (From Johnson, 1987.)

6. OTHER COMPONENTS OF AGING

Many other processes change over the life span of the nematode (Johnson and Simpson, 1985). These include the accumulation of lipofuscin, an increase in lysosomal enzyme activity, and the loss of general motor ability. A tentative relationship between several of these various physiological events can be drawn, based on an analysis of the long-lived strains (Fig. 7).

7. CONCLUSION

The simplest interpretation of the mode of action of *age-1* is that the wild-type gene product is responsible for a fivefold increase in reproductive fitness and also causes a loss of life to only 60% of the potential life span in the absence of *age-1*+. This pleiotropic action of this locus is consistent with widely accepted notions concerning the evolution of senescence (Charlesworth, 1980): that senescence is nonadaptive and that senescence arises by the failure to select against genes that are either neutral early in life (mutation accumulation) or advantageous early in life (antagonistic pleiotropy) but negative later. The phenotype of *age-1* suggests that this locus is one whose mode of action is consistent with the model of antagonistic pleiotropy.

ACKNOWLEDGMENTS. This work was supported by grant AG05720 from the National Institutes of Health, grant 8208652 from the National Science Foundation, and a Charles A. Dana Award from the American Federation for Aging Research. Some stocks were supplied by, and are available through, the Caenorhabditis Genetics Center, which is supported by contract NO1-AG-9-2113 between the National Institutes of Health (NIH) and the curators of the University of Missouri. The author thanks N. L. Foltz, D. B. Friedman, P. A. Fitzpatrick, W. L. Conley, and J. E. Shoemaker for permission to cite unpublished data.

REFERENCES

Botstein, D., and Mauer, R., 1982, Genetic approaches to the analysis of microbial development, *Annu. Rev. Genet.* **16**:61–83.
Charlesworth, B., 1980, *Evolution in Age-Structured Populations*, Cambridge University Press, Cambridge, England.

Foltz, N. L., Brooks, A., and Johnson, T. E., Genetic specification of life span and self-fertility in wild-type *Caenorhabditis elegans*, submitted.

Friedman, D. B., and Johnson, T. E., 1988a, A mutation in the *age-1* gene in *Caenorhabditis elegans* lengthens life and reduces hermaphrodite fertility, *Genetics* **118**:75–86.

Friedman, D. B., and Johnson, T. E., 1988b, Three mutants that extend both mean and maximum life span of the nematode, *Caenorhabditis elegans*, define the *age-1* gene, *J. Gerontol.* **43**:8102–8109.

Johnson, T. E., 1986, Molecular and genetic analyses of a multivariate system specifying behavior and life span. *Behav. Genet.* **16**:221–235.

Johnson, T. E., No heterosis effects are observed in *Caenorhabditis elegans*, submitted.

Johnson, T. E., and Simpson, V. J., 1985, Aging studies in *Caenorhabditis elegans* and other nematodes, in: *CRC Handbook of Cell Biology of Aging* (V. Cristolfalo, ed.), CRC Press, Boca Raton, Florida, pp. 481–495.

Johnson, T. E., and Wood, W. B., 1982, Genetic analysis of life-span in *Caenorhabditis elegans*, *Proc. Natl. Acad. Sci. USA* **79**:6603–6607.

Klass, M. R., 1983, A method for the isolation of longevity mutants in the nematode *Caenorhabditis elegans* and initial results, *Mech. Aging Dev.* **22**:279–286.

Lints, F. A., 1978, *Genetics and Ageing, Interdisciplinary Topics in Gerontology*, Vol. 14, S. Karger, Basel.

Rose, M. R., 1984, Genetic covariation in *Drosophila* life history: untangling the data, *Am. Nat.* **123**:565–569.

5

Alzheimer's Disease
Enter Protein Chemistry

GEORGE G. GLENNER

1. INTRODUCTION

With the evidence that autopsies of demented individuals over the age of 65 demonstrate a predominance of lesions normally associated with Alzheimer's disease, i.e., neurofibrillary tangles and "senile" (neuritic plaques) (Tomlinson *et al.*, 1968, 1970), the significance of Alzheimer's disease as a public health problem became evident. The correlation of plaque count with the degree of dementia further established the relationship of this pathologic lesion with clinical manifestations (Blessed *et al.*, 1968). Another interesting and significant correlation was the pathologic evidence that Down's syndrome individuals over the age of 40 had all the pathologic lesions of Alzheimer's disease as well as many of the clinical manifestations (Jervis, 1948).

Cerebrovascular amyloidosis was first described in the leptomeninges and intracortices (Fischer, 1910). This lesion was also designated as amyloid (Divry and Florkin, 1927). Although early investigators noted its association with dementia and/or plaques (Pantelakis, 1954; Surbeck, 1961), it was more often related to normal aging than to Alzheimer's disease until an extensive study of more than 400 Alzheimer's disease autopsies revealed its presence in 92% of Alzheimer's disease cases and relative absence in non-Alzheimer's disease patients (Glenner, 1983; Glenner *et al.*, 1981). It has also been associated with intracortical and leptomeningial hemorrhage (Torack, 1975), usually in conjunction with Alzheimer's disease. A condition known as hereditary Congophilic angiopathy with hemorrhage (HCHWA-I) has been reported from Iceland (Gudmundsson *et al.*, 1972), in which the victims die of cerebral hemorrhage, usually at age 20–30 years. The amyloid protein from these cases has been found to be homologous with a serum protein, cystatin C (gamma trace) (Cohen *et al.*, 1983). In this study, our objective was to define the chemical nature of the amyloid fibers of plaques and cerebral vessels in Alzheimer's disease in order to decipher the nature of these lesions

GEORGE G. GLENNER • Department of Pathology, University of California–San Diego, School of Medicine, La Jolla, California 92093.

and their role in its pathogenesis. We describe here the characteristics and localization of the amyloid β-protein, a marker protein for Alzheimer's disease.

2. MATERIALS AND METHODS

2.1. Amyloid Fibril Concentration, Purification, and Analysis

Human brains of Alzheimer's disease victims obtained at autopsy were frozen at $-70°C$. Histological sections were taken and stained for amyloid; only those with extensive cerebrovascular amyloidosis were selected for amyloid fibril isolation. The brains of two patients, aged 61 and 62 years, diagnosed as having Down's syndrome were similarly processed. Age-matched normal brains were used for controls. The leptomeninges were stripped and gross cortex contaminants removed. Concentrates of the amyloid fibrils from amyloid-laden leptomeningeal vessels were obtained by previously described methods (Glenner et al., 1972). Samples of the amyloid fibril concentrate were prepared for X-ray diffraction (XRD) by suspending small pieces of the fresh amyloid in distilled water and concentrating the suspension into the tip of a 0.17-mm-diameter thin-walled quartz capillary by centrifugation ($1000g$) (Eanes and Glenner, 1968).

The collagenase-treated pellet was solubilized in 6 M guanidine–HCl, 0.1 M Tris–HCl, 24 mM dithiothreitol, 0.34 mM EDTA, at pH 8.0 (22% w/v), and stirred at room temperature for 48 hr. After 48 hr, the solution was centrifuged in a Beckman L-5-50B ultracentrifuge at $105,000g$ for 60 min at 4°C. The pellet was separated from the supernatant. The supernatant was placed into 1000-M_r cutoff dialysis tubing (Spectra/Por 6, Fisher Scientific) and dialyzed and lyophilized; the resulting powder was stored dessicated at $-70°C$. Sodium dodecyl sulfate (SDS–urea polyacrylamide gel electrophoresis (PAGE) (Laemmli, 1970) was modified only by the addition of 8 M urea in the stacking and resolving gel. Slab gels (15%) were made 0.75 mm thick and run at 10-mA constant current. After electrophoresis, gels were stained with Coomassie Brilliant Blue.

G-100 Sephadex column chromatography was employed (Glenner et al., 1972), using a 2.5 × 100-cm G-100 calibrated Sephadex column (Pharmacia) equilibrated with 5 M guanidine–HCl, 1 N acetic acid. The column was calibrated with cytochrome C (horse heart), 12,384 M_r and glucagon, 3485 M_r. The protein elution profile was monitored at 280 nm with a Beckman 35 spectrophotometer. The protein peak centered at 4200 M_r was pooled and dialyzed against deionized water, lyophilized, and stored dessicated at $-70°C$; 100 μg of the lyophilized protein from peak fractions of the Sephadex column was solubilized into 25 μl of 5 M guanidine–HCl, 1 N acetic acid. This was injected into a Waters high-performance liquid chromatography (HPLC) system. The mobile phases were solvent A: 0.1% trifluoroacetic acid/H_2O, solvent B: 100% acetonitrile. The gradient was linear from 10% to 50% solvent B over 60 min. The flow rate was 0.8 ml/min, and the protein peaks were detected at 229 nm with 2.0 AUFS. The stationary phase was a Vydac 214TP54 C_4 peptide column. Three major protein peaks were found that had no correspondence with control samples. These protein peaks were pooled separately, lyophilized, and stored at $-70°C$. HPLC-purified samples were dissolved in heptofluorobutyric acid and loaded in a Beckman 890 C spinning cup sequencer for amino acid sequencing. The collected anilothiazolone amino acids were converted to phenylthiohydantoin amino acids (PTH-amino acids) with 1 N HCl/MeOH at 50°C for 10 min. The PTH-amino acids were dried and redissolved in MeOH. The PTH-amino acids were analyzed on a Beckman 322 system fitted with an ETH–Permaphase guard column and an IBM 6μ CN column in line. The eluent was monitored at 254 nm.

2.2. Immunochemistry

A synthetic peptide (OPl) with the sequence consisting of the first 10 residues of the β-protein (Asp-Ala-Glu-Phe-Arg-His-Asp-Ser-Gly-Tyr) was synthesized according to Marglin and Merrifield (1970). A cysteine residue was added to the carboxyl terminal for coupling the peptide to a carrier protein. OPl was coupled to keyhole limpet hemocyanin (KLH) through the cysteine with m-maleimidobenzolyl-N-hydroxysuccinimide ester (Sigma). Five 10-week-old female BALB/c mice were injected intraperitoneally (IP) with 4 μg OPl coupled to KLH (OPl–KLH) in Freund's complete adjuvant (Sigma). The mice were boosted 14 days later with 4 μg OPl–KLH in Freund's incomplete adjuvant (Sigma). Three weeks after initial immunization, the mice were boosted once more with 1.0 μg OPl–KLH in 10 mM Tris, 150 mM NaCl, at pH 8.0. Serum was obtained 7 days after the final boost. The mice immune sera were assayed for anti-OPl activity by solid-phase enzyme-linked immunosorbent assay (ELISA) (Walter and Doolittle, 1983). Each mouse serum was diluted 1 : 10,000–1 : 32,000 in 0.1% ovalbumin, 20 mM Tris, 150 mM NaCl, 0.2% Tween-20, 0.01% Thimerosal, at pH 8.0. Assays were performed on polyvinyl chloride microtiter plates (Dynatech) in which 0.05 μg F82B or 0.1 μg KLH had been dried in the wells. Bound antibodies were detected with peroxidase-conjugated goat antimouse IgG at 1 : 1000 dilution (Cappel). O-Phenylenediamine was used as the substrate, and quantitation was done with a Multiskan Microplate Reader (Flow Laboratories) at 492 nm. All five immunized mice sera were found immunoreactive to β-protein, OPl, and KLH, and were unreactive to F82B. Normal mouse serum was unreactive to all antigens tested. The mouse serum with the highest titer against β-protein was designated OPlMSl and used for all further work in this investigation. The specificity of antiserum OPlMSl for β-protein and OPl was tested. A limiting dilution of OPlMSl (1 : 6000) was preincubated with varying concentrations of inhibitors OPl and F82B (an unrelated 17-amino acid peptide) at 4°C for 12 hr and then reacted in a solid-phase ELISA.

2.3. Immunohistochemistry

Localization of amyloid deposits was demonstrated with mouse anti-OPl serum (OPlMSl) by the peroxidase–antiperoxidase (PAP) method (Sternberger, 1979; Fujihara et al., 1980). Formalin-fixed sections of autopsied brain tissues were obtained from Alzheimer's disease, adult Down's syndrome, HCHWA-I, and age-matched control cases. Tissue sections were cut 6.0 μm thick and fixed to glass slides. The sections were then challenged with the following series of antibodies with wash steps in between each: (1) OPlMSl (experimental) or normal mouse serum (control) at 1 : 2500 dilution or 1.0% ovalbumin–PBS (blank), (2) rabbit antimouse immunoglobulin G (IgG) at 1 : 1000, (3) swine anti rabbit IgG at 1 : 100, and (4) rabbit peroxidase–antiperoxidase at 1 : 1000 (Dakopatts). Positive immunoreaction was detected with 3,3'-diaminobenzidine (Sigma). Congo red (Kodak) staining followed, and Mayer's hematoxylin (MCB Chemicals) was used as a counterstain. For inhibition experiments, a 1 : 500 dilution of OPlMSl was preincubated with 1.0% OPl or KLH in 20 mM Tris, 150 mM NaCl, 0.2% Tween-20, 0.01% Thimerosal, at pH 8.0, for 12 hr at 4°C prior to use in the procedure just outlined. A Leitz Orthoplan polarizing microscope was employed for visualization and photomicroscopy.

3. RESULTS

The amyloid fibril concentrates of cerebrovascular amyloid gave unoriented X-ray crystallographic patterns having a 4.75 Å outer and 10 Å inner d spacing. This pattern is indicative of the β-pleated sheet conformation characteristic of all amyloid fibrils (Eanes and Glenner, 1968). Six Alzheimer's disease cases and three age-matched control cases were examined by SDS–urea PAGE. The lyophilized material revealed a unique band of protein, β-protein, that was not seen in control samples prepared in identical fashion. This protein could be consistently fractionated on a calibrated G-100 Sephadex column with its peak fraction centered at 4200 M_r. Because of its uniqueness to amyloid fibril preparations, it was assumed, as shown in numerous previous studies (Glenner et al., 1972), to be a major protein constituent of amyloid fibrils. HPLC fractionated three peaks from the G-100 preparation of both the Alzheimer's disease and adult Down's syndrome β-protein, and these were found to have almost identical amino acid compositions. Two other cases of Alzheimer's disease and one case of adult Down's syndrome gave identical HPLC profiles.

Our studies show that the HPLC elution profiles of β-protein from the cerebrovascular amyloid fibrils of Alzheimer's disease (Glenner and Wong, 1984a) and adult Down's syndrome (Glenner and Wong, 1984b) are almost identical. The amino acid sequence analysis of the Down's and Alzheimer's disease β-protein fraction to residue 28 is presented in Table I.

The Down's protein was found to have an amino acid sequence identical to that of the Alzheimer's disease protein (Glenner and Wong, 1984b) through position 28, with the exception of a repeatedly confirmed substitution of Glu for Gln residue at position 11 (Table I). The retention of Gln[15] strongly suggests that Glu[11] is a true substitution and is not due to an artificial deamidation; however, the latter possibility cannot be ruled out. This substitution most likely indicates the existence of polymorphism. The β-protein is not homologous to the serum protein cystatin C (Cohen et al., 1983) found to compose the cerebrovascular amyloid protein of the HCHWA-I or to any other known sequenced protein.

The preparation from the second Down's case gave an HPLC profile with an identical major peak at 35% acetonitrile, but inadequate material was available for sequencing. These findings indicate that, of the three disease processes most often characterized by cerebrovascular amyloidosis, i.e., Alzheimer's disease, adult Down's syndrome, and HGHWA-I, only Alzheimer's disease and adult Down's syndrome share a homologous amyloid protein. This is the first chemical evidence of a relationship between Alzheimer's disease and Down's syndrome (Glenner and Wong, 1984a,b; Wong et al., 1985).

There is no known spontaneous or experimental animal model for Alzheimer's disease. There are mouse models for Down's syndrome (Epstein, 1983) but, since the trisomic fetuses

TABLE I. Amino Acid Sequence Analysis of β-Protein[a]

	1	2	3	4	5	6	7	8	9	10	11	12	13	14
AD	Asp	Ala	Glu	Phe	Arg	His	Asp	Ser	Gly	Tyr	Gln	Val	His	His
DS	Asp	Ala	Glu	Phe	Arg	His	Asp	Ser	Gly	Tyr	*Glu*	Val	His	His

	15	16	17	18	19	20	21	22	23	24	25	26	27	28
AD	Gln	Lys	Leu	Val	Phe	Phe	Ala	Glu	Asp	Val	Gly	Ser	Asn	Lys
DS	Gln	Lys	Leu	Val	Phe	Phe	Ala	Glu	Asp	Val	Gly	Ser	Asn	Lys

[a]From cerebrovascular amyloid fibrils obtained from Alzheimer's disease (AD) and adult Down's syndrome (DS). Variant residue is in italic type.

do not survive beyond term, their value for the study of Alzheimer's disease is limited. The human familial cases of Alzheimer's disease tend to follow an autosomal-dominant pattern of inheritance (Heston, 1976) with the usual statistical prediction of affected progeny. However, the great similarity in the cerebral lesions between adult Down's syndrome and Alzheimer's disease (Burger and Vogel, 1973; Glenner, 1983) and the demonstration of chemical homology in the pathologic amyloid fibril β-protein strongly suggest that Down's syndrome may represent the first truly predictable model for Alzheimer's disease. Since 100% of adult Down's syndrome individuals have cerebrovascular amyloid deposits composed of β-protein, it was initially suggested by us that the β-protein in these amyloid deposits is a phenotypic protein for Down's syndrome and that the gene encoding for it is localized, as with other Down's phenotypic genes, on chromosome 21 (Glenner and Wong, 1984b).

Tissue from six cases of Alzheimer's disease, two cases of adult Down's syndrome, one case of HCHWA-I, and three age-matched normal brains were immunohistochemically studied by the Sternberger (1979) PAP method (Fujihara et al., 1980) using OPlMSl. Amyloid-laden vascular sites in the leptomeningial and intracortical areas in Alzheimer's disease and adult Down's syndrome cases immunostained intensely and corresponded precisely to the areas of Congo red polarization birefringence. This birefringence resulting from Congo red staining is an accepted histochemical marker for the β-pleated sheet structure of amyloid (Glenner et al., 1974).

In addition, both diffuse ("primitive") and compact ("mature") neuritic plaques reacted with OPlMSl in the PAP procedure in Alzheimer's disease and adult Down's syndrome tissue sections. There were rare instances in Alzheimer's disease and adult Down's syndrome tissue in which localized PAP staining of sites resembling small diffuse plaques did not have corresponding Congo red birefringence. This could be because of the ability of the PAP procedure to detect localized deposits of β-protein that were not in the β-pleated sheet conformation and were therefore nonbirefringent. PAP staining of CVA and neuritic plaques could be completely inhibited if OPlMSl was preincubated with OPl. Preincubation of OPlMSl with a concentration of KLH that eliminated all anti-KLH activity as detected by ELISA had no effect on the PAP staining of cerebrovascular amyloidosis and neuritic plaques. The specific inhibition with OPl strongly indicates that the specific PAP staining by OPlMSl was entirely attributable to antibodies to OPl.

The normal brain tissues examined showed no significant PAP staining beyond the very slight background also obtained when normal mouse serum was used in place of OPlMSl. This finding confirms the observation by SDS–PAGE and HPLC of the uniqueness of the β-protein in cerebral tissues to Alzheimer's disease and adult Down's syndrome (Glenner and Wong, 1984a,b). The HCHWA-I case, although heavily laden with cerebrovascular amyloid as detected by Congo red birefringence, was also unreactive to PAP staining.

No PAP staining was seen associated with neurofibrillary tangles. This finding suggests that the etiology and source of neurofibrillary tangles is either distinct from that of cerebrovascular amyloidosis and neuritic plaques or that the anti-OPl determinants of neurofibrillary tangles are sterically inaccessible.

4. DISCUSSION

The present studies confirm in part our initial hypothesis (Glenner, 1979) as to the pathogenesis of Alzheimer's disease. It is evident from the XRD data that the amyloid of the cerebral vessels (cerebrovascular amyloidosis) is a fibril composed of proteins in a twisted β-pleated sheet conformation (Glenner, 1983; Eanes and Glenner, 1968). The physical nature of the amyloid cores of the neuritic plaques and the paired helical filaments (PHF) of the neurofibrillary tangles is also believed to be that of a β-pleated sheet protein (Glenner *et al.*, 1974; Kirschner *et al.*, 1986). The relative absence of the cerebrovascular amyloid protein, β-protein, in vessels of normal individuals and HCHWA-I indicates that β-protein is a unique marker protein for Alzheimer's disease. While having common cerebral lesions, the almost identical amino acid sequence of β-protein of the cerebrovascular fibrils in both Alzheimer's disease and adult Down's syndrome is the first chemical evidence that Down's syndrome is a pathologic model for Alzheimer's disease. Immunohistochemical studies further substantiate the relative uniqueness of β-protein for Alzheimer's disease.

The HCHWA-I case, although heavily laden with cerebrovascular amyloid as detected by Congo red staining, was unreactive by PAP staining. This was expected, since HCHWA-I cerebrovascular amyloid fibrils are composed of cystatin C protein (Cohen *et al.*, 1983) which has no homology with the β protein. The experiment with the HCHWA-I case was included as an additional control to demonstrate the specificity of OPlMSl for β-amyloid protein. HCHWA-I was thought to be the only other neuropathologic process known to have cerebrovascular amyloidosis as a significant lesion. However, a case of Dutch HCHWA (HCHWA-D) was recently found to have β-protein comprising the cerebrovascular amyloid deposits (van Duinen *et al.*, 1987). Since our isolation and purification scheme for β-protein eliminated contamination by intracerebral tissue, it eliminated contamination of our original preparations of cerebrovascular amyloidosis by plaques and tangles. Localization of β-protein antibodies to amyloid deposits in cerebral vessels of both Alzheimer's disease and Down's syndrome (Wong *et al.*, 1985) was expected in view of the similarity in amino acid sequence of their β-protein. Not only was the intended target, cerebrovascular amyloidosis, stained by OPlMSl, but so were the neuritic plaques in both Alzheimer's disease and adult Down's syndrome. Localization of the β-protein antibodies to neuritic plaques in both Alzheimer's disease and Down's syndrome indicates that the source of amyloid in both plaques and vessels is the same. It further supports the concept that Down's syndrome is a chemical model for Alzheimer's disease.

What distinguishes our immunohistochemical work from earlier reports (Ishii *et al.*, 1975; Powers *et al.*, 1981) is that we used antibodies raised to a well-defined, pure, synthetic peptide whose sequence was derived from the first 10 residues of a purified protein that appears by three different criteria to be relatively unique to Alzheimer's disease and adult Down's syndrome. We now know from ultrastructural studies that the immunohistochemical reaction with OPlMSl detects β-protein as intimately associated with the amyloid fibril component of the vessels and plaques (Ikeda *et al.*, 1987).

The amino acid compositions of plaque amyloid "cores" and cerebrovascular amyloidosis are similar (Kidd *et al.*, 1978; Allsop *et al.*, 1986). Therefore, it is likely that plaque amyloid fibrils also would be found to consist of β-protein. Masters *et al.* (1985b) reported the amino acid sequencing of the amyloid core of plaques obtained from cases of Alzheimer's disease and Down's syndrome. These workers obtained an inseparable series of at least four polypeptides by HPLC fractionation that had progressive deletions of their N-terminal amino acids. Masters *et al.* ordered these according to the amino acid sequence of β-protein and obtained homology with it except for discrepancies in positions 27 (Ser for Asn) and 28 (Ala for Lys) to that of β-protein. It is doubtful that these polypeptides could have been ordered into sequence without the known sequence of β-protein, since at each cycle at least four amino acids would have been detected. Sequence analysis by these investigators of Down's syndrome plaque core amyloid revealed complete homology with that in Alzheimer's disease. Partial confirmation of these sequence analyses (except for positions 27 and 28) of the plaque core amyloid β-protein have been presented (Selkoe *et al.*, 1986; Kang *et al.*, 1987).

Using antibodies to peptide 1–11 and 11–23 of β-protein, Masters *et al.* (1985a) claimed that not only did antibodies to peptides 11–23 react with cerebrovascular amyloid and amyloid plaque core in Alzheimer's disease, but, contrary to the findings of Wong *et al.* (1985), their antibodies to peptide 1–11 reacted with neurofibrillary tangles. The findings of cerebrovascular wall and plaque amyloid reacting to antibodies to β-protein (Wong *et al.*, 1985) have been confirmed by several investigators (Allsop *et al.*, 1986; Selkoe *et al.*, 1986); in agreement with our observations, no reactivity of neurofibrillary tangles with anti-β-protein antibodies was found. However, Kidd *et al.* (1978) and Allsop (1986) noted that the amino acid compositions of neuritic plaques, neurofibrillary tangles, and cerebrovascular amyloidosis are similar and suggested that they are all composed of the same protein. Masters *et al.* (1985a) provided amino acid sequence evidence that the protein of the PHF and β-protein were homologous and Guiroy *et al.* (1987), analyzing the PHF obtained from cases of Guam–Parkinson's dementia, came to a similar conclusion. Thus, current evidence suggests that the fibrillar (amyloid) component of all three pathognomonic lesions of Alzheimer's disease are formed from β-protein.

Characterization of β-protein provided definitive proof that the plaques of Alzheimer's disease have no chemical identity with those of the infectious Creutzfeldt–Jakob disease, as originally proposed on empirical grounds (Prusiner, 1984), since the amino acid sequences of the constituent amyloid fibril proteins (the "prion" of Creutzfeldt–Jakob disease and the β-protein of Alzheimer's disease) are distinctly different. Thus, the strongest argument thus far proposed for Alzheimer's disease being an infectious process cannot be confirmed.

Earlier reports suggested that the formation of neuritic plaques is the result of breaks in the blood–brain barrier (Glenner, 1979; Glenner *et al.*, 1981). Miyakawa *et al.* (1982) found that all neuritic plaques are associated with at least one degenerating amyloidotic capillary. We presented evidence that the β-protein found in cerebral vessel amyloid is also found in the neuritic plaques. We therefore proposed, as a working hypothesis, that cerebrovascular amyloidosis derives from an isotypic variant of a serum protein precursor (Glenner, 1980; Glenner *et al.*, 1984), e.g., the variant prealbumin in familial amyloidotic polyneuropathy (FAP) (Dwulet and Benson, 1984). Cerebrovascular amyloidosis damages capillary walls (Glenner, 1979), causing seepage of β-protein precursor, among other plasma substances, into the neuropil, leading to the formation of the amyloid of the neuritic plaque via lysosomal (Glenner *et al.*, 1984) enzymatic activity of microglia degrading the precursor of β-protein (Glenner, 1980; Glenner *et al.*, 1971). We suggested that an abnormal degradative product of β-protein is also neurotoxic, blocking strategic receptors of specific cortical neurons, perturbing their environment, and leading to PHF formation, presumably from endogenous neuronal material (Glenner *et al.*, 1984).

Four years after the discovery of β-protein, and based on its amino acid sequence, oligonucleotide probes were used to screen normal human brain complementary DNA (cDNA) libraries in order to identify and characterize the gene coding for β-protein. Through the use of somatic cell hybrids, the gene was localized, as predicted (Glenner and Wong, 1984b), to chromosome 21 by four independent groups (Goldgaber *et al.*, 1987; Kang *et al.*, 1987; Robakis *et al.*, 1987; Tanzi *et al.*, 1987). The gene contains an open reading frame coding for 695 amino acids. It was deduced that the sequence of this β-protein precursor has the characteristics of a cell membrane receptor (Kang *et al.*, 1987). Since an internal sequence is identical with that of the β-protein found in amyloid deposits in the brain, conversion of the precursor protein to the amyloid protein probably occurs by proteolysis. Thus, similarities to epidermal growth factor and the endorphins are apparent; i.e., proteolysis may yield a variety of physiologically active peptides (Allsop et al., 1988).

The inherited form of Alzheimer's disease is also associated with a familial Alzheimer's disease genetic marker, FAD (St. George-Hyslop et al., 1987). The β-protein gene appears not to be linked to the FAD marker (Van Broeckhoven et al., 1987) and appears not to be abnormal in quality or quantity and not the cause of Alzheimer's disease per se. This would argue against the amyloid β-protein precursor being an isotypic variant as we earlier surmised based on precedent (Dwulet and Benson, 1984). An inconstant insert has been found in the sequence of the β-protein gene that codes for a Kunitz-type inhibitor (Ponte et al., 1988; Tanzi et al., 1988). Thus far, its presence or absence has not been correlated with the presence of Alzheimer's disease. In addition, immunohistochemical evidence indicates that a segment of β-protein binds to presumptive receptors on adrenocortical and pancreatic islet β-cells (Allsop et al., 1988), perhaps with regulator or hormonal activity. The ubiquity of the β-protein has been demonstrated by histochemical hybridization methods. A significant production of β-protein messenger RNA (mRNA) could be demonstrated in many organs, with the highest levels observed in brain tissue (Bahmanyar et al., 1987). The variety of species synthesizing β-protein indicates that it is highly conserved in nature. Using the mouse model for Down's syndrome, trisomy 16 (Epstein, 1983), the β-protein gene was identified on chromosome 16 (Lovett et al., 1987), thus supporting its validity as a model for Down's syndrome.

5. A PATHOGENIC MECHANISM

These findings make possible new approaches to the pathogenesis of Alzheimer's disease. The vast majority of amyloid fibril proteins result from the deposition of β-pleated sheet twisted fibrils. This structure is created by proteolysis or other physicochemical alteration of an amyloidogenic protein, e.g., usually an isotypic variant of a normal protein such as prealbumin (Dwulet and Benson, 1984). Since Alzheimer's disease is a pathologic process, there must be an abnormality in either the chemical composition of the amyloid β-protein precursor or its proteolytic processing that distinguishes its metabolism from that in normal individuals. Abnormalities in chemical composition may arise at many points during the post-translational cascade of events that lead to protein modification and eventually to amyloid fibril deposition, e.g., in glycosylation of the nascent protein or in the proteolytic processing of the 695-amino acid precursor to its final, minimal 28-amino acid amyloid fibril product.

The FAD marker could include a gene coding for an abnormal hydrolytic or anhydrolytic lysosomal enzyme. Alternatively, it may code for an abnormal enzyme inhibitor. In either case, the present focus in Alzheimer's disease is on the β-protein precursor and abnormalities in either its native form or its degradation, or both. The demonstration in one case of an FAD genetic marker on chromosome 9 (Jenkins et al., 1987) may indicate that a protein (enzyme or inhibitor) related in function to that encoded by the FAD marker on chromosome 21 is involved in abnormal β-protein precursor processing in this specific family. Clues to the pathogenesis of Alzheimer's disease from the study of Down's syndrome and its models (Lovett et al., 1987) are problematic, since only in the latter can an increase in the β-protein gene dosage be demonstrated. Although the chemical end product of β-protein precursor metabolism, the amyloid fibril, is identical in Down's syndrome and Alzheimer's disease, the pathogenic mechanism leading to accumulation of the end product may not be.

The possible relationship of a lysosomal or other proteolytic enzyme defect to Alzheimer's disease is intriguing because lysosomal enzyme differences have been implicated (Glenner and Wong, 1987) in the preferential localization of Alzheimer's amyloid fibrils solely to the cerebral vasculature (and not to peripheral vessels) and in the variable size of β-protein between vessel and plaque deposits (Glenner and Wong, 1987; Kang et al., 1987). This signifies quantitative or qualitative differences in the proteolytic enzyme and/or inhibitor complement, between the cerebral and peripheral vasculature, possibly of endothelial cells, and between cerebral endothelial cells and microglia. Abnormalities of the cerebral proteolytic and/or inhibitor systems in Alzheimer's disease will probably be found to lead to the classic pathologic cerebral lesions of Alzheimer's disease. Approaches both to diagnostic methods and to therapy, e.g., specific enzyme inhibition, should soon follow.

6. SUMMARY

The discovery of the amyloid β-protein in cerebrovascular amyloid fibrils and the cores of senile ("neuritic") plaques in the lesions of Alzheimer's disease and in the corresponding lesions of adult Down's syndrome has laid the groundwork for molecular biological studies in this disease. Down's syndrome may be the first chemical model for Alzheimer's disease, since the β-protein gene has been localized to chromosome 21 and, although apparently normal, appears to be associated with an abnormal familial Alzheimer's disease genetic marker, also on chromosomal 21. This marker may include a gene encoding for an abnormal proteolytic enzyme or enzyme inhibitor. If this is the case, definition of this gene product may lead to an *in vivo* diagnostic test and therapeutic approaches, e.g., development of a specific enzyme inhibitor preventing amyloid fibril formation.

ACKNOWLEDGMENTS. This research was supported by grant AG-05683 from the National Institute on Aging, National Institutes of Health, and grant 86-89625 from the California State Department of Health Services. All tissues from Alzheimer's disease patients and most control brain tissues were obtained from the National Alzheimer's Disease Brain Bank (University of California, San Diego), supported in part by the national Alzheimer's Disease and Related Disorders Association.

REFERENCES

Allsop, D., 1986, Biochemistry of cerebral amyloid in Alzheimer's disease, the unconventional slow virus diseases and Icelandic cerebrovascular amyloidosis, in: *Amyloidosis* (J. Marrink and M. H. Van Rijswijk, eds.), Martinus Nijhoff, Dordrecht, pp. 243–253.

Allsop, D., Landon, M., Kidd, M., Lowe, J. S., Reynolds, G. P., and Gardner, A., 1986, Monoclonal antibodies raised against a subsequence of senile plaque core protein react with plaque cores, plaque periphery and cerebrovascular amyloid in Alzheimer's disease, *Neurosci. Lett.* 68:252–256.

Allsop, D., Wong, C. W., Ikeda, S., Landon, M., Kidd, M., and Glenner, G. G., 1988, Immunohistochemical evidence for the derivation of a peptide ligand from the amyloid β-protein precursor of Alzheimer disease, *Proc. Natl. Acad. Sci. USA* 85:2790–2794.

Bahmanyar, S., Higgins, G. A., Goldgaber, D., Lewis, D. A., Morrison, J. H., Wilson, M. C., Shankar, S. K., and Gajdusek, D. C., 1987, Localization of amyloid β protein messenger RNA in brains from patients with Alzheimer's disease, *Science* 237:77–80.

Blessed, G., Tomlinson, B. E., and Roth, M., 1968, The association between quantitative measures of dementia and of senile change in the cerebral grey matter of elderly subjects, *Br. J. Psychiatry* **114:**797–811.

Burger, P. C., and Vogel, F. S., 1973, The development of the pathologic changes of Alzheimer's disease and senile dementia in patients with Down's syndrome, *Am. J. Pathol.* **73:**457–476.

Cohen, D. E., Feiner, H., Jensson, O., and Frangione, B., 1983, Amyloid fibril in hereditary cerebral hemorrhage with amyloidosis (HCHWA) is related to the gastroenteropancreatic neuroendocrine protein, gamma trace, *J. Exp. Med.* **158:**623–628.

Divry, P., and Florkin, M., 1927, Sur les propriétés optiques de l'amyloide, *C. R. Soc. Biol.* **97:**1808–1810.

Dwulet, F. E., and Benson, M. D., 1984, Primary structure of an amyloid prealbumin and its plasma precursor in a heredofamilial polyneuropathy of Swedish origin, *Proc. Natl. Acad. Sci. USA* **81:**694–698.

Eanes, E. D., and Glenner, G. G., 1968, X-ray diffraction studies of amyloid filaments, *J. Histochem. Cytochem.* **16:**673–677.

Epstein, C. J., 1983, Down's syndrome and Alzheimer's disease: Implications and approaches, in: *Banbury Report 15: Biological Aspects of Alzheimer's Disease* (R. Katzman, ed.), Cold Spring Harbor Laboratory, Cold Spring Harbor, New York, pp. 169–182.

Fischer, O., 1910, Die presbyophrene Demenz deren anatomische Gründlage und klinische Abgrenzung, *Z. Ges. Neurol. Psychiatry* **3:**371–471.

Fujihara, S., Balow, J. E., Costa, J. C., and Glenner, G. G., 1980, Identification and classification of amyloid in formalin-fixed, paraffin-embedded tissue sections by the unlabeled immunoperoxidase method, *Lab. Invest.* **43:**358–365.

Glenner, G. G., 1979, Congophilic microangiopathy in the pathogenesis of Alzheimer's syndrome (presenile dementia), *Med. Hypoth.* **5:**1231–1236.

Glenner, G. G., 1980, Amyloid deposits and amyloidosis: The β-fibrilloses (Medical Progress Report), *N. Engl. J. Med.* **302:**1283–1292, 1333–1343.

Glenner, G. G., 1983, Alzheimer's disease: Multiple cerebral amyloidosis, in: *Banbury Report 15: Biological Aspects of Alzheimer's Disease, Cold Spring Harbor Symposium* (R. Katzman, ed.), Cold Spring Harbor Laboratory, Cold Spring Harbor, New York, pp. 137–144.

Glenner, G. G., and Wong, C. W., 1984a, Alzheimer's disease: Initial report of the purification and characterization of a novel cerebrovascular amyloid protein, *Biochem. Biophys. Res. Commun.* **120:**885–890.

Glenner, G. G., and Wong, C. W., 1984b, Alzheimer's disease and Down's syndrome sharing of a unique cerebrovascular amyloid fibril protein, *Biochem. Biophys. Res. Commun.* **122:**1131–1135.

Glenner, G. G., and Wong, C., 1987, Amyloidosis in Alzheimer's disease and Down's syndrome, in: *Banbury Report 27: Molecular Neuropathology of Aging* (P. Davies and C. E. Finch, eds.), Cold Spring Harbor Laboratory, Cold Spring Harbor, New York, pp. 253–265.

Glenner, G. G., Ein, D., Eanes, E. D., Bladen, H. A., Terry, W., and Page, D., 1971, The creation of "amyloid" fibrils from Bence Jones proteins *in vitro*, *Science* **174:**712–714.

Glenner, G. G., Harada, M., and Isersky, C., 1972, The purification of amyloid fibril proteins, *Prep. Biochem.* **2:**39–51.

Glenner, G. G., Eanes, E. D., Bladen, H. A., Linke, R. P., and Termine, J. D., 1974, β-pleated sheet fibrils: A comparison of native amyloid with synthetic protein fibrils, *J. Histochem. Cytochem.* **22:**1141–1158.

Glenner, G. G., Henry, J. H., and Fujihara, S., 1981, Congophilic angiopathy in the pathogenesis of Alzheimer's degeneration, *Ann. Pathol.* **1:**120–129.

Glenner, G. G., Wong, C. W., Quaranta, V., and Eanes, E. D., 1984, The amyloid deposits in Alzheimer's disease: Their nature and pathogenesis, *Appl. Pathol.* **83:**7908–7912.

Goldgaber, D., Lerman, M. I., McBride, O. W., Saffiotti, U., and Gadjdusek, D. C., 1987, Characterization and chromosomal localization of a cDNA encoding brain amyloid of Alzheimer's disease, *Science* **23:**877–880.

Gudmundsson, G., Hallgrimasson, J., Johasson, T. A., Bjarnason, O., 1972, Hereditary cerebral hemorrhage with amyloidosis, *Brain* **95**:387–404.

Guiroy, D. C., Miyazaki, M., Multhaup, G., Fischer, P., Garruto, R. M., Beyreuther, K., Masters, C. L., Simms, G., Gibbs, C. J., Jr., and Gajdusek, D. C., 1987, Amyloid of neurofibrillary tangles of Guamanian parkinsonism-dementia and Alzheimer disease share identical amino acid sequence, *Proc. Natl. Acad. Sci. USA* **84**:2073–2077.

Heston, L. L., 1976, Alzheimer's disease, trisomy 21, and myeloproliferative disorders: Associations suggesting a genetic diathesis, *Science* **196**:322–323.

Ikeda, S., Wong, C. W., Allsop, D., Landon, M., Kidd, M., and Glenner, G. G., 1987, Immunogold labeling of cerebrovascular and neuritic plaque amyloid fibrils in Alzheimer's disease with an anti-β-protein monoclonal antibody, *Lab Invest.* **57**:446–449.

Ishii, T., Haga, S., and Shimizu, F., 1975, Idnetification of components of immunoglobulins in senile plaques by means of fluorescent antibody technique, *Acta Neuropathol. (Berl.)* **32**:157–162.

Jenkins, E. C., Devine-Gage, E. A., Yao, X. L., Nouck, G. E., Jr., Brown, W. T., Wisniewski, H. M., and Robakis, N. K., 1987, In-situ hybridization of the beta-amyloid protein probe to chromosome 9 in patients with familial Alzheimer's disease (Letter), *Lancet* **2**:1155–1156.

Jervis, G. A., 1948, Early senile dementia in mongoloid idocy, *Am. J. Psychiatry* **105**:102–106.

Kang, J., Lemaire, H.-G., Unterbeck, A., Salbaum, J. M., Masters, C. L., Grzeschik, K.-H., Multhaup, G., Beyreuther, K., and Müller-Hill, B., 1987, The precursor of Alzheimer's disease amyloid A4 protein resembles a cell-surface receptor, *Nature (Lond.)* **325**:733–736.

Kidd, M., Allsop, D., and London, M., 1978, Senile plaque amyloid, paired helical filaments, and cerebrovascular amyloid in Alzheimer's disease are all deposits of the same protein, (Letter), *Lancet* **i**:278.

Kirschner, D. A., Abraham, C., and Selkoe, D. J., 1986, X-ray diffraction from intraneuronal paired helical filaments and extraneuronal amyloid fibers in Alzheimer disease indicates cross-β conformation, *Proc. Natl. Acad. Sci. USA* **83**:503–507.

Laemmli, U. D., 1970, Cleavage of structural proteins during the assembly of the head of bacteriophage T, *Nature (Lond.)* **227**:680–685.

Lovett, M., Goldgaber, D., Ashley, P., Cox, D. R., Gajdusek, D. C., and Epstein, C. J., 1987, The mouse homolog of the human amyloid β protein (AD-AP) gene is located on the distal end of mouse chromosome 16: Further extension of the homology between human chromosome 21 and mouse chromosome 16, *Biochem. Biophys. Res. Commun.* **144**:1069–1075.

Marglin, A., and Merrifield, R. B., 1970, Chemical synthesis of peptides and proteins, *Annu. Rev. Biochem.* **39**:841–866.

Masters, C. L., Multhaup, G., Simms, G., Pottgiesser, J., Martins, R. N., and Beyreuther, K., 1985a, Neuronal origin of a cerebral amyloid: Neurofibrillary tangles of Alzheimer's disease contain the same protein as the amyloid of plaque cores and blood vessels, *EMBO J.* **4**:2757–2763.

Masters, C. L., Simms, G., Weinman, N. A., Multhaup, G., McDonald, B. L., and Beyreuther, K., 1985b, Amyloid plaque core protein in Alzheimer disease and Down syndrome, *Proc. Natl. Acad. Sci. USA* **82**:4245–4249.

Miyakawa, T., Shimoji, A., Kuramoto, R. and Higuchi, Y., 1982, The relationship between senile plaques and cerebral blood vessels in Alzheimer's disease and senile dementia: Morphological mechanisms of senile plaque production, *Virchows Arch. [Cell Pathol.]* **40**:121–129.

Pantelakis, S., 1954, Un type particulier d'angiopathie sénile du système nerveux central: l'angiopathie Congophile. Topographie et fréquence, *Monatsschr. Psychiat. Neurol.* **128**:219–256.

Ponte, P., Gonzalez-DeWhitt, P., Schilling, J., Miller, J., Hsu, D., Greenberg, B., Davis, K., Wallace, W., Lieberburg, I., Fuller, F., and Cordell, B., 1988, A new A4 amyloid mRNA contains a domain homologous to serine proteinase inhibitors, *Nature (Lond.)* **331**:525–527.

Powers, J. M., Schlaeffer, W. W., Willingham, M. C., and Hall, B. J., 1981, An immunoperoxidase study of senile plaque amyloid, *J. Neuropathol. (Berl.)* **39**:311 (abst.).

Prusiner, S. B., 1984, Some speculations about prions, amyloid, and Alzheimer's disease, *N. Engl. J. Med.* **310**:661–663.

Robakis, N. K., Wisniewski, H. M., Jenkins, E. C., Devine-Gage, E. A., Houck, G. E., Yao, X.-L., Ramakrishna, N., Wolfe, G., Silverman, W. P., and Brown, W. T., 1987, Chromosome 21q21 sublocalisation of gene encoding beta-amyloid peptide in cerebral vessels and neuritic (senile) plaques of people with Alzheimer disease and Down syndrome (Letter), *Lancet* **1:**384–385.

Selkoe, D. J., Abraham, C. R., Podlisny, M. B., and Duffy, L. K., 1986, Isolation of low-molecular-weight proteins from amyloid plaque fibers in Alzheimer's disease, *J. Neurochem.* **46:**1820–1834.

St. George-Hyslop, P. H., Tanzi, R. E., Polinsky, R. J., Haines, J. L., Nee, L., Watkins, P. C., Myers, R. H., Feldman, R. G., Pollen, D., Drachman, D., Growdon, J., Bruni, A., Foncin, J.-F., Salmon, D., Frommelt, P., Amaducci, L., Sorbi, S., Piacentini, S., Stewart, G. D., Hobbs, W. J., Conneally, P. M., and Gusella, J. F., 1987, The genetic defect causing familial Alzheimer's disease maps on chromosom 21, *Science* **235:**885–890.

Sternberger, L. A., 1979, *Immunocytochemistry,* 2nd ed., Wiley, New York, 104–169.

Surbeck, E. B., 1961, L'angiopathie dyshorique (Morel) de l'écorce cérébrale: étude anatomoclinique el statistique: aspect génétique, *Acta Neuropathol. (Berl.)* **1:**168–197.

Tanzi, R. E., Gusella, J. F., Watkins, P. C., Bruns, G. A. P., St.-George-Hyslop, P., Van Keuren, M. L., Patterson, D., Pagan, S., Kurnit, D. M., and Neve, R. L., 1987, Amyloid β protein gene: cDNA, mRNA distribution, and genetic linkage near the Alzheimer locus, *Science* **235:**880–884.

Tanzi, R. E., McClatchey, A. I., Lamperti, E. D., Villa-Komaroff, L., Gusella, J. F., and Neve, R. L., 1988, Protease inhibitor domain encoded by an amyloid protein precursor mRNA associated with Alzheimer's disease, *Nature (Lond.)* **331:**528–532.

Tomlinson, B. E., Blessed, G., and Roth, M., 1968, Observations on the brains of non-demented old people, *J. Neurol. Sci.* **7:**331–356.

Tomlinson, B. E., Blessed, G., and Roth, M., 1970, Observations on the brains of demented old people, *J. Neurol. Sci.* **11:**205–242.

Torack, R. M., 1975, Congophilic angiopathy complicated by surgery and massive hemorrhage, *Am. J. Pathol.* **81:**349–366.

Van Broeckhoven, C., Genthe, A. M., Vandenberghe, A., Horsthemke, B., Backhovens, H., Raeymaekers, P., Van Hul, W., Wehnert, A., Gheuens, J., Cras, P., Bruyland, M., Martin, J. J., Salbaum, M., Multhaup, G., Masters, C. L., Beyreuther, K., Gurling, H. M. D., Mullan, M. J., Holland, A., Barton, A., Irving, N., Williamson, R., Richards, S. J., and Hardy, J. A., 1987, Failure of familial Alzheimer's disease to segregate with the A4-amyloid gene in several European families, *Nature (Lond.)* **329:**153–155.

van Duinen, S. G., Castano, E. M., Prelli, F., Bots, G. T. A. B., Luyendijk, W., and Frangione, B., 1987, Hereditary cerebral hemorrhage with amyloidosis in patients of Dutch origin is related to Alzheimer disease, *Proc. Natl. Acad. Sci. USA* **84:**5991–5994.

Walter, G., and Doolittle, R. R., 1983, Antibodies against synthetic peptides, in: *Genetic Engineering: Principles and Methods,* Vol. 5 (J. K. Setlow, and A. Hollaender, eds.), Plenum, New York, pp. 61–91.

Wong, C. W., Quaranta, W. V., and Glenner, G. G., 1985, Neuritic plaques and cerebrovascular amyloid in Alzheimer disease are antigenically related, *Proc. Natl. Acad. Sci. USA* **82:**8729–8732.

6

Evidence for the Molecular Basis of Aging and Sequestration of Mammalian Erythrocytes

DAVID AMINOFF

1. INTRODUCTION

This chapter represents a progress report—a story that relates the interplay of blood groups and red blood cell (RBC) survival to culminate in our current hypothesis for the molecular basis of aging and sequestration of mammalian senescent RBC from circulation. It was Ashby who, in 1919, demonstrated that RBC have a definite life span in the circulation. He accomplished this by the transfusion of RBC of blood group O into individuals of blood types A or B. He noted that, despite the compatibility of the blood transfusion, the RBC did not survive indefinitely. His data suggested an average life span of 83 days.

Since that observation, the limited life span of RBC has been demonstrated by a number of different techniques, some of which permitted a more accurate assessment of the duration of this life span—120 days in man (Berlin *et al.*, 1959). This involves the turnover of the equivalent of 2×10^{11} RBC/day in a normal adult (Bocci, 1981) and 1.6×10^5 of recirculations of a given RBC before its ultimate sequestration from the circulation (Allison, 1960).

The increase in density associated with increasing age of RBC provided a suitable physical method to separate RBC of different age (Piomelli *et al.*, 1967). That made it possible to observe many time-dependent changes in RBC involving size, deformability,

---

Abbreviations used in this chapter: aRBC, enzymatically desialated RBC; CMP–NAN, cytidine monophosphate derivative of sialic acid; Endoglycosidase, endo-*N*-acetyl-α-D-galactosaminidase; FITC–LFA, fluorescein isothiocyanate-labeled LFA; FITC–PNA, fluorescein isothiocyanate-labeled PNA; FITC–WGA, fluorescein isothiocyanate-labeled WGA; Gal, D-galactose; GalNac, D-*N*-acetylgalactosamine; GlcNAc; D-N-acetylglucosamine; GOST, galactose oxidase, *sialyltransferase* reactive sites; IgG, immunoglobulin; LFA, *Limax flavus* agglutinin; NAN, *N*-acetylneuraminic acid; PNA, peanut agglutinin; RBC, red blood cells; SFG(s), senescence factor glycopeptide(s); SRBC, senescent RBC, the densest fraction of RBC; WGA, wheat germ agglutinin; YRBC, young RBC, the lightest fraction of RBC.

DAVID AMINOFF • Institute of Gerontology, Department of Biological Chemistry, University of Michigan, Ann Arbor, Michigan 48109-2007.

osmotic fragility, and enzymatic activity. These observations raised the intriguing question of whether the life span of RBC is programmed or stochastic, depending on which of the many changing parameters became the critical factor at any given set of circumstances. Extensive studies have been undertaken on the biochemical changes occurring during the life span of RBC (Fornaini, 1967; Prankerd, 1969). A recent symposium, "The Cellular and Molecular Aspects of Aging: The Red Cell as a Model," updated many of these observations (Eaton *et al.*, 1985). The major difficulties, however, have been the unraveling of the complexities involved and the assignment of the primary signal for the sequestration of senescent RBC. In other words, which of the many changes involved also could be responsible for the ultimate sequestration of the senescent RBC?

Serendipity provided us with a plausible solution to the problem. We had long been interested in the conversion of red blood cells of A, B to the O(H) type to provide a universal blood donor type suitable for transfusion. This appeared feasible from the known chemical structures of the blood group substances (Watkins, 1972). We were successful in enzymatically converting RBC of type B to type H in rabbits, rats, and gibbons using the α-galactosidase from coffee beans and from *Clostridium sporogenes* (Maebashi) (Dybus and Aminoff, 1983). Autologous transfusions in rats and rabbits of the RBC treated with α-galactosidase resulted in no significant change in the life span of RBC in circulation.

We were successful also in enzymatically converting blood type A cells to O(H) (Levy and Aminoff, 1980), but the resulting transformed RBC did not survive in the corresponding autologous transfusion. This we attributed to the presence of a contaminating sialidase present in the *C-perfringens* extract used as the source of the α-N-acetylgalactosaminidase, as we and others had shown previously that treatment of RBC with sialidase results in their rapid sequestration from the circulation (Aminoff *et al.*, 1976). This was typical of all mammalian but not avian species tested (Aminoff *et al.*, 1976; Perret *et al.*, 1978, 1981).

Asialoerythrocytes appear to be removed from circulation by the liver and spleen in the same way as senescent RBC (Aminoff *et al.*, 1976). Removal of only 12% of total sialic acid with sialidase was sufficient for definitive sequestration to occur (Aminoff *et al.*, 1976). These observations, taken together with the report of 10–15% less sialic acid in old as compared with young RBC (Danon, 1966; Baxter and Beeley, 1975), gave rise to an intriguing speculation: Could the natural physiological decrease in sialic acid content of RBC in circulation be a signal responsible for the removal of the old erythrocytes from circulation?

We were lured further into this controversy—and away from our initial objective of preparation of a universal blood donor RBC from type A cells—by two arguments presented to us against the acceptability of such a hypothesis: (1) the then current belief that the sequestration of senescent RBC can be attributed primarily to the rigidity of their cell membrane and their inability to negotiate the intricate capillaries successfully, especially in the spleen; and (2) that the decrease in the sialic acid content of RBC with *in vivo* aging could be accounted for by a loss of cell-surface carbohydrates as the membrane of RBC buds off as vesicles (Prankerd, 1969; Gattegno *et al.*, 1976).

Our successful response to both contentions brought us greater confidence in our line of investigation and irrevocably involved us as active participants in this area of controversy. First, we demonstrated that liver and spleen macrophages can distinguish between normal RBC and those experimentally desialated with sialidase, whereas the hepatocytes could not (Aminoff *et al.*, 1977). This emphasized the potential involvement of highly specific cell–cell interaction, i.e., that a chemical, and not necessarily a change in physical property of the aging RBC, could be involved.

Our response to the second challenge (Aminoff *et al.*, 1981) demonstrated that over and above the loss of sialic acid as part of the glycoprotein membrane lost as vesicles, there is a loss of covalently bound sialic acid with the exposure of the penultimate sugar galactose. This sugar was detected and quantified by (1) oxidation with galactose oxidase followed by reduction with tritiated borohydride (Gahmberg and Hakomori, 1973), identified as GO substrate sites; and (2) direct resialation with sialyl transferase and CMP-[^{14}C]-NAN, similarly identified as ST substrate sites. Thus, we were able to show the presence of more GOST substrate receptor sites in old as compared with young RBC (Aminoff et al., 1981). This would be an appropriate point at which to jump ahead to outline what our current hypothesis is for the aging and sequestration of senescent mammalian RBC from circulation. This discussion then proceeds to develop the evidence for the molecular basis of aging.

2. CURRENT WORKING HYPOTHESIS

The model that emerges from all these studies is as follows (Fig. 1). RBC senescence is accompanied by a contraction of the cell volume due to a loss of cell membrane (Prankerd, 1969). This results in an overall loss of surface carbohydrate components such that all the constituent sugars of cell membrane are lost in the same proportions (Gattegno et al., 1976). Over and above this general loss of carbohydrates and other membrane components, there is a specific loss of covalently bound sialic acid residues near the end of the life span of RBC in circulation, the "twilight zone."

The sialic acid residues that are lost, we believe, are derived from the oligosaccharide chains of glycophorin molecules on the surface of RBC (Fig. 2), which is responsible for blood groups M and N activity of RBC. This involves both the 15 O-glycosyl, and one N-glycosyl oligosaccharide chains of human glycophorin A (Tomita and Marchesi, 1975) or rat glycophorin (Edge et al., 1981, 1986). The removal of sialic acid residues results in the unmasking of β-galactosyl residues, in the predominant O-glycosyl oligosaccharide chains, to result in exposure of the disaccharide Gal-(1,3) GalNAc residues. These are recognized by an autoimmune antigalactosyl IgG (Alderman et al., 1981; Galili et al., 1983) as well as by lectin-like receptors on monocytes and macrophages (Schlepper-Schafer et al., 1983; Vaysse

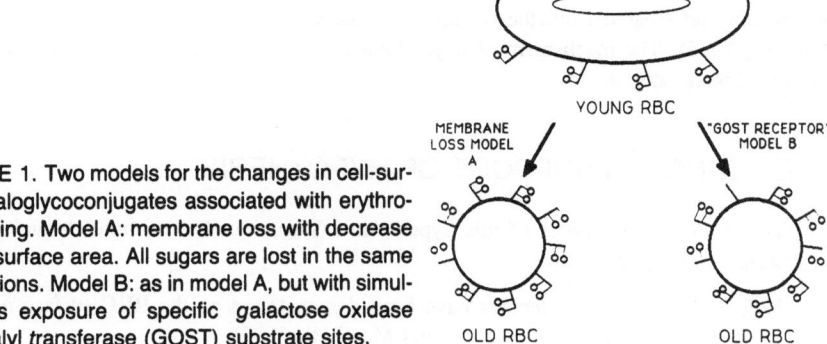

FIGURE 1. Two models for the changes in cell-surface sialoglycoconjugates associated with erythrocyte aging. Model A: membrane loss with decrease in cell-surface area. All sugars are lost in the same proportions. Model B: as in model A, but with simultaneous exposure of specific galactose oxidase and sialyl transferase (GOST) substrate sites.

YOUNG RBC

MEMBRANE LOSS MODEL A

"GOST RECEPTOR" MODEL B

OLD RBC

OLD RBC

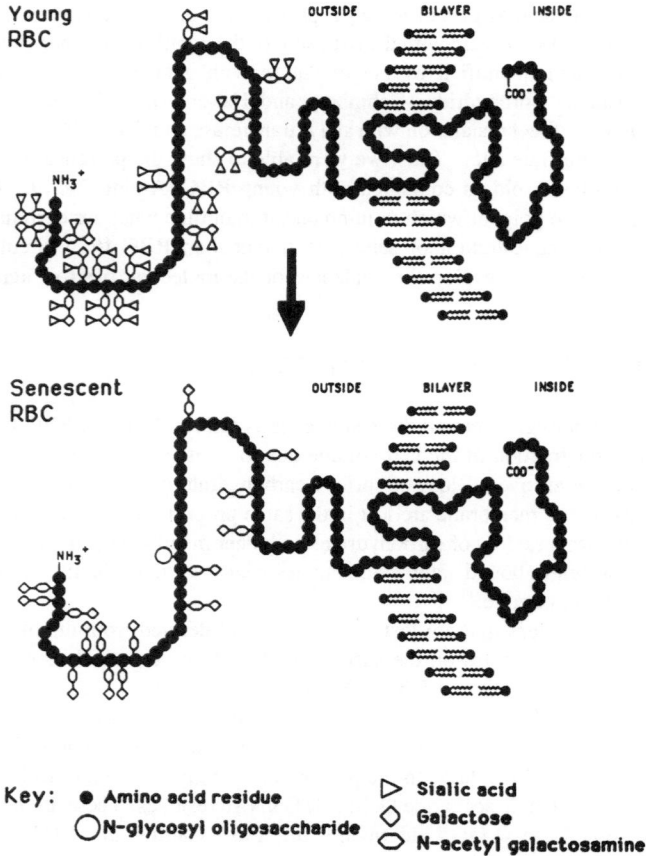

FIGURE 2. Loss of sialic acid residues from the oligosaccharide chains of glycophorin from young RBC near the end of the "twilight zone," just before the sequestration of the senescent RBC.

et al., 1986). The senescent RBC, with their exposed specific galactosyl residues, thus are recognized and cleared from the circulation, predominantly in the spleen (Smedsrod and Aminoff, 1985). The mechanism of physiological desialation that leads to all these events still remains an enigma.

3. EVIDENCE IN SUPPORT OF HYPOTHESIS

The evidence in support of this hypothesis has continued to accumulate and can be summarized briefly as follows:

1. Glycophorin-like molecules have been demonstrated on the RBC surface of most mammalian species (Furthmayr and Marchesi, 1983).

2. Careful chemical analysis of the carbohydrate moiety of these molecules has demonstrated the preponderance of O-glycosyl tetrasaccharides with small quantities of the two isoforms of the trisaccharide; there is little or no evidence for the presence of disaccharide or monosaccharide chains (Lisowska et al., 1980) (Fig. 3).

3. We have demonstrated the presence of more galactose oxidase and sialyl transferase (GOST) reactive sites on senescent, as compared with young, RBC (Aminoff et al., 1981) (Figs. 1 and 4).

4. On the basis of our knowledge of the structures of these oligosaccharide chains in glycophorin, we devised a procedure to isolate these GOST sites as senescence factor glycopeptides SFG(s) from human senescent RBC. Moreover, we have shown that the same isolation procedure when applied to young RBC did not result in the isolation of SFG(s) (Henrich and Aminoff, 1983) (Figs. 5 and 6).

5. The SFG(s) are recognized by spleen monocytes. This recognition is destroyed by treatment with β-galactosidase (Henrich and Aminoff, 1983) (Fig. 7).

6. The SFG(s) are very potent inhibitors of autologous erythrophagocytosis, inhibiting at nanomolar concentrations (Vaysse et al., 1986; Fig. 8).

7. Treatment of rat RBC with various glycosidases has demonstrated the potential of:
   a. "Artificial aging" of RBC by treatment with sialidase.
   b. "Rejuvenation" of the artificially aged RBC by the appropriate enzymatic removal of either the terminal β-Gal, or the Gal-β-(1–3)GalNAc residues (Aminoff et al., 1987; Gutowski et al., 1988) (Fig. 9).

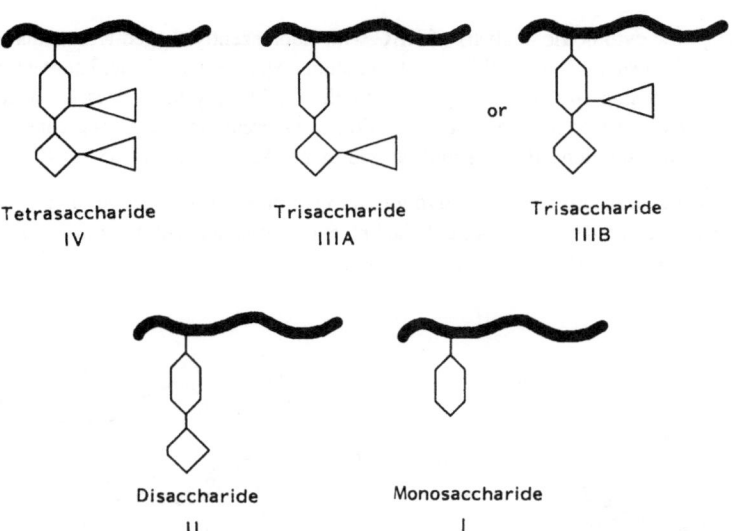

FIGURE 3. Tetrasaccharide and two trisaccharide structures found in native human RBC glycophorin are shown in the top row. The disaccharide and monosaccharide structures that have not been detected are shown in lower row. Lisowska et al. (1980) found the oligosaccharides present in human glycophorin in the proportions IV : IIIA : IIIB, 8 : 3 : 1 with no II or I.

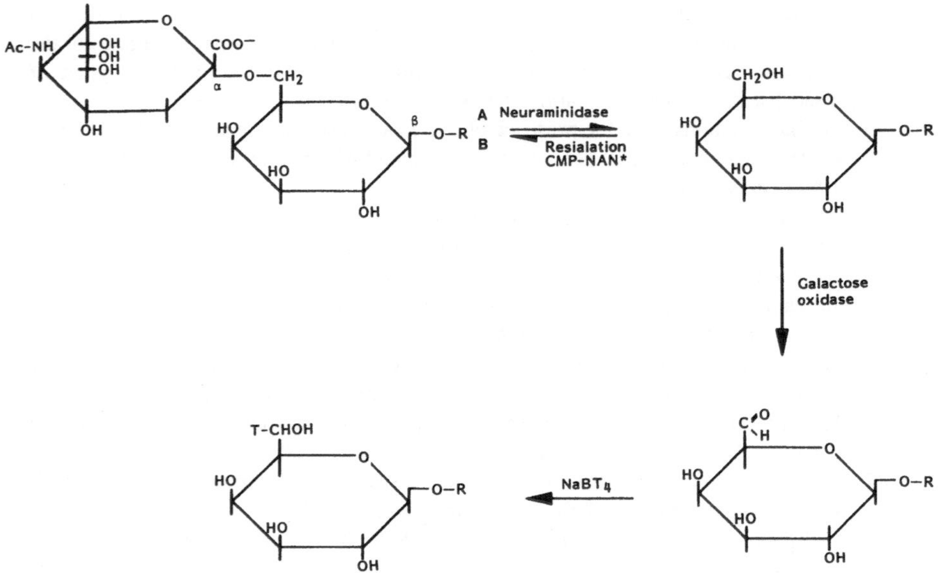

FIGURE 4. Detection of galactose oxidase and sialyl transferase (GOST) sites on senescent or asialo RBC involves treatment of SRBC or aRBC with (A) galactose oxidase, followed by reduction with tritiated borohydride to radioactively label the GO sites; (B) radioactively tagged CMP-[^{14}C]-NAN and (2->3 and 2->6) sialyl transferases, to radioactively label the ST sites.

8. Flow cytometric analysis of RBC with fluorescently tagged lectins that detect sialic acid residues have indicated (a) a gradual decrease in sialic acid content of RBC with decreasing size (increasing age) of cells, and a very rapid decrease at the "twilight zone" just prior to their sequestration from circulation; and (b) greater susceptibility of the smaller RBC to sialidase treatment (Aminoff et al., 1988) (Fig. 10).

A more detailed discussion of our hypothesis, incorporating 1–8 above, and the evidence for and against our model has been published recently, together with the criticism of this model by two reviewers and our response to this criticism (Aminoff, 1988).

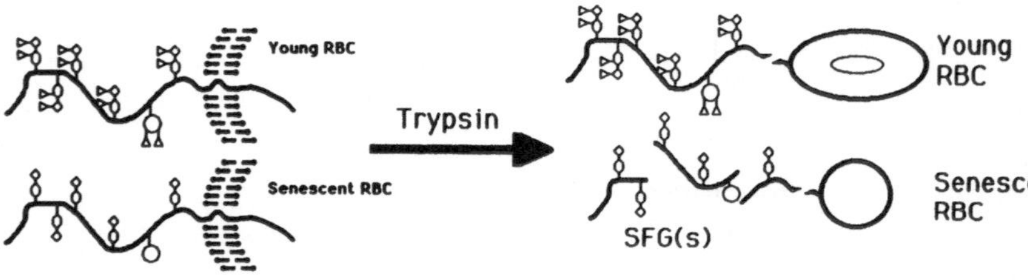

FIGURE 5. Trypsinization of YRBC or SRBC results in the release of a mixture of sialoglycopeptides and glycopeptides, respectively. The sialic acid residues protect some of the susceptible peptide bonds, such that YRBC give fewer glycopeptides than SRBC or aRBC.

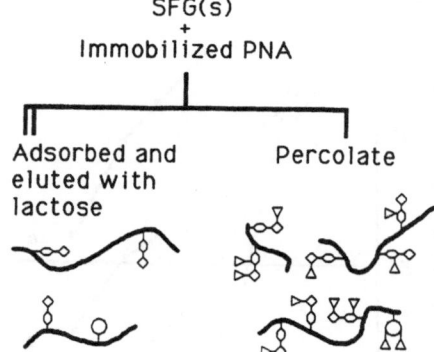

SFG(s)
+
Immobilized PNA

Adsorbed and   Percolate
eluted with
lactose

FIGURE 6. Separation of the sialoglycopeptides from the glycopeptides is achieved on a
column of immobilized peanut agglutinin
(PNA). Only the sialic acid-free glycopeptides
are adsorbed, and these are subsequently
eluted with lactose.

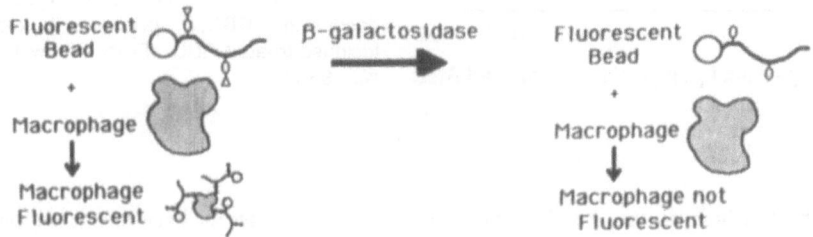

FIGURE 7. The senescent factor glycopeptides SFG(s) are covalently bound to fluorescent microspheres. These are recognized by the macrophages, adsorbed, and subsequently phagocytized. Treatment of the covalently bound SFG(s) microspheres with β-galactosidase removes the recognition signal, and the microspheres do not attach to the macrophages.

FIGURE 8. Blood monocytes adhere
to slides and, upon culturing for 24 hr,
transform to macrophages. These
macrophages will adhere to and pha-
gocytize autologous senescent RBC.
This adhesion and phagocytosis is inhibited by nanomolar concentrations
of SFG(s) in contrast to galactose at
millimolar, and galactose-containing
neoglycoproteins at micromolar concentrations—all concentrations are
based on total galactose content.
(From Vaysse et al., 1986.)

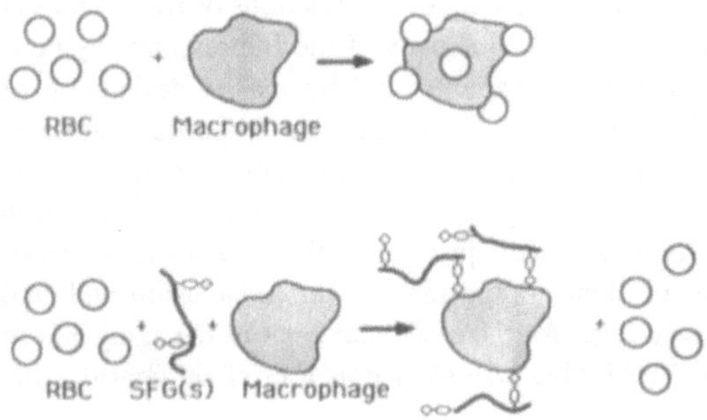

RBC   Macrophage

RBC   SFG(s)   Macrophage

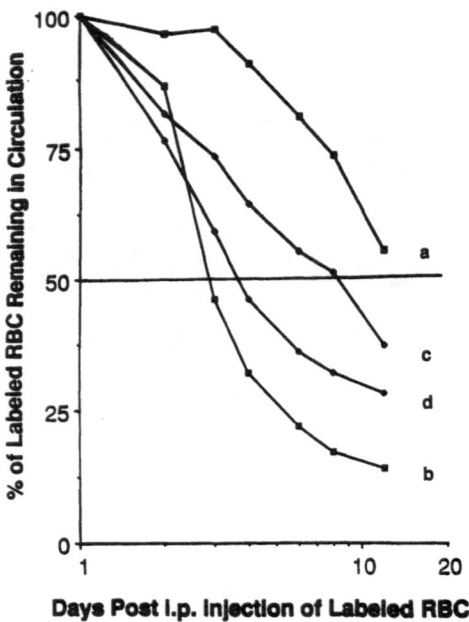

FIGURE 9. Survival of enzymatically treated rat RBC in circulation. a, Control, RBC, incubated in isotonic saline; b, sialidase-treated RBC; c, sialidase + endoglycosidase-treated RBC; d, sialidase + β-galactosidase-treated RBC. (From Gutowski *et al.*, 1988.)

The last item on the list (8) is the result of some very recent experiments we have undertaken using flow cytometric analysis of human RBC (Fig. 10a,b). We followed the fluorescence profile of RBC given by their interactions with miscellaneous fluorescently labeled lectins, such as wheat germ agglutinin (FITC–WGA), *Limax flavus* agglutinin (FITC–LFA), and peanut agglutinin (FITC–PNA) (Fig. 10c). These results indicate that as a first approximation, the intensity of fluorescence/RBC with the two lectins, WGA and LFA, appears to remain unchanged for RBC throughout most of their life span (as reflected by the size distribution). However, at the two extremes of cell size, corresponding to the two extremes in RBC *in vivo* age, where fewer RBC are available for statistical analysis, the results would appear to suggest that the younger (larger) RBC have more fluorescence than do the older (smaller) RBC. Using the same scale for comparison, there is no apparent reactivity of the human RBC with FITC–PNA.

The specificity of the reactions of RBC with FITC–WGA is demonstrated by the ability to decrease the intensity of the fluorescence by both a competitive inhibitor of the reaction, *N*-acetylglucosamine, and by partial desialation of RBC with sialidase (Fig. 10d). The fluorescence profile given with the partially desialated RBC is of interest in that it suggests that the smaller cells lose their sialic acid more rapidly than the larger cells. This would imply that a change in cell size could be responsible for the more rapid desialation of RBC at the "twilight zone" just before their sequestration from circulation. Obviously, more work has to be done to substantiate this conclusion and, indeed, to unequivocally substantiate our hypothesis for the molecular basis of the aging and sequestration of RBC. For the time being, the following will suffice as a brief summary of the present state of the art.

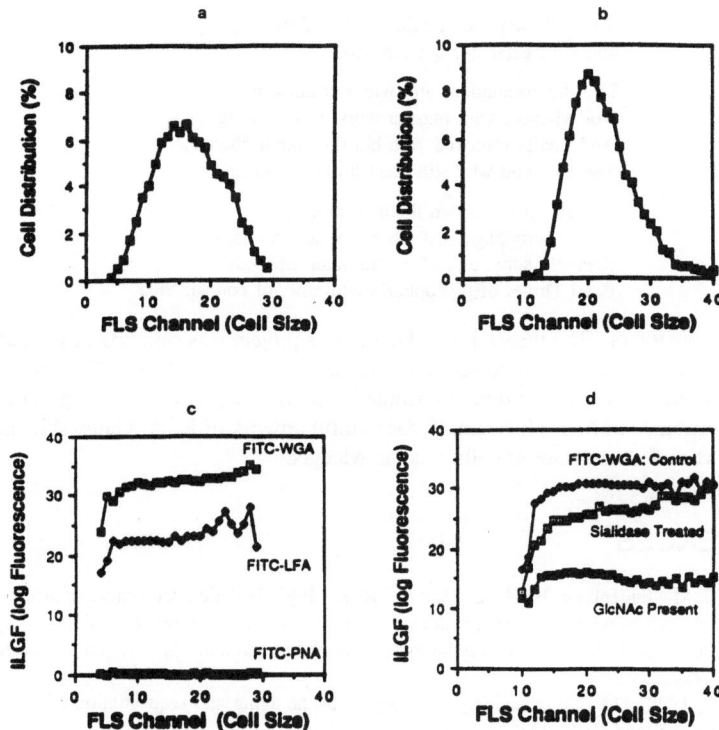

FIGURE 10. Flow cytometric analyses of RBC. (a,b) Typical size distribution of RBC as determined by lightscatter with two different samples of human RBC. (c) RBC in (a) treated with FITC–WGA, FITC–LFA, and FITC–PNA. (d) RBC in (b) treated with FITC–WGA alone and in the presence of 0.2 M N-acetylglucosamine, GlcNAc, or after partial removal of sialic acid residues following treatment with sialidase from *Vibrio cholerae*. (From Aminoff *et al.*, 1988.)

4. QUINTESSENCE OF ERYTHROCYTE SENESCENCE
(with Apologies to Omar Khayyam's Rubaiyat)

Oh come with Dave Aminoff, and leave the wise
To talk, one thing is certain, that RBC die,
One thing is certain and the rest is a lie;
The red cell, having reached 120 days, forever dies.

Myself when young did eagerly experiment
with RBC and sialidase, observing a great event
The red cell that once danced and pranced,
Now struggles within a macrophage without a chance.

With you the seed of wisdom did I sow,
And with all our hands labored it to grow,
And this was the harvest that we reaped—

Red cells with sialic acid, in they flow,
and with galactose out they go.

Into the circulation, and why not knowing
Nor whence, with plasma willy nilly flowing.
And finally removed with but this minor change,
The how and why still need further exploring.

Is it an IgG to which there is no key,
Or a macrophage past which we still cannot see?
Recently some talk of autoimmune antibody
Band Three, of glycophorin and now, of course, SFG.

ACKNOWLEDGMENTS. The research involved in this project was supported by grant HL AM 17881 from the National Institutes of Health and AG 08018 from NIA. Permission to reproduce some of the text and figures (Aminoff, 1988) was granted by Springer-Verlag. The editorial assistance of Mrs. H. Aminoff, the skillful artwork of K. A. Gutowski, and careful typing of Miss F. Gruda are gratefully acknowledged.

REFERENCES

Alderman, E. M., Fudenberg, H. H., and Lovins, R. E., 1981, Isolation and characterization of an age-related antigen present on senescent human red blood cells, *Blood* **58**:341–349.
Allison, A. C., 1960, Turnover of erythrocytes and plasma proteins in mammals, *Nature (Lond.)* **188**:37–40.
Aminoff, D., 1988, The role of sialoglycoconjugates in the aging and sequestration of red cells from circulation, *Blood Cells,* **14**:229–257.
Aminoff, D., Ghalambor, M. A., and Henrich, C. J., 1981, GOST, galactose oxidase and sialyl transferase, substrate and receptor sites in erythrocyte senescence, in: *Erythrocyte Membranes*. Vol. 2: *Recent Clinical Experimental Advances* (W. C. Kruckeberg, J. W. Eaton, and G. J. Brewer, eds.), Liss, New York, pp. 269–278.
Aminoff, D., VorderBruegge, W. F., Bell, W. C., Sarpolis, K., and Williams, R., 1977, Role of sialic acid in survival of erythrocytes in circulation: Interaction of neuraminidase-treated and untreated erythrocytes with spleen and liver at the cellular level, *Proc. Natl. Acad. Sci. USA* **74**:1521–1524.
Aminoff, D., Bell, W. C., Fulton, I., and Ingebrigtsen, N., 1976, Effect of sialidase on the viability of erythrocytes in circulation, *Am. J. Hermatol.* **1**:419–432.
Aminoff, D., Gutowski, K. A., and Linseman, D. A., 1987, The effect of glycosidases on the survival of red blood cells in circulation, *Biochem. Soc. Trans.* **15**:394.
Aminoff, D., Gutowski, K. A., Brede, D. E., and Hudson, J. L., 1988, Flow cytometric analysis of human erythrocytes probed with FITC-labelled lectins, in: *Sialic Acid,* Proceedings of Japanese–German Symposium on Sialic Acid, West Berlin, May 18–21 (R. Schauer and T. Yamakawa, eds.), Kieler Verlag Wissenschaft and Bildung, Kiel, pp. 224–225.
Ashby, W., 1919, Determination of length of life of transfusion blood corpuscles in man, *J. Exp. Med.* **29**:267–281.
Baxter, A., and Beeley, J. G., 1975, Changes in surface carbohydrate of human erythrocytes aged *in vivo, Biochem Soc. Trans.* **3**:134–136.
Berlin, N. I., Waldman,, T. A., and Weissman, S. M., 1959, Life span of red blood cells, *Physiol. Rev.* **39**:577–616.
Bocci, V., 1981, Annotation. Determinants of erythrocyte ageing: A reappraisal, *Br. J. Haematol.* **48**:515–522.
Danon, D., 1966, Biophysical aspects of red cell ageing, Eleventh Congress of International Society of Hematology, pp. 394–405.

Dybus, S., and Aminoff, D., 1983, Action of alpha-galactosidase from *Clostridium sporogenes* and coffee beans on blood group antigens or erythrocytes and their effect on the viability of erythrocytes in circulation, *Transfusion* **23:**244–247.

Eaton, J. W., Konzen, D. K., and White, J. G., 1985, *Cellular and Molecular Aspects of Aging: The Red Cell as a Model*, Liss, New York.

Edge, A. S. B., and Weber, P., 1981, Purification and characterization of the major sialoglyoproteins, of the rat erythrocyte membrane, *Arch. Biochem. Biophys.* **209:**697–705.

Edge, A. S. B., VanLangenhove, A., Reinhold, V., and Weber, P., 1986, Characterization of O-glycosidically linked oligosaccharides of rat erythrocyte membrane sialoglycoproteins, *Biochemistry* **25:**8017–8024.

Fornaini, G., 1967, Biochemical modifications during the life span of the erythrocyte, *Ital. J. Biochem.* **16:**257–330.

Furthmayr, H., and Marchesi, V. T., 1983, Glycophorins: Isolation, orientation, and localization of specific domains, *Methods Enzymol.* **96:**268–280.

Gahmberg, C. G., and Hakomori, S.-I., 1973, External labelling of cell surface galactose and galactosamine in glycolipid and glycoprotein of human erythrocyte, *J. Biol. Chem.* **248:**4311–4317.

Galili, U., Korkesh, A., Kahane, I., and Rachmilewitz, E. A., 1983, Demonstration of a natural antigalactosyl IgG antibody on thalassemic red blood cells, *Blood* **61:**1258–1264.

Gattegno, L., Bladier, D., Garnier, M., and Cornillot, P., 1976, Changes in carbohydrate content of surface membranes of human erythrocytes during ageing, *Carbohydr. Res.* **52:**197–208.

Gutowski, K. A., Linseman, D. A., and Aminoff, D., 1988, The effect of glycosidases on the survival of rat-erythrocytes in circulation, *Carbohydr. Res.* **178:**307–313.

Henrich, C. J., and Aminoff, D., 1983, Isolation and characterization of a glycopeptide from human senescent erythrocytes, *Carbohydr. Res.* **120:**55–66.

Levy, G. N., and Aminoff, D., 1980, Purification and properties of an alpha-*N*-acetylgalactosaminidase from *Clostridium perfringens*, *J. Biol. Chem.* **255:**11737–11742.

Lisowska, E., Duk, M., and Dahr, W., 1980, Comparisons of alkali-labile oligosaccharide chains of M and N blood-group glycopeptides from human erythrocyte membrane, *Carbohydr. Res.* **79:**103–113.

Perret, G., Bladier, D., Pre, J., and Cornillot, P., 1978, Comparison of nucleated and enucleated asialylated erythrocytes survival time. Possible role of T-agglutinin, *Comp. Biochem. Physiol.* **60A:**417–420.

Perret, G., Bladier, D., Vassy, R., and Cornillot, P., 1981, Desialosylation of mammalian and nonmammalian red blood cells: Effect on *in vivo* survival in relation to the number of unmasked T-sites on VCN treated erythrocytes and serum T-agglutinin titers, *Comp. Biochem. Physiol.* **69A:**59–63.

Piomelli, S., Lurinsky, G., and Wasserman, L. R., 1967, The mechanism of red cell aging. I. Relationship between cell age and specific gravity evaluated by ultracentrifugation in a discontinuous density gradient, *J. Lab. Clin. Med.* **69:**659–674.

Prankerd, T. A. J., 1969, Nonimmunological mechanisms of red cell destruction, *Ser. Hematol.* **2:**53–58.

Schlepper-Schafer, J., Kolb-Bachofen, V., and Kolb, H., 1983, Identification of a receptor for senescent erythrocytes on liver macrophages, *Biochem. Biophys. Res. Commun.* **115:**551–559.

Smedsrod, B., and Aminoff, D., 1985, Use of ^{75}Se-labeled methionine to study the sequestration of senescent red blood cells, *Am. J. Hematol.* **18:**31–40.

Tomita, M., and Marchesi, V. T., 1975, Amino-acid sequence and oligosaccharide attachment sites of human erythrocyte glycophorin, *Proc. Natl. Acad. Sci. USA* **72:**2964–2968.

Vaysse, J., Gattegno, L., and Bladier, D., 1986, Adhesion and erythrophagocytosis of human senescent erythrocytes by autologous monocytes and their inhibition by beta-galactosyl derivatives, *Proc. Natl. Acad. Sci. USA.* **18:**1339–1343.

Watkins, W. M., 1972, Blood group specific substances, in: *Glycoproteins: Their Composition Structure and Function* (A. Gottschalk, ed.), Elsevier, Amsterdam, pp. 830–891.

7

α_1-Antichymotrypsin

The Role of Proteases and Their Inhibitors in the Amyloid Deposition of Alzheimer's Disease and Normal Brain Aging

HUNTINGTON POTTER and CARMELA R. ABRAHAM

1. INTRODUCTION

Normal brain aging, Alzheimer's disease, and Down's syndrome are all characterized by similar neuropathological lesions. Such neuropathology is much more severe and occurs at much earlier ages in Alzheimer's disease and Down's syndrome than in normal aging and suggests that these diseases should be studied as model systems of a more widespread problem. In addition, the fact that Alzheimer's disease arises repeatedly in certain families in which it appears to be passed down from generation to generation as an autosomal-dominant trait indicates that mutation in a single gene *can* lead to the disease (Heston *et al.*, 1981; for reviews, Matsuyama *et al.*, 1985; Jarvik and Matsuyama, 1986). The same neurodegeneration, loss of memory, and neuropathological lesions characterize both these familial and the more common sporadic cases of Alzheimer's disease (Terry 1978a,b; Heston *et al.*, 1981; McKahnn *et al.*, 1984). Therefore, the study of an aberrant protein in inherited Alzheimer's disease might lead to an understanding of the biochemical mechanism for the generation of the disease in certain families, and by extension, perhaps all other cases as well. Furthermore, an understanding of the physiological basis of the disorder should be directly relevant to understanding the process of normal aging.

    The approach we have taken to studying the biochemical basis of Alzheimer's disease and normal aging is to isolate the genes that code for key proteins involved in the neurodegenerative process. It may then be possible to deduce the functions of the proteins encoded by these genes from their derived amino acid sequence. The fact that inherited cases of Alzheimer's indicate that a single protein that is abnormal in structure or amount is alone sufficient to cause disease makes isolating the gene for such a protein of particular interest.

HUNTINGTON POTTER and CARMELA R. ABRAHAM • Department of Neurobiology, Harvard Medical School, Boston, Massachusetts 02115. *Present address for C.R.A.:* Arthritis Center, Boston University School of Medicine, Boston, Massachusetts 02118.

As a basis for cloning genes related to Alzheimer's disease, one approach is first to identify proteins that appear to be altered in the disease. The most apparent pathological characteristics of the brains of Alzheimer's disease victims is the presence of large numbers of abnormal proteinaceous deposits, whose prevalence is highly correlated to the degree of neurological dysfunction (Roth *et al.*, 1966; Tomlinson *et al.*, 1968; Terry, 1978a,b). These lesions are the intraneuronal aggregates of helically wound pairs of intermediate-sized filaments, called neurofibrillary tangles (for review, see Price *et al.*, 1986; Selkoe, 1986), and the extraneuronal amyloid-like deposits. These latter occur in the walls of meningeal and intracortical blood vessels (Glenner, 1983; Miyakawa *et al.*, 1982) and in the cores of neuritic or senile plaques (Scholz, 1938; Mandybur, 1975; Mountjoy *et al.*, 1982; Merz *et al.*, 1983). Several lines of evidence suggest that, of the two types of lesions, the amyloid deposits may be more specifically characteristic of normal aging and Alzheimer's disease. For example, neurofibrillary tangles and neuronal cell death can arise in other situations besides Alzheimer's disease, such as after chronic trauma, dementia pugilistica, or Guam Parkinson dementia, where there is no evidence for vascular amyloid or neuritic plaques (Gajdusek and Salazar, 1982; Wisniewski *et al.*, 1979). Furthermore, aged monkeys also suffer neurological degeneration and accumulate neuritic plaques, but not neurofibrillary tangles (Struble *et al.*, 1985).

The first identified constituent of Alzheimer amyloid deposits was 4- to 5-kDa peptide, designated the β-protein. This protein was originally isolated from meningeal blood vessels and sequenced by Glenner and Wong (1984), and was also shown to be present in the amyloid of neuritic plaque cores (Masters *et al.*, 1985; Wong *et al.*, 1985; Gorevic *et al.*, 1986; Selkoe *et al.*, 1986). Several groups have recently isolated complementary DNA (cDNA) clones coding for the amyloid β-protein precursor, using oligonucleotide probes (Goldgaber *et al.*, 1987; Kang *et al.*, 1987; Tanzi *et al.*, 1987a; Robakis *et al.*, 1987). Analysis of an apparently full-length clone showed the precursor of the β-protein to be a 695-amino acid protein that resembles a cell-surface receptor (Kang *et al.*, 1987). The β-protein is a small portion of this polypeptide near its carboxy terminal and includes part of the putative membrane spanning region and part of the adjacent extracellular domain. The messenger RNA (mRNA) for the β-protein is expressed in several cell types within the brain and is also found in high abundance in other tissues, especially spleen, heart, and kidney (Bahmanyar *et al.*, 1987; Tanzi *et al.*, 1987a).

In a second and parallel approach, we have used antisera raised against the Alzheimer's amyloid fibers as a handle for cloning the relevant gene(s) coding for these proteins. To this end, we first used the antisera to search for cells expressing the protein(s) present in the Alzheimer's disease lesions. The tissue so identified was liver. The antisera were then used to screen a cDNA library made from human liver mRNA and to identify the particular bacterium whose resident member of the library was expressing the Alzheimer's amyloid protein.

2. RESULTS

2.1. Serine Protease Inhibitor α_1-Antichymotrypsin is a Component of Alzheimer's Amyloid Deposits

The first gene we isolated proved, upon sequence analysis, to encode the serine protease inhibitor, α_1-antichymotrypsin (Abraham *et al.*, 1988). Several lines of analysis were then initiated to prove that this protein was indeed a specific component of the Alzheimer's amyloid deposits. First, we showed that several independently prepared antisera to purified α_1-antichymotrypsin were able specifically to label the amyloid deposits in the cores of neuritic plaques and in the walls of cerebral and meningeal blood vessels in Alzheimer's disease brain (Fig. 1). Furthermore, we demonstrated that the amyloid plaque cores contain at least two, and probably more, independent epitopes of α_1-antichymotrypsin. Proteolytic fragments released by the cleavage of α_1-antichymotrypsin with lysylendopeptidase were separated by reverse-phase high-performance liquid chromatography (RP-HPLC). The various antisera, both to purified α_1-antichymotrypsin and to the amyloid plaque cores, were then tested on dot blots containing each of the 26 distinguishable peptides from the HPLC column. Two of the antisera to pure α_1-antichymotrypsin recognized different, partially overlapping, sets of the peptides. Within each set there was a single very strongly staining peptide that was different for each antiserum. Thus, lysylendopeptidase digestion of pure α_1-antichymotrypsin released at least two distinct epitopes from the α_1-antichymotrypsin. The amyloid antiserum that we used to isolate our clone of α_1-antichymotrypsin recognized many of the HPLC-separated fragments that the two antisera to pure α_1-antichymotrypsin do (including the two strongly staining peptides), as well as a few others. Thus, the antiserum made directly against the amyloid from Alzheimer's disease brain recognized at least two epitopes of α_1-antichymotrypsin and very likely more. These data indicate that it is α_1-antichymotrypsin itself, and not an immunologically related protein, that is a component of the Alzheimer's amyloid deposits (Abraham et al., 1988).

Another issue was whether the α_1-antichymotrypsin is a structural component of the

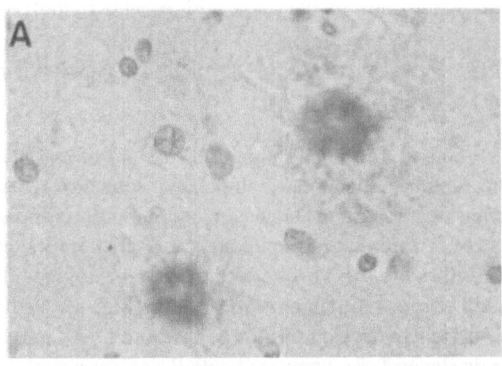

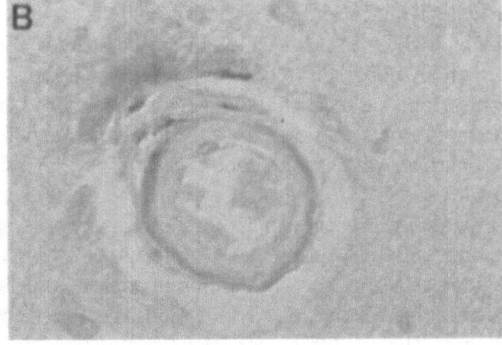

FIGURE 1. Antibodies against pure α_1-antichymotrypsin label amyloid deposits in Alzheimer's disease. Paraffin sections of Alzheimer's disease brain immunolabeled with antisera to α_1-antichymotrypsin as described. Both the cores of neuritic plaques (A) and the amyloid deposits associated with blood vessels (B) are labeled by α_1-antichymotrypsin antibodies.

amyloid deposits or a serum protein that leaks into the neuropil from the circulation and becomes nonspecifically absorbed to pre-existing deposits. Several aspects of our data argue that α_1-antichymotrypsin is a specific, integral component of the Alzheimer's amyloid deposits. First, that the α_1-antichymotrypsin is very tightly bound to or integral to the amyloid deposits is argued by our inability to remove it by harsh treatment, such as boiling in sodium dodecyl sulfate (SDS) and β-mercaptoethanol. Furthermore, several independently prepared commercial antisera to α_1-antichymotrypsin recognize purified amyloid plaque cores that have also been extracted extensively by boiling in SDS and β-mercaptoethanol. When such core preparations are examined in the electron microscope, they are seen to consist entirely of aggregated amyloid filaments without associated debris. Finally, immunogold staining and electron microscopic analysis of these purified amyloid filaments indicates that α_1-antichymotrypsin is intimately associated with the β-protein in the filaments (Fig. 2).

With respect to the specificity of α_1-antichymotrypsin in the amyloid deposits, as compared with other serum components, we also carried out an immunologic analysis of the Alzheimer's brain tissue sections for the presence of other serum components (IgG, prealbumin, antithrombin III, α_1-antitrypsin) and failed to find any evidence for these proteins in the Alzheimer's amyloid deposits. Two of these tests (those for antithrombin III and α_1-antitrypsin) are particularly interesting because these proteins are closely related, structurally and functionally, to α_1-antichymotrypsin. The presence of the other two serum proteins we tested for (IgG and prealbumin) was reported some years ago in amyloid deposits of Alzheimer's disease brain tissue sections. We have not been able to reproduce this finding, nor have other researchers (Gorevic et al., 1986; Ihara, 1986). We have carried out a similar immunochemical analysis on the purified preparations of Alzheimer's neuritic plaque cores and again find labeling only with α_1-antichymotrypsin antisera.

2.2. Enhanced Expression of α_1-Antichymotrypsin in Alzheimer's Disease Brain

The high concentration (250 μg/ml) of α_1-antichymotrypsin in the serum suggests that the inhibitor specifically associated with the Alzheimer amyloid deposits may be derived from the circulation. However, the inhibitor is found in many types of cells besides hepatocytes: macrophages, epithelial and endothelial cells, mast cells, and histiocytes (Papadimitriou et al., 1980). We therefore examined the expression of α_1-antichymotrypsin in brain tissue. (Abraham et al., 1988) (Fig. 3). Figure 3a shows a Northern blot analysis of α_1-antichymotrypsin mRNA in newborn liver (lane 1) and in Alzheimer's disease and normal brain (lanes 2–7), compared with β-actin as a control probe in the lower blot. Liver expressed α_1-antichymotrypsin RNA, as expected. In lanes 2–4, RNA samples from three areas of a single Alzheimer's disease brain are compared. Hippocampus (lane 4) contained the most α_1-antichymotrypsin RNA, inferior temporal gyrus (lane 3) showed an intermediate level of expression, and precentral gyrus (lane 2) contained the least, compared with β-actin RNA, on the same blot. Lanes 5–7 show the level of α_1-antichymotrypsin RNA in the same three areas of a normal, 74-year-old, control brain. The expression in each normal sample is beneath the low level found in precentral gyrus of the Alzheimer's disease brain, while the actin RNA is substantially higher than in the Alzheimer's disease brain, despite the loading of equal amounts of RNA on the gel. The level of α_1-antichymotrypsin RNA in the three different regions of Alzheimer's disease brain appears to parallel the pathological involvement (indicated by the density of amyloid deposits) of these brain areas in most cases of Alzheimer's disease. That is, the hippocampus and inferior temporal gyrus generally contain abundant

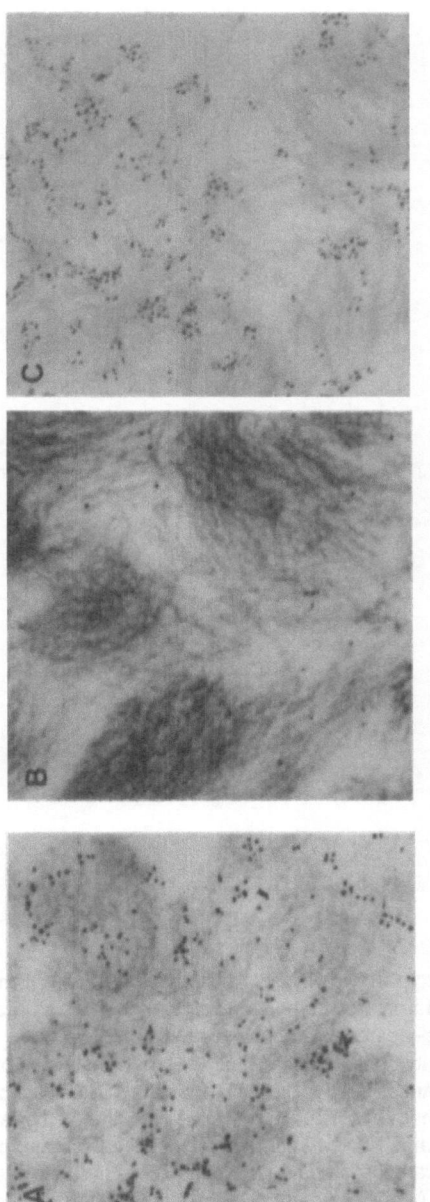

FIGURE 2. Immunogold electron microscopy of α_1-antichymotrypsin and β-protein in isolated Alzheimer amyloid filaments. Amyloid cores of neuritic plaques were isolated by the procedure of Selkoe and Abraham (1986), which included extraction by boiling in SDS and β-mercaptoethanol and sucrose-density centrifugation. Purified cores were labeled in aqueous suspension with an antiserum to either α_1-antichymotrypsin or β-protein, followed by colloidal gold-labeled secondary antisera, as described. After labeling and washing, the cores were recovered by centrifugation, embedded, and sectioned. (A) Electron micrograph of a sectioned amyloid core in which the individual filaments are seen and the α_1-antichymotrypsin has been decorated with antibody-linked 5-nm gold spheres. (B,C) Electron micrographs of the same preparation of amyloid cores reacted with a rabbit preimmune serum (B), or an antiserum to the native β-protein (C), followed by gold-secondary antibody. Electron micrograph of immunogold labeling of α_1-antichymotrypsin in amyloid filaments could be accomplished with either of the two antisera shown to recognize different sets of epitopes released from pure α_1-antichymotrypsin by lysylendopeptidase digestion.

a

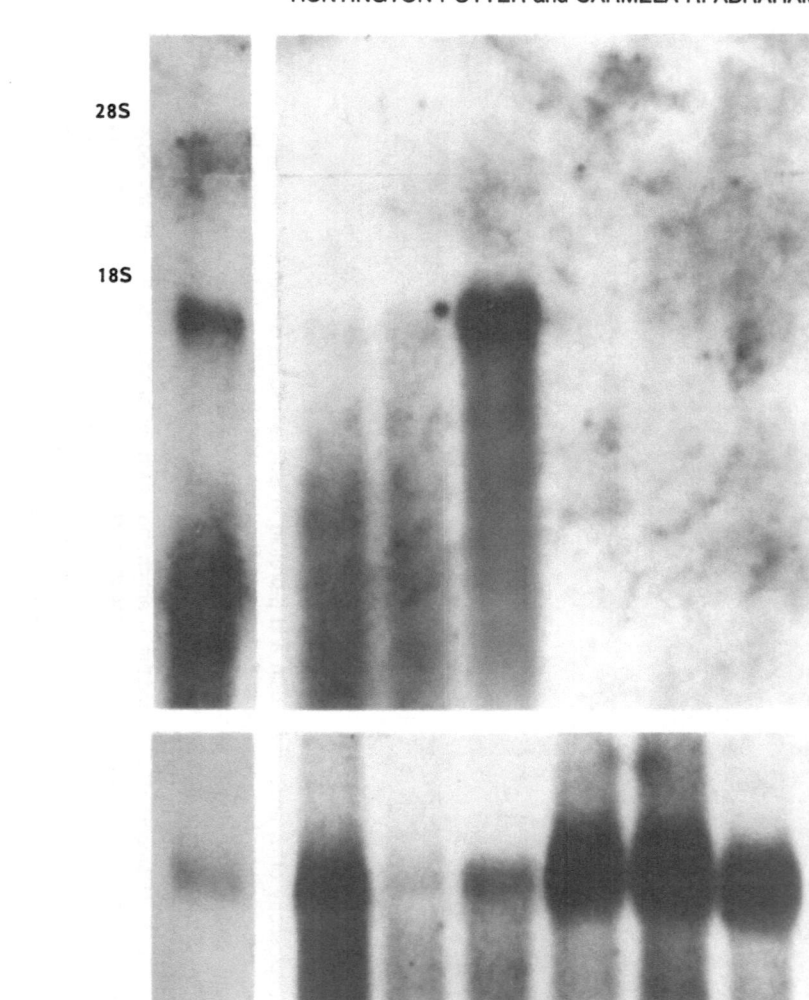

FIGURE 3. Expression of α_1-antichymotrypsin. (a) Northern blot analysis of α_1-antichymotrypsin RNA. Whole cell RNA was prepared from newborn liver and from normal and Alzheimer's brain, electrophoresed on formaldehyde–agarose gels, and blotted to nitrocellulose filters as described. The yield of RNA by 260-nm absorption and by ethidium bromide staining of the gels was the same for all tissue samples. α_1-Antichymotrypsin cDNA from the pGEM 4 subclone was radiolabeled and used to probe the Northern blot. Lane 1: newborn liver RNA, 3 μg; lanes 2–4: 30 μg of RNA from three areas of the same 86 year-old Alzheimer's disease brain: percentral gyrus, inferior temporal gyrus and hippocampus; lanes 5–7: 30 μg of RNA from the same areas of a normal, 74-year-old, control cortex. As expected, the liver expressed large amounts of the mRNA coding for α_1-antichymotrypsin. In addition, Alzheimer's disease brain contains α_1-antichymotrypsin RNA, particularly in hippocampus, an area generally having large numbers of amyloid deposits. Other newborn tissues (kidney, thymus, gut, adrenal, muscle, and spleen) were similarly analyzed and found to lack detectable α_1-antichymotrypsin RNA (not shown). The

b

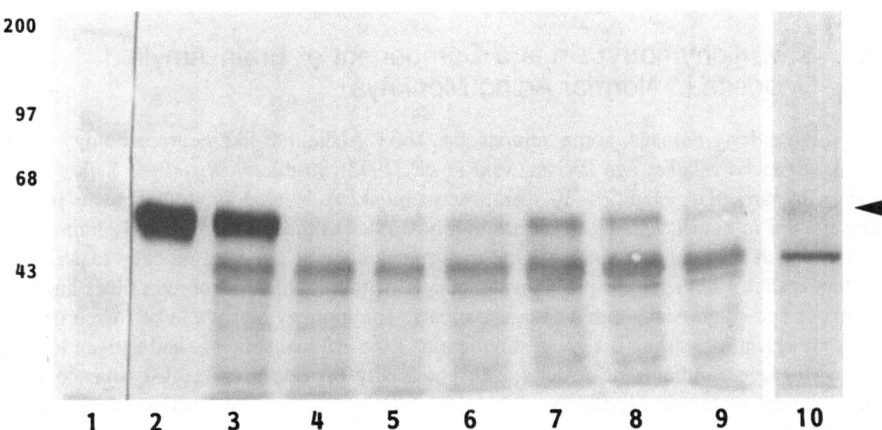

same blot was reprobed with radiolabeled human β-actin cDNA as a control. The Alzheimer's brain samples are seen to have less intact β-actin mRNA than does the control brain, while containing more α_1-antichymotrypsin RNA. A second control probe (for glycerol-3 phosphate dehydrogenase) was performed on this and other Northern blots and also showed reduced RNA in the Alzheimer's compared with the normal brain (not shown). (b) Western blot analysis of α_1-antichymotrypsin from normal and Alzheimer's disease brain and from normal liver. Lane 1: MW standards. Lane 2: 0.5 μg of purified α_1-antichymotrypsin. Lane 3: 0.5 μg of purified α_1-antichymotrypsin immunoprecipitated prior to loading on the gel. The arrow indicates the immunoprecipitated α_1-antichymotrypsin. The lower bands in this and subsequent lanes are the IgG used in the immunoprecipitation. For lanes 4–10, 20 μg of protein from a high-speed supernatant of homogenized tissue was immunoprecipitated with a rabbit antiserum to α_1-antichymotrypsin, and the precipitate solubilized, electrophoresed on SDS-polyacrylamide gels, and blotted as described. Lane 4: Occipital lobe of a normal, aged control brain. This brain region usually contains amyloid deposits in Alzheimer's disease. Lanes 5–7: Frontal cortex (precentral gyrus), temporal cortex (inferior temporal gyrus), and hippocampus from the same Alzheimer's disease brain analyzed in Fig. 3a. Lanes 8, 9: Temporal cortex (inferior temporal gyrus) from two additional Alzheimer's disease brains. Lane 10: Normal human liver. The results indicate that the amount of soluble α_1-antichymotrypsin (besides that found in the insoluble amyloid deposits) appears greater in the areas of Alzheimer's disease brain known to be affected by the disease, as was the α_1-antichymotrypsin RNA (cf. Fig. 3a).

neuritic plaques and neurofibrillary tangles and, in the case studied here, contained the most α_1-antichymotrypsin RNA. By contrast, the precentral gyrus (primary motor cortex), which is often unaffected in Alzheimer's disease, contained a low level of α_1-antichymotrypsin mRNA.

The increase in α_1-antichymotrypsin RNA in affected areas of Alzheimer's disease brain is paralleled by a corresponding increase in the level of protein. Figure 3B shows a Western blot analysis of α_1-antichymotrypsin immunoprecipitated from tissue homogenates. Compared with normal brain (lane 4), Alzheimer brain (lanes 5–9) showed enhanced levels of soluble α_1-antichymotrypsin protein in those areas that contain abundant amyloid deposits.

This immunoprecipitable protein is in addition to the α_1-antichymotrypsin protein in the insoluble amyloid deposits.

2.3. α_1-Antichymotrypsin is a Component of Brain Amyloid Deposits in Normal Aging Monkeys

Like elderly humans, some animals also show Alzheimer-like neuropathology as they reach advanced relative age (Wisniewski et al., 1973; Struble et al., 1985; Selkoe et al., 1987). In particular, aged (20–30 years) rhesus monkeys develop amyloid deposits in blood vessels and in neuritic plaques that are highly similar to those seen in elderly humans and patients with Alzheimer's disease. One major advantage of the aged monkey experimental system is that it obviates the problems associated with variable postmortem times and treatments of end-stage Alzheimer's disease patients. The monkey brains can be frozen immediately after death, ensuring the greatest retention of the original structure and antigen localization. Moreover, animals of various ages potentially provide a controlled time course of development of the neuropathology; thus, the relative protein composition of the amyloid (β-protein, α_1-antichymotrypsin, and other potential components) may be followed over time, throwing light on possible mechanisms of amyloid deposition. Finally, the fact that aged monkeys do not develop neurofibrillary tangles indicates that they may provide a clean system for studying the mechanism of amyloid deposition, unalloyed with the intracellular neuropathology that also characterizes the human disease.

The finding of the serine protease inhibitor, α_1-antichymotrypsin, as a component of the amyloid deposits in Alzheimer's disease and normal aged human brain (Abraham et al., 1988) prompted us to ask whether the amyloid deposits in normal aged monkey brain, previously shown to be similar to the human deposits by a number of criteria, also contained α_1-antichymotrypsin. Specifically, amyloid deposition associated with neuritic plaques and with the brain vasculature was analyzed in aged monkeys using three probes: thioflavin S, the cytochemical stain classically used to identify amyloid and believed to recognize β-pleated sheet conformation; and specific antibodies recognizing α_1-antichymotrypsin or the β-protein, respectively (Abraham et al., 1989). Several conclusions were reached: (1) α_1-antichymotrypsin is a specific component of the amyloid deposits arising in aged rhesus monkey brain, as it is in similar deposits in Alzheimer's disease and normal aged human brain; (2) amyloid deposition in the meningeal vessels and the cores of neuritic plaques arises approximately contemporaneously (about age 25 years), but within an individual animal, plaques may be present in the absence of detectable blood vessel amyloid; (3) amyloid deposition in the cortical vasculature is detected only in the oldest rhesus monkeys (31 years), and by all three criteria; and (4) white matter vasculature appears to be free of amyloid neuropathology.

3. DISCUSSION

Proteases and their inhibitors appear to play important complementary roles in the nervous system. Thus, for example, sympathetic and sensory neurons in culture release various proteases as they extend processes, presumably to serve a ground-breaking role in growth cone elongation (Pittman, 1984, 1985; Krystosek and Seeds, 1984; Patterson, 1985; Pittman and Patterson, 1987). Whereas the neurons secrete proteases, their target cells often secrete protease inhibitors, possibly needed to end process extensions and promote the formation of stable synapses (Pittman, 1984, 1985). Proteases and their inhibitors are also involved in glial function; i.e., actively proliferating Schwann cells secrete a protease (Kalderon *et al.*, 1984), and rat glioma cells secrete a neurite-promoting factor that is a potent serine protease inhibitor (Monard *et al.*, 1983; Guenther *et al.*, 1985), the mRNA of which is found almost exclusively in brain tissue (Gloor *et al.*, 1986). Given the delicate balance in the organism between proteases and their inhibitors, any alteration in activity, amount, or location of a protease or a protease inhibitor could seriously disrupt the dynamic maintenance of the local architecture or function of a tissue such as brain.

Although the fact that both the β-protein gene and the inherited disease locus in some Alzheimer's families have been localized on chromosome 21 (St. George-Hyslop *et al.*, 1987; Tanzi *et al.*, 1987a; Goldgaber *et al.*, 1987; Kang *et al.*, 1987; Robakis *et al.*, 1987) initially suggested that the two genes might be one and the same, it has now become clear that the Alzheimer's disease locus in the families in which it is linked to chromosome 21 is actually quite far away from the β-protein gene; therefore, a genetically altered β-protein or its precursor cannot be the explanation for Alzheimer's disease in these families (Van Broekhoven *et al.*, 1987; Tanzi *et al.*, 1987b). Rather, it seems likely that the processing of the β-protein precursor to yield the amyloidogenic β-protein is the key event in amyloid deposition. Such processing would be carried out and modulated by brain proteases and their respective inhibitors. Because the two key requirements for Alzheimer amyloid deposition— the proteolytic processing of the β-protein precursor to release the amyloidogenic β-protein and the failure of the brain to digest and clear away the developing deposits—are both dependent on the relative activity of proteases and their inhibitors in the brain, the search for such proteins is currently under way.

We were initially surprised to find that α₁-antichymotrypsin is a component of the amyloid deposits of Alzheimer's disease and normal aging, although it had long been suspected that the protein(s) of the amyloid might be derived from the serum (Miyakawa *et al.*, 1982; Glenner, 1983). However, consideration of other amyloid diseases and the fact that the β-protein is a peptide fragment derived from a much larger precursor indicated several ways in which α₁-antichymotrypsin might contribute to the formation of amyloid deposits, either directly or in its capacity as a protease inhibitor. These are outlined in Fig. 4.

Perhaps the simplest role that α₁-antichymotrypsin might play in amyloid deposition would be as a direct structural component of the amyloid fibers. The results of immunogold electron microscopy, and the fact that α₁-antichymotrypsin cannot be selectively removed from the amyloid deposits, support such a hypothesis. Thus, for example, a mutation in the gene for α₁-antichymotrypsin, or an altered post-translational modification, might lead to a protein that has a greater-than-normal tendency to aggregate and form filaments by itself. Alternatively, α₁-antichymotrypsin may be especially adherent in Alzheimer brain and irreversibly associates with other proteins, such as β-protein, to form the amyloid filaments more rapidly than occurs during normal aging.

There is ample precedent for serum (and other) proteins becoming insoluble and depositing as amyloid fibers because of mutations in their structural genes (Abraham *et al.*, 1988). For example, the inherited form of cerebral amyloid angiopathy is characterized by deposits of amyloid in the arteries and arterioles of the brain and the meninges (for review, see Vanley *et al.*, 1981). Recently, Ghiso and Frangione and colleagues (Ghiso *et al.*, 1986a,b) showed that a familial form of cerebral amyloid angiopathy, inherited as an autosomal-dominant disease endemic to a certain region of Iceland (Gudmundsson, 1972), is characterized by a variant of the protease inhibitor, cystatin C (also called γ trace).

Another example in which a variant protein forms amyloid fibers in the nervous system,

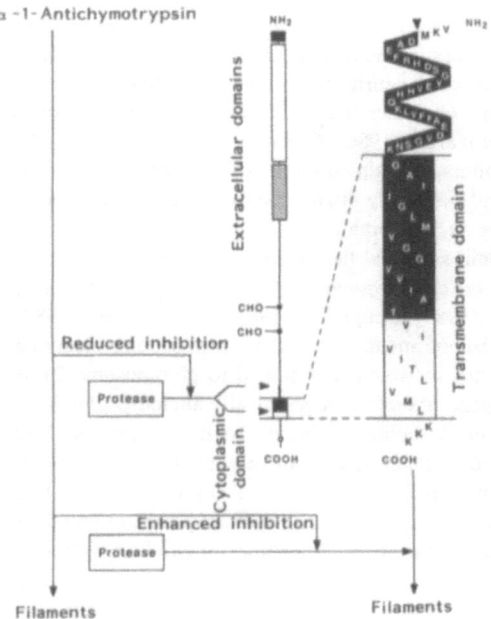

FIGURE 4. Model of the potential involvement of α_1-antichymotrypsin to Alzheimer amyloid deposition. As discussed in the text, α_1-antichymotrypsin may contribute to Alzheimer amyloid deposits in one of several ways. First, the α_1-antichymotrypsin protein may be an important physical component of the amyloid filaments (left-hand diagram). Such a possibility is suggested by the protein's very tight association with the filaments (see Fig. 2). A more likely class of models build on the protease inhibitory function of α_1-antichymotrypsin (right-hand diagram). In one model, the reduction of this activity in Alzheimer brain is seen as allowing more proteolytic release of the β-protein from its precursor (top right). In the second model, an increase of α_1-antichymotrypsin in Alzheimer's disease or normal aging is seen as inhibiting the proteolytic breakdown and subsequent clearing of developing amyloid deposits.

apparently due to a single genetic mutation, occurs in the autosomal-dominant neural disease familial amyloidotic polyneuropathy. In this case, the amyloidogenic polypeptide is the thyroxine-binding protein, transthyretin (also called prealbumin) (Skinner and Cohen, 1981), in which amino acid substitution can occur at positions 49 and 30, respectively (Pras *et al.*, 1983; Dwulet and Benson, 1984).

With respect to the possibility that α_1-antichymotrypsin may be altered in Alzheimer's disease, it is interesting to note that the gene for this protein resides on chromosome 14, band q32 (Rabin *et al.*, 1986)—the position of the immunoglobulin locus. Weitkamp and colleagues (1983) reported the genetic lesion in one Alzheimer family to be weakly linked to the immunoglobulin (Ig) locus.

In contrast to the possibility of forming insoluble filaments and contributing directly to the formation of amyloid, α_1-antichymotrypsin may instead play an indirect role in the formation of the amyloid deposits by virtue of its function as a serine protease inhibitor. Despite its name, α_1-antichymotrypsin is actually a relatively weak inhibitor of chymotrypsin itself, and its true physiological role is unknown (for review, see Travis and Salvesen, 1982). Thus, it is reasonable to consider the potential roles that α_1-antichymotrypsin may play as a protease inhibitor in the development of the amyloid in the light of the recent information obtained that the β-protein is a 42–43-amino acid fragment of a larger precursor protein (see Fig. 4). For example, a local excess of α_1-antichymotrypsin might prevent a normal brain protease from clearing deposits of the β-protein. Alternatively, insufficient protease inhibitor might allow more of the precursor protein to be converted into the self-aggregating β-peptide, again leading to amyloid deposition. In this regard, it is interesting to note that the N-terminal cleavage site that generates the β-peptide is bordered by a methionine (Kang *et al.*, 1987) and would therefore be expected to be recognized by a chymotrypsin-like protease.

Recently, it was found that the β-protein precursor itself may also be a protease inhibitor

(Kitaguchi *et al.*, 1988, Tanzi *et al.*, 1988: Ponte *et al.*, 1988). Specifically, at least three alternatively spliced versions of the mRNA of the β-protein precursor have been cloned, two of which include a previously unsuspected exon that encodes an additional protein domain with striking homology to the Kunitz-type protease inhibitor. There is no evidence that any portion of the β-protein precursor (other than the β-protein itself) is present in the amyloid deposits. Nonetheless, this extra protein domain may serve some function (e.g., in protecting the membrane-bound β-protein precursor from proteolytic digestion) that is also relevant to the deposition of the β-protein itself into amyloid filaments.

Recently we have examined the molecular basis for the association of α_1-antichymotrypsin and the β-protein. A radioiodine-labeled peptide corresponding to amino acids 1–28 of the β-peptide becomes bound to ACT in an SDS-resistant complex. The use of cross-linking agents stabilizes even a greater amount of the peptide onto ACT. Other experiments suggest that the 1–28 peptide may bind to the ACT protein at its active protease-inhibitory site: (1) The addition of chymotrypsin to ACT prior to the addition of the peptide prevents the association, and (2) The peptide reduces ACT's ability to subsequently inhibit chymotrypsin. An examination of the amino acid sequence of the β-peptide reveals a region near the N-terminus that shows striking homology to the active site of serine proteases. Studies with peptides having specific amino acids changed in this region are underway to test whether this protease-like region is the basis for the specific association of ACT and the β-protein. The detergent-stable complex we have detected provides an attractive basis for the formation of the insoluble protein filaments that comprise the amyloid deposits of Alzheimer's disease.

4. SUMMARY

There is increasing theoretical and experimental evidence for the involvement of proteases and/or their inhibitors in the amyloid deposition in Alzheimer's disease. Thus far, two protease inhibitors have been implicated—α_1-antichymotrypsin and the β-protein precursor—but it remains to identify their respective target proteases.

REFERENCES

Abraham, C. R., Selkoe, D. J., and Potter, H., 1988, Immunochemical identification of the serine protease inhibitor α_1-antichymotrypsin in the brain amyloid deposits of Alzheimer's disease, *Cell* **52**:487–501.

Bahmanyar, S., Higgins, G. A., Goldgaber, D., Lewis D. A., Morrison, J. H., Wilson, M. C., Shankar, S. K., and Gajdusek, D. C., 1987, Localization of amyloid β-protein messenger RNA in brains from patients with Alzheimer's disease, *Science* **237**:77–80.

Dwulet, F. E., and Benson, M. D., 1984, Primary structure of an amyloid prealbumin and its plasma precursor in a heredofamilial polyneuropathy of Swedish origin, *Proc. Natl. Acad. Sci. USA* **81**:694–698.

Gadjusek, D. C., and Salazar, A., 1982, Amyotrophic lateral sclerosis and Parkinsonian syndromes in high incidence among Anga and Jakai peoples of West New Guinea, *Neurology (NY)* **32**:107–126.

Ghiso, J., Jensson, O., and Frangione, B., 1986, Amyloid fibrils in hereditary cerebral hemorrhage with amyloidosis of Icelandic type is a variant of γ-trace basic protein (Cystatin C), *Proc. Natl. Acad. Sci. USA* **83**:2974–2978.

Ghiso, J., Pons-Estel, B., and Frangione, B., 1986, Hereditary cerebral amyloid angiopathy: The amyloid fibrils contain a protein which is a variant of Cystatin C, an inhibitor of lysosomal cysteine proteases, *Biochem. Biophys. Res. Commun.* **136**:548–554.

Glenner, G. G., 1983, Alzheimer's Disease: Multiple cerebral amyloidosis, *Banbury Rep.* **15**:137–144.

Glenner, G. G., and Wong, C. G., 1984, Initial report of the purification and characterization of a novel cerebrovascular amyloid protein, *Biochem. Biophys. Res. Commun.* **120**:885–890.

Gloor, S., Odink, K., Guenther, J., Nick, H., and Monard, D., 1986, A glia-derived neurite promoting factor with protease inhibitory activity belongs to the protease nexins, *Cell* **47**:687–693.

Goldgaber, D., Lerman, M. I., McBride, O. W., Saffiotti, U., and Gajdusek, D. C., 1987, Characterization and chromosomal localization of a c-DNA encoding brain amyloid of Alzheimer's disease, *Science* **235**:877–880.

Gorevic, P. D., Goni, F., Pons-Estel, B., Alvarez, F., Peress, N. S., and Frangione, B., 1986, Isolation and partial characterization of neurofibrillary tangles and amyloid plaque core in Alzheimer's disease: Immunohistological studies, *J. Neuropathol. Exp. Neurol.* **45**:647–664.

Gudmundsson, G., Hallgrimsson, J., Jonasson, T. A., and Bjarnason, O., 1972, Hereditary cerebral hemorrhage with amyloidosis, *Brain* **95**:387–404.

Guenther, J., Nick, H., and Monard, D., 1985, A glia-derived neurite-promoting factor with protease inhibitory activity, *EMBO J.* **4**:1963–1966.

Heston, L. L., Mastri, A. R., Anderson, V. E., and White, J., 1981, Dementia of the Alzheimer type. Clinical genetics, natural history, and associated conditions, *Arch. Gen. Psychiatry* **38**:1085–1090.

Ihara, Y., 1986, A critical comment of imunocytochemistry of amyloid core in Alzheimer's disease, *Neuropathology* 3 (Suppl.):59–66.

Jarvik, L. F., and Matsuyama, S. S., 1986, Dementia of the Alzheimer type: Genetic aspects, in: *The Biological Substrates of Alzheimer's Disease* (A. B. Scheibel and A. F. Wechslev, eds.), Academic, Orlando, Florida, pp. 17–20.

Jervis, G. A., 1948, Early senile dementia in mongoloid idiocy, *Am. J. Psychiatry* **105**:102–106.

Kalderon, N., 1984, Schwann cell proliferation and localized proteolysis: Expression of plasminogen-activator activity predominates in the proliferating cell populations, *Proc. Natl. Acad. Sci. USA* **81**:7216–7220.

Kang, J., Lemaire, H.-G., Unterbeck, A., Salbaum, J. M., Masters, C. L., Grzeschik, K.-H., Multhaup, G., Beyreuther, K., and Muller-Hill, B., 1987, The precursor of Alzheimer's disease amyloid A4 protein resembles a cell-surface receptor, *Nature (Lond.)* **325**:733–736.

Kitaguchi, N., Takahashi, Y., Tokushima, Y., Shiojiri, S., and Ito, H., 1988, Novel precursor of Alzheimer's disease amyloid protein shows protease inhibitory activity, *Nature (Lond.)* **331**:530–532.

Krystosek, A., and Seeds, N. W., 1984, Peripheral neurons and Schwann cells secrete plasminogen activator, *J. Cell. Biol.* B98:773–776.

Mandybur, T. I., 1975, The incidence of cerebral amyloid angiopathy in Alzheimer's disease, *Neurology (NY)* **25**:120–126.

Masters, C. L., Simms, G., Weinman, N. A., Multhaup, G., McDonald, B. L., and Beyreuther, K., 1985, Amyloid plaque core protein in Alzheimer disease and Down syndrome, *Proc. Natl. Acad. Sci. USA* **82**:4245–4249.

Matsuyama, S. S., Jarvik, L. F., and Kumar, V., 1985, Dementia: Genetics, in: *Recent Advances in Psychogeriatrics* (T. Arie, ed.), Churchill-Livingstone, Edinburgh, pp. 45–69.

McKahnn, G., Drachman, D., Folstein, M., Katzman, R., and Price, D., 1984, Clinical diagnosis of Alzheimer's disease, *Neurology (NY)* **34**:939–944.

Merz, P. A., Wisniewski, H. M., Somerville, R. A., Bobin, S. A., Iqbal, K., and Masters, C. L., 1983, Ultrastructure of amyloid fibrils from neuritic and amyloid plaques, *Acta Neuropathol. (Berl.)* **60**:113–124.

Miyakawa, T., Shimoji, A., Kuramoto, R., and Higuchi, Y., 1982, The relationship between senile plaques and cerebral blood vessels in Alzheimer's disease and senile dementia, *Virchows Arch. [Cell Pathol.]* **40**:121–129.

Monard, D., Niday, E., Limat, A., and Solomon, F., 1983, Inhibition of protease activity can lead to neurite extension in neuroblastoma cells, *Prog. Brain Res.* **58**:359–364.

Mountjoy, C. Q., Tomlinson, B. E., and Gibson, R. H., 1982, Amyloid and senile plaques and cerebral blood vessels. A semiquantitative investigation of a possible relationship, *J. Neurol. Sci.* **57**:89–103.

Papadimitriou, C. S., Stein, H., and Papacharalampous, N. X., 1980, Presence of α$_1$-antichymotrypsin and α$_1$-antitrypsin in haematopoietic and lymphoid tissue cells as revealed by the immunoperoxidase method, *Pathol. Res. Pract.* **169**:287–297.

Patterson, P. H., 1985, On the role of proteases, their inhibitors and the extracellular matrix in promoting neurite outgrowth, *J. Physiol. (Paris)* **80**:207–211.

Pittman, R. N., 1984, Neuron–target cell interactions may involve protease–inhibitor interactions, *Soc. Neurosci.* **10**:194.5.

Pittman, R. N., 1985, Release of plasminogen activator and a calcium-dependent metalloprotease from culture sympathetic and sensory neurons, *Dev. Biol.* **110**:91–101.

Pittman, R. N., and Patterson, P. H., 1987, Characterization of an inhibitor of neuronal plasminogen activator released by heart cells, *J. Neurosci.* **7**:2664–2673.

Ponte, P., Gonzales-DeWhitt, P., Schilling, J., Miller, J., Hsu, D., Greenberg, B., Davis, K., Wallace, W., Lieberburg, I., Fuller, F., and Cordell, B., 1988, A new A4 amyloid mRNA contains a domain homologous to serine protease inhibitors, *Nature (Lond.)* **331**:525–527.

Pras, M., Prelli, F., Franklin, E. C., and Frangione, B., 1983, Primary structure of an amyloid prealbumin variant in familial polyneuropathy of Jewish origin, *Proc. Natl. Acad. Sci. USA* **80**:539–542.

Price, D. L., 1986, New perspectives in Alzheimer's disease, *Annu. Rev. Neurosci.* **9**:489–512.

Rabin, M., Watson, M., Kidd, V., Woo, S. L. C., Breg, W. R., and Ruddle, F. H., 1986, Regional location of α$_1$-antichymotrypsin and α$_1$-antitrypsin genes on human chromosome 14, *Somatic Cell. Genet.* **12**:209–214.

Robakis, N. D., Wisniewski, H. M., Jenkins, E. C., Devine-Gage, E. A., Houck, G. E., Yao, X.-L., Ramakrishna, N., Wolfe, G., Silverman, W. P., and Brown, W. T., 1987, Chromosome 21q21 sublocalisation of gene encoding β-amyloid peptide in cerebral vessels and neuritic (senile) plaques of people with Alzheimer disease and Down syndrome, *Lancet* **i**:384–385.

Roth, M., Tomlinson, B. E., and Blessed, G., 1966, Correlation between scores for dementia and counts of "senile plaques" in cerebral grey matter of elderly subjects, *Nature (Lond.)* **209**:109–110.

St. George-Hyslop, P. H., Tanzi, R. E., Polinsky, R. J., Haines, J. L., Nee, L., Watkins, P. C., Myers, R., Feldman, R., Pollen, D., Drachman, D., Growdon, J., Bruni, A., Foncin, J.-F., Frommelt, P., Amaducci, L., Sorbi, S., Piacentini, S., Stewart, G. D., Hobbs, W. J., Conneally, P. M., and Gusella, J. F., 1987, The genetic defect causing familial Alzheimer's disease maps on chromosome 21, *Science* **235**:885–889.

Scholz, W., 1938, Studien zur Pathologie der Hirngefasse II: Die drusige Entartung der Hirnarterien und Capillaren, *Z. Ges. Neurol. Psychiatry* **162**:694–702.

Selkoe, D. J., 1986, altered structural proteins in plaques and tangles: What do they tell us about the biology of Alzheimer's disease?, *Neurobiol. Aging* **7**:425–432.

Selkoe, D. J., Abraham, C. R., Podlisny, M. B., and Duffy, L. K., 1986, Isolation of low-molecular weight proteins from amyloid plaque fibers in Alzheimer's disease, *J. Neurochem.* **46**:1820–1834.

Selkoe, D. J., Bell, D. S., Podlisny, M. B., Price, D. L., and Cork, L. C., 1987a, Conservation of brain amyloid proteins in aged mammals and humans with Alzheimer's disease, *Science* **235**:873–877.

Skinner, M., and Cohen, A. S., 1981, The prealbumin nature of the amyloid protein in familial amyloid polyneuropathy (FAP)-Swedish variety, *Biochem. Biophys. Res. Commun.* **99**:1326–1332.

Struble, R. G., Price, D. L., Jr., Cork, L. C., and Price, D. L., 1985, Senile plaques in cortex of aged normal monkeys, *Brain Res.* **361**:267–275.

Tanzi, R. E., Gusella, J. F., Watkins, P. C., Bruns, G. A. P., St. George-Hyslop, P., Van Keuren, M. L., Patterson, D., Pagan, S., Kurnit, D. M., and Neve, R. L., 1987a, Amyloid β protein gene: cDNA, mRNA distribution, and genetic linkage near the Alzheimer locus, *Science* **235**:880–884.

Tanzi, R. E., St. George-Hyslop, P. H., Haines, J. L., Polinsky, R. J., Nee, L., Foncin, J.-F., Neve, R. L., McClatchey, A. I., Conneally, P. M., and Gusella, J. F., 1987b, The genetic defect in familial Alzheimer's disease is not tightly linked to the amyloid β-protein gene, *Nature (Lond.)* **329:**156–157.

Tanzi, R. E., McClatchey, A. I., Lamperti, E. D., Villa-Komaroff, L., Gusella, J. F., and Neve, R. L., 1988, Protease inhibitor domain encoded by an amyloid protein precursor mRNA associated with Alzheimer's disease, *Nature (Lond.)* **331:**528–530.

Terry, R. D., 1978a, Aging, senile dementia and Alzheimer's disease, in: *Aging,* Vol. 7: *Alzheimer's Disease: Senile Dementia and Related Disorders,* R. Katzman, R. D. Terry, and K. L. Bick, eds.), Raven Press, New York, pp. 11–14.

Terry, R. D., 1978b, Ultrastructural alterations in senile dementia, in: Aging, Vol. 7: *Alzheimer's Disease: Senile Dementia and Related Disorders* (R. Katzman, R. D. Terry, and K. L. Bick, eds.), Raven Press, New York, pp. 375–382.

Tomlinson, B. E., Blessed, G., and Roth, M., 1968, Observations on the brains of non-demented old people, *J. Neurol. Sci.* **7:**331–356.

Travis, J., and Salvesen, G. S., 1983, Human plasma proteinase inhibitors, *Annu. Rev. Biochem.* **52:**655–709.

Van Broekhoven, C., Genthe, A. M., Vandenberghe, A., Horsthemke, B., Backhovens, H., Raey-maekers, P., Van Hul, W., Wehnert, A., Gheuens, J., Cras, P., Bruyland, M., Martin, J. J., Salbaum, M., Multhaup, G., Masters, C. L., Beyreuther, K., Gurling, H. M. D., Mullan, M. J., Holland, A., Barton, A., Irving, N., Williamson, R., Richards, S. J., and Hardy, J. A., 1987, Failure of familial Alzheimer's disease to segregate with the A4-amyloid gene in several European families, *Nature (Lond.)* **329:**153–155.

Vanley, C. T., Aguilar, M. J., Kleinhenz, R. J., and Lagios, M. D., 1981, Cerebral amyloid angiopathy, *Hum. Pathol.* **12:**609–616.

Weitkamp, L. R., Nee, L., Keats, B., Polinsky, R. J., and Guttormsen, S., 1983, Alzheimer disease: Evidence for susceptibility loci on chromosomes 6 and 14, *Am. J. Hum. Genet.* **35:**443–453.

Wisniewski, H. M., Ghetti, B., and Terry, R. D., 1973, Neuritic (senile) plaques and filamentous changes in aged rhesus monkeys, *J. Neuropathol. Exp. Neurol.* **32:**566–584.

Wisniewski, K. E., Jervis, G. A., Moretz, R. C., and Wisniewski, H. M., 1979, Alzheimer neurofibrillary tangles in diseases other than senile and presenile dementia, *Ann. Neurol.* **5:**288–294.

Wong, C. W., Quaranta, V., and Glenner, G., 1985, Neuritic plaques and cerebrovascular amyloid in Alzheimer disease are antigenically related, *Proc. Natl. Acad. Sci. USA* **82:**8729–8732.

8

Replication of Adenovirus 2 and Adeno-Associated Virus 2 in Young and Senescent Human Diploid Fibroblasts

PIRUZ NAHREINI and ARUN SRIVASTAVA

1. INTRODUCTION

Aging has been known since antiquity and, despite being one of mankind's most inevitable consequences, the molecular basis of aging remains virtually unknown. Although aging research has become a focus of intensive study in recent years and has attracted global attention, there is no unified theory of the origin of aging. The obscure origin of aging has been the subject of a great deal of elegant experimentation and equally good amount of imaginative speculations.

The seminal studies of Hayflick and Moorehead (1961) first documented the limited proliferative potential of cultured human diploid fibroblasts *in vitro;* these cultures continue to be excellent model systems for cellular aging *in vitro* (Finch and Hayflick, 1977). Although a number of attractive mechanisms have been proposed by several investigators (Orgel, 1963; Bell *et al.*, 1978; Smith and Lumpkin, 1980; Bunn and Tarrant, 1980; Burmer *et al.*, 1982; Macieira-Coelho, 1984; Hayflick, 1984), the molecular correlates between the limited replicative potential (senescence) of human fibroblasts and the impaired DNA replication observed in these cells have become particularly increasingly clear. For example, it has been shown that a great majority of senescent cells fail to enter S phase of the cell cycle and are unable to initiate cellular DNA synthesis (Cristofalo and Sharf, 1973; Olashaw *et al.*, 1983). Whether the senescent phenotype is a direct consequence of impaired S-phase entry and subsequent cellular DNA replication remains unknown. Despite the accumulation of a wealth of information on this aspect of cellular senescence, the following two fundamental questions remain unanswered: (1) whether the impaired S-phase entry observed in senescent cells is reversible, and (2) if so, whether senescent cells are capable of supporting S-phase-dependent DNA replication.

PIRUZ NAHREINI and ARUN SRIVASTAVA • Division of Hematology and Oncology, Departments of Medicine, Microbiology and Immunology, Indiana University School of Medicine, Indianapolis, Indiana 46202.

Because of the enormous complexity of the cellular genome, we have used DNA-containing viruses of human origin, the adenovirus and the adeno-associated virus, which have proved useful models for studies on eukaryotic genome organization and function (Berk, 1986; Berns and Bohenzky, 1987). For example, productive infection of permissive host cells by adenovirus results in the suppression of host-cell DNA synthesis under conditions of active cell growth (Hodge and Scharff, 1969; Pina and Green, 1969), but adenovirus infection of both permissive and nonpermissive cells has been shown to result in an induction of host-cell DNA synthesis, provided the cells are infected in a quiescent state (Yamashita and Shimojo, 1969; Spindler et al., 1985). By contrast, adeno-associated virus is completely dependent on the host cell for its replication (Yakobson et al., 1987). We exploited these features of the two viruses to address the following two questions: (1) Can S phase be induced in senescent fibroblasts?, and (2) Is the host cell DNA replication machinery functionally intact in senescent cells?

Here we report the response of nondividing cultured human diploid fibroblasts during experimental infection by adenovirus (Ad) as well as by adeno-associated virus (AAV), an unrelated but adenovirus-dependent human parvovirus. We document that the cellular components involved in S-phase entry as well as cellular DNA replication are intact in senescent cells but may become nonfunctional during cellular senescence. We also postulate that the impaired S-phase entry observed in senescent cells may not be a sufficient condition to create and/or maintain the senescent phenotype.

2. ADENOVIRUS 2 REPLICATION IN CULTURED HUMAN DIPLOID FIBROBLASTS

Productive infection of quiescent human embryonic kidney (HEK) cells and human embryonic lung fibroblasts (WI-38) by adenovirus has been reported by Yamashita and Shimojo (1969) and Spindler et al. (1985), respectively, but it was unclear what percentage of the in vitro replicative life span of these human diploid fibroblast (HDF) cultures had already been consumed in these studies. Since both groups detected induction of cellular DNA synthesis after Ad infection, it was of significant interest to examine whether senescent fibroblasts could also support Ad replication, because in contrast to early-passage quiescent cells, late-passage senescent cells are incapable of cellular DNA synthesis (Cristofalo and Sharf, 1973; Olashaw et al., 1983).

Figure 1 depicts the kinetics of production of the cytopathic effect (CPE) observed after Ad2 infection of representative cultures of early-passage quiescent cells (Fig. 1a–d) and late-passage senescent cells (Fig. 1e–h) after mock infection and at 0, 24, and 48 hr p.i., respectively. That the CPE was observed in senescent cultures suggested the possibility that these cells also supported Ad2 replication. Similar results were obtained with senescent cultures of normal HDF strains WI-38 and IMR-90. All subsequent experiments were carried out with early- and late-passage diploid fibroblast strain IMR-90 cells.

2.1. Induction of S Phase in HDF

We next examined whether Ad2 infection of senescent cultures also resulted in an induction of cellular DNA synthesis. To this end, the percentage of cells in each phase of the cell cycle was measured by flow cytometry of propidium iodide-stained nuclei from early-passage quiescent and late-passage senescent cells with mock infection and with Ad2 infec-

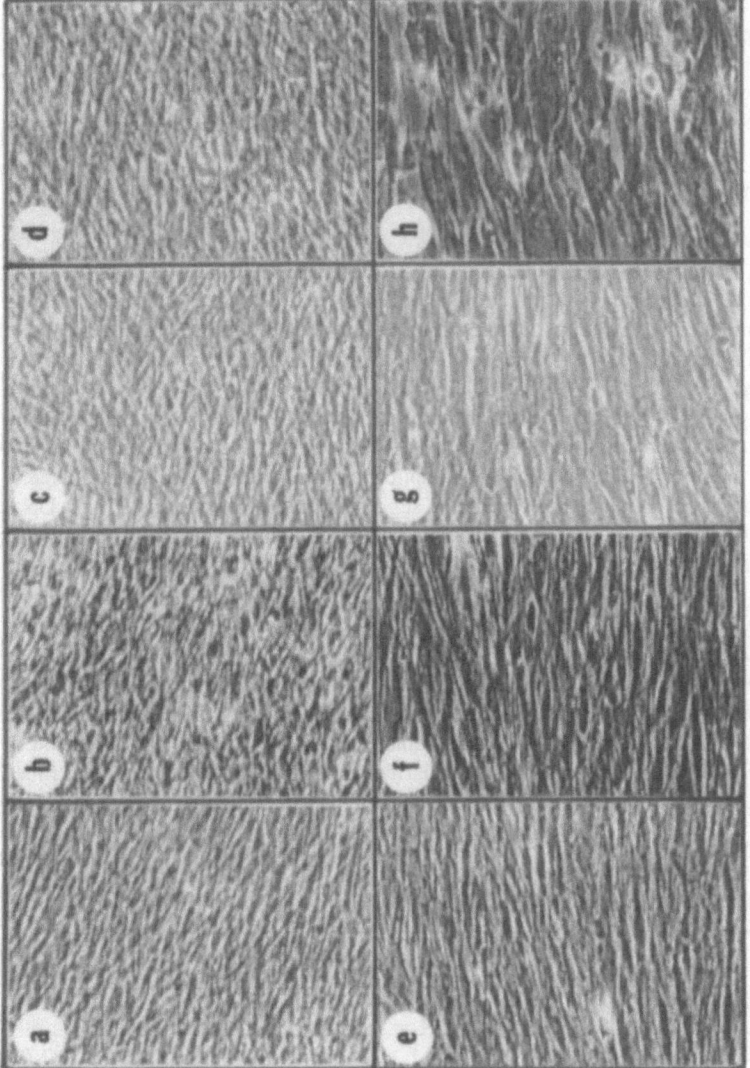

FIGURE 1. Morphology of early-passage (MPD = 20) quiescent human diploid fibroblast strain WI-38 (a) and late-passage (MPD = 51) senescent cells (e). (b–d) Ad2-infected quiescent cells at 0 hr p.i., 24 hr p.i., and 48 hr p.i., respectively. (f–h) Ad2-infected senescent cells at 0 hr p.i., 24 hr p.i., and 48 hr p.i., respectively. p.i., postinfection. (From Srivastava and Naherini, 1989.) (×100)

tion at various times, as shown in Fig. 2. Area integration from the data representing cell-cycle distribution of these cells is also presented in Table I.

It is interesting to note that while most of the uninfected early-passage quiescent and late-passage senescent cells were indeed arrested in G_0/G_1 phase (>85%), and only about 2–3% were in S phase at 0 hr p.i., as expected, the cell-cycle distribution was clearly altered to include approximately 10–15% cells in S phase, and a decline to approximately 60% in cells in G_0/G_1 phase 48 hr p.i. in both quiescent and senescent cultures. A two- to threefold increase in cells in the G_2/M phase was also noted. These results strongly suggested that Ad2 infection resulted in induction of cellular DNA synthesis in senescent cells, the extent of which was comparable to that observed in quiescent cells (Spindler et al., 1985).

2.2. Adenovirus DNA Replication in HDF

We next wished to document the efficiency of viral DNA replication in these two cultures, which was carried out by Southern blotting (Southern, 1975). Total genomic DNA isolated at various times after Ad2 infection of quiescent and senescent IMR-90 cells was digested to completion with the restriction endonuclease Kpn I; equivalent amounts were electrophoresed on agarose gels and probed with the total Ad2 DNA probe on a Southern blot as shown in Fig. 3.

Little Ad2-hybridization signal could be detected 0 hr p.i. in quiescent and senescent IMR-90 cells (lanes 1 and 4, respectively), but by 24 hr p.i. (lanes 2 and 5) and 48 hr p.i. (lanes 3 and 6), significant levels of viral DNA replication were evident. The nearly identical extent of hybridization intensities observed also suggested that the efficiency of Ad2 DNA replication was comparable in quiescent and senescent HDF. Similar results were obtained with other strains of fibroblast cultures (data not shown).

2.3. Production of Progeny Adenovirus by HDF

It was also of interest to examine whether senescent fibroblast cultures were capable of producing progeny virus particles as an index of normal intracellular viral RNA and protein synthesis observed in quiescent WI-38 cells by Spindler et al. (1985). This was measured as the amount of Ad2 DNA-hybridizable signal in clarified culture supernatants at various times p.i. on a quantitative DNA dot blot (Srivastava and Lu, 1988), as shown in Fig. 4.

TABLE I. Effect of Adenovirus Infection on Cell-Cycle Distribution of Normal Human Diploid Quiescent and Senescent Fibroblasts[a,b]

Mean population doublings (MPD)	Percent distribution of cells[c]											
	Mock infected			0 hr p.i.			24 hr p.i.			48 hr p.i.		
	G_0/G_1	S	G_2/M	G_0/G_1	S	G_2/M	G_0/G_1	S	G_2/M	G_0/G_1	S	G_2/M
14	87.5	2.8	9.7	89.7	2.3	8.0	61.1	9.8	29.1	58.8	11.1	30.1
49	85.5	1.7	12.8	84.4	2.1	13.5	73.8	8.3	17.9	60.8	15.5	23.7

[a]From Srivastava and Nahreini (1989).
[b]p.i., postinfection.
[c]Approximately 20,000 cells were analyzed for each sample as previously described (Jackson et al., 1984; Yen and Guernsey, 1986).

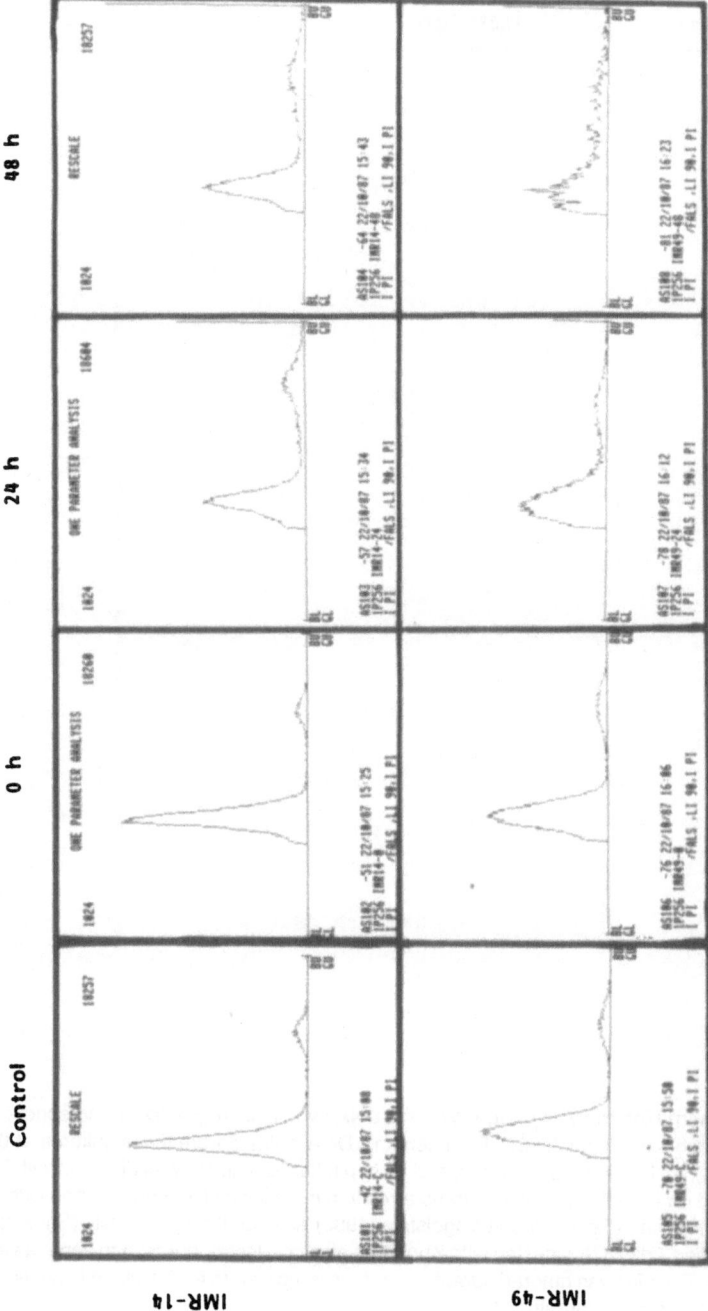

FIGURE 2. DNA histograms of mock-infected and Ad2-infected quiescent (top) and senescent (bottom) IMR-90 cells at 0 hr, 24 hr, and 48 hr, p.i., respectively, fractionated by fluorescence-activated cell sorting as described by Jackson et al. (1984) and Yen and Guernsey (1986). p.i., postinfection. (From Srivastava and Nahreini, 1989.)

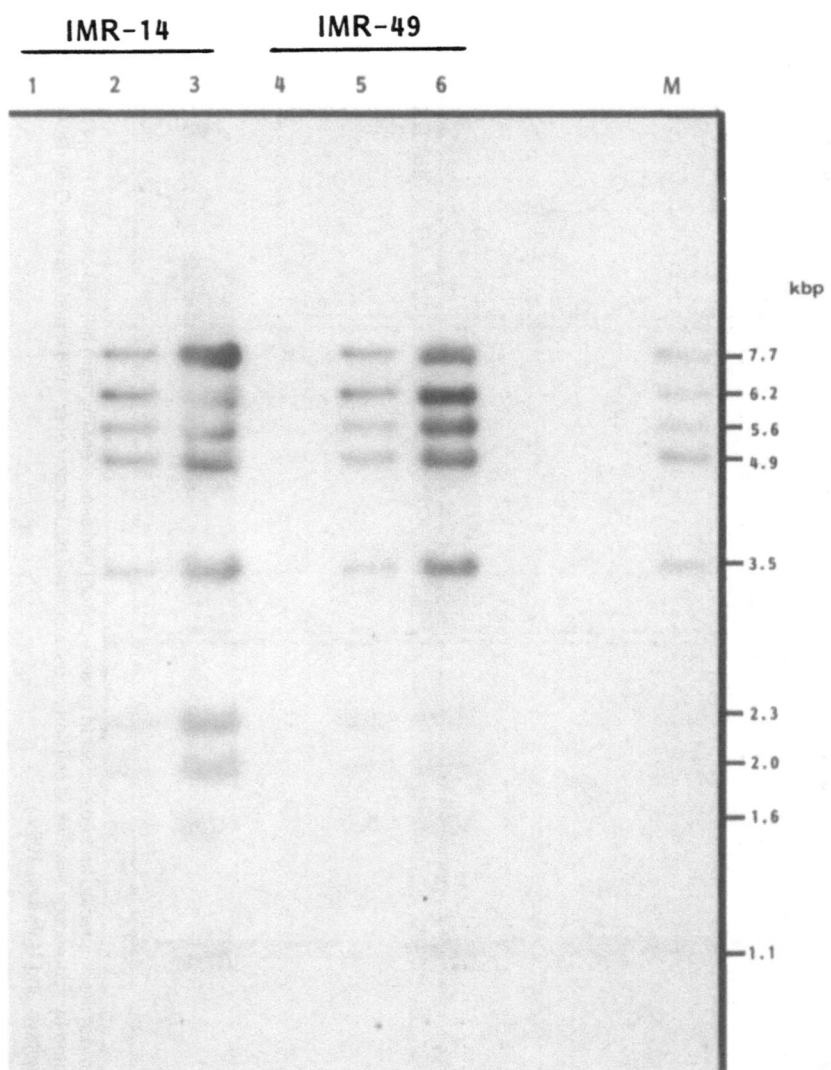

FIGURE 3. Southern blot analysis of adenovirus 2 DNA synthesis in quiescent and senescent human diploid fibroblast strain IMR-90. Total genomic DNA isolated from these cultures at 0 hr p.i. (lanes 1 and 4), 24 hr p.i. (lanes 2 and 5), and 48 hr p.i. (lanes 3 and 6) was digested with Kpn I, electrophoresed on a 1.2% agarose gel, transferred to nitrocellulose filter, and probed with the total Ad2 DNA ^{32}P-probe (Feinberg and Vogelstein, 1983) as described previously (Srivastava et al., 1985). Purified Ad2 DNA digested with Kpn I was also co-electrophoresed to serve as size markers (lane M). The blot was autoradiographed at room temperature for 30 min. p.i., postinfection. (From Srivastava and Nahreini, 1989.)

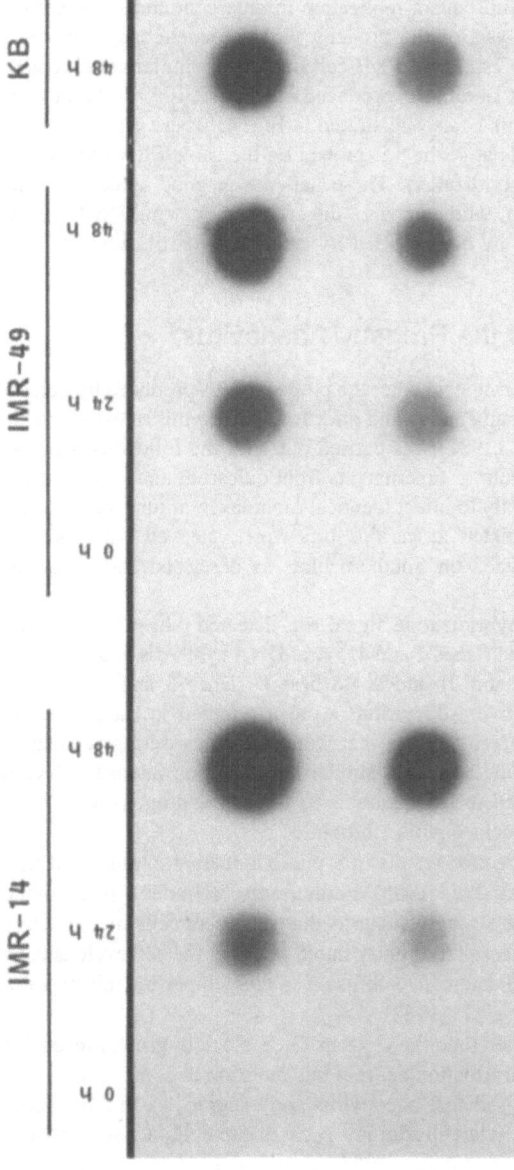

FIGURE 4. Dot blot analysis of the progeny adenovirus 2 DNA in infected cell culture supernatants. Clarified culture supernatants (1-ml aliquots) from Ad2-infected quiescent and senescent IMR-90 cells were collected at 0 hr p.i., 24 hr p.i., and 48 hr p.i.; deproteinized, denatured, and filtered through a nitrocellulose filter; and probed with the total Ad2 DNA probe as described by Srivastava and Lu (1988). A culture supernatant (100-μl aliquot) from Ad2-infected KB cells at 48 hr p.i. was also included in this experiment. The blot was autoradiographed for 16 hr at −70°C. p.i., postinfection. (From Srivastava and Nahreini, 1989.)

It is evident that while no hybridization signal was detected 0 hr p.i., by 24 hr p.i., progeny adenovirus particles were released into the culture medium and the total amount of the progeny virus increased more than twofold by 48 hr p.i. from both quiescent and senescent fibroblast cultures. These results also corroborate the data from Fig. 3 that the efficiency of Ad2 infection and subsequent replication in quiescent and senescent cells was comparable. A comparative analysis of the progeny virus production by cultured normal diploid fibroblasts and that by an established KB cell line under similar conditions revealed that both quiescent and senescent fibroblasts produced only about 10% of the progeny virus as that produced by KB cells. This is also illustrated in Fig. 4, where only one tenth of the culture supernatant from KB cells at 48 hr p.i. probed on the same filter produced approximately the same intensity of hybridization. These data are in good agreement with those reported by Spindler et al. (1985), who compared the efficiency of viral DNA replication in quiescent WI-38 and HeLa cells by buoyant-density centrifugation of radiolabeled cellular and viral nucleic acids.

2.4. Biological Activity of the Progeny Adenovirus

It was then of interest to determine whether the progeny virus produced by quiescent and senescent fibroblasts was biologically active and infectious. To do this, a two-cycle infection assay described by Lavery et al. (1987) was carried out with the following modifications. Equivalent amounts of clarified culture supernatants from quiescent and senescent fibroblast cultures 48 hr p.i. were used directly to infect identical monolayer cultures of KB cells. Total KB cell genomic DNA was isolated at various times p.i., cleaved with the restriction endonuclease HindIII, and analyzed on Southern blots as described above, as shown in Fig. 5.

Once again, while no Ad2-hybridization signal was detected 0 hr p.i. from both quiescent and senescent cultures inocula (lanes 1 and 4), viral DNA synthesis could be detected in KB cells at 24 hr p.i. (lanes 2 and 5) and at 48 hr p.i. (lanes 3 and 6). These results documented that biologically active Ad2 virions were assembled in, and released from, cultured fibroblasts during primary infections that were infectious during secondary infections of KB cells. Furthermore, the relatively similar hybridization intensity of viral DNA observed in KB cells substantiated that comparable levels of the progeny virus titers were produced by quiescent and senescent diploid fibroblasts.

Our observation that Ad2 infection results in S-phase induction in quiescent fibroblasts corroborates the results of Spindler et al. (1985). Furthermore, a similar S-phase induction in Ad2-infected senescent fibroblasts strongly suggests that senescent cells may be physiologically very similar to quiescent cells as far as entry into S phase of the cell cycle is concerned. A cogent example of experimental data with cell fusion studies supporting this hypothesis has recently been presented by Stein et al. (1982).

How might Ad2 infection overcome the G_0/S or G_1/S block in growth-restricted cells? Two recently published sets of information address this question to some extent. For example, Spindler et al. (1985) proposed that adenovirus early region 1A that encodes a 243-amino acid protein alters the cellular physiology such that the G_0-arrested population is driven into S phase. By contrast, Liu et al. (1985) identified a set of cell-cycle-dependent genes that are activated by adenovirus infection, expression of which reaches a maximum in the late G_1/S phase of the cell cycle. A direct comparison of the two systems is difficult, however, because different cell strains and cell lines were used in these studies.

Although we did not examine the viral life cycle at various stages during infection of

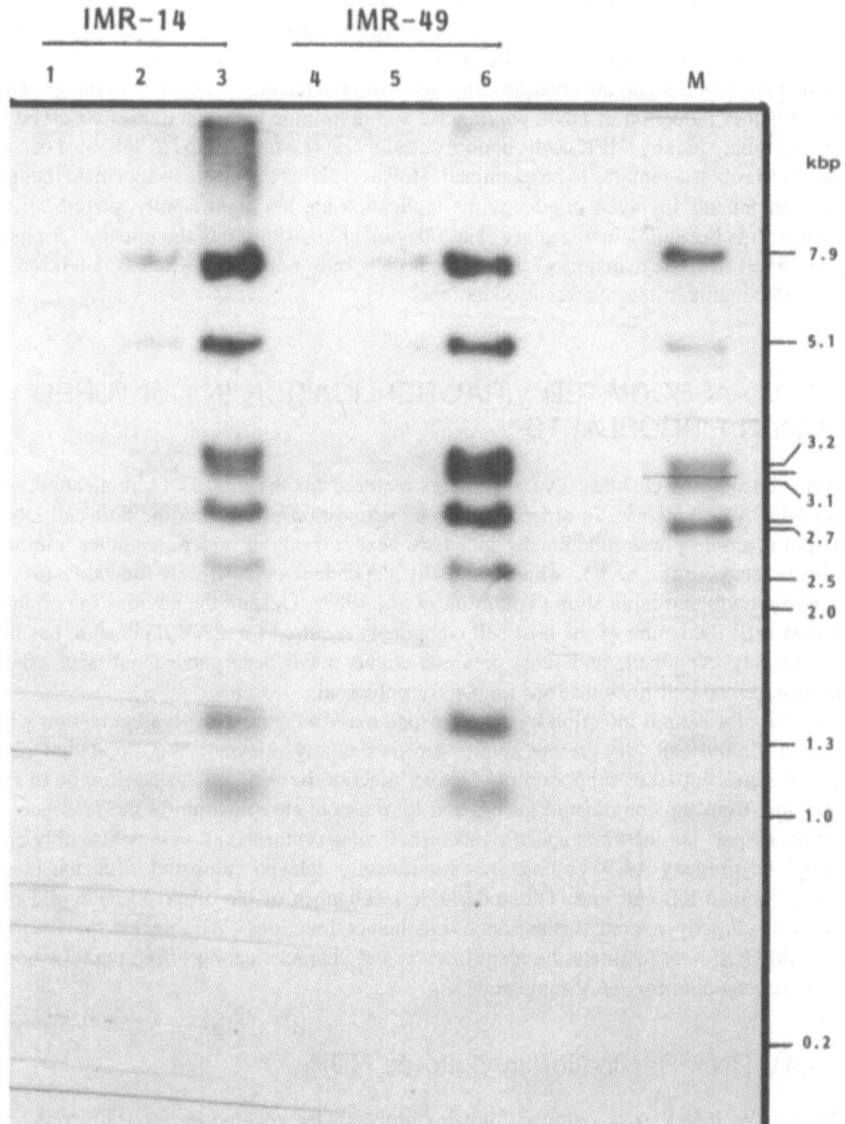

FIGURE 5. Southern blot analysis of adenovirus 2 DNA synthesis in secondary infections of KB cells at 0 hr p.i. (lanes 1 and 4), 24 hr p.i. (lanes 2 and 5), and 48 hr p.i. (lanes 3 and 6) by progeny virus produced by quiescent and senescent IMR-90 cells. Total genomic DNA samples isolated from KB cells were digested with *Hind*III and equivalent amounts were analyzed on Southern blots. *Hind*III-digested purified Ad2 DNA was also co-electrophoresed to serve as size markers (lane M). The blot was autoradiographed at room temperature for 4 hr. p.i., postinfection. (From Srivastava and Nahreini, 1989.)

senescent fibroblasts, it is unlikely that major qualitative or quantitative differences exist between quiescent and senescent cells. It is intriguing that the efficiency of viral infection and production of progeny virus was significantly lower in cultured fibroblasts than that in an established KB cell line, an observation consistent with the results obtained by Spindler *et al.* (1985). Whether induction of DNA polymerase and thymidine kinase activities observed in human embryonic kidney (HEK) cells upon Ad2-infection (Ledinko, 1967, 1968) also occurs in cultured fibroblasts remains to be examined. However, it is reasonable to speculate that the cellular components involved in adenovirus replication are not significantly altered during senescence. It is becoming increasingly clear (Dayton *et al.*, 1989) that the impaired S-phase entry observed in a great majority of senescent cells may not be a sufficient condition to create and/or maintain the senescent phenotype.

3. ADENO-ASSOCIATED VIRAL REPLICATION IN CULTURED HUMAN FIBROBLASTS

Since adenovirus encodes several proteins required for the viral DNA replication, including a DNA polymerase, in order to address the question of whether the host-cell DNA replication machinery was functionally intact we next carried out infection studies with the adeno-associated virus (AAV), which is totally dependent on host cell functions for its productive growth and replication (Yakobson *et al.*, 1987). Despite the obvious importance of the host cell, the nature of the host-cell component required for AAV replication has not been rigorously examined, and most previous studies have been carried out with established/transformed cell lines that are frequently polyploid.

In view of a natural infection by AAV, which may frequently involve interaction with the normal diploid cell, the present studies are particularly relevant. We report that both young and senescent HDF supported productive infection by AAV as well as rescue of the viral genome from a recombinant plasmid and its subsequent replication in the presence of adenovirus helper, but the virus-specific macromolecular synthesis, as well as assembly and release of the progeny AAV virions, was significantly delayed compared with that in an established human KB cell line. The underlying mechanism of the observed delay did not appear to be directly related to the adenovirus-helper functions. We suggest that further studies with HDF may facilitate the identification and characterization of the putative host-cell function essential for AAV replication.

3.1. AAV DNA Replication in Cultured HDF

Productive infection of cultured human fibroblasts by adenovirus was observed previously by Yamashita and Shimojo (1969) and by Spindler *et al.*, (1985). We recently extended these studies and documented that both quiescent and senescent HDF are equally efficient in supporting Ad2 replication (Srivastava and Nahreini, 1989). In view of these studies, it was of significant interest to examine whether HDF could also support AAV replication. Co-infection of early- and late-passage HDF with Ad2 and AAV was therefore carried out in parallel with that of an established human KB cell line. Low-molecular-weight DNA was isolated from these cultures at various times p.i., and equivalent amounts of DNA samples were analyzed on Southern blots for the characteristic AAV DNA replicative intermediates, as shown in Fig. 6.

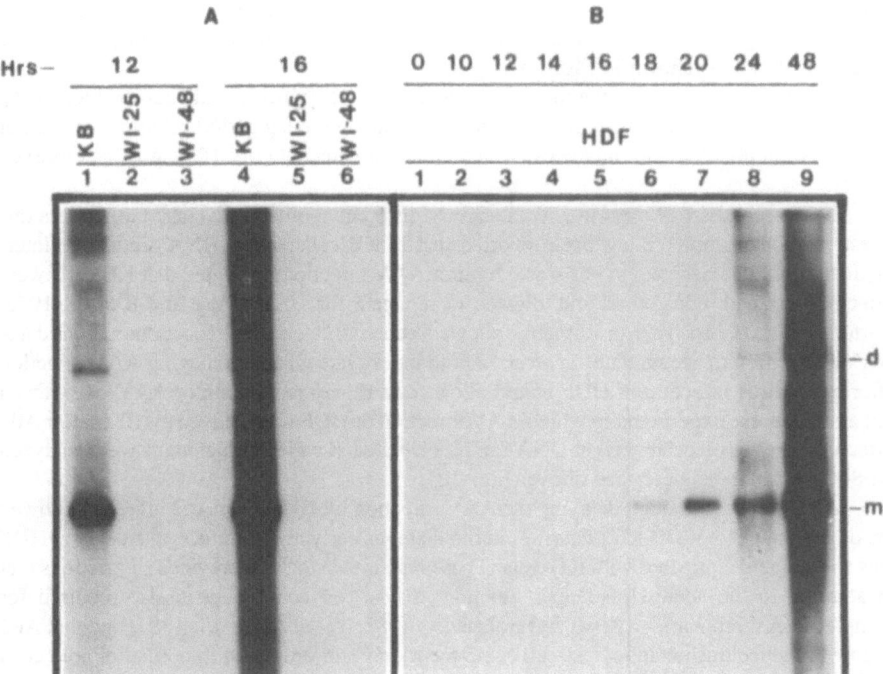

FIGURE 6. Southern blot analysis of AAV DNA replication in KB and HDF cells. Approximately 70% confluent monolayer cultures were co-infected with AAV and Ad2 at 37°C for 1 hr; equivalent amounts of low-molecular-weight DNA isolated at various indicated times were analyzed on Southern blots using a ^{32}P-labeled AAV viral DNA probe as described for Fig. 2. (A) AAV DNA replication in KB (lanes 1 and 4), and HDF at early (WI-38 at 25 MPD; lanes 2 and 5) and late (WI-38 at 48 MPD; lanes 3 and 6) cells 12 and 16 hr p.i. (B) Kinetics of AAV DNA replication in HDF (WI-38 at 32 MPD) cells. *m* and *d* denote the monomeric and dimeric forms, respectively, of the AAV DNA replicative intermediates. p.i., postinfection. (From Nahreini and Srivastava, 1989.)

It is interesting to note that while AAV DNA replication occurred in KB cells in a timely manner (Fig. 6A, lanes 1 and 4) as observed by other investigators, under identical conditions, both early- (lanes 2 and 5), and late- (lanes 3 and 6) passage HDF failed to support AAV DNA replication during this time frame. However, AAV DNA replicative intermediates could be observed upon prolonged incubation of 18–20 hr p.i., in early-passage HDF (Fig. 6B). Similar results were obtained with late-passage HDF (data not shown). These results document that normal HDF cells are capable of supporting AAV DNA replication, albeit after a significant delay, compared with KB cells.

We next wished to investigate whether the observed delay in the accumulation of AAV DNA replicative intermediates in HDF was a direct consequence of a less likely possibility of limiting amounts of infecting Ad2/AAV virions or, alternatively, due to reduced amounts of Ad2-encoded and/or induced polypeptides required for AAV DNA replication. The following two sets of experiments were carried out. In the first, the ratio of infecting Ad2/AAV input virus inocula was increased progressively during primary infections of HDF, and low-molecular-weight DNA isolated at various times p.i., was analyzed on Southern blots as described above, as shown in Fig. 7A.

It is evident that neither the increase in the titers of the virus inocula nor the increase in the Ad2/AAV ratio had any significant effect in reducing the lag period prior to detection of AAV DNA replicative intermediates, which could be detected only 18 hr p.i., as observed before.

In the second set of experiments, a slightly different approach was taken to address this question. For example, it has been reported that in KB cells, AAV DNA replicative inter-mediates could be detected as early as 3 hr after AAV infection, provided that KB cells were infected first with adenovirus and allowed to replicate for 10 hr (Rose and Koczot, 1972; Carter et al., 1973). This presumably allowed adenovirus-encoded functions required for AAV replication to accumulate. In an attempt to investigate whether delaying AAV infection after adenovirus infection of HDF would allow for a timely replication of AAV, we carried out a time-course experiment in which AAV infection of HDF was delayed by 10 hr after Ad2 infection. Low-molecular-weight DNA samples isolated at various time points were analyzed on Southern blots as described above (Fig. 7B).

It is clear that although delaying the AAV infection by 10 hr after Ad2 infection allowed the detection of AAV DNA replicative intermediates as early as 6–8 hr p.i., the delay in HDF was still evident compared with KB cells. These results substantiate previous suggestions that in addition to the adenovirus-helper function, a host-cell component is also required for complete AAV replication (Berns and Bohenzky, 1987; Yakobson et al., 1987) and that Ad2 is able to induce this putative host-cell component only sub-optimally in normal diploid cells as compared with KB cells.

3.2. Assembly and Release of AAV Progeny Virions in HDF

It was then of interest to examine whether the observed delay in AAV DNA replication in HDF also resulted in delayed production of the progeny AAV virions as an index of intracellular viral RNA and protein synthesis and assembly of mature virions. This was measured as the amount of AAV DNA-hybridizable signal in clarified culture supernatants, at various times after co-infection of HDF with Ad2 and AAV, on a quantitative DNA dot blot described previously (Srivastava and Lu, 1988), as shown in Fig. 8.

It is evident that no AAV-hybridization signal could be detected up to 30 hr p.i. in culture supernatants from HDF, while, under identical conditions, AAV progeny virions could be detected 24 hr p.i. in KB cells. AAV progeny virions were, however, released into the culture medium of HDF 48 hr p.i., and both early- and late-passage HDF produced approximately equivalent amounts of the virus. These results thus document a general overall delay in all aspects of AAV replication in HDF; they also substantiate our earlier observations that senescent HDF can be induced to undergo S phase of the cell cycle and that the DNA replication machinery in these cells is functionally intact (Srivastava and Nahreini, 1989).

3.3. Rescue/Replication of the AAV Genome in HDF

Previous studies have documented the excision of the AAV genome in latently infected Detroit 6 cells (Cheung et al., 1980) upon infection with adenovirus (Ostrove and Berns, 1980; Laughlin et al., 1986). The AAV genome can also be rescued from recombinant plasmids transfected into adenovirus-infected HeLa cells (Samulski et al., 1982, 1983;

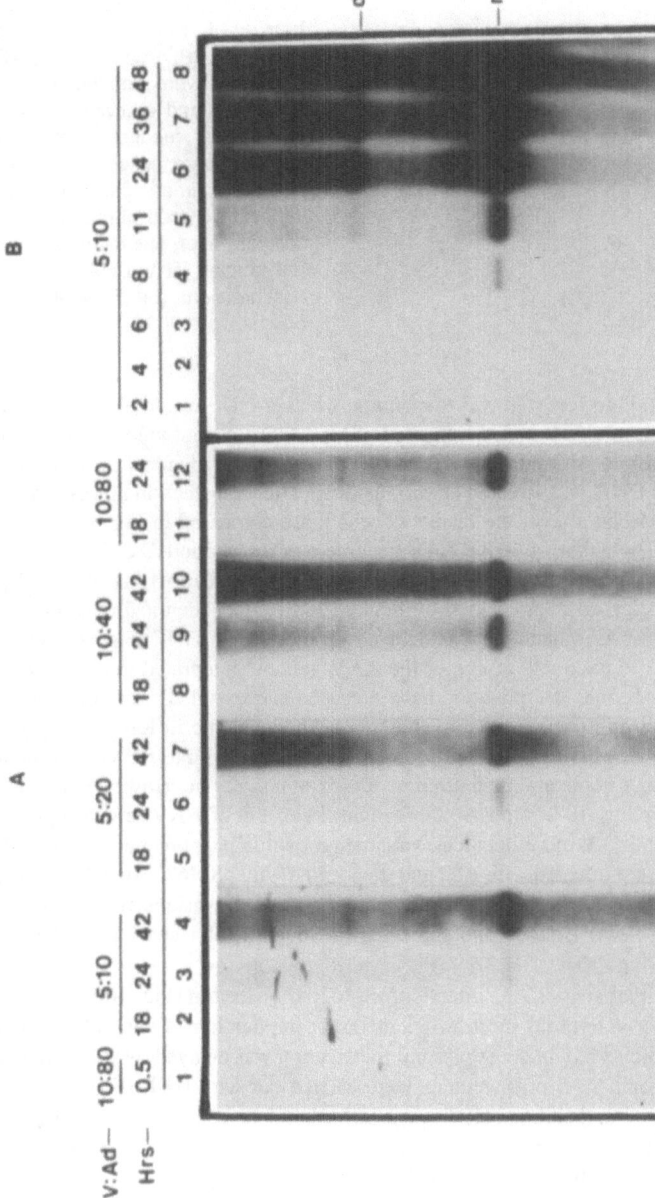

FIGURE 7. Southern blot analysis of AAV DNA replication in HDF (WI-38 at 25 MPD) cells. (A) Cells were infected with indicated ratios of the $TCID_{50}$ of AAV/Ad2 virus stocks as described by Srivastava et al. (1983), and low-molecular-weight DNA samples isolated at various times p.i. were analyzed for the AAV DNA replicative intermediates. (B) Influence of infection of HDF by Ad2 for 10 hr prior to AAV infection on the accumulation of AAV DNA replicative intermediates. Low-molecular-weight DNA samples isolated at various indicated times after AAV-infection were analyzed. p.i., postinfection. (From Nahreini and Srivastava, 1989.)

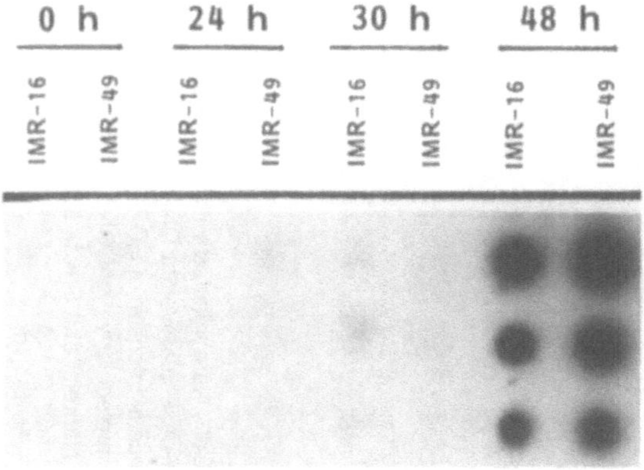

FIGURE 8. Dot blot analysis for the release of the progeny AAV virions from HDF. Strain IMR-90 cells at early (16 MPD) and late (49 MPD) passage were co-infected with AAV/Ad2, and equivalent amounts of culture medium from these cultures were collected at various indicated times p.i. and deproteinized, filtered through a nitrocellulose filter, and hybridized with a ^{32}P-labeled AAV DNA probe. p.i., postinfection. (From Nahreini and Srivastava, 1989.)

Laughlin *et al.*, 1983). Our next step was to examine whether HDF would also allow rescue of the AAV genome from a recombinant plasmid pSM620. Equivalent amounts of pSM620 DNA were transfected into Ad2-infected KB and HDF cells under identical conditions, and low-molecular weight DNA was isolated at various times after transfection and analyzed on Southern blots as described above, the results of which are compared in Fig. 9.

It is interesting to note that while the AAV genome was rescued in KB cells followed by DNA replication approximately 24 hr post-transfection (Fig. 9A, lane 4) as observed previously by other investigators (Samulski and Shenk, 1988), under identical conditions, the rescue/replication of the AAV genome was delayed up to 48 hr in HDF (Fig. 9B, lane 6).

Previous attempts to uncouple rescue of the AAV genome integrated into the host-cell chromosome and its subsequent replication have not been successful. During the course of these studies, using pSM620 as a source of the latent AAV genome in KB cells, we were intrigued to note that when the recombinant plasmid was transfected into KB cells soon after Ad2 infection, the rescue/replication occurred at approximately 20 hr. However, if plasmid transfection was delayed by 10 hr after Ad2 infection, the extent of AAV rescue/replication was reduced significantly. A more detailed examination of this phenomenon was therefore carried out. KB cells were infected with Ad2 and transfected with pSM620 soon thereafter, or transfection was delayed by 10 hr after Ad2 infection, and at various times p.i., low-molecular-weight DNA was isolated and subjected to Southern blot analysis as described above, as depicted in Fig. 10.

As can be seen, simultaneous Ad2 infection/pSM620 transfection (Fig. 10A, lanes 1, 3, and 5) resulted in nearly fivefold more efficient rescue/replication of the AAV genome compared with experiments in which the plasmid transfection was delayed by 10 hr after Ad2 infection (lanes 2, 4, and 6). Similar studies were carried out with HDF (Fig. 10B). It is evident that AAV rescue/replication in HDF was also further delayed as observed before. It is noteworthy that in HDF also, prior infection with Ad2 did not significantly alter the extent of AAV rescue/replication as observed in KB cells.

These results suggest that adenovirus-encoded functions may not be required for rescue of the AAV genome, although they are clearly required for subsequent DNA replication. These results also indicate that a certain amount of time must elapse while the plasmid DNA is within the cell, regardless of the state of infection, before the rescue. The other possibility is that rescue occurs independent of the Ad2 functions but escapes detection primarily

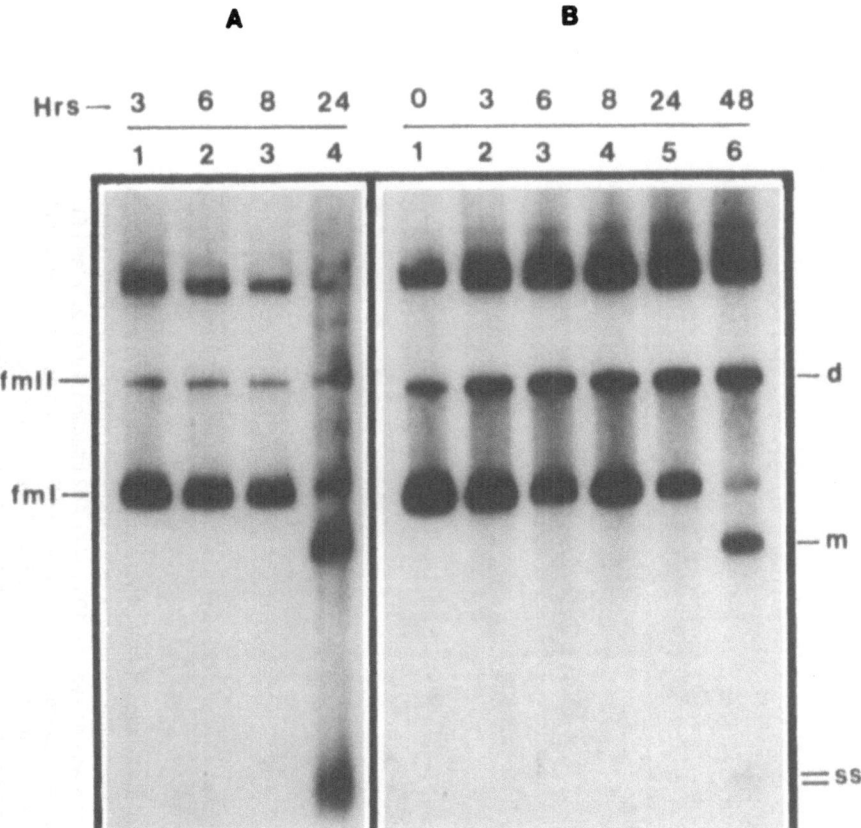

FIGURE 9. Southern blot analysis of rescue and replication of the AAV genome from a recombinant plasmid in KB and HDF cells. Ad2-infected KB (A) and HDF (B) cells were transfected with 1 μg of pSM620 DNA, and equivalent amounts of low-molecular-weight DNA isolated at various-indicated times post-transfection were analyzed. *fm*I and *fm*II denote the covalently closed, supercoiled, and relaxed circular forms, respectively, of the plasmid DNA. *ss*, single-stranded AAV DNA molecules. p.i., postinfection. (From Nahreini and Srivastava, 1989.)

because a critical threshold concentration of the replicated AAV DNA must accumulate, a phenomenon clearly dependent on Ad2-encoded and/or Ad2-induced putative host-cell components.

In sum, we examined normal human diploid fibroblasts for productive infection by AAV for two reasons. First, AAV replication studies have traditionally been carried out with established/transformed cell lines, whereas HDF are normal diploid cells with a limited proliferative potential and might thus be a reasonable model system for a natural AAV infection. Second, it is possible that further studies to characterize the host-cell component required for productive replication/rescue of AAV may be more amenable because of the diploid nature of these cells.

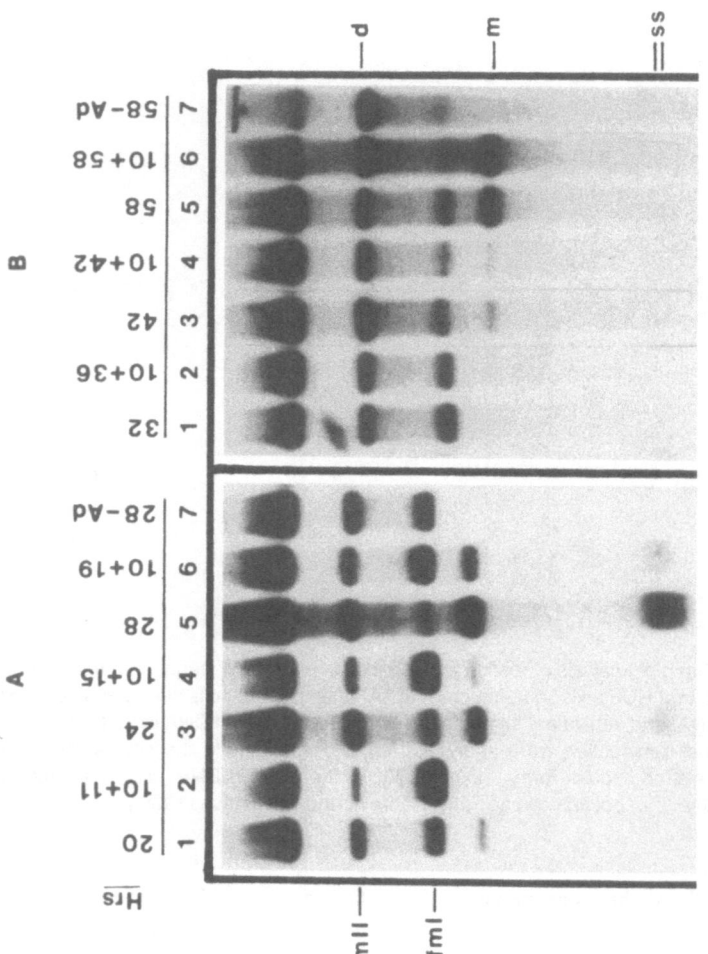

FIGURE 10. Southern blot analysis of the kinetics of AAV DNA rescue/replication in KB and HDF cells. Ad2-infected KB (A) and HDF (B) cells were either simultaneously transfected with pSM620 DNA (lanes 1, 3, and 5) or the plasmid transfection was delayed for 10 hr after Ad2 infection (lanes 2, 4, and 6). Low-molecular-weight DNA samples were isolated at various indicated times, and equivalent amounts were analyzed. Lane 7 (A,B) indicates low-molecular-weight DNA isolated from mock-infected cells transfected with pSM620 DNA. p.i., postinfection. (From Nahreini and Srivastava, 1989.)

Our initial attempts to demonstrate AAV DNA replication in HDF in the absence of a helper virus did not succeed. A variety of physical (ultraviolet irradiation) and chemical (hydroxyurea, thymidine) treatments (Yakobson et al., 1987) also failed to elicit a positive response (data not shown). Co-infection by adenovirus, however, did support productive infection of HDF by AAV, but there was a significant delay in accumulation of AAV DNA replicative intermediates as well as assembly and release of mature progeny virions compared with that in an established human KB cell line. The delay did not appear to be the result of limiting adenovirus functions because HDF could be productively infected with adenovirus (Spindler et al., 1985; Srivastava and Nahreini, 1989).

Perhaps the most interesting observation from these studies is that rescue of the AAV genome from a recombinant plasmid appeared to be independent of adenovirus-helper functions. This was true both for KB and for HDF cells, although the delay in rescue/replication of the AAV genome in HDF was still apparent. These studies thus lend support to the observation by Yakobson et al. (1987), who documented AAV genome rescue/replication in the absence of adenovirus-encoded polypeptides. The precise mechanism by which the latent AAV genome is excised remains an open question, but our recent studies indicate that excision may involve nonspecific nicking (Nahreini and Srivastava, in preparation), a putative nuclease activity augmented during cellular senescence in vitro (Dayton et al., 1989). It is tempting to speculate that although the excision mechanisms in both KB and HDF cells may share certain common features, subtle differences may exist as well. It is now of significant interest to pursue studies with HDF to characterize the putative host-cell components required for the productive infection and rescue/replication of AAV.

4. CONCLUSIONS

Mammalian DNA viruses, by virtue of their much less complex nature, compared with that of eukaryotic cells, have continued to provide powerful model systems to explore the underlying mechanisms of eukaryotic genome organization and function. Beyond the basic understanding of the molecular correlates of eukaryotic cellular and viral DNA replication, further studies with cultured human diploid fibroblasts and DNA viruses of human origin promise to lead to the detection and identification of putative host-cell components crucial for DNA biosynthesis that have hitherto remained unknown. At the very least, cultured human fibroblasts offer a very useful model system for either a natural adeno-infection or AAV infection, or both.

ACKNOWLEDGMENTS. This research was supported in part by grant AI-26323 from the National Institutes of Health, and by grants from the American Heart Association, Indiana Affiliate, Inc., and the Phi Beta Psi Sorority (A.S.). The authors wish to thank Sandra Jackson for expert technical assistance and Stephanie Moore for her excellent secretarial assistance during the preparation of this manuscript.

REFERENCES

Bell, E., Marek, L. F., Levinstone, D. S., Merrill, C., Sher, S., Young, I. T., and Eden, M., 1978, Loss of division potential in vitro: Aging or differentiation?, Science 202:1158–1163.
Berk, A. J., 1986, Adenovirus promoters and E1A transactivation, Annu. Rev. Genet. 20:45–79.

Berns, K. I., and Bohenzky, R., 1987, Adeno-associated viruses: An update, *Adv. Virus Res.* **32:**243–307.

Bunn, C. L., and Tarrant, G. M., 1980, Limited lifespan in somatic cell hybrids and cybrids, *Exp. Cell Res.* **127:**385–396.

Burmer, G. C., Zeigler, C. J., and Norwood, T. H. 1982, Evidence for endogenous polypeptide-mediated inhibition of cell-cycle transit in human diploid cells, *J. Cell Biol.* **94:**187–192.

Carter, B. J., Koczot, F. J., Garrison, J., Rose, J. A., and Dolin, R., 1973, Separate function provided by adenovirus for adeno-associated virus multiplication, *Nature (Lond.)* **244:**71–73.

Cheung, A. K. M., Hoggan, M. D., Hauswirth, W. W., and Berns, K. I., 1980, Integration of the adeno-associated virus genome into cellular DNA in latently infected Detroit 6 cells, *J. Virol.* **33:**739–748.

Cristofalo, V. J., and Sharf, B. B., 1973, Cellular senescence and DNA synthesis, *Exp. Cell. Res.* **76:**419–427.

Dayton, M. A., Nahreini, P., and Srivastava, A., 1989, Augmented nuclease activity during cellular senescence *in vitro, J. Cell. Biochem.* **39:**75–85.

Feinberg, A. P., and Vogelstein, B., 1983, A technique for radiolabeling DNA restriction endonuclease fragments to high specific activity, *Anal. Biochem.* **132:**6–13.

Finch, C. E., and Hayflick, L. E., 1977, *Handbook of the Biology of Aging,* Van Nostrand–Reinhold, New York, pp. 101–189.

Hayflick, L. E., 1984, Intracellular determinants of cell aging, *Mech. Aging Dev.* **28:**177–185.

Hayflick, L. E., and Moorehead, P. S., 1961, The serial cultivation of human diploid cell strains, *Exp. Cell Res.* **25:**585–621.

Hodge, L. D., and Scharff, M. D., 1969, Effect of adenovirus on host cell DNA synthesis in synchronized cells, *Virology* **37:**554–564.

Jackson, C. W., Brown, L. K., Somerville, B. C., Lyles, S. A., and Look, A. T., 1984, Two-color flow cytometric measurement of DNA distribution of rat megakaryocytes in unfixed, ultrafractionated marrow cell suspensions, *Blood* **63:**768–772.

Laughlin, C. A., Tratshin, J.-D., Coon, H., and Carter, B. J., 1983, Cloning of infectious adeno-associated virus genomes in bacterial plasmids, *Gene* **23:**65–73.

Laughlin, C. A., Cardellichio, C. B., and Coon, H. C., 1986, Latent infection of KB cells with adeno-associated virus type 2, *J. Virol.* **60:**515–524.

Lavery, D., Fu, S. M., Lufkin, T., and Chen-Kiang, S., 1987, Productive infection of cultured human lymphoid cells by adenovirus, *J. Virol.* **61:**1466–1472.

Ledinko, N., 1967, Stimulation of DNA synthesis and thymidine kinase activity in human embryonic kidney cells infected by adenovirus 2 or 12. *Cancer Res.* **27:**1459–1469.

Ledinko, N., 1968, Enhanced deoxyribonucleic acid polymerase activity in human embryonic kidney cultures infected with adenovirus 2 or 12, *J. Virol.* **2:**89–98.

Liu, H. T., Baserga, R., and Mercer, W. E., 1985, Adenovirus type 2 activates cell cycle-dependent genes that are a subset of those activated by serum, *Mol. Cell. Biol.* **5:**2936–2942.

Macieira-Coelho, A., 1984, Genome reorganization during cellular senescence, *Mech. Aging Dev.* **27:**257–262.

Nahreini, P., and Srivastava, A., 1989, Rescue and replication of the adeno-associated virus genome in mortal and immortal human cells, *Intervirology.* **30:**74–85.

Olashaw, N. E., Kress, E. D., and Cristofalo, V. J., 1983, Thymidine triphosphate synthesis in senescent WI-38 cells, *Exp. Cell Res.* **149:**547–554.

Orgel, L. E., 1963, The maintenance of the accuracy of protein synthesis and its relevance to aging, *Proc. Natl. Acad. Sci. USA* **49:**517–521.

Ostrove, J. M., and Berns, K. I., 1980, Adenovirus early region lb gene function required for rescue of latent adeno-associated virus, *Virology* **104:**502–505.

Pina, M., and Green, M., 1969, Biochemical studies on adenovirus multiplication. XIV. Macromolecule and enzyme synthesis in cells replicating oncogenic and non-oncogenic human adenovirus, *Virology* **38:**573–586.

Rose, J. A., and Koczot, F. J., 1972, Adenovirus-associated virus multiplication. VII. Helper requirement for viral deoxyribonucleic and ribonucleic acid synthesis, *J. Virol.* **10**:1–8.

Samulski, R. J., and Shenk, T., 1988, Adenovirus E1B 55-M$_r$ polypeptide facilitates timely cytoplasmic accumulation of adeno-associated virus mRNAs, *J. Virol.* **62**:206–210.

Samulski, R. J., Berns, K. I., Tan, M., and Muzyczka, N., 1982, Cloning of adeno-associated virus into pBR322: Rescue of intact virus from recombinant plasmid in human cells, *Proc. Natl. Acad. Sci. USA* **79**:2077–2081.

Samulski, R. J., Srivastava, A., Berns, K. I., and Muzyczka, N., 1983, Rescue of adeno-associated virus from recombinant plasmids: Gene correction within the terminal repeats of AAV, *Cell* **33**:135–143.

Smith, J. R., and Lumpkin, C. K. L., Jr., 1980, Loss of gene repression activity: A theory of cellular senescence, *Mech. Aging Dev.* **13**:387–392.

Southern, E. M., 1975, Detection of specific sequences among DNA fragments separated by gel electrophoresis, *J. Mol. Biol.* **98**:503–517.

Spindler, K. R., Eng, C. Y., and Berk, A. J., 1985, An adenovirus early region 1A protein is required for maximal viral DNA replication in growth-arrested human cells, *J. Virol.* **53**:742–750.

Srivastava, A., 1987, Repication of the adeno-associated virus DNA termini *in vitro, Intervirology* **27**:138–147.

Srivastava, A., and Lu, L., 1988, Replication of the B19 parvovirus in highly enriched hematopoietic progenitor cells from normal human bone marrow, *J. Virol.* **62**:3505–3509.

Srivastava, A., and Nahreini, P., 1989, Productive infection of quiescent and senescent human diploid fibroblasts by adenovirus 2, Submitted for publication.

Srivastava, A., Lusby, E. W., and Berns, K. I., 1983, Nucleotide sequence and organization of the adeno-associated virus 2 genome, *J. Virol.* **45**:555–564.

Srivastava, A., Norris, J. S., Reis, R. J. S., and Goldstein, S., 1985, c-Ha-*ras*-1 proto-oncogene amplification and over-expression during the limited replicative lifespan of normal human fibroblasts, *J. Biol. Chem.* **260**:6404–6409.

Stein, G. H., Yanishevsky, R. M., Gordon, L., and Beeson, M., 1982, Carcinogen-transformed human cells are inhibited from entry into S-phase by fusion to senescent cells but cells tansformed by DNA tumor viruses overcome the inhibition, *Proc. Natl. Acad. Sci. USA* **79**:5287–5291.

Yakobson, B., Koch, T., and Winocour, E., 1987, Replication of adeno-associated virus in synchronized cells without the addition of a helper virus, *J. Virol.* **61**:972–981.

Yamashita, T., and Shimojo, H., 1969, Induction of cellular DNA synthesis by adenovirus 12 in human embryo kidney cells, *Virology* **36**:351–355.

Yen, A., and Guernsey, D. L., 1986, Increased c-*myc* RNA levels associated with the precommitment state during HL-60 myeloid differentiation, *Cancer Res.* **46**:4156–4161.

9

Lactoferrin Immunoreactivity and Binding Sites in Neurons, Neuritic Plaques, and Neurofibrillary Tangles in Alzheimer's Disease

ALEXANDER P. OSMAND and ROBERT C. SWITZER III

1. INTRODUCTION

Alzheimer's disease (AD) is the major cause of dementia in the elderly and afflicts between two and four million persons in the United States alone (Cook-Deegan and Whitehouse, 1987). Although considerable advances in understanding the molecular biology of the principal molecular constituents of the characteristic brain lesions of this disorder have recently been made, little is formally known about the etiology and pathogenesis of AD. Previous evidence suggesting that aluminum or its compounds are causally involved (Crapper et al., 1973) or that a loss of cholinergic neurons is the primary neuropathologic feature (Davies and Maloney, 1976) has not been confirmed. It is generally accepted, however, that an understanding of the mechanisms involved in the initiation and formation of the pathognomic features of AD, the neuritic (amyloid) plaques (NP) and neurofibrillary tangles (NFT), will provide the essential basis for a rational approach to the treatment and prevention of this disease. The observations described here arise from a study of potential etiologic factors involved in the generation of NP and NFT.

1.1. Pathophysiology of Alzheimer's Disease

Alzheimer's disease is characterized by a dementia with an insidious onset and a progressive deterioration of cognitive functions; diagnosis of the disorder is confirmed by histopathological evidence of the presence of large numbers of neuritic plaques and neurofibrillary tangles obtained at autopsy or biopsy (McKhann et al., 1984). A typical medical history would establish a loss of memory and other cognitive deficits early in the course of the

ALEXANDER P. OSMAND • Department of Medicine, University of Tennessee Medical Center, Knoxville, Tennessee 37920.   ROBERT C. SWITZER III • Department of Pathology, University of Tennessee Medical Center, Knoxville, Tennessee 37920.

disease, although patients rarely present for diagnosis before the development of a significant impairment of the activities of daily living. Considerable heterogeneity in the course of the disease has been documented, and this has been reflected in diverse histopathologic features (Bondareff *et al.*, 1987); however, correlations between subtyping based on pathologic features and the clinical course of the disease in specific patients have not been made in this latter or other studies. The presence of significant numbers of NP and NFT in the normal aging brain is most logically interpreted as subclinical or incipient AD (Ulrich, 1985; Katzman *et al.*, 1988).

1.1.1. Histopathology and Neurochemistry of Alzheimer's Disease

Alzheimer's disease is characterized by the presence of large numbers of NP and NFT in multiple regions of the brain. The highest numbers of NFT are found in entorhinal cortex, the amygdaloid nucleus, and the subiculum; considerable numbers are also seen in several regions of the neocortex, most notably the frontal, parietal, and temporal association regions. With the exception of the olfactory cortex, NP and NFT are less common in all primary sensory and motor regions of cortex. Plaques tend to follow a similar distribution but do not necessarily correlate in specific cases (Terry, 1985). A moderate to severe cortical deficiency of acetylcholine (ACh) and choline acetyltransferase is present in AD; loss of cholinergic activity correlates with plaque count and cognitive deficits (Terry, 1985). Reduced neuronal cell counts have also been found in the nucleus basalis of Meynert (nbM), the major source of cortical cholinergic innervation (Whitehouse *et al.*, 1981); additional nuclei that provide major projections to the cortex, the locus ceruleus, and the dorsal raphe may contain NFT and show considerable loss of neurons (Bondareff *et al.*, 1982; Yamamoto and Hirano, 1985). Significant variations in neuronal loss in subcortical nuclei that supply extrinsic (nonpeptide) neurotransmitters could account for conflicting descriptions of cortical deficits in these transmitters in AD.

1.1.2. Biochemical Properties of Neuritic Plaques and Neurofibrillary Tangles

Amyloid has long been recognized as a major component of neuritic plaques and, despite several claims for the presence of amyloid proteins characteristic of systemic amyloid, a protein unique to the amyloid of neurodegenerative diseases has been characterized and the sequence of the amyloid protein and its presumptive precursor identified from a complementary DNA (cDNA) clone (Kang *et al.*, 1987). The amyloid protein is composed of a 42-amino acid residue sequence near (and including part of) the C-terminal putative transmembrane segment of a 695-residue precursor. This sequence lacks homology with known proteins; however, a region of the molecule rich in acidic amino acids can be shown to have some similarity to the yeast mitochondrial ubiquinone–cytochrome c reductase subunit VI (A. P. Osmand, unpublished observations). The recent unexpected finding of an additional domain of 56 residues variably interpolated immediately following this acidic region suggests that this may be a distinct domain; the homology of the 56-residue insert to the Kunitz family of protease inhibitors adds an intriguing dimension to the functional role of the precursor (Ponte *et al.*, 1988; Tanzi *et al.*, 1988; Kitaguchi *et al.*, 1988).

The complex filamentous structure of neurofibrillary tangles has been interpreted as distinct from that of amyloid, which is generally composed of paired fibrils; however, NFT share the birefringent congophilia characteristic of amyloid, and recently the size and amino acid sequence of the protein subunits of highly purified NFT were shown to be identical with the A4 amyloid protein, although with a variable degree of N-terminal heterogeneity due to truncation (Guiroy et al., 1987).

1.1.3. Immunochemical Markers in Alzheimer's Disease

Numerous components, of the neuronal cytoskeleton and cytoplasm and of extra-neuronal origin, have been detected in association with NFT and NP, largely by immu-nohistochemical methods. The definition of molecules that either decorate or become incorporated into these structures, e.g., by transglutaminase activation (C. C. Miller and Anderton, 1986), would be expected to provide some understanding of the mechanisms of their formation; those uniquely found in the brain in AD should provide the greatest insight. Of the multiple components described to date, the reactivity of neuropathologic features of AD with certain monoclonal antibodies and the presence and redistribution of the micro-tubule-associated protein (MAP), τ, are the most outstanding. A monoclonal antibody termed Alz-50 appears to react with a 68,000-dalton protein (A68) believed to be associated with an early cytological change in AD, based on its reactivity with morphologically normal neurons in AD as well as large numbers of NFT and NP (Wolozin et al., 1986; Hyman et al., 1988). Initial studies have indicated that, although traces of Alz-50 reactivity may be found in association with other neurodegenerative diseases, the presence of large quantities of A68 is unique to AD (Wolozin and Davies, 1987). Alz-50 immunoreactivity may overlap with the determinants identified by a set of monoclonal antibodies that appear also to react selectively with cortical neurons that are damaged in AD; one of these, monoclonal antibody 3A4, appears to follow closely the pathological sequence of cortical involvement and may react with a phosphorylated epitope (C. A. Miller et al., 1987). Initial suggestions that the paired helical filaments in NFT may be derived from neurofilaments, based on immunoreactivity with certain antisera, have been discounted owing to the reactivity of these antisera with phosphorylated epitopes, principally with the protein τ (Nukina et al., 1987). Reactivity of NFT and NP with antibody to nonphosphorylated epitopes of τ has been shown (Wood et al., 1986); additional data (Kowall and Kosik, 1987) confirm that both phosphorylation and axonal cytoskeletal integrity are disrupted in cortical neurons in AD.

1.2. Neuroanatomical Associations of Lesions in Alzheimer's Disease

Current concepts of the structure and role of certain corticocortical pathways and cor-ticolimbic connectivities have led several investigators to suggest an anatomical correlation between the regional pathology in AD and the symptomatology of this disorder. Van Hoesen and colleagues have pointed out that the cell pathology observed in the entorhinal cortex in AD isolates the hippocampus from both input and output pathways essential for memory (Hyman et al., 1984). This study was extended to demonstrate the involvement of the perforant pathway (a principal route of cortical input to hippocampus) and the depletion of the neurotransmitter, glutamate, at the terminal zone of this pathway (Hyman et al., 1986, 1987). It has long been appreciated that the maximal involvement of cortical and subcortical regions in AD is found in the entorhinal cortex, the medial amygdala, and the hippocampal formation; the former two and the prepyriform cortex, which is also involved extensively in AD (Reyes et al., 1987), receive most of the output from the olfactory bulb and are considered primary and secondary olfactory cortex. Arguing that the pathological process in AD could be expected to progress along certain corticocortical fibers, either orthograde or retrograde, from some origin, Pearson *et al.* (1985) suggested that the distribution of pathologic features reflected this connectivity and that the maximal severity in olfactory regions indicated a primary involvement of the olfactory pathway in this disorder. The occurrence of NFT in the olfactory bulb in AD (Esiri and Wilcock, 1984) and the existence of olfactory deficits in AD (Serby *et al.*, 1985; Rezek, 1987) further support this contention. That AD may well begin in the nose was the subject of a speculative review by Roberts (1986).

1.3. Iron and Iron Transport Proteins in Neurodegenerative Diseases

A role of oxygen-derived radicals in processes involved in both aging and neurodegenerative disorders has long been considered, and the participation of catalytic forms of iron in such phenomena is generally assumed (for a review of mechanisms and substrates, see Halliwell and Gutteridge, 1986). A redistribution of iron in the cerebral cortex in AD, specifically into glia associated with NP, has been reported (Hallgren and Sourander, 1960) and recently confirmed (Switzer *et al.*, 1986). The contribution of iron and free radicals as major pathogenetic factors in the initiation or formation of NFT and/or NP does not seem to have been further considered; the high level of oxidative activity in neuritic plaques and the presence of iron would be expected to favor such reactions. The initial purpose of the present study was to investigate the role of iron and of iron-transport and iron-storage proteins in the pathogenesis of AD. The unexpected finding of large quantities of the iron-binding protein of external secretions, lactoferrin, in specific association with NFT and NP in the AD brain (Osmand and Switzer, 1987), has been further characterized and is the subject of this report.

2. METHODS

2.1. Patients, Tissue Sources, and Routine Histological Methods

Brains from AD and control cases were perfused at autopsy and stored in buffered formalin before sectioning. Diagnosis of AD was based on the presence of premortem dementia and postmortem histopathological evaluation, using established criteria (McKhann *et al.*, 1984); control cases were from nondemented individuals without significant numbers of NFT or NP (Table I). In addition, two Down's syndrome (DS) cases that had been confirmed cytogenetically and two DS cases obtained from the University of Virginia Brain Bank were studied.

Coronally cut slabs of tissue from the left hemisphere were taken to include the region between the anterior commissure and the mamillary bodies; blocks were cut to include portions of temporal, entorhinal, and insular cortex and of amygdala, hippocampal formation, thalamus, hypothalamus, and basal ganglia. These blocks were equilibrated with 10% ethanol in 10% formalin and 40-μm sections cut on a freezing microtome. Near adjacent sections were stained for NP and NFT with thioflavin S and a modified silver stain (Campbell *et al.*, 1987), iron was detected with a modified Perls stain (Hill and Switzer, 1984), and neurons were stained with thionin.

TABLE I. Lactoferrin Immunoreactivity in Normal
and Alzheimer's Disease Brain Tissue

Group	Sex	N	Age (years)	Postmortem interval (hr)	Lactoferrin immunoreactivity[a]
Alzheimer's disease	M	12	76 ± 5	16.2 ± 6	11/12
	F	19	75 ± 9	15.7 ± 7	17/19
Controls	M	8	72 ± 6	10.5 ± 6	3/8[b]
	F	8	75 ± 12	18.5 ± 9	0/8
Down's syndrome		4	17,21,24,59	—	1/4[c]

[a]As defined in text.
[b]Weak neuronal or glial staining in atypical regions; no NP or NFT.
[c]59-year-old patient: dense staining limited to amygdala.

2.2. Immunohistochemical Staining of Brain Tissue

The following antisera were obtained from commercial sources and used as described below at the indicated dilution: affinity-purified rabbit antihuman lactoferrin (Jackson ImmunoResearch Laboratories, West Grove, Pennsylvania), 1:500; rabbit antihuman ferritin (Accurate Chemical and Scientific, Westbury, New York), 1:10,000; rabbit antiglial fibrillary acidic protein (Dako Corporation, Santa Barbara, California), 1:5000; species-specific biotinylated affinity-purified anti-immunoglobulin antibodies and Vectastain avidin–biotin-complex kits were obtained from Vector Laboratories (Burlingame, California); alkaline phosphatase and horseradish peroxidase (HRP)-conjugated antibodies to mouse IgM were obtained from BioRad Laboratories (Richmond, California). The monoclonal mouse IgM antibody, Alz-50 (Wolozin et al., 1986), was generously provided by Dr. P. Davies as a cell-free culture supernatant and was used at a dilution of 1:20 to 1:50.

All steps were performed on free-floating sections with gentle rotatory agitation. Tissue sections were incubated briefly in 0.2% Triton X-100 and 3% hydrogen peroxide to permeabilize the tissue and limit endogenous peroxidase activity. Sections were incubated for 24–48 hr at 0–4°C with appropriate dilutions of polyclonal antibodies in a 0.01 M phosphate-buffered saline (PBS), at pH 7.4, containing 0.3% Triton X-100, 2.5 mg/ml λ-carrageenan and 0.5 mg/ml sodium azide. After extensive washing with PBS, bound primary antibodies were detected with the Vectastain ABC method using alkaline phosphatase (blue) or HRP (red-brown) reagent kits exactly as described by the manufacturer. After further washes, sections were mounted and dried and processed for light microscopy. Detection of the A68 protein with the Alz-50 monoclonal antibody was performed as described by Wolozin et al. (1986).

Immunochemical specificity was confirmed where possible by inhibition with purified antigen and implied by the sensitivity of the reactivity of all antisera at high dilution; additional controls included the substitution of normal sera at the first step or the exclusion of any single immunochemical reagent at subsequent steps.

2.3. Lactoferrin Binding to Brain Sections

To demonstrate the presence of lactoferrin binding sites in AD and normal brain tissue, 40-μm sections were incubated with highly purified lactoferrin at 1–100 μg/ml for 1 hr in 0.15 M sodium chloride containing 0.01 M Tris (pH 7.4), 0.2% Triton-X100, and 5% normal goat serum; washed three times with buffer; and stained for lactoferrin as described above.

3. RESULTS

3.1. Lactoferrin and Markers of AD Brain

During a study of the distribution of iron and of iron-storage and iron-transport proteins in the brain in AD, the unexpected presence of lactoferrin immunoreactivity was observed. This study has been extended to include more than 30 AD cases, 16 control cases, and 4 Down's brain samples (see Table I). In 28 of 31 AD cases, reactivity with antilactoferrin antibody was seen to various degrees. Prominent laminar staining of NFT and granular staining of NP in entorhinal cortex and medial amygdala (Fig. 1) was seen in most cases. In several cases, staining of the lesions approached the density of silver stains of near adjacent sections and detected an equal number of NP; however, many neurons appeared to contain lactoferrin-positive tangles but failed to react with selective silver stains (Fig. 1). Weak reactivity with thioflavin S confirmed the neurofibrillary nature of these tangled cells.

Some cases showed reactions in other cortical regions examined; where present, lactoferrin immunoreactivity with NFT and NP in temporal and insular cortex was mostly limited to occasional staining of NP, particularly at the base of the collateral and other temporal and insular sulci. Dense staining of NFT in entorhinal cortex occurred both in the clusters of tangled stellate cells in layer II and in the smaller tangled pyramidal cells in layer IV. No correlations were noted between the apparent density of staining and the age of the patient or the duration of the disease; each of the cases depicted in Fig. 1 had a history of dementia before death, spanning 2–12 years.

Except in three cases of weak atypical staining of a few cortical neurons and glia, normal human tissue failed to exhibit immunoreactivity for lactoferrin in brain parenchyma (data not shown). Additional immunochemical controls, excluding or substituting reagents, were uniformly negative; antigenic inhibition with purified lactoferrin was complicated by the ability of lactoferrin–antilactoferrin immune complexes to bind to brain tissue; however, following preincubation of brain tissue with excess lactoferrin and thorough washing, a stoichiometric amount of pure lactoferrin was adequate to provide specific inhibition of affinity-purified rabbit antibody. In all cases studied thus far, the presence of iron in plaques closely followed the distribution of ferritin and was largely seen in microglia associated with NP; the astrogliosis

$\longrightarrow$

FIGURE 1. Lactoferrin (b,d,f) and silver (a,c,e) staining of amygdala and entorhinal cortex of AD brain. Case 1 (a,b) demonstrated lactoferrin immunoreactivity in NP in amygdala and adjacent cortex and in clusters of stellate neurons in entorhinal cortex (b, arrows). Case 2 (c,d) showed diffuse staining for lactoferrin of neurons throughout amygdala with an approximately equivalent number of NP in both fields. Case 3 (e,f) demonstrated pronounced lactoferrin immunoreactivity in stellate cell clusters (f) that were unreactive with silver stain (e); a few tangled neurons were visible in this field (arrows); NP were present in both layers I and IV. NP, neuritic plaques. (a–d) Bars = 1000 μm. (e,f) Bars = 200 μm.

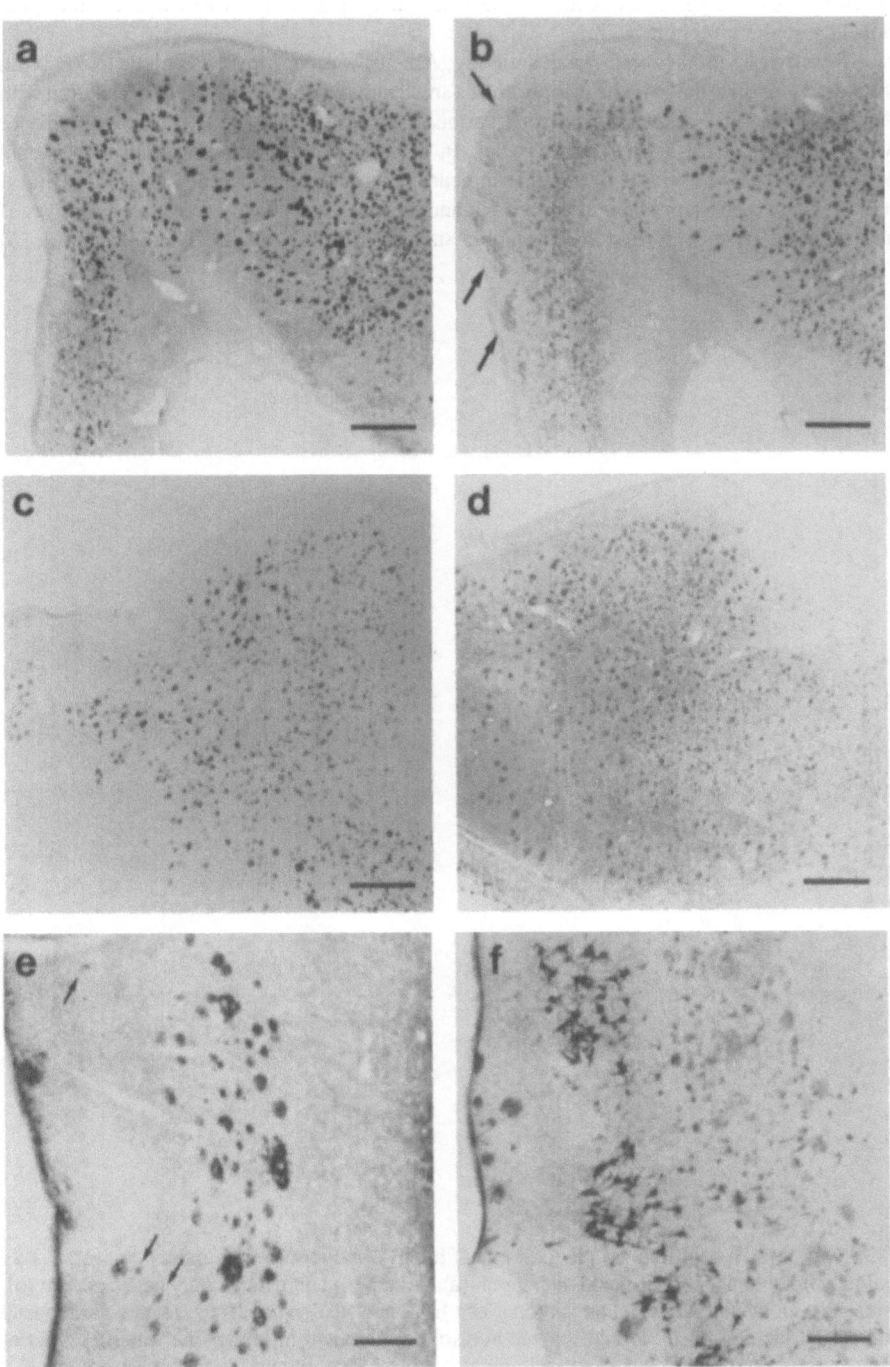

investing the outer perimeter of mature NP was readily demonstrated with antiserum to glial fibrillary acidic protein (Fig. 2).

Reactivity with the monoclonal antibody, Alz-50, was confirmed as unique to AD brain tissue and was distributed in the cytoplasm of a small number of neurons and in association with the tangles in NFT-containing neurons variously in cortex, amygdala, nucleus basalis of Meynert, and certain hypothalamic nuclei. In contrast to the limited staining of neuronal perikarya, Alz-50 reactivity was visible in neurites throughout temporal and insular cortex, with frequent aggregation in and around NP and an apparent laminar preference for layers II and IV/V of most regions studied. Double staining with Alz-50 and Lactoferrin (Fig. 3)

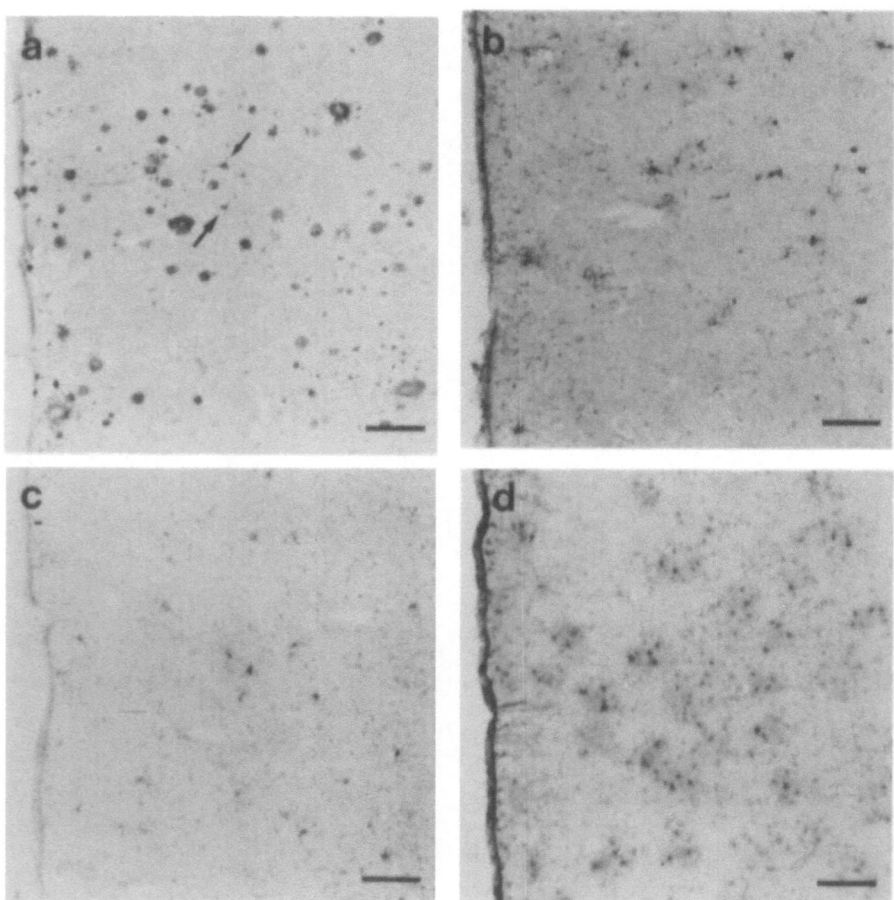

FIGURE 2. Markers of neuritic plaques in AD brain. Parahippocampal cortex in case 3 was stained immunohistochemically for lactoferrin (a), ferritin (b), and glial fibrillary acidic protein (d), and with a modified Perls reaction for iron (Fe^{3+}). NP and NFT (arrows) in all layers were readily stained for lactoferrin (a); ferritin (b) and iron (c) codistributed in (micro)glia within NP; astrogliosis was evident in all layers (d) with large astrocytes appearing to surround plaques. AD, Alzheimer's disease; NFT, neurofibrillary tangles; NP, neuritic plaques. Bars = 200 μm.

indicated that very few NFT reactive with antilactoferrin antibody also stained for Alz-50. The Alz-50-reactive neurites in NP appeared distinct from the distribution of lactoferrin.

Four cases of Down's syndrome were also studied. One (from a 59-year-old) reacted significantly with antibody to lactoferrin and with Alz-50 (see Table I; Fig. 4). In this case, only a limited sample of temporal lobe was available and lactoferrin immunoreactivity was restricted to plaques in the amygdala and adjacent pyriform cortex, while Alz-50 reactivity extended to parahippocampal cortex. Of the three other cases studied, none contained features immunoreactive for lactoferrin, although two (21 and 24 years) were shown by silver staining to contain immature plaques throughout the temporal lobe.

3.2. Lactoferrin Binding in Normal and AD Brain Tissue

The presence of high-affinity binding sites in pyramidal neurons in cortex was revealed by preincubation of sections of normal and AD brain with low concentrations of lactoferrin. Binding occurred at concentrations as low as 1 μg/ml in the presence of both exogenous (serum) protein and nonionic detergent and was resistant to extensive washing. Apparent saturation of binding was not observed at the highest concentrations tested (100 μg/ml), suggesting considerable heterogeneity of binding sites. As shown in Fig. 5, association was primarily selective for the perikarya of pyramidal neurons and maximal to larger neurons, notably in layer II of entorhinal cortex and in the nucleus basalis. An increased immunoreactivity with antibody was not seen in NP or NFT in AD brain after preincubation with lactoferrin, although binding of lactoferrin to residual intact neurons was present (Fig. 5).

4. DISCUSSION

These studies demonstrate for the first time the concomitant occurrence of lactoferrin immunoreactivity within the lesions of AD; without a comprehensive study of brain tissue from patients with other neurodegenerative disorders, the specificity of this association cannot be established. Age-matched controls included two cases of parkinsonism, one of which was weakly reactive. Although the presence of intact lactoferrin *per se* has not been formally proved, the reactivity with multiple antisera at high dilution, stoichiometric inhibition with pure lactoferrin, and the demonstration of high-affinity binding sites in normal neurons argue strongly for the presence of this protein. The use of monoclonal or polyclonal antibodies to different epitopes or regions of lactoferrin and direct immunoassay of native or extracted tissue should provide the necessary verification. In this discussion, the presence of native lactoferrin will be assumed, although neither fragmentation during deposition nor spurious antigenic cross-reactivity can be precluded.

Lactoferrin (lactotransferrin) and serum transferrin (serotransferrin) are homologous proteins of 75,000–80,000 M_r with two metal binding sites on each molecule, and the three-dimensional structure of lactoferrin has been determined at 3.2-Å resolution (Anderson *et al.*, 1987), comparative studies indicate that the magnitude of the iron binding constant of lactoferrin is more than 200 times greater than that of transferrin (Aisen and Liebman, 1972). It is therefore considered unlikely that lactoferrin functions as an iron-transport protein, although it has been shown to mediate iron uptake by cells of the reticuloendothelial system (RES) (Moguilevsky *et al.*, 1987). However, iron taken up in this manner is incorporated into ferritin following intralysosomal degradation, rather than entering the cytoplasmic pool of available iron. Lactoferrin is a principal protein of mucosecretory surfaces (Masson *et al.*,

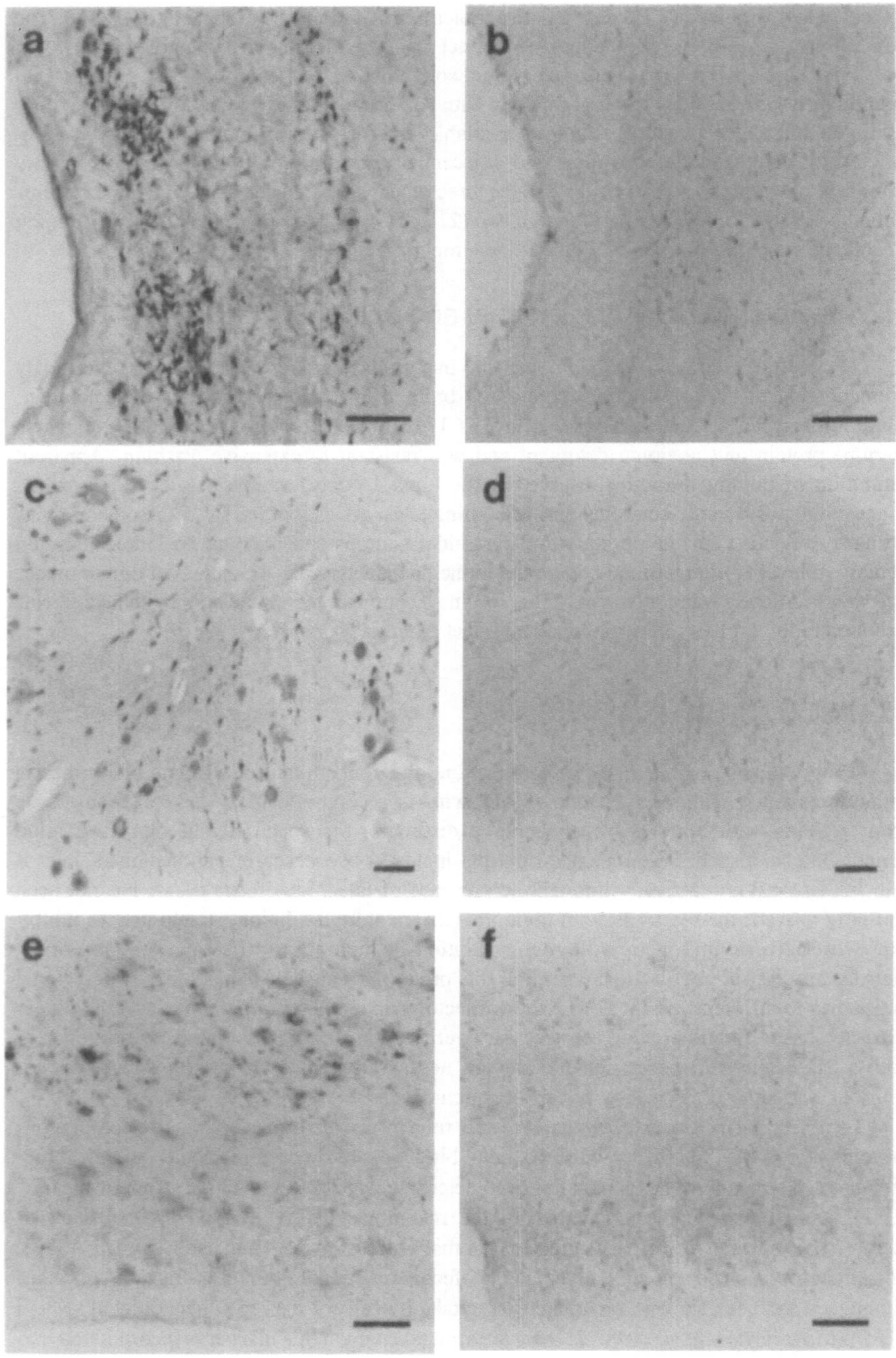

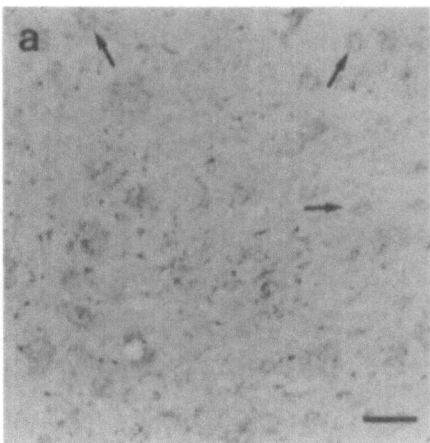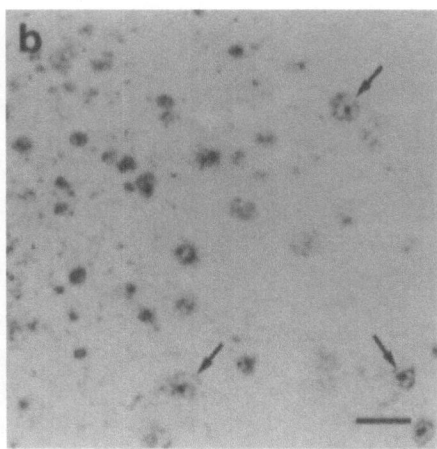

FIGURE 4. Alz-50 (a) and lactoferrin (b) in the amygdala of a 59-year-old patient (case 5) with Down's syndrome. Alz-50 was seen in neurons and neurites throughout the medial amygdala, with an apparent accumulation in the periphery of NP (a, arrows). Lactoferrin was present in both NP and NFT, but NP stained with an uncharacteristic granular distribution (b, arrows). NFT, neurofibrillary tangles; NP, neuritic plaques. Bars = 200 μm.

1966) and is only otherwise found in the specific granules of polymorphonuclear leukocytes (Masson *et al.*, 1969). In secretions, apolactoferrin is believed to function as a bacteriostatic agent by depriving micro-organisms of essential iron, while in neutrophils there is direct evidence for a critical role for lactoferrin in radical-dependent cytotoxic mechanisms (Ambruso and Johnston, 1981; Vercellotti *et al.*, 1985). The expression of neutrophil lactoferrin appears to be developmentally regulated and unique to this hematopoietic cell lineage (Rado *et al.*, 1987); synthesis of lactoferrin in the mouse uterus has been shown to be inducible by estrogens (Pentecost and Teng, 1987).

4.1. Neuroanatomical Distribution of Lactoferrin

The presence of lactoferrin immunoreactivity in neuritic plaques and neurofibrillary tangles in AD could arise by several mechanisms. First, lactoferrin may be synthesized in pyramidal neurons, either by induction of transcription and translation of lactoferrin mes-

←——

FIGURE 3. Relative distribution of lactoferrin (a,c,e) and Alz-50 (b,d,f) in three cases of AD were distinctive. In the entorhinal cortex of case 1, the characteristically lactoferrin-positive stellate cells in layer II and NFT in layer IV (a) were rarely reactive for Alz-50; both layers, however, contain numerous Alz-50-positive neurites (b). The CA1 region of hippocampus in case 3 contained numerous cells and NP immunoreactive for both lactoferrin (c) and Alz-50 (d); double immunohistochemical staining of these regions showed that these were different cell populations (data not shown). NP and NFT in temporal cortex of case 4 showed weaker staining for lactoferrin (e); the characteristic laminar distribution of Alz-50-positive neurites and few Alz-50 reactive neurons were also visible (f). AD, Alzheimer's disease; NFT, neurofibrillary tangles; NP, neuritic plaques. Bars = 200 μm.

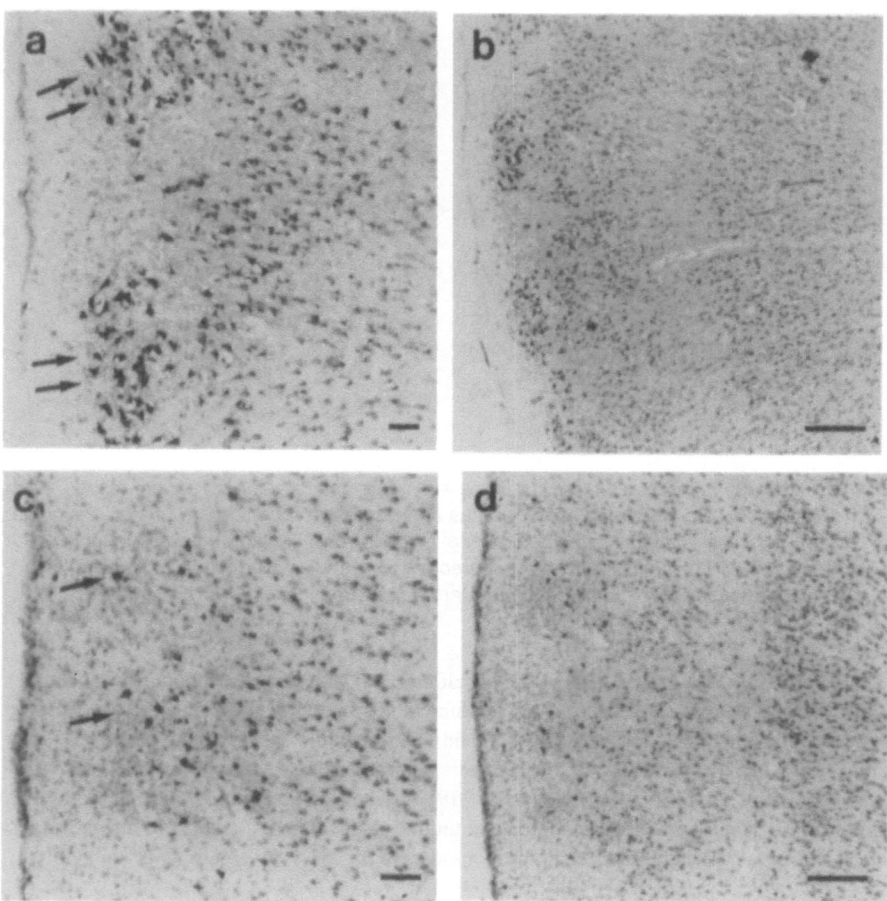

FIGURE 5. Preincubation of normal (a,b) and AD brain (c,d) tissue with lactoferrin demonstrated widespread uptake by pyramidal neurons and a weak reactivity with glia. Case 6, a 78-year-old normal patient, showed dense staining of clusters of stellate cells in entorhinal cortex (a, double arrows). In AD (63-year-old patient), uptake is reduced, as fewer neurons are present in outer layers of cortex (d); a few surviving stellate cells in layer II of entorhinal cortex were able to bind lactoferrin (c, arrows). AD, Alzheimer's disease. Bars = 200 μm.

senger RNA (mRNA) or by translation of exogenous mRNA taken up from transsynaptic transport; these are considered unlikely as cytoplasmic staining of neuronal perikarya has not been detected. Second, lactoferrin may be taken up by neurons or NP and NFT from plasma-derived protein diffusing into brain; indeed, lactoferrin is present in plasma, although at very low concentrations, exceeding 10 ng/ml only during episodes of neutrophil degranulation associated with systemic inflammatory reactions. Although staining for lactoferrin of the endothelium of blood vessels was occasionally observed, the avid uptake of this protein by cells of the RES (Moguilevsky *et al.*, 1987) makes this an improbable source. Finally, lactoferrin may be transported, presumably transynaptically, to certain neurons during a critical stage of their degeneration; tight interaction of this protein with structural elements involved in the formation of NFT and in the matrix of NP would facilitate the incorporation of lactoferrin as a "decorative" component of these lesions. The detection of high-avidity binding sites for lactoferrin in the large pyramidal cells involved in AD and the neuroanatomical distribution of the NFT and NP that contain lactoferrin strongly support this hypothesis.

The cogent arguments placed by Pearson *et al.* (1985) concerning the relevance of the regional involvement and connectivities of the pathological changes in AD to the sequential pathogenesis of the disease are particularly relevant here. The presence of lactoferrin in NP and NFT in basal nuclei of amygdala and pyriform cortex, in NFT of stellate neurons in layer II of entorhinal cortex, and in NP in entorhinal cortex and hippocampal formation can be logically accounted for by retrograde transport from the olfactory mucosa where the protein is present at high concentrations (Masson *et al.*, 1966). The regions in AD brain in which lactoferrin is regularly detectable receive most of the primary and secondary projections of the olfactory bulb. Additional regions of the brain that have been indicated as primary targets of pathology in AD, including the nucleus basalis, the dorsal raphe, and the locus ceruleus, each have major projections to the areas of lactoferrin involvement, and some have additional projections to the olfactory formation. Most importantly, the corticocortical input and output fibers of the entorhinal cortex pass from and to precisely those areas of temporal, parietal, frontal, and cingulate cortex that are secondarily involved in AD (Pearson *et al.*, 1985).

4.2. Implications for the Etiology of Alzheimer's Disease

Implicit in these assertions is a potential role for an intrinsic or extrinsic dysfunction of the olfactory tract as a principal component of AD. Interestingly, asymmetries have been recently described in the distribution of NFTs in hippocampus and entorhinal cortex (Moossy *et al.*, 1988), precisely as would be expected if the disease progressed along certain fiber pathways from some focus in the olfactory system. The presence of quantities of lactoferrin in the lesions of AD patients independent of the duration of clinical disease would suggest an early participation of this pathway. It is possible that the presence of lactoferrin demonstrates a general breakdown in the integrity of transport mechanisms within and between neurons of the olfactory tract and cortex, beginning perhaps in sensory neurons of the olfactory epithelium. If this sequence is initiated in the olfactory mucosa, the presence of characteristic morphological changes might provide a valuable marker (and diagnostic) for an early stage in AD.

4.3. Potential Role for Lactoferrin in the Pathogenesis of Alzheimer's Disease

The absence of lactoferrin from the plaques and NFT in many regions of brain indicates that this protein is clearly not essential for their formation; however, the ability of lactoferrin to participate in oxygen radical production raises the possibility that iron and lactoferrin may be involved in early and possibly critical steps in the pathogenesis of AD. Such reactivity would be independent of whether the lactoferrin was exogenously derived or had been synthesized within the neurons. It has not escaped our notice that the metal ion binding functions of lactoferrin and its apparent redistribution in AD could provide a transport mechanism for aluminum or other metal ions or their compounds from the environment to those regions of brain initially involved in AD. The uptake of aluminum from the nasal cavity, apparently via the olfactory tract, has been experimentally demonstrated (Perl and Good, 1987).

ACKNOWLEDGMENTS. This work was supported by grants from the Robert H. and Monica Cole Foundation and the Alzheimer's Disease and Related Disorders Association (ADRDA) and by grant NS-23634 from the National Institutes of Health (NINCDS). We are grateful to the staff and residents of the Department of Pathology, University of Tennessee Medical Center, to the Cole Foundation and to the Eastern Tennessee chapter of the ADRDA for support of the AD autopsy program. Additional tissue was generously provided by the University of Virginia Brain Bank. Dr. Peter Davies, Albert Einstein College of Medicine, New York, kindly provided Alz-50 monoclonal antibody. The excellent technical assistance of S. K. Campbell, J. A. Donovan, and S. Karné is gratefully acknowledged.

REFERENCES

Aisen, P., and Liebman, A., 1972, Lactoferrin and transferrin: A comparative study, *Biochim. Biophys. Acta* **257:**314–323.

Ambruso, D. R., and Johnston, R. B., Jr., 1981, Lactoferrin enhances hydroxyl radical production by human neutrophils, neutrophil particulate fractions, and an enzymatic generating system, *J. Clin. Invest.* **67:**352–360.

Anderson, B. F., Baker, H. M., Dodson, E. J., Norris, G. E., Rumball, S. V., Waters, J. M., and Baker, E. N., 1987, Structure of human lactoferrin at 3.2-Å resolution, *Proc. Natl. Acad. Sci. USA* **84:**1769–1773.

Bondareff, W., Mountjoy, C. Q., and Roth, M., 1982, Loss of neurons of origin of the adrenergic projection to cerebral cortex (nucleus locus ceruleus) in senile dementia, *Neurology (NY)* **32:**164–168.

Bondareff, W., Mountjoy, C. Q., Roth, M., Rossor, M. N., Iversen, L. L., and Reynolds, G. P., 1987, Age and histopathologic heterogeneity in Alzheimer's disease, *Arch Gen. Psychiatry* **44:**412–417.

Campbell, S. K., Switzer, R. C. III, and Martin, T. L., 1987, Alzheimer's plaques and tangles: A controlled and enhanced method, *Soc. Neurosci. Abst.* **13:**678.

Cook-Deegan, R. M., and Whitehouse, P. J., 1987, Alzheimer's disease and dementia: The looming crisis, *Issues Sci. Technol.* **1987:**52–63.

Crapper, D. R., Krishnan, S. S., and Dalton, A. J., 1973, Brain aluminum distribution in Alzheimer's disease and experimental neurofibrillary degeneration, *Science* **180:**511–513.

Davies, P., and Maloney, A. J. F., 1976, Selective loss of central cholinergic neurons in Alzheimer's disease (Letter to the editor), *Lancet* **2:**1403.

Esiri, M. M., and Wilcock, G. K., 1984, The olfactory bulbs in Alzheimer's disease, *J. Neurol. Neurosurg. Psychiatry* **47:**56–60.

Guiroy, D. C., Miyazaki, M., Multhaup, G., Fischer, P., Garruto, R. M., Beyreuther, K., Masters, C. L., Simms, G., Gibbs, C. J., Jr., and Gajdusek, D. C., 1987, Amyloid of neurofibrillary tangles of Guamanian parkinsonism-dementia and Alzheimer disease share identical amino acid sequence, *Proc. Natl. Acad. Sci. USA* **84:**2073–2077.

Hallgren, B., and Sourander, P., 1960, The non-haem iron in the cerebral cortex in Alzheimer's disease, *J. Neurochem.* **5:**307–310.

Halliwell, B., and Gutteridge, J. M., 1986, Oxygen free radicals and iron in relation to biology and medicine: Some problems and concepts (Invited paper), *Arch. Biochem. Biophys.* **246:**501–514.

Hill, J. M., and Switzer, R. C. III, 1984, The regional distribution and cellular localization of iron in the rat brain, *Neuroscience* **11:**595–603.

Hyman, B. T., Van Hoesen, G. W., Damasio, A. R., and Barnes, C. L., 1984, Alzheimer's disease: Cell-specific pathology isolates the hippocampal formation, *Science* **225:**1168–1170.

Hyman, B. T., Van Hoesen, G. W., Kromer, L. J., and Damasio, A. R., 1986, Perforant pathway changes and the memory impairment of Alzheimer's disease, *Ann. Neurol.* **20**:472–481.

Hyman, B. T., Van Hoesen, G. W., and Damasio, A. R., 1987, Alzheimer's disease: Glutamate depletion in the hippocampal perforant pathway zone, *Ann. Neurol.* **22**:37–40.

Hyman, B. T., Van Hoesen, G. W., Wolozin, B. L., Davies, P., Kromer, L. J., and Damasio, A. R., 1988, Alz-50 antibody recognizes Alzheimer-related neuronal changes, *Ann. Neurol.* **23**:371–379.

Kang, J., Lemaire, H.-G., Unterbeck, A., Salbaum, J. M., Masters, C. L., Grzeschik, K.-H., Multhaup, G., Beyreuther, K., and Müller-Hill, B., 1987, The precursor of Alzheimer's disease amyloid A4 protein resembles a cell-surface receptor, *Nature (Lond.)* **325**:733–736.

Katzman, R., Terry, R., DeTeresa, R., Brown, T., Davies, P., Fuld, P., Renbing, X., and Peck, A., 1988, Clinical, pathological, and neurochemical changes in dementia: A subgroup with preserved mental status and numerous neocortical plaques, *Ann. Neurol.* **23**:138–144.

Kitaguchi, N., Takahashi, Y., Tokushima, Y., Shiojiri, S., and Ito, H., 1988, Novel precursor of Alzheimer's disease amyloid protein shows protease inhibitory activity, *Nature (Lond.)* **331**:530–532.

Kowall, N. W., and Kosik, K. S., 1987, Axonal disruption and aberrant localization of tau protein characterize the neuropil pathology of Alzheimer's disease, *Ann. Neurol.* **22**:639–643.

Masson, P. L., Heremans, J. F., and Dive, C., 1966, An iron-binding protein common to many external secretions, *Clin. Chim. Acta* **14**:735–739.

Masson, P. L., Heremans, J. F., and Schonne, E., 1969, Lactoferrin, an iron-binding protein in neutrophilic leukocytes, *J. Exp. Med.* **130**:643–658.

McKhann, G., Drachman, D., Folstein, M., Katzman, R., Price, D., and Stadlan, E. M., 1984, Clinical diagnosis of Alzheimer's disease: Report of the NINCDS–ADRDA work group under the auspices of Department of Health and Human Services Task Force on Alzheimer's disease, *Neurology (NY)* **34**:939–944.

Miller, C. A., Rudnicka, M., Hinton, D. R., Blanks, J. C., and Kozlowski, M., 1987, Monoclonal antibody identification of subpopulations of cerebral cortical neurons affected in Alzheimer disease, *Proc. Natl. Acad. Sci. USA* **84**:8657–8661.

Miller, C. C., and Anderton, B. H., 1986, Transglutaminase and the neuronal cytoskeleton in Alzheimer's disease, *J. Neurochem.* **46**:1912–1922.

Moguilevsky, N., Masson, P.-L., and Courtoy, P.-J., 1987, Lactoferrin uptake and iron processing into macrophages: A study in familial haemochromatosis, *Br. J. Haematol.* **66**:129–136.

Moossy, J., Zubenko, G. S., Martinez, A. J., and Rao, G. R., 1988, Bilateral symmetry of morphologic lesions in Alzheimer's disease, *Arch. Neurol.* **45**:251–254.

Nukina, N., Kosik, K. S., and Selkoe, D. J., 1987, Recognition of Alzheimer paired helical filaments by monoclonal neurofilament antibodies is due to crossreaction with tau protein, *Proc. Natl. Acad. Sci. USA* **84**:3415–3419.

Osmand, A. P., and Switzer, R. C. III, 1987, Lactoferrin immunoreactivity in neuritic plaques and neurofibrillary tangles in Alzheimer's disease: Localization to the rhinencephalon and adjacent cortex, *Soc. Neurosci. Abst.* **13**:1149.

Pearson, R. C. A., Esiri, M. M., Hiorns, R. W., Wilcock, G. K., and Powell, T. P. S., 1985, Anatomical correlates of the distribution of the pathological changes in the neocortex in Alzheimer disease, *Proc. Natl. Acad. Sci. USA* **82**:4531–4534.

Pentecost, B. T., and Teng, C. T., 1987, Lactotransferrin is the major estrogen inducible protein of mouse uterine secretions, *J. Biol. Chem.* **262**:10134–10139.

Perl, D. P., and Good, P. F., 1987, Uptake of aluminum into central nervous system along nasal-olfactory pathways, *Lancet* **1**:1028.

Ponte, P., Gonzalez-DeWhitt, P., Schilling, J., Miller, J., Hsu, D., Greenberg, B., Davis, K., Wallace, W., Lieberburg, I., Fuller, F., and Cordell, B., 1988, A new A4 amyloid mRNA contains a domain homologous to serine proteinase inhibitors, *Nature (Lond.)* **331**:525–527.

Rado, T. A., Wei, X., and Benz, E. J., Jr., 1987, Isolation of lactoferrin cDNA from a human myeloid library and expression of mRNA during normal and leukemic myelopoiesis, *Blood* **70**:989–993.

Reyes, P. F., Golden, G. T., Fagel, P. L., Fariello, R. G., Katz, L., and Carner, E., 1987, The prepiriform cortex in dementia of the Alzheimer type, *Arch. Neurol.* **44:**644–645.

Rezek, D. L., 1987, Olfactory deficits as a neurologic sign in dementia of the Alzheimer type, *Arch. Neurol.* **44:**1030–1032.

Roberts, E., 1986, Alzheimer's disease may begin in the nose and may be caused by alumniosilicates, *Neurobiol. Aging* **7:**561–567.

Serby, M., Corwin, J., Conrad, P., and Rotrosen, J., 1985, Olfactory dysfunction in Alzheimer's disease and Parkinson's disease (Letter to the editor), *Am. J. Psychiatry* **142:**781–782.

Switzer, R. C. III, Martin, T. L., Campbell, S. K., Parker, J. C., and Caldwell, E. D., 1986, Iron and ferritin in the neuritic plaques of Alzheimer's disease, *Soc. Neurosci. Abst.* **12:**100.

Tanzi, R. E., McClatchey, A. I., Lamperti, E. D., Villa-Komaroff, L., Gusella, J. F., and Neve, R. L., 1988, Protease inhibitor domain encoded by an amyloid protein precursor mRNA associated with Alzheimer's disease, *Nature (Lond.)* **331:**528–530.

Terry, R. D., 1985, Alzheimer's disease, in: *Textbook of Neuropathology* (R. L. Davis and D. M. Robertson, eds.), Williams & Wilkins, Baltimore, pp. 824–841.

Ulrich, J., 1985, Alzheimer changes in nondemented patients younger than sixty-five: Possible early stages of Alzheimer's disease and senile dementia of Alzheimer type, *Ann. Neurol.* **17:**273–277.

Vercellotti, G. M., van Asbeck, B. S., and Jacob, H. S., 1985, Oxygen radical-induced erythrocyte hemolysis by neutrophils. Critical role of iron and lactoferrin, *J. Clin. Invest.* **76:**956–962.

Whitehouse, P. J., Price, D. L., Clark, A. W., Coyle, J. T., and DeLong, M. R., 1981, Alzheimer's disease: Evidence for selective loss of cholinergic neurons in the nucleus basalis, *Ann. Neurol.* **10:**122–126.

Wolozin, B., and Davies, P., 1987, Alzheimer-related neuronal protein A68: Specificity and distribution, *Ann. Neurol.* **22:**521–526.

Wolozin, B. L., Pruchnicki, A., Dickson, D. W., and Davies, P., 1986, A neuronal antigen in the brains of Alzheimer patients, *Science* **232:**648–650.

Wood, J. G., Mirra, S. S., Pollock, N. J., and Binder, L. I., 1986, Neurofibrillary tangles of Alzheimer disease share antigenic determinants with the axonal microtubule-associated protein tau (τ), *Proc. Natl. Acad. Sci. USA* **83:**4040–4043.

Yamamoto, T., and Hirano, A., 1985, Nucleus raphe dorsalis in Alzheimer's disease: Neurofibrillary tangles and loss of large neurons, *Ann. Neurol.* **17:**573–577.

10

Immunological Investigation of Thymic-Dependent Immunity in Normal Aging and in Patients with Senile Dementia of Alzheimer Type

GIANCARLO SAVORANI, GABRIELE SARTI, AFRO SALSI,
FRANCESCO CAVAZZUTI, LUCIO ZANICHELLI,
GIUSEPPE TUCCI, EUGENIO MOCCHEGIANI,
NICOLA FABRIS, MARIELLA CHIRICOLO,
and FEDERICO LICASTRO

1. INTRODUCTION

Alzheimer's disease (AD) is a primary degenerative and progressive form of dementia with an insidious onset (Amaducci and Sorbi, 1985; Gottfries, 1985). With advancing age, an increasing prevalence of AD has been observed. In industrialized countries, approximately 6% of people over 65 years, 22% of those over 80 years, and 40% of the elderly over 90 years of age are affected by this debilitating illness (Henderson, 1986).

In Italy, according to a recent survey, an increase of about 40% in the prevalence of the disease has been calculated for 1980–2000 (from 419,000 to 586,000 persons) (Amaducci *et al.*, 1986). This increment is very close to that expected in the United States, where this figure reaches 42%. In Japan, projections for the increment of AD prevalence are even more dramatic, reaching 72% (Amaducci and Sorbi, 1985).

These figures have complex and serious social implications, since dementia is the main cause of disability in old age. In fact, patients with AD show a gradual memory loss and

GIANCARLO SAVORANI, GABRIELE SARTI, AFRO SALSI, FRANCESCO CAVAZZUTI, LU-CIO ZANICHELLI, and GIUSEPPE TUCCI • Department of Geriatric Medicine, Malpighi Hospital USL 28, 40138 Bologna, Italy.   EUGENIO MOCCHEGIANI • Gerontology Research Depart-ment, Italian National Research Center on Aging, 60100 Ancona, Italy.   NICOLA FABRIS • Ger-ontology Research Department, Italian National Research Center on Aging, 60100 Ancona, Italy.   MARIELLA CHIRICOLO and FEDERICO LICASTRO • Department of Experimental Pa-thology, University of Bologna, 40126 Bologna, Italy.

intellectual failure with cognitive impairment, as well as changes in personality and behavior that interfere with previous social and working activities (McKhann et al., 1984). However, no changes in consciousness have been reported in this form of dementia (DSM III) (American Psychiatric Association, 1980; McKhann et al., 1984). Clinical diagnosis of AD is very difficult and is only presumptive in vivo (Hollander et al., 1986; Roth, 1986). However, the accuracy in diagnosis has increased considerably after the introduction of more sensitive screening protocols (Nerl et al., 1984; Amaducci and Sorbi, 1985; Wade et al., 1987). Such diagnostic difficulties stem partially from the heterogeneity of this disease. In fact, AD most probably is not a single clinical entity, but rather a complex syndrome that can be divided in different subtypes showing different clinical, neurophysiological, histological, and neurochemical features (Rossor et al., 1984; Mayeux et al., 1985; Roth, 1986; Forte et al., 1988). For instance, it is possible to distinguish an AD form of early onset (AD2) that has an accelerated clinical course with stronger speaking disturbances and a higher deficit of cholinergic neurotransmitters. Also detectable is a second form of AD characterized by late onset (Seltzer and Sherwin, 1983; Rossor et al., 1984). Other identified AD clinical subtypes show the presence of myoclonus or alterations of extrapyramidal neurons (Mayeux et al., 1985). For these reasons, several studies have focused on possible ante mortem markers to improve the accuracy of diagnosis (Nerl et al., 1984; Hollander et al., 1986; Savorani et al., 1986). Some alterations of the immune system have been reported in AD (Tavolato and Argentiero, 1980; MacDonald et al., 1982; Pouplard et al., 1983; Savorani et al., 1986; Gaskin et al., 1987). However, published results on the immune system are discordant, and several discrepancies appear in the literature on this topic (Miller et al., 1981; Skias et al., 1985). This chapter presents data regarding some immune functions of the thymic branch of the immune system in a group of nonfamilial AD patients, and age- and sex-matched controls.

2. MATERIALS AND METHODS

2.1. Subjects

Thirteen patients with senile dementia of Alzheimer type (mean age 74 ± 3 years) and 13 age- and sex-matched controls (mean age 77 ± 3 years) were studied. The controls consisted of either healthy elderly persons living in a retirement home, and/or elderly patients hospitalized with minor pathological alterations that did not interfere with brain or immune functions.

The diagnosis of dementia of Alzheimer type was carried out after careful analysis of patients' personal and familiar records and clinical examination according to the recommendations of DSM III (APA, 1980). Only patients who presented with mental impairment for a period longer than 6 months and scored less than 5 on Hachinski's ischemic score (Hachinski et al., 1975) were selected. Concomitant diseases were excluded after evaluation of results from metabolic parameters, including red blood cell (RBC), white blood cell (WBC) count, hemoglobin (Hb), platelet number, blood urea nitrogen (BUN), glucose, uric acid, creatine, cholesterol, tryglycerides, Na, K, Cl, total protein bilirubin, GOT, GPT, and alkaline phosphatase; electrocardiographs (EKG), chest radiographs, and computed tomography (CT) scans were also evaluated. Hormonal status was evaluated by measuring thyroid-stimulating hormone (TSH), triiodothyronine (T3), thyroxine (T4), oestradiol (OD), luteinizing hormone (LH) follicle-stimulating hormone (FSH), and prolactin (PRL) by commercial radioimmunoassay (RIA) (ARE, Serono Diagnostica Italy).

2.2. Intellectual Performance Tests

Alzheimer's disease patients were examined by performing the Mini Mental State (MMS) test (Folstein *et al.*, 1975). Memory and attention were also evaluated.

2.3. Plasmic Zinc Level

Venous blood was collected in fluorinated plastic tubes in the presence of EDTA. After centrifugation at 4°C and 2000 rpm plasma were collected and samples stored at −80°C. Zinc concentration was measured by atomic adsorption as previously described (Fabris *et al.*, 1984).

2.4. Plasmic Thymulin Level

Thymulin concentration in the plasma was determined by a bioassay as previously described (Fabris *et al.*, 1984). Levels of active and inactive thymulin were measured by the bioassay after the addition of exogenous zinc to plasma samples as described elsewhere (Fabris *et al.*, 1984).

2.5. Isolation of Peripheral Blood Lymphocytes

Blood was collected by venous puncture in plastic tubes containing EDTA. Peripheral blood lymphocytes (PBL) were purified by Ficoll gradient centrifugation (Boyum, 1968). PBL cultures were performed as previously described (Licastro *et al.*, 1983a). Briefly, 1×10^5 lymphocytes were cultured in complete medium consisting of RPMI 1640 containing 10% heat-inactivated pooled AB human serum, 100 U penicillin, 100 μg/ml streptomycin, and 2 mM glutamine (Flow lab). Stimulated lymphocytes were activated by phytohemagglutinin (PHA-P) (Difco: final concentration in complete medium 0.1 or 1 μl/ml) and cultured in a CO_2 incubator for 3 or 4 days. Some lymphocyte cultures were treated with human recombinant interleukin-2 (IL-2) (Boehringwerke: final concentration in complete medium 20 U/ml).

Cell proliferation was assessed by pulsing lymphocytes with tritiated thymidine, ([³H]methylthymidine ([³H]-TdR) (Amersham, England: spec. act. = 5 Ci/mmole) for the last 6 hr of culture.

2.6. Lymphocyte Harvesting and Radioactivity Measurement

At the end of the culture period, lymphocyte cultures were harvested, washed on glass fiber filters with the aid of a multiple cell harvester (Skatron), and [³H]-TdR incorporation measured by liquid scintillation counting as previously described (Franceschi *et al.*, 1981).

3. RESULTS

Results regarding the hormonal profile of AD patients and sex- and age-matched controls are reported in Table I. No statistical differences were found in the two groups studied. Plasma levels of zinc and thymulin in AD patients and controls were also studied; the results are reported in Table II. We did not find any difference in the plasmic concentration of zinc

TABLE I. Hormonal Profile in Healthy
Elderly Patients and in Patients with Senile
Dementia of Alzheimer's Type[a]

		Controls	AD patients
T3	(ng/ml)	1.08 ± 0.2	0.95 ± 0.2
T4	(ng/ml)	64.3 ± 15.3	75.7 ± 14.1
TSH	(μU/ml)	1.7 ± 1.2	2.0 ± 1.6
OD	(pg/ml)	9.1 ± 9.8	4.1 ± 1.1
LH	(mU/ml)	8.1 ± 6.6	7.1 ± 4.9
FSH	(mU/ml)	24.4 ± 25.3	17.3 ± 17.5
PRL	(ng/ml)	2.8 ± 1.3	2.8 ± 1.3

[a]Data are expressed as mean ±1 SD.

between AD patients and controls. The basal levels of thymulin were also comparable in the two groups studied. However, after the addition of exogenous zinc to the plasma samples, the increase in the biological activity of thymulin was higher in controls than in AD patients (Table III). The proliferative activity of circulating lymphocytes after PHA activation was measured. Lymphocyte responses to suboptimal or optimal PHA concentrations were comparable in the two groups (Table IV).

Addition of exogenous human recombinant IL-2 increased suboptimal PHA response of lymphocytes from controls and AD patients as well. No difference was detected in the two groups (Table IV). By contrast, supplementation with IL-2 did not affect lymphocyte responses to optimal PHA dose in both groups (Table IV). However, IL-2 alone was able to induce a small but significant proliferation of peripheral blood lymphocytes. Once again, no differences were observed between the two groups (Table IV).

4. DISCUSSION

A survey of AD mortality data has shown an increased incidence of infectious diseases in the terminal phase of the diseases (Chandra *et al.*, 1986), suggesting an involvement of the immune system in the pathogenesis of this disease (Fudenbergh *et al.*, 1984). An imbalance

TABLE II. Plasma Levels of Zinc
and Thymulin in Healthy Elderly Patients
and in Patients with Senile Dementia
of Alzheimer's Type[a]

Group	N	Zinc (μg/dl)	Thymulin Log$_2$
Controls	13	71 ± 4	2.1 ± 0.24
AD patients	13	76 ± 3	2.6 ± 0.17

[a]Data are expressed as mean ±1 SD.

TABLE III. Biological Activity of Thymulin in Plasma
Samples from Healthy Elderly Patients
and from Patients with Senile Dementia of Alzheimer's
Type after Addition of Exogenous Zinc[a]

Group		Thymulin after zinc addition	
		Log_2	% increase SI[b]
Controls	13	4 ± 0.25	2.10 ± 0.23[c]
AD patients	13	3 ± 0.24	1.25 ± 0.08[c]

[a]Data are expressed as mean ± 1 SD.
[b]SI (stimulation index) = thymulin activity with zinc/thymulin activity without zinc.
[c]$p < 0.01$: Statistical significance according to Student's t-test.

in serum immunoglobulins has been observed in AD patients (Behan and Feldman, 1970; Kalter and Kelly, 1975; Tavolato and Argentiero, 1980), and a decreased responsiveness to polyclonal mitogens has also been reported (Miller et al., 1981; Singh et al., 1987); however, this decreased responsiveness has not been found in other studies (Kalter and Kelly, 1975; MacDonald et al., 1982; Leffell et al., 1985). Contradictory results concerning also T-suppressor cell activity have been found (Miller et al., 1981; Leffell et al., 1985; Skias et al., 1985). More recently, autoantibodies specific for brain antigens have been found in either the sera or the cerebrospinal fluid (CSF) of AD patients (Pouplard et al., 1983; Singh et al., 1986; Gaskin et al., 1987). Interestingly, some of these antibodies appear to react against cells of hypophysis (Pouplard et al., 1983). A recent epidemiological analysis in Italy did not find an increased incidence of viral infectious diseases associated with AD (Amaducci et al., 1986).

The role of the immune system in the pathogenesis of AD is not clearly established; the presence of different clinical groups of the disease may imply a differential involvement of the immune system.

TABLE IV. Proliferative Activity of Peripheral Blood Lymphocytes
from Five Healthy Elderly and Six Patients with Senile Dementia
of Alzheimer's Type after Activation with PHA, with or without
Addition of Exogenous Human Recombinant IL-2

	Controls	AD patients
No mitogen	262 ± 30[a]	266 ± 118
PHA 0.1 μl/ml	13,762 ± 2,290	16,367 ± 6,547
+ IL-2[b]	25,336 ± 3,763	30,724 ± 3,084
PHA 1 μl/ml	30,636 ± 2,147	47,505 ± 8,132
+ IL-2[b]	29,633 ± 6,429	42,354 ± 7,880
IL-2	7,657 ± 692	10,267 ± 2,744

[a]Data refer to incorporation of [^{3}H]-TdR measured as cpm (mean of four replicas ±1 SD).
[b]IL-2 final concentration: 20 U/ml.

Immune functions, particularly those belonging to the thymus branch of the immunity, decrease with advancing age in normal elderly persons (Licastro et al., 1983b; Fabris et al., 1984). Therefore, it is more difficult to determine an immune impairment specifically associated with AD.

We have investigated the endocrine function of the thymus gland, studying the plasmic level of a zinc-dependent thymic hormone—a nonapeptide called thymulin (Dardenne et al., 1982). Thymulin has been shown to promote T-cell differentiation and maturation (Dardenne et al., 1982). This hormone decreases dramatically in the plasma of elderly people and in young subjects with Down's syndrome (Fabris et al., 1984). Furthermore, thymulin requires a zinc molecule to exert its biological activity on lymphocytes (Dardenne et al., 1982).

We did not find any difference in the plasmic level of zinc and in the basal plasmic level of thymulin between normal elderly and AD patients. In both cases, zinc and thymulin were low as expected for subjects in this age range. However, in AD patients, the biological activity of thymulin after the addition of zinc in vitro increased less than in normal elderly subjects. These results suggest that in AD, the thymus gland may release a reduced amount of thymulin, as compared with the amount released in normal elderly persons. An alternative hypothesis explaining the ineffectiveness of zinc addition may be that the thymulin molecule has a reduced capacity to bind the zinc atom.

By contrast, we found that the mitogen response of lymphocytes from AD patients was within the age range. The addition of IL-2 to PHA-stimulated cultures showed the same moderate positive effect on lymphocytes from either normal elderly or AD patients. These data are at variance with other data showing a decrement of mitogen responsiveness in AD patients (Miller et al., 1981; Singh et al., 1987). Such a discrepancy may be related to the heterogeneity of AD; i.e., only some clinical subgroups may show a further impairment of T-cell proliferation after in vitro activation. Furthermore, the AD patients evaluated in our investigation showed no signs of infectious disease; also, immunological screening was performed soon after the diagnosis. Some conditions not directly related to the biology of AD, but that may affect immune parameters, are listed in Table V. A random distribution of patients according to the criteria listed in Table V might at least in part explain the confusing results regarding some immune functions in AD. In conclusion, the increased impairment of the endocrine portion of the thymus gland might be an early sign of immune impairment in AD, since no other immunological disfunctions were present.

5. SUMMARY

We studied some immune parameters in old normal donors and in patients with dementia of Alzheimer type (AD). The plasma level of zinc and of a zinc-dependent hormone (thy-

TABLE V. Conditions Not Directly Related
to the Biology of Alzheimer's Disease That May Affect
Degree of Immunological Deterioration

1. Age of patient at onset of the disease
2. Time lag between onset of disease and diagnosis
3. Time lag for onset of disease, time of diagnosis, and time of immunological screening

mulin) was studied in the two groups. AD patients and age-and sex-matched controls showed low but comparable levels of plasmic zinc, and no difference was found in the basal levels of thymulin. The biological activity of this thymic hormone was partially restored in plasma from healthy donors by the *in vitro* addition of zinc; however, this effect was not observed in most plasma samples from AD patients.

The proliferative activity of peripheral blood lymphocytes stimulated by PHA after 3 days of culture was also studied. In the two groups studied, no statistical difference was found in lymphocyte PHA responses. The addition of human recombinant IL-2 to stimulated culture increased lymphocyte responses to a suboptimal PHA dose but not to an optimal PHA dose. No difference were detected between the two groups. These data indicate that only a few immune parameters are more impaired in AD patients than in normal elderly subjects. In particular, these patients show a stronger imbalance in endocrine thymic function.

ACKNOWLEDGMENTS. This chapter was supported by research grants from the Ministero della Pubblica Istruzione Italiane and partly by the Regione Emilia Romagna. We thank Dr. L. J. Davis for helping us in the preparation of the manuscript and A. DiPietro for technical assistance.

REFERENCES

Amaducci, L., and Sorbi, S., 1985, L'invecchiamento cerebrale: Definizione ed inquadramento nosologico, *G. Gerontol.* **33**:1033–1054.

Amaducci, L. A., Fratiglioni, L., Rocca, W., Fieschi, C., Livrea, P., Pedone, D., Bracco, L., Lippi, A., Gandolfo, C., Bino, G., Prencipe, M., Bonatti, M., Girotti, F., Carella, F., Tavolato, B., Ferla, S., Lenzi, G. L., Carolei, A., Gambi, A., Grigoletto, F., and Schoenberg, B., 1986, Risk factors for clinically diagnosed Alzheimer's disease: A case-control study for an Italian population, *Neurology (NY)* **36**:922–931.

American Psychiatric Association, 1980, *Diagnostic and Statistical Manual of Mental Disorders*, 3rd ed., American Psychiatric Association, Washington, D.C.

Behan, P. O., and Feldman, R. G., 1970, Serum protein, amyloid and Alzheimer's disease, *J. Am. Geriatr. Soc.* **18**:792–797.

Boyum, 1968, Separation of leukocytes from blood and bone marrow, *Scand. J. Clin. Lab. Invest.* **21**(suppl. 97):77–89.

Chandra, V., Bharucha, N. E., and Schoenberg, B. S., 1986, Conditions associated with Alzheimer's disease at death: Case-control study, *Neurology (NY)* **36**:209–211.

Dardenne, M., Pleau, J. M., Nabama, B., Lefancier, P., Denierr, P., Chosy, M., and Bach, J. F., 1982, Contributions of zinc and other metal to the biological activity of serum thymic factor, *Proc. Natl. Acad. Sci. USA* **79**:5370–5373.

Fabris, N., Mocchegiani, E., Amadio, L., Zannotti, M., Licastro, F., and Franceschi, C., 1984, Thymic hormone deficiency in normal ageing and Down's syndrome: Is there a primary failure of the thymus?, *Lancet* **1**:983–986.

Folstein, M., Folstein, S., and McHugh, P. R., 1975, Mini Mental state: A practical method for grading the cognitive state of patients for the clinician, *J. Psychiatr. Res.* **12**:189–198.

Forte, P. L., Crimi, G., and Beltramello, A., 1988, Correlazioni cliniche, neuropsicologiche e neu-roradiologiche nella involuzione cerebrale senile, *G. Gerontol.* **36**:45–57.

Franceschi, C., Licastro, F., Chiricolo, M., Bonetti, F., Zannotti, M., Fabris, N., Mocchegiani, E., Fantini, M. P., Paolucci, P., and Masi, M., 1981, Deficiency of autologous mixed lymphocyte reactions and serum thymic factor level in Down's syndrome, *J. Immunol.* **126**:2161–2164.

Fudenbergh, H. H., Whitten, H. D., Arnaud, P., and Khansari, N., 1984, Is Alzheimer's disease an immunological disorder? Observations and speculations, Clin. Immunol. Immunopathol. 32:127–131.

Gaskin, F., Kingsley, B. S., and Fu, S. M., 1987, Autoantibodies to neurofibrillary tangles and brain tissue in Alzheimer's disease, J. Exp. Med. 165:245–250.

Gottfries, C. G., 1985, Definition of normal ageing senile dementia and Alzheimer's disease, in Normal Ageing, Alzheimer's Disease and Senile Dementia (G. G. Gottfries ed.), Editions Université Bruxelles, Brussels, pp. 11–17.

Hachinski, V. C., Iliff, L. D., Zilhka, E., Dubolay, G. H., McAllister, V., Marshall, J., Ross-Russel, R. W., and Symon, L., 1975, Cerebral blood flow in dementia, Arch. Neurol. 32:632–637.

Henderson, A. S., 1986, The epidemiology of Alzheimer's disease, Br. Med. Bull. 42:3–10.

Hollander, E., Mohs, R. C., and Davis, K. L., 1986, Antemortem markers of Alzheimer's disease, Neurobiol. Aging 7:367–387.

Kalter, S., and Kelly, S., 1975, Alzheimer's disease: Evaluation of immunological indeces, NY State J. Med. 75:1222–1225.

Leffell, M. S., Lumsden, L., and Steiger, W. A., 1985, An analysis of T lymphocyte subpopulations in patients with Alzheimer's disease, J. Am. Geriatr. Soc. 33:4–8.

Licastro, F., Chiricolo, M., Tabacchi, L., Barboni, F., Zannotti, M., and Franceschi, C., 1983a, Enhacing effect of lithium and potassium ions on lectin-induced lymphocyte proliferation in ageing and Down's syndrome subjects, Cell. Immunol. 75:111–121.

Licastro, F., Tabacchi, L., Chiricolo, M., Parente, R., Cenci, M., Barboni, F., and Franceschi, C., 1983b, Defective self-recognition in subjects of far advanced age, Gerontology 29:64–72.

Macdonald, S. M., Goldstone, A. H., Morris, J. E., Exton-Smith, A. N., and Callard, R. E., 1982, Immunological parameters in the aged and in Alzheimer's disease, Clin. Exp. Immunol. 49:123–128.

Mayeux, R., Stern, Y., and Spaton, S., 1985, Heterogeneity in dementia of the Alzheimer type: Evidence of subgroups, Neurology (NY) 35:453–461.

McKhann, G., Drachman, D., Folstein, M., Katzman, R., Price, D., and Stadlan, E., 1984, Clinical diagnosis of Alzheimer's disease: Report of the NINCDS-ADRDA work group under the auspices of Department of Health and human services Task Force on Alzheimer's disease, Neurology (NY) 34:939–944.

Miller, A. E., Neighbour, A., Katzman, R., Arouson, M., and Lipkowiz, R., 1981, Immunological studies in senile dementia of the Alzheimer type: Evidence for enhanced suppressor cell activity, Ann. Neurol. 10:506–510.

Nerl, C., Mayeux, R., and O'Neill, G. J., 1984, HLA-linked complement markers in Alzheimer's and Parkinson's disease: C variant (C4B2)—a possible marker for senile dementia of the Alzheimer type, Neurology (NY) 34:310–314.

Pouplard, A., Emile, J., and Vincent-Pineau, F., 1983, Autoanticorps circulants anti cellules à prolectine de l'hipophyse humaine et maladie d'Alzheimer, Rev. Neurol. (Paris) 139:187–191.

Rossor, M. N., Iversen, L. L., Reynolds, G. P., Mountjoy, C. P., and Roth, M., 1984, Neurochemical characteristics of early and late onset types of Alzheimer's disease, Br. Med. J. 288:961–964.

Roth, M., 1986, The association of clinical and neurological findings and its bearing on the classification and aetiology of Alzheimer's disease, Br. Med. Bull. 42:42–50.

Savorani, G., Salsi, A., De vinci, C., Piazzi, S., Sarti, G., Corneli, M., Palmirani, R., Tupone, A., Tolomelli, M., and Cavazzuti, F., 1986, Studies on the possible role of zinc and immune response in Alzheimer's disease, in: Immunoregulation in Aging EURAGE, 9, (A. Facchini, J. J. Haaijmann, and G. Labò, eds.), Rijswijk, The Netherlands, pp. 197–203.

Seltzer, B., and Sherwin, I., 1983, A comparison of clinical features in early and late-onset primary degenerative dementia. One entity or two?, Arch. Neurol. 40:143–146.

Singh, V. K., Fudenberg, H. H., and Brown, F. R. III, 1987, Immunologic dysfunction: Simultaneous study of Alzheimer's and older Down's patients, Mech. Ageing Dev. 37:257–264.

Skias, D., Bania, M., Reder, A. T., Luchins D., and Antel, J. P., 1985, Senile dementia of Alzheimer type (SDAT): Reduced T_6 cell-mediated suppressor activity, *Neurology (NY)* **35:**1635–1638.

Tavolato, B., and Argentiero, V., 1980, Immunological indices in presenile Alzheimer's disease, *J. Neurol. Sci.* **46:**325–331.

Wade, J. P. H., Mirsen, T. R., Hachinski, V. C., Fisman, M., Lau, C., and Merskey, H., 1987, The clinical diagnosis of Alzheimer's disease, *Arch. Neurol.* **44:**24–29.

II

Metabolic, Membrane, and Cellular
Markers and Models

11

Chronic Diseases and Disorders
A Hypothesis Suggesting an Age-Dependent versus an Age-Related Class

JACOB A. BRODY

1. INTRODUCTION

Two classes of age-associated diseases and disorders, one age-dependent and the other age-related, are suggested to provide a utilitarian hypothesis with research preventive and therapeutic implications. Molecular and immunological mechanisms pertinent to causality and progression are likely to be distinctive for these two classes. Age-dependent diseases and disorders are defined as those whose pathogenesis directly involves the aging of the host; thus, morbidity and mortality related to these diseases follows the age-specific death rate, which increases exponentially from about 35 years on (Fig. 1). Age-related diseases and disorders are those which have specific temporal patterns for their occurrence but after a certain time in life, new cases cease to occur. Thus, the body appears to have become resistant to this class.

In 1900, only 25% of all deaths occurred in people aged 65 and over, while by 1985, more than 75% of all deaths occurred after age 65. Currently, 30% of deaths occur in people over age 80, and almost 20% occur in people over age 85; it is generally accepted that the percentage of deaths in the older age groups will increase in proportion during the next few decades (Siegel, 1980; Taeuber, 1983; USNCHS, 1983; Schneider and Brody, 1983).

The hypothesis is being advanced now because chronic diseases and disorders of old age have gradually replaced the acute diseases of younger years. Therefore, an emerging issue is the separation of those diseases associated with older ages from the aging process (Brody and Schneider, 1986).

JACOB A. BRODY • School of Public Health, University of Illinois at Chicago, Chicago, Illinois 60680.

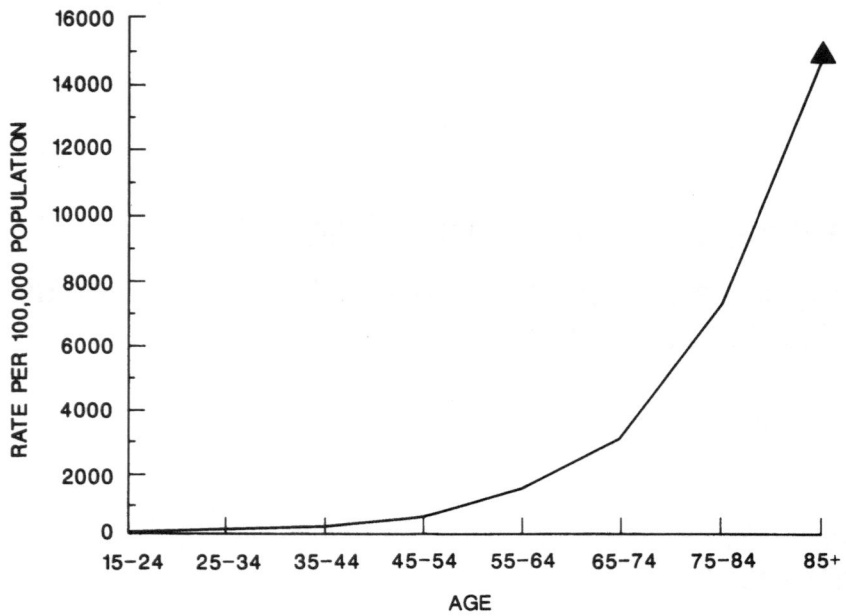

FIGURE 1. Mortality rates for all causes by age group, 1978. (From USNCHS, 1978.)

2. AGE-DEPENDENT DISEASES AND DISORDERS

By far, the most common age-dependent disease is coronary heart disease whose mortality parallels overall age-specific mortality (shown in Fig. 2 with All Cause Mortality in the background). Cerebrovascular disease behaves in a similar way with age. The mortality rates from these diseases double approximately every 5–10 years from about age 35 onward. Blindness and deafness have similar patterns, as do type II diabetes and altered glucose metabolism and deaths from certain infectious diseases, particularly pneumococcal pneumonia. Hip fracture and attendant osteoporosis follow similar patterns; two common neurologic diseases, Alzheimer's disease and Parkinson's disease, also appear to parallel age-specific mortality.

Age-dependent diseases and conditions seem to be intimately related to the normal aging of the host. They require a fertile soil, which seems to be the background accumulation of normal aging. Neurofibrillary tangles and amyloid plaques, for example, are thought, perhaps, to be a process associated with normal aging. In certain instances, however, a remarkable proliferation occurs that becomes the diagnostic entity, Alzheimer's disease. The clinical onset of the disease is dependent on an array of threshold phenomena accruing with age. Once reached, the host becomes susceptible.

3. AGE-RELATED DISEASES AND DISORDERS

This class of conditions occurs at a particular time in life and frequently in later life, but after a specific age, these diseases and disorders typically decline in frequency or increase at a

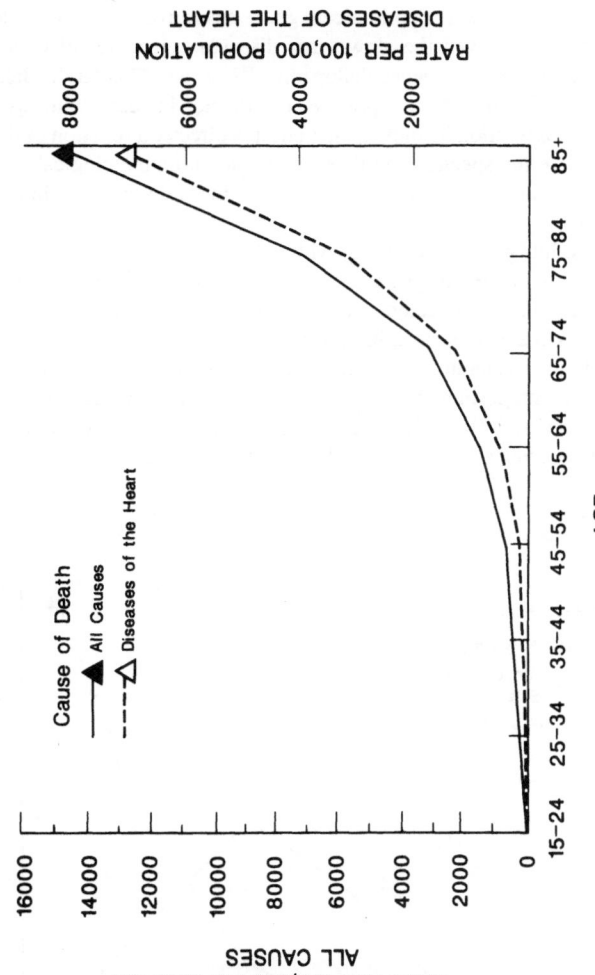

FIGURE 2. Mortality rates for selected causes by age group, 1978: diseases of the heart. (From USNCHS, 1978.)

less than exponential rate. Thus, these diseases and conditions have an important temporal relationship with the host, but the critical factors do not appear to be related to normal aging. Several neurologic diseases are prototypic of this class. Amyotrophic lateral sclerosis almost never occurs before age 40, and new cases are rare after age 55 or 60, (shown in Fig. 3 with All Cause Mortality in the background). Multiple sclerosis rarely occurs before age 20 and is extremely unlikely to have its onset after age 50. Schizophrenia appears occasionally during the first decade of life and then with increasing frequency until the third decade. After about age 25–35, new cases do not appear. Peptic ulcer, gout, ulcerative colitis, and alcoholism rarely have onset in later life. Even the slow virus diseases, subacute sclerosing panencephalitis, progressive multifocal leukoencephalopathy, Kuru, and Creutzfeld–Jakob's disease, display different ranges of age susceptibility but do not increase with age. This is surprising in view of the observation in animals that onset is directly a function of duration of time following exposure for the species, and there is no known immunological component. Thus, it would be assumed that with continuous exposure, these disease should accumulate with age, but they do not.

The cancers have an intriguing relationship with age. Most cancers have widely differing age ranges but, almost without exception, they occur at a certain time in life and beyond that time, most cancers decline. Considered as an aggregate, the median age for diagnosis is about 65 years. Mortality rises in a linear fashion from age 40 through about age 70, when the rate of the disease starts to decelerate. There are recent data available for the first time on people in their tenth decade suggesting that the actual incidence of cancer declines very late in life. From age 65 to 69, about 30% of all deaths are from cancer, while at age 85 and over, only 1 in 10 deaths is from cancer. There is considerable evidence that mutagenesis measured

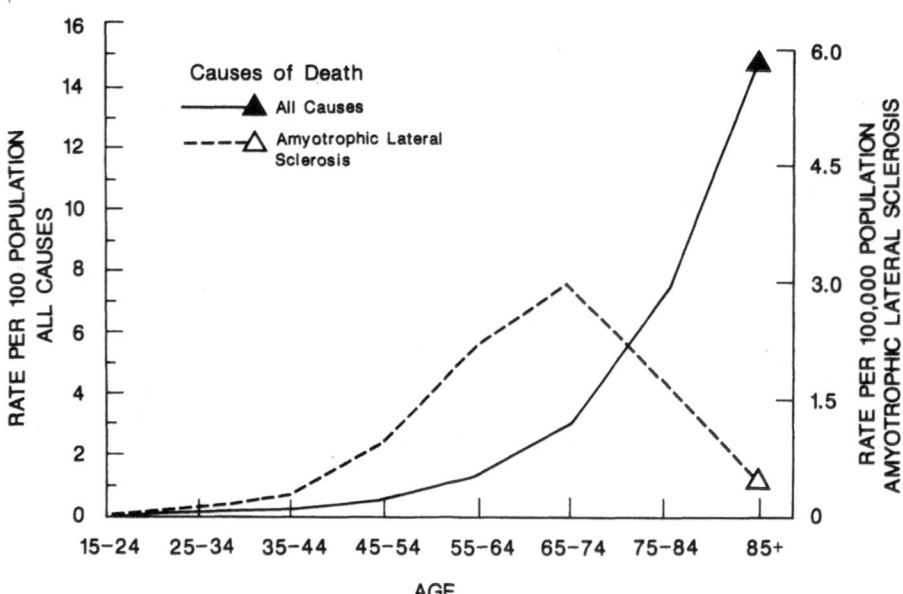

FIGURE 3. Mortality rates for selected causes by age group, 1978: amyotrophic lateral sclerosis. (From USNCHS, 1978.)

in different human cells increases with age. Thus, it is surprising that cancers do not show an age-dependent pattern. It is widely accepted that most immune parameters decline with age and this could explain the obvious inconsistency between rate of mutagenesis and cancers. It is possible that in later years, the body's immune defenses are insufficient to mount a full carcinogenic reaction even in the presence of higher numbers of mutations.

4. IMPLICATIONS

The age-related group is essentially opportunistic upon the host and will be expressed only if a combination of factors are present in a proper sequence at a certain age. If the factors which initiate age-related diseases and disorders can be determined and methods developed to prevent or successfully treat them, the disease or disorder is unlikely to occur beyond a certain fixed age. Thus, the impact of these disorders would be reduced by successfully shepherding the individual through the specific age period of susceptibility; either through prevention or successful therapy. The important point is that once the age of susceptibility is past, the disease will not occur again and is thus eliminated as a source of morbidity or mortality.

It is unlikely for most age-related diseases and disorders that they fail to occur beyond a certain age because of exhaustion of susceptibles. To exhaust susceptibles, it is necessary either to produce a universal immunity for all those who do not develop the condition or to arrive at the state where maximum genetic penetrance is achieved. This would not appear to be the case with diverse conditions including gout, glioblastoma, amyotrophic lateral sclerosis, slow virus diseases, or ulcerative colitis, all of which disappear with advancing age. In none of these diseases is there evidence of solid immunity or of a driving genetic pattern.

Thus research efforts should be oriented at understanding the intrinsic or extrinsic factors which put an individual at risk during a specific age window. If it could be determined why altered purine metabolism in late life does not produce clinical gout, we might use that information to prevent gout in the earlier susceptible years. If we understood the relationship of geographic influence, measles virus antibody, and certain HLA types with multiple sclerosis, it might be possible to prevent this disease. If we could gain insight into why having one's first child at an early age protects against subsequent breast cancer, effective preventive strategies might be formulated.

Age-dependent diseases and conditions are gradually emerging as the major source of disability, and we can expect that age-related problems will exert less and less effect on either morbidity or mortality. Age-dependent conditions accumulate with aging. Therapeutic interventions in age-dependent diseases may have limited success because the organ is already compromised and because at advanced old age, relatively minor insults may cause death. This does not suggest that death is the result of normal or natural processes, since death will still result from a specific pathologic insult, albeit a lesser pathological insult would then produce the same result in a younger individual.

I must emphasize my own view that no age-dependent disease or disorder is inevitable. The specific phenomenon will manifest itself differently in different people. The class all shares the common factor that their manifestation is dependent on natural aging.

Aging is not the individual age-dependent diseases and disorders that rise exponentially with age. It is, in fact, the coexistence of more than one condition coupled with an array of age-dependent social and economic factors, including loneliness, widowhood, and poverty, which, as a group, rise at a rate far greater than exponential. This results in the wide range of physical and social disabilities that concentrate in later years.

5. CONCLUSIONS

The most burdensome problems of aging increasingly are age-dependent conditions that are nonfatal, such as blindness, deafness, osteoarthritis and other joint problems, and dementia. Better understanding of these and other age-dependent situations could lead to effective prevention strategies. The strategy, in fact, is postponement of various age-dependent biological phenomena. A good example of this approach is related to osteoporosis and hip fracture. In the United States, there are about 150,000 new cases of hip fracture per year among white women. The rate of hip fracture increases exponentially, doubling every 5–6 years from about age 40. Parallel information exists about the progression of osteoporosis from age 20 through age 90. Insights into the mechanisms involved in demineralization of bone that could delay the process for only 6 years should lower the rate of hip fracture by almost 50%. The key is to find the appropriate age and mechanism in a vulnerable structure whose pathology will be manifest only late in life and postpone the onset of the aging process (in the above instance, osteoporosis). Ultimately, we would like to postpone the occurrence of hip fracture to an age beyond death. This would be true prevention indeed.

The study of events at the molecular and immunological level might benefit from keeping in mind the separation of, but dependence on, normal aging and the threshold in which age-dependent events can become manifest. These should show distinctive patterns from the events associated with age-related diseases that are likely to require knowledge of a specific pattern of serial events prior to a given age.

REFERENCES

Brody, J. A., and Schneider, E. L., 1986, Diseases and disorders of aging: an hypothesis, *J. Chron. Dis.* **39:**871–876.

Schneider, E. L., and Brody, J. A., 1983, Aging, natural death, and compression of morbidity: Another view, *N. Engl. J. Med.* **309:**854–856.

Siegel, J. S., 1980, Recent and prospective demographic trends for the elderly population and some implications for health care, in: *Proceedings of the Second Conference on the Epidemiology of Aging*, NIH Publication No. 80-969, U.S. Government Printing Office, Washington, D.C.

Taeuber, C. M., 1983, *America in Transition: An Aging Society, Current Population Reports*, Special Studies, Series P-23, No. 128, U.S. Department of Commerce, Bureau of the Census, Washington, D.C.

United States National Center for Health Statistics, 1980, *Vital Statistics of the United States*, Vol. II: *Mortality*, Part A, Advance Report on Final Mortality Statistics, 1978. Hyattsville, Maryland, Vol. 29, No. 6 (Suppl.), DHHS Publication No. (PHS)-F-80-1120.

United States National Center for Health Statistics, 1983, *Changing Mortality Patterns, Health Services Utilization, and Health Care Expenditures. United States, 1978–2003*. Hyattsville, Maryland, NCHS Analytical and Epidemiological Studies, Vital and Health Statistics, Series 3, No. 23, DHHS publication No. (PHS)83-1407).

12

Changes in Receptors and Signal Transduction Events during Aging

GEORGE S. ROTH

1. INTRODUCTION

Physiological and behavioral responses to many classes of stimuli are altered during aging. Best studied among these have been hormone and neurotransmitter signal transduction sequences. Age-related alterations in these processes have been grouped into receptor and postreceptor changes. Our laboratory has focused on three systems that exhibit representative age-associated alterations in signal transduction mechanisms: (1) dopaminergic regulation of motor function, (2) estrogenic regulation of uterine anabolic function, and (3) α-adrenergic regulation of parotid secretory function (for review, see Roth, 1985).

In the former two systems, age-related loss of receptors is at least partially responsible for impaired responsiveness. For example, decreases in striatal D_2-dopamine receptors have now been demonstrated in aged mice, rats, rabbits, monkeys, and humans. These reductions have been closely correlated with impaired motor performance, such as wire and rod walking, rotational behavior, inclined screen performance, and various tasks involving proper balance, gait, and so forth.

Loss of uterine estrogen receptors has been reported in a number of mouse and rat strains; these reductions have been closely correlated with impaired estrogenic regulation of gene expression, including induction of enzymes required for energy metabolism, cellular hypertrophy, and division. In addition, an age-related reduction in the association of receptor—estrogen complexes with the genome also contributes to impaired activation of RNA polymerase II, the enzyme required for messenger RNA (mRNA) transcription and resultant gene expression.

In the case of α-adrenergic-stimulated parotid gland secretion, functional deterioration is not caused by changes at the receptor level. α_1-Adrenergic receptors, which mediate secretory responsiveness, are not lost with age, and there are no reductions in their interaction with α-adrenergic agonists. Instead, aged rat parotid cells exhibit an impaired ability to mobilize

GEORGE S. ROTH • Molecular Physiology and Genetics Section, Gerontology Research Center, National Institute on Aging, National Institutes of Health, Francis Scott Key Medical Center, Baltimore, Maryland 21224.

TABLE I. Systems Exhibiting Impaired Stimulation of Calcium Mobilization
during Aging

Stimulus	Species	Tissue	Response	References
α-Adrenergic	Rat	Parotid	Electrolyte secretion	Ito *et al.* (1982); Bodner *et al.* (1983)
	Rat	Parotid	Glucose oxidation	Ito *et al.* (1981); Gee *et al.* (1986)
	Rat	Aorta	Contraction	Cohen and Berkowitz (1976)
β-Adrenergic	Rat	Heart	Contraction	Guarnieri *et al.* (1980)
Cholinergic	Rat	Brain (striatum)	Dopamine release	Joseph *et al.* (1988)
Depolarization	Rat	Heart	Contraction	Elfellah *et al.* (1986)
	Rat	Brain (forebrain and cortex)	Acetylcholine release	Meyer *et al.* (1986); Peterson and Gibson (1983a)
	Mouse	Brain (forebrain)	Acetylcholine release	Peterson *et al.* (1985)
	Mouse	Whole animal	Motor function	Peterson and Gibson (1983b)
	Rat	Whole animal	Maze learning	Davis *et al.* (1983)
Serotonin	Rat	Aorta	Contraction	Cohen and Berkowitz (1976)
Gonadotropin-releasing hormone	Rat	Pituitary	Gonadotropin secretion	Chuknyiska *et al.* (1987)
Lectin	Rat	Lymphocyte	Mitogenesis	Wu *et al.* (1985); Segal (1986)
	Mouse	Lymphocyte	Mitogenesis	Miller *et al.* (1987); Proust *et al.* (1987)
	Human	Lymphocyte	Mitogenesis	Chopra *et al.* (1987)
Compound 48–80	Rat	Mast cell	Histamine release	Orida and Feldman (1982)
Formyl-methionyl-leucyl-phenyl	Human	Neutrophil	Superoxide generation	Lipschitz *et al.* (1987, 1988)
Thyroid hormones	Human	Erythrocyte	Activation of calcium ATPase	Davis *et al.* (1987)
Low-density lipoprotein	Human	Polymorphonuclear leukocytes	Release of β-glucuronidase	Fulop *et al.* (1985)
Cytochalasin B	Human	Polymorphonuclear leukocytes	Release of β-glucuronidase	Fulop *et al.* (1985)
Immune complexes	Human	Polymorphonuclear leukocytes	Release of β-glucuronidase	Fulop *et al.* (1985)
Phosphatidylserine	Rat	Brain	Protein kinase activation	Calderini *et al.* (1986)

calcium in response to α_1-adrenergic stimulation, resulting in reduced water and electrolyte secretion. This impairment appears to be due to a decreased responsiveness of intracellular calcium stores to inositol trisphosphate, the second messenger in this signal transduction sequence. Generation of ionositol trisphosphate is not significantly reduced with age.

Even more interesting is the fact that similar age-related impairments in calcium-dependent responses have been reported in many other systems, some of which mobilize this ion in very different ways. For example, β-adrenergic stimulated cardiac muscle contraction is at least partially dependent on extracellular calcium and elevation of intracellular cyclic adenosine monophosphate (cAMP) levels. Yet, stimulation of contraction is also impaired with age. Other systems exhibiting similar phenomena include mitogen-stimulated lymphocyte DNA synthesis, cholinergic regulation of acetylcholine (ACh) release and motor and learning/memory performance, formyl–methionyl–leucyl–phenylalanine (FMLP) activation of neutrophil superoxide generation and phagocytic function, α-adrenergic and serotonergic-stimulated aortic contraction, and luteinizing hormone-releasing hormone (LHRH) stimulation of pituitary gonodotropin secretion, among many others (Table I).

Most remarkable is the fact that in all these systems, age-related impairments in responsiveness can be at least partially reversed if sufficient calcium can be delivered to its intracellular site of action. Thus, aging appears to influence diverse mechanisms of calcium flow with a common result, i.e., impaired movement. Despite this deterioration, many old cells maintain an innate capacity to function as well as young cells if the impaired calcium movement can be overcome. The widespread manifestation of this particular phenomenon offers hope of novel therapeutic strategies for many age-related dysfunctions in calcium-dependent processes.

REFERENCES

Bodner, L., Hoopers, M. T., Gee, M., Ito, H., Roth, G. S., and Baum, B. J., 1983, Multiple transduction mechanisms are likely involved in calcium mediated exocrine secretory events in rat parotid cells, *J. Biol. Chem.* **258:**2774–2777.

Calderini, G., Bellini, F., Bonetti, A. C., Galbaiti, E., Teoloto, S., and Toffano, G., 1986, Effect of aging on phospholipid senestitive Ca^{++} dependent protein kinase in the rat brain, *Abst. Soc. Neurosci.* **12:**275.

Chopra, R., Nagel, J., and Adler, W., 1987, Decreased response of T cells from elderly individuals to phytohemogglutinin (PHA) stimulation can be augmented by phorbol myristate acetate (PMA) in conjunction with Ca-ionophore A23187, *Gerontologist* **27:**204A.

Chuknyiska, R. S., Blackman, M. R., and Roth, G. S., 1987, Ionophore A23187 partially reverses LH secretory defect of pituitary cells from old rats, *Am. J. Physiol.* **258:**E233–E237.

Cohen, M. L., and Berkowitz, B. A., 1976, Vascular contraction: Effect of age and extracellular calcium, *Blood Vessels* **67:**139–149.

Davis, H. P., Idowu, A., and Gibson, G. E., 1983, Improvement of 8-arm maze performance in aged Fischer 344 rats with 3, 4-diaminopyridine, *Exp. Aging Res.* **9:**211–214.

Davis, P. J., Davis, F. B., Blas, S. D., Schoenl, M., and Edwards, L., 1987, Donor age-dependent decline in response of human red cell Ca^{++}-ATPase activity to thyroid hormone *in vitro*, *J. Clin. Endocrinol. Metab.* **64:**921–925.

Elfellah, M. S., Johns, A., and Shepherd, A. M. M., 1986, Effect of age on responsiveness of isolated rat atria to carbachol and on binding characteristics of atria muscarinic receptors, *J. Cardiovasc. Pharmacol.* **8:**873–877.

Fulop, T., Faris, G., Worcum, I., Paragh, G., and Leovey, A., 1985, Age related variations of some polymorphonuclear leukocyte functions, *Mech. Aging Dev.* **29:**1–8.

Gee, M. V., Ishikawa, Y., Baum, B. J., and Roth, G. S., 1986, Impaired adrenergic stimulation of rat parotid cell glucose oxidation during aging: the role of calcium, *J. Gerontol.* **41:**331–335.

Guarnieri, T., Filburn, C. E., Zitnick, G., Roth, G. S., and Lakatta, E. G., 1980, Mechanisms of altered cardiac isotropic responsiveness during aging in the rat, *Am. J. Physiol.* **239:**H501–H508.

Ito, H., Hoopes, M. T., Roth, G. S., and Baum, B. J., 1981, Adrenergic and cholinergic mediated glucose oxidation by rat parotid gland acinar cells during aging, *Biochem. Biophys. Res. Commun.* **98:**275–282.

Ito, H., Baum, B. J., Uchida, T., Hoopes, M. T., Bodner, L., and Roth, G. S., 1982, Modulation of rat parotid cell α-adrenergic responsiveness at a step subsequent to receptor activation, *J. Biol. Chem.* **257:**9532–9538.

Joseph, J. A., Dalton, T. K., Roth, G. S., and Hunt, W. A., 1988, Alterations in muscarinic control of striatal dopamine autoreceptors in senescence: A deficit at the ligand–muscarinic receptor interface?, *Brain Res.* **454:**149–155.

Lipschitz, D. A., Udupa, K. B., and Boxer, L. A., 1987, Evidence that microenvironmental factors account for the age-related decline in neutrophil function, *Blood* **70:**1131–1135.

Lipschitz, D. A., Udupa, K. B., and Boxer, L. A., 1989, The role of calcium in the age related decline of neutrophil function, *Blood* (in press).

Meyer, E. M., Crews, F. T., Otero, D. H., and Larson, K., 1986, Aging decreases the sensitivity of rat cortical synaptosomes to calcium ionophore-induced acetylcholine release, *J. Neurochem.* **47:**1244–1246.

Miller, R. A., 1986, Immunodeficiency of aging: Restorative effects of phorbol ester combined with calcium ionophore, *J. Immunol.* **137:**805–808.

Miller, R. A., Jacobson, B., Weil, G., and Simons, E. R., 1987, Diminished calcium influx in lectin-stimulated T cells from old mice, *J. Cell. Physiol.* **132:**337–342.

Orida, N., and Feldman, J. D., 1982, Age related deficiency in calcium uptake by mast cells, *Fed. Proc.* **41:**822.

Peterson, C., and Gibson, G. E., 1983a, Aging and 3,4-diaminopyridine alter synaptosomal calcium uptake, *J. Biol. Chem.* **258:**11482–11486.

Peterson, C., and Gibson, G. E., 1983b, Amelioration of age-related neurochemical and behavioral deficits by 3,4-diaminopyridine, *Neurobiol. Aging* **4:**25–30.

Peterson, C., Nicholls, D. G., and Gibson, G. E., 1985, subsynaptosomal distribution of calcium during aging and 3,4-diaminopyridine treatment, *Neurobiol. Aging* **6:**297–304.

Proust, J. J., Filburn, C. R., Harrison, S. A., Buchholz, M. A., and Nordin, A. A., 1987, Age-related defect in signal transduction during lectin activation of murine T lymphocytes, *J. Immunol.* **139:**1472–1478.

Roth, G. S., 1985, Effects of aging on mechanisms of α-adrenergic and dopaminergic action, *Fed. Proc.* **45:**60–64.

Wu, W., Pahlavani, M., Richardson, A., and Cheung, H. T., 1985, Effect of maturation and age on lymphocyte proliferation induced by A23187 through an interleukin independent pathway, *J. Leukocyte Biol.* **38:**531–540.

13

Molecular Aging of Membrane Molecules and Cellular Removal

MARGUERITE M. B. KAY

1. INTRODUCTION

Investigations into mechanisms by which macrophages distinguish mature from senescent calf cells showed that a glycoprotein, senescent cell antigen, a terminal differentiation antigen, appears on the surface of senescent cells (Kay, 1974, 1975, 1978, 1981a–c, 1982a; Bennett and Kay, 1981; Kay and Bennett, 1982; Kay et al., 1982). It is recognized by the antigen-binding Fab region (Kay, 1978) of a specific immunoglobulin G (IgG) autoantibody in serum that attaches to cells carrying senescent cell antigen and initiates their removal by marcophages (Kay, 1975, 1978). Senescent cell antigen was first observed on the surface of senescent human erythrocytes (Kay, 1974, 1975) but has since been demonstrated on the surface of lymphocytes, polymorphonuclear leukocytes, platelets, embryonic kidney cells, and adult liver cells (Kay, 1981a).

The first hint that a neo-antigen appeared on senescent cells came from studies showing that IgG autoantibodies selectively bind to old human red blood cells (RBC) aged *in situ* (Kay, 1974, 1975) during investigations of the mechanism by which macrophages distinguish between senescent and other "self" cells. Human red blood cells (RBC) were used as a model for these studies because of the ready availability of these cells and the ease with which populations of different ages can be separated (Kay, 1974, 1975).

2. IGG IS PRESENT ON OLD BUT NOT YOUNG CELLS

It was hypothesized that Ig in normal human serum attaches to the surface of senescent RBC until a critical level is reached that results in phagocytosis. The results of these studies demonstrated that Ig is required to initiate phagocytosis of senescent and stored cells and that IgG attaches *in situ* to senescent human RBC (Kay, 1975). Old RBC separated by density

MARGUERITE M. B. KAY • Departments of Medicine, and Medical Biochemistry and Genetics, and Medical Microbiology and Immunology, Texas A&M University, and Teague Veterans Center, Temple, Texas 76504.

centrifugation from freshly drawn blood had IgG but no IgA or IgM on their surface, as determined by scanning immunoelectron microscopy (SEM) (Kay, 1975). Young RBC did not have Ig on their surface. Incubation of old RBC with autologous macrophages resulted in their phagocytosis regardless of whether incubations were performed in medium with serum, autologous Ig-depleted serum, or whole serum (Kay, 1975). Young RBC were not phagocytized under any of these conditions. Thus, it appeared that the IgG attached *in situ* to senescent human RBC and rendered them vulnerable to phagocytosis by macrophages. The presence of IgG autoantibodies on the surface of old cells indicates that a new antigen has appeared that is not present on other cells. This was the first indication that a neo-antigen appears on senescent cells.

3. RED CELL LIFE-SPAN STUDIES

These results were confirmed *in vivo* using mice bred and maintained in a maximum security barrier devoid of viruses, *Mycoplasma,* and pathogenic bacteria, thereby excluding an exogenous source for the senescent cell antigen (Bennett and Kay, 1981). RBC were labeled *in situ* with ^{59}Fe, which labels the newly synthesized hemoglobin (Hb) in young cells. Red cells were separated on Percoll gradients, 1 or 40 days after radioactive iron injection, into young and old populations, and injected into separate groups of syngeneic mice. Kinetic studies demonstrated that <90% of the ^{59}Fe-labeled young RBC were removed from the circulation within 45 days. By contrast, >90% of the ^{59}Fe-labeled old RBC were removed within 20 days. The difference in the rate of removal of young and old RBC was statistically significant ($p \leq 0.001$). Kinetic studies on density-separated spleen cell populations showed that the radioactivity decreased in the RBC fraction concomitantly with an increase in radioactivity in the splenic macrophage fraction. The radioactivity was found to be inside macrophages (Bennett and Kay, 1981).

Studies performed *in vitro* with mouse splenic macrophages and autologous young and old RBC showed that mouse macrophages phagocytized senescent but not young RBC ($p \leq 0.001$). The phagocytosis of middle-aged RBC ($\sim$23%) was intermediate between that of young RBC (5%) and old RBC ($\sim$50%). This suggested that the appearance of the senescent cell antigen, and therefore molecular aging of membranes, was a cumulative process.

Returning senescent cells stripped of IgG to the circulation has not been tried because senescent cell IgG (association constant: 1×10^{14} M^{-1}) cannot be eluted from old RBC without destroying them. Even if this could be done, the life span of the RBC would not be increased after being returned to the circulation because more IgG autoantibodies would bind to the red cells as soon as they were injected. This would occur because the basic membrane lesion, appearance of the senescent cell antigen, which initiated IgG binding would not be altered by removal of IgG.

4. SENESCENT CELL IGG IS AN AUTOANTIBODY

Immunoglobulin G attached to senescent cells *in situ* was shown to be an autoantibody (Kay, 1978). The antibodies could be dissociated from senescent cells. The dissociated antibodies specifically reattached via the antigen-binding (Fab) portion of the IgG molecule to homologous senescent, but not mature cells (Kay, 1978). Fab binding was demonstrated by antigen blockade studies, SIEM, and ^{125}I-labeled protein A binding to the Fc region of

IgG bound to senescent cells and vesicles (Kay, 1978; Kay et al., 1982; Lutz and Kay, 1981). Thus, the antibody to the senescent cell antigen is an autoantibody and not a nonspecific or a cytophilic antibody (Kay, 1978). It exhibited specific immunologic binding via the Fab region. Binding of an IgG autoantibody to senescent RBC through immunological mechanisms indicated that antigenic determinants recognized by these IgG autoantibodies appeared on the membrane surface as RBC aged.

5. ISOLATION OF SENESCENT CELL ANTIGEN

Senescent cell antigen was isolated from sialoglycoprotein mixtures with affinity columns prepared with IgG eluted from senescent cells (Kay, 1981a). Material specifically bound by the column was eluted with glycine–HCl buffer, at pH 2.3. Both glycoprotein and protein stains of gels of the eluted material showed a band migrating at a relative molecular weight of 62,000 in the component 4.5 region. These experiments suggested that the 62,000-M_r glycopeptide carried the antigenic determinants recognized by IgG obtained from freshly isolated senescent cells. The 62,000-M_r peptide, but not the remaining sialoglycoprotein mixture from which it was isolated, abolished the phagocytosis-inducing ability of IgG eluted from senescent RBC in the erythrophagocytosis assay (Kay, 1981a,b, 1982a). This indicated that the 62,000-M_r peptide was the antigen that appeared on the membrane of cells as they aged.

6. SENESCENT CELL ANTIGEN IS PRESENT ON NUCLEATED CELLS

Examination of other somatic cells for the antigen that appears on senescent RBC demonstrated its presence on lymphocytes, platelets, neutrophils, and cultured human adult liver cells and primary cultures of human embryonic kidney cells as determined by a phagocytosis inhibition assay (Kay, 1981a). The senescent cell antigen was isolated from lymphocytes (Kay, 1981a, 1982a) with the senescent RBC IgG affinity column. Gel electrophoresis of the material obtained from the column revealed a band migrating at a molecular weight of 62,000 at the same position as the antigen isolated from senescent RBC. This finding confirmed the results obtained from the phagocytosis inhibition assay, indicating that the antigen which appeared on senescent RBC also appeared on other somatic cells.

Appearance of the 62,000-M_r antigen on RBC initiates binding of IgG autoantibodies *in situ* and phagocytosis of senescent cells by macrophages (Kay, 1974, 1975, 1978). The antigen is present on stored human lymphocytes, platelets, and neutrophils and on cultured liver and kidney cells. In addition, IgG autoantibodies in normal serum have been shown to bind to senescent RBC *in situ* in humans (Kay, 1975), mice (Bennett and Kay, 1981), rats (Glass et al., 1983), cows (Bartosz et al., 1982), and rabbits (Khansari and Fudenberg, 1984; Vomel and Platt, 1981). Thus, the immunological mechanism for removing senescent and damaged RBC appears to be a general physiological process for removing cells programmed for death in mammals and, possibly, other vertebrates (Kay, 1974, 1975, 1981a).

Other groups, extrapolating from the classic experiments of Ashwell and co-workers, who showed that the lifetime of serum glycoproteins could be drastically shortened by removal of external carbohydrates (Ashwell and Morrell, 1974), have suggested that binding and phagocytosis of old erythrocytes requires disappearance of terminal sialic acid residues and subsequent exposure of penultimate galactose residues (Aminoff and Vorder Bruegge, 1978; Aminoff et al., 1977). Proponents of this theory have presented the results of experiments in which IgG molecules were eluted from intact thalassemic erythrocytes by incubation with various carbohydrates, to support the view that the IgG molecules responsible for the removal of senescent erythrocytes bind specifically to newly exposed galactose residues (Galili et al., 1983).

In order to determine what role, if any, galactose has in the physiological removal of old erythrocytes, we tried to elute IgG from intact senescent erythrocytes, as well as from their membranes, with buffer containing galactose (Kay and Bosman, 1985). Incubation of senescent RBC with galactose did not inhibit their phagocytosis by macrophages indicating that galactose did not displace senescent cell IgG. Incubation with galactose did not elute senescent cell IgG from the membranes of RBC. In addition, absorption of senescent cell IgG with the carbohydrate portion of band 3 did not alter binding to band 3 in immunoblots. The fraction specifically eluted from affinity columns containing the carbohydrate portion of band 3 did not bind to erythrocyte membranes in immunoblots. These results suggest that the IgG binding specifically to senescent erythrocytes is not directed against galactose residues.

7. SENESCENT CELL ANTIGEN APPEARS TO BE DERIVED FROM BAND 3

Since mature erythrocytes cannot synthesize proteins, senescent cell antigen is probably generated by modification of a pre-existing protein of higher molecular weight (Kay, 1981b, 1982a). It was postulated that senescent cell antigen is a component of the 4.5 region derived from band 3 (Kay and Bennett, 1982) based on both extraction and isolation conditions, relative molecular weight, and its characterization as a glycosylated peptide (Kay 1981a).

Experiments designed to test this hypothesis showed that senescent cell antigen is immunologically related to band 3 and may represent a physiologically significant breakdown product of the parent molecule (Kay et al., 1982; Kay, 1981b). Both band 3 and senescent cell antigen abolished the phagocytosis-inducing ability of IgG eluted from senescent cells, whereas spectrin, bands 2.1, 4.1, actin, glycophorin A, periodic acid-Schiff (PAS)-staining bands 1–4, and desialylated PAS-staining bands 1–4 did not. In addition, rabbit antibodies to both purified band 3 and senescent cell antigen and IgG eluted from senescent cells reacted with band 3 and its breakdown products as determined by immunoautoradiography of RBC membranes, indicating that these molecules share common antigenic determinants not possessed by other RBC membrane components (Kay, 1981c; Kay et al., 1982, 1983).

These results confirmed those obtained with the erythrophagocytosis assay by indicating that band 3 carries the antigenic determinants of senescent cell antigen. Thus, senescent cell antigen is immunologically related to band 3 and may be derived from it.

Senescent cell antigen was mapped along the band 3 molecule using topographically defined fragments of band 3. Both binding of IgG eluted from senescent RBC (senescent cell IgG) to defined proteolytic fragments of band 3 in immunoblots, and two-dimensional peptide mapping of senescent cell antigen, band 3, and defined proteolytic fragments of band 3 were used to localize senescent cell antigen along the band 3 molecule (Kay, 1984b). Peptide mapping was performed using the procedure of Elder et al. (1977) wherein the purified protein is subjected to sodium dodecyl sulfate polyacrylamide gel electrophoresis (SDS–PAGE) and then cut from the gel as a single thin slice. The gel slice is then iodinated and used for analysis. Use of this procedure avoids mapping of "contaminants." The data suggested that the antigenic determinants of senescent cell antigen that are recognized by physiologic IgG autoantibodies reside on an external portion of a naturally occurring transmembrane fragment of band 3 that has lost an 40,000-M_r cytoplasmic (NH_2-terminal) segment and part of the anion-transport region. A critical cell age-specific cleavage of a band 3 appears to occur in the transmembrane, anion transport region of band 3.

Band 3, the major anion-transport protein, mediates the exchange of anions (chloride and bicarbonate) across the membrane (Cabantchik and Rothstein, 1974; Lepke et al., 1976) and is binding site for the glycolytic enzymes aldolase (Strapazon and Steck, 1977), phosphofructokinase (Karadsheh, 1977), glyceraldehyde-3-phosphate-dehydrogenase (G3PD) (Kliman and Steck, 1975) and for hemoglobin (Salhany and Shaklai, 1979). Water transfer across the membrane has been attributed to band 3 (Brown et al., 1975). Structurally, the ~95,000-M_r band 3 molecule crosses the membrane between 3 and 12 times (Mueckler et al., 1985; Steck, 1978; Ramjeesingh and Rothstein, 1982). A cytoplasmic segment containing the amino-terminal binds to band 2.1 (ankyrin), which attaches to the internal filamentous cytoskeleton through band 2.1 (ankyrin) (Bennett and Stenbuck, 1979). Band 3 has been found in all cells examined, including neurons (Kay et al., 1983; Drenckhahn, 1984; Drenckhahn et al., 1985). Degradation of band 3 generates senescent cell antigen (Kay, 1974, 1975, 1978, 1981a–c, 1982a,b, 1984a,b, 1985a,b, 1986; Bennett and Kay, 1981; Kay and Bennett, 1982; Kay et al., 1982, 1986; Bosman et al., 1988; Bosman and Kay, 1988). Appearance of senescent cell antigen results in the removal of old cells (Kay, 1974, 1975, 1978, 1981a–c, 1982a,b, 1984a,b, 1985a,b, 1986; Bennett and Kay, 1981; Kay and Bennett, 1982; Kay et al., 1982a,b, 1986; Bosman et al., 1988; Bosman and Kay, 1988). Thus, band 3 is a crucial molecule involved in a cellular aging.

8. BAND 3 UNDERGOES DEGRADATION AS CELLS AGE

Since senescent cell antigen and band 3 share antigenic determinants, the effect of cellular age on the accumulation of band 3 breakdown products was investigated using the immunoblotting technique (Kay, 1982b, 1984a,b). Freshly isolated cells were used, and membranes were prepared in the presence of protease inhibitors, including diisopropylfluorosphosphate (DFP), EDTA, and EGTA. Antibodies to band 3 and senescent cell antigen were used to determine the relative amount of band 3 breakdown products in the membranes of young, middle-aged, and old cells by immunoautoradiography using the gel overlay and immunoblotting procedures (Kay, 1982b, 1984a,b). Results revealed binding of both antibodies to band 3 and IgG eluted from senescent cells to a polypeptide migrating at 62,000 M_r in membranes of old but not young cells. The results indicated that band 3 breakdown products increase with cell age and that antigenic determinants recognized by the IgG eluted from senescent cells reside on a 62,000-M_r fragment of band 3.

Since our previous studies indicated that senescent cell antigen is derived from band 3 by cleavage in the transmembrane anion-transport region (Kay, 1981b, 1982a,b, 1984a,b; Kay and Bosman, 1985), we suspected that anion transport might be altered with cellular aging (Kay et al., 1986). If this suspicion proved correct, we would have a functional assay for aging of band 3, the major anion-transport protein of the erythrocyte membrane.

Transport studies on age-separated rat erythrocytes indicated that anion transport decreased with age (Kay et al., 1986). The Michaelis constant (K_m) increased, and the maximal velocity (V_{max}) decreased in old erythrocytes as compared with middle-aged erythrocytes.

These data provided us with another assay of cellular function to use to determine whether erythrocytes are senescent. However, it is doubtful that the number of molecules of band 3 to which IgG is bound (100 per cell) is adequate to account for the magnitude of change in anion transport. Therefore, we suspect that another as yet unidentified change precedes events initiating IgG binding and is responsible for the changes observed in anion transport.

The strongest piece of evidence supporting proteolysis of band 3 as an event initiating IgG binding, but not band 3 aging, is the finding that a senescent cell IgG column does not bind intact nondenatured band 3 (Kay, 1981a,b, 1982a). It only binds a 62,000-M_r product of band 3. However, senescent cell IgG will bind band 3 denatured by NaDodSO$_4$ (Kay et al., 1983; Kay, 1984a,b). We believe that proteolysis is not the primary aging change in band 3, although data suggest that it may be required to initiate IgG binding. Data supporting this include the finding that RBC with other changes (e.g., an altered V_{max} but with all other parameters normal) and no increased breakdown products of band 3 do not have increased IgG binding. Although we have not been able to demonstrate crosslinking, we still consider it a possibility for an aging event that may precede proteolysis and IgG binding.

Although band 3 comprises 25% of the erythrocyte membrane protein, circulating, naturally occurring autoantibodies to band 3 in normal human serum (Kay et al., 1982) do not bind to RBC unless they are senescent, stored, or damaged (Kay, 1975, 1978). However, anti-band 3 autoantibodies will bind to band 3 denatured by SDS treatment (Kay et al., 1982, 1983). Since the Fab region of the IgG molecule is 9 nm across, we suspected that IgG could not bind to native band 3 in erythrocyte membranes due to steric considerations. In order to test the hypothesis that band 3 is shielded from antibodies in the membranes of intact RBC, we investigated binding of rabbit IgG antibodies to band 3 and to senescent cell antigen in membranes of intact erythrocytes, as well as erythrocytes treated with either trypsin or chymotrypsin (Kay and Goodman, 1984). Mild trypsinization of whole RBC cleaves glycophorin A and C but spares band 3 (Steck, 1974; Furthmayer, 1978). Digestion of whole RBC with chymotrypsin yields an ~60,000-M_r transmembrane fragment of band 3 and an ~38,000-M_r fragment containing the carboxyl terminal (Steck et al., 1976).

Human RBC were incubated in phosphate-buffered saline + glucose (PBS-G) containing ATP either without any enzyme or with trypsin (100 μg/ml). After washing, cells were incubated with anti-band 3, anti-senescent cell antigen, anti-human RBC, or without antibody. Cells were washed and incubated with Fab anti-rabbit IgG–gold colloid. The results showed that anti-band 3 did not bind to red cells that had not been treated with trypsin (Kay and Goodman, 1984). However, it did bind to RBC treated with trypsin before incubation with antibodies to band 3. Binding of anti-senescent cell antigen to untreated or trypsin treated RBC was negligible. Antibodies to human RBC, which were used as a positive control, bound to both untreated and treated RBC. An additional positive control consisted of incubating RBC ghosts prepared by hypotonic lysis with antibodies to band 3 followed by Fab anti-rabbit IgG–gold colloid. Heavy labeling of RBC membranes was observed. Negative controls consisted of incubation of untreated or treated RBC with antibodies from unimmunized rabbits or Fab anti-rabbit IgG–gold colloid with prior incubation with antibodies. Binding to negative controls was not observed.

This experiment was repeated using chymotrypsin instead of trypsin. Similar results were obtained except that binding of anti-band 3 to chymotrypsin-treated cells was less than that observed following trypsin treatment (Kay and Goodman, 1984).

These results indicate that antibodies to band 3 do not bind to untreated intact RBC. Since trypsin treatment of intact RBC, which digests glycophorins A and C, permits binding of antibodies to band 3, results suggest that band 3 is shielded in the membrane by glycophorins.

Trypsinization of RBC did *not* result in binding of antibodies to the senescent cell antigen to RBC. Therefore, binding of antibodies to the senescent cell antigen to RBC membrane is not attributable to a simple exposure of the antigen but must require other changes in the membrane. Other experiments suggest that degradation of band 3 may be required to initiate binding (Kay, 1984a,b).

Results of the chymotrypsin experiments suggest that proteolytic cleavage of band 3 at the outside is not sufficient to permit binding of antibodies to band 3 or initiate binding of antibodies to the senescent cell antigen. Lack of binding or antibodies to band 3 in this case may result from steric hindrance. Failure of antibodies to the senescent cell antigen to bind to chymotrypsin-treated RBC suggests that cleavage at a site other than that attacked by chymotrypsin may be required to generate the senescent cell antigen.

9. BAND 3 IS PRESENT IN NUCLEATED CELLS

We suspected that band 3 was present in nucleated somatic cells as well as in RBC because the senescent cell antigen, which is immunologically related to band 3 (Kay *et al.*, 1982, 1983), is present on lymphocytes, platelets, adult liver cells, and embryonic kidney cells (Kay, 1981a,b). Furthermore, antibodies prepared against the senescent cell antigen isolated from white blood cells (WBC) react with erythrocyte band 3 (Kay *et al.*, 1983), and other cells are known to transport anions (Cheng and Levy, 1980).

As a test of this hypothesis, primary cultures of human fibroblasts, lung cells, neutrophils, mononuclear WBC, squamous epithelial (mouth) cells, lung squamous epithelial carcinoma, rhabdomyosarcoma, mouse neuroblastoma cells, and rat hepatocytes were examined for the presence of immunoreactive forms of band 3 by immunofluorescence, immunoelectron microscopy, and immunoautoradiography (Kay *et al.*, 1983). Band 3-related polypeptides were demonstrated in all these cells. Peptide mapping indicated that these polypeptides share peptide homology with erythrocyte band 3.

Antibodies to erythrocyte band 3 bind to the surface of nucleated somatic cells as determined by surface immunofluorescence and immunoelectron microscopy studies. Immunofluorescence studies indicate that the band 3-like proteins in nucleated cells are mobile because they participate in anti-band 3-induced cell-surface patching and capping (Kay *et al.*, 1983).

Immunoautoradiographic analysis showed that antibodies to band 3 react with a 95,000-M_r polypeptide in membranes of freshly isolated WBC; in polypeptides of 60,000, 48,000, and 38,000 M_r in cultured human lung cells; and in polypeptides of 69,000 and 60,000 M_r in cultured neoplastic cells. These polypeptides were present in cell membranes prepared with DFP, EDTA, and EGTA to avoid artifactual proteolysis. Therefore, these lower-molecular-weight immunoreactive forms of band 3 may be present in the membranes of normal and neoplastic cells *in vivo*. Electron paramagnetic resonance spectroscopy (EPR) of neoplastic cells incubated with spin-labeled (SL) SITS indicated that membranes of nucleated cells have an anion transporter that is accessible from the outside and that behaves similar to RBC band 3 (M. M. B. Kay and L. R. Dalton, preliminary data). Thus, polypeptides related to erythrocyte senescent cell antigen (Kay, 1981a) and erythrocyte band 3 (Kay *et al.*, 1983; Kay and Dalton, preliminary data; Drenckhahn *et al.*, 1984) have been demonstrated in nucleated cells, including neurons.

Other investigators have confirmed the presence of band 3 in other cell types and tissues (Low *et al.*, 1985; Cox *et al.*, 1985) and have presented evidence indicating that band 3 in other cell types does bind to the cytoskeletal network (Low *et al.*, 1985). Furthermore, evidence indicates that large amounts of band 3 are found in the basolateral plasma membrane of the intercalated cells of renal distal tubules and collecting ducts (Low *et al.*, 1985; Cox *et al.*, 1985). These results were anticipated based on the premise that band 3 performs anion transport in nonerythroid cells just as it does in erythroid cells (Cheng and Levy, 1980). Thus, transport of chlorine, bicarbonate, and so forth, in the collecting ducts of the kidney would be mediated by the same mechanism as in erythrocytes.

Cox *et al.* (1985) were able to demonstrate the presence of band 3-like peptides in avian (chicken) kidney by immunofluorescence, peptide mapping, and complementary DNA (cDNA) probe. However, these workers state that they were unable to demonstrate band 3 in any other tissues in contrast to the results of other investigators in the field (Kay *et al.*, 1983; M. M. B. Kay and L. R. Dalton, preliminary data; Drenckhan, 1984; Low *et al.*, 1985). This discrepancy may simply be a matter of sensitivity or quality of biological preparations or may be related to the quality, specificity, or other characteristics of the antisera. For example, Cox *et al.* (1985) used $NaDodSO_4$-denatured band 3 obtained from polyacrylamide slab gels to produce antisera. This treatment can destroy antigenic determinants and alter antigenic characteristics. Furthermore, the antibodies appeared weak as determined by immunoblots. Methionine-labeled rather than unlabeled polypeptides were used to characterize binding of the antisera. Both RBC and renal proximal tubule cells have large amounts of band 3 relative to other cells (e.g., 25% of membrane protein for RBC of 1.2×10^6 copies/cell) because anion transport represents one of their major functions. This undoubtedly facilitated detection of band 3 by Cox *et al.* (1985) in these cells types.

It is interesting that the band 3 polypeptides detected in avian kidneys had slightly higher molecular weights (100,000 and 105,000) than did those detected by erythrocytes.

We postulated that generation of senescent cell antigen may result from oxidation-induced crosslinking followed by proteolysis (Kay *et al.*, 1982, 1983, 1986). In evaluating oxidation as a possible mechanism responsible for generation of senescent cell antigen, we studied erythrocytes from vitamin E-deficient rats (Kay *et al.*, 1986). The importance of vitamin E as an antioxidant, providing protection against free radical-induced membrane damage, has been well documented (McCay and King, 1980; Menzel, 1980; Farrell *et al.*, 1977). Vitamin E is localized primarily in cellular membranes, and a major role of vitamin E is the termination of free-radical chain reactions propagated by the polyunsaturated fatty acids of membrane phospholipids. Vitamin E-deficient erythrocytes are defective in their ability to scavenge free radicals (Farrell *et al.*, 1977; Dodge *et al.*, 1967). Specific biochemical alterations in the membrane erythrocytes from vitamin E-deficient rhesus monkeys have been described (Shapiro *et al.*, 1982a,b). Furthermore, vitamin E deficiency represents a "physiological" method for rendering cells susceptible to free-radical damage and may simulate conditions encountered *in situ*.

Red cells from vitamin E-deficient rats behaved like old erythrocytes in the phagocytosis assay and in anion transport and G3PD activity. In addition, increased breakdown products of band 3 were observed in erythrocyte membranes from vitamin E-deficient rats. Vitamin E-deficient rats developed a compensated hemolytic anemia, as observed in vitamin E-deficient humans (Kay *et al.*, 1986).

In this phagocytosis assay, old erythrocytes obtained from rats fed a diet containing normal amounts of vitamin E were phagocytized, whereas young and middle-aged erythrocytes were not. By contrast, young and middle-aged as well as old erythrocytes were phagocytized when obtained from vitamin E-deficient rats. There was a significant difference in phagocytosis between erythrocytes obtained from normal rats and vitamin E-deficient rats, even when unfractionated erythrocytes were used for the assay (Kay et al., 1986). IgG was present on young and middle-aged cells from vitamin E-deficient rats (Kay et al., 1986). Anion-transport studies on erythrocytes from vitamin E-deficient rats revealed that their anion transport was impaired, as was transport in old erythrocytes (Kay et al., 1986).

Differences were not detected in protein or glycoprotein composition of erythrocyte membranes from control and vitamin E-deficient rats. Although high-molecular-weight polypeptides or polymers were detected with Coomassie blue staining of 2–16% polyacrylamide gels, there were no differences in the number or amount of these polypeptides between control and experimental samples.

Immunoblotting studies demonstrated the presence of increased breakdown products of band 3 in cells from vitamin E-deficient rats as is observed in old cells (Kay et al., 1986). Thus, vitamin E deficiency leads to accelerated RBC aging, presumably through oxidation.

We have not observed high-molecular-weight complexes containing band 3 in membranes from vitamin E-deficient rats or old cells aged in situ, except under conditions that precipitate IgG (unpublished observations). Similar results were obtained with RBC from copper-deficient chickens (G. Bosman, E. Harris, and M. M. B. Kay, unpublished data). This suggests that any oxidative system may cause premature aging of erythrocytes.

Several different laboratories agree that appearance of senescent cell antigen initiates IgG binding and destruction of RBC (Kay, 1974, 1975, 1978, 1981a–c, 1982a, 1984b, 1985a; Bennett and Kay, 1981; Kay and Bennett, 1982; Kay et al., 1982, 1986; Wegner et al., 1980; Glass et al., 1983; Bartosz et al., 1982a,b; Khansari and Fudenberg, 1984; Galili et al., 1983; Kay and Bosman, 1985; Singer et al., 1986; Alderman et al., 1980; Tannert, 1978; Smalley and Tucker, 1983; Khansari et al., 1983; Walker et al., 1984; Halhuber et al., 1980; Hebbell and Miller, 1984; Khansari and Fudenberg, 1983). However, the molecular changes responsible for generating the antigen have yet to be elucidated. Preliminary studies suggest that senescent cell antigen is derived from band 3, probably by degradation (Kay et al., 1982, 1983; Kay, 1982, 1984b). Lutz and colleagues have suggested that senescent cell antigen is a dimer of band 3 (Lutz and Stringaro-wipf, 1984; Lutz et al., 1984; Lutz, 1983). Sayare et al. (1982) showed that band 3 can crosslink with hemoglobin under oxidative conditions. Low et al. (1985) suggested that clustered band 3 can generate senescent cell antigen. It was once thought that a galactose might represent an antigenic site on senescent cell antigen (Galili et al., 1984, 1985). However, it has been shown that Galili et al. were studying a different antigen that is restricted to primates (Galili et al., 1987).

As an approach to elucidating mechanisms of band 3 aging, we investigated "experiments of nature." During these investigations, we discovered two unique defects in band 3. One of the defects, high-molecular-weight band 3, is characterized by a band 3 molecule that migrates in gels as though it were $\approx 98,500\, M_r$ instead of $\approx 95,000\, M_r$, as does normal band 3 (Kay et al., 1987, 1989). Thus, it behaves as though there were an addition of $3500\, M_r$ to the band 3 molecule. The other defect is fast-aging band 3, which appears to be more susceptible to proteolysis than normal band 3 molecule (Kay et al., 1989). Cells from individuals with the latter defect have a significantly shortened life span and behave in many ways like old RBC (Vomel and Platt, 1981; Kay, 1975, 1982b, 1984a,b; Aminoff and Vorder Bruegge, 1978; Aminoff et al., 1977; Galili et al., 1983; Kay et al., 1983, 1986; Kay and Goodman, 1984).

Viable defects in the band 4 molecule appear to be quite rare because there are no reported band 3 defects in the literature. A variant of band 3 has been reported following artificial treatment *in vitro* (Mueller and Morrison, 1977; Morrison *et al.*, 1981). However, no functional defects were described in association with this band 3 doublet (Mueller and Morrison, 1977). One defect, reported by Agre *et al.* (1981), was initially thought to represent a band 3 defect because it was associated with a reduction in high-affinity ankyrin-binding sites. However, erythrocytes from affected family members had a spectrin, not a band 3, abnormality. No abnormalities in molecular weight were observed.

Recently, we studied a family with a structural alteration of band 3 associated with acanthocytosis, as well as functional RBC aberrations (Kay *et al.*, 1987, 1988). One of three siblings was completely normal, while the RBC of the other two had a band 3 that migrated as though it were ~2000–4000 M_r larger than normal band 3 molecule. This change in migration was not due to carbohydrate changes because it still migrated slower than normal band 3 following treatment with endoglycosidase F. High-molecular-weight band 3 was associated with the following changes: acanthocytosis (21% and 25%), restriction of rotational diffusion of band 3 in the membrane as determined by electron paramagnetic resonance (EPR) spectroscopy, increased anion transport, decreased glucose efflux, and decreased number of high-affinity ankyrin-binding sites (Table I). EPR spectroscopy and cleavage studies with trypsin and chymotrypsin and two-dimensional peptide maps indicate that the addition is in the anion-transport region. RBC of each parent exhibited anion and glucose transport abnormalities, and small numbers of acanthocytes were seen. Abnormalities in erythrocyte IgG binding, fluorescence polarization, and other membrane proteins as determined by gel electrophoresis were not detected in the cells by any family members. Thus, a specific structural change in the anion-transport region of band 3 is associated with functional and morphological changes. The functional changes were not due to the morphological changes (acanthocytosis) because cells from a patient with abeta-lipoproteinemia with 84% acanthocytes exhibited changes opposite those of cells with high-molecular-weight band 3.

Another family that we are studying has a band 3 that appears to be more susceptible to proteolysis than normal with increased breakdown products in the 4.5 region (Kay *et al.*,

TABLE I. Changes Associated with High-Molecular-Weight and Fast-Aging Band 3 and Senescent (Old) Erythrocytes[a,b]

Individual	BD3	Morph	Transport		Ankyrin-binding sites	Rotational correction time	IgG
			Anion	glu			
HMW propositus	↑ MW	acan	↑	↓	↓	↑	nl
HMW sibling 1	nl	nl	nl	nl	nl	nl	nl
HMW sibling 2	↑ MW	acan	↑	↓	↓	↑	nl
Abeta-Liproprotein	nl	acan	↓	↓	↑	ND	
Fast-aging	↑ BRK	poik	↓	↓	nl		↑
Old cells	↑ BRK	nl	↓	↓	ND	ND	↑

[a]HMW, high-molecular-weight; BD3, band 3; MW, molecular weight; BRK, breakdown products of band 3 present on immunoblots; Morph, erythrocyte morphology; acan, acanthocytes; poik, poikilocytosis; trans, transport (V_{max}); glu, glucose influx; IgG, IgG binding determined by ^{125}I-protein A binding.
[b] ↑, increase; ↓, decrease.

1989). Structural and functional studies performed on this fast-aging band 3 included anion transport, EPR spectroscopy using a spin-label specific for the anion-transport region, and ankyrin-binding assays. Fast-aging band 3 RBC showed increased IgG binding, decreased anion and glucose transport, decreased G3PD activity, and degradation of band 3. These functional changes are the same as those observed during normal RBC aging *in situ* (Kay, 1974, 1975, 1978, 1981a–c, 1982a, 1982b, 1985a; Bennett and Kay, 1981; Kay and Bennett, 1982; Kay *et al.*, 1982, 1983, 1986; Wegner *et al.*, 1980; Glass *et al.*, 1983; Bartosz *et al.*, 1982a,b; Khansari and Fudenberg, 1985; Galili *et al.*, 1983; Singer *et al.*, 1986; Alderman *et al.*, 1980; Tannert, 1978; Smalley and Tucker, 1983; Khansari *et al.*, 1983; Walker *et al.*, 1984; Halhuber *et al.*, 1980; Hebbell and Miller, 1984; Khansari and Fudenberg, 1983). Affected individuals have reticulocyte counts of 20% indicating rapid destruction of RBC. The accelerated destruction of cells *in situ* is consistent with our experimental findings.

Our present detailed knowledge of the RBC membrane combined with the new techniques available for probing erythrocyte structure and function should permit identification of the primary locus of the genetic defect in families and kindreds with band 3 defects. We are currently mapping the functional and dysfunctional binding domains of band 3 membrane proteins in these mutants (Kay *et al.*, 1987, 1988). The technology is available to define the precise molecular alterations in terms of DNA changes, and these studies are in progress. We anticipate that band 3 mutants will allow us to identify specific band 3 functions with specific sequences and to map the aging "command center" of the molecule.

REFERENCES

Agre, P., Orringer, E. P., Chui, D., and Bennett, V., 1981, A molecular defect in two families with hemolytic poikilocytic anemia. Reduction of high affinity membrane binding sites of ankyrin, *J. Clin. Invest.* **68:**1566–1576.

Alderman, E. M., Fudenberg, H. H., and Lovins, R. E., 1980, Binding of immunoglobulin classes to subpopulations of human red blood cells separated by density-gradient centrifugation, *Blood* **55:**817–822.

Aminoff, D., and VorderBruegge, W., 1978, Viability of erythrocytes in circulation and its dependence on cell surface glycoconjugates, in: *Glycoconjugates Research*, Vol. II, *Proceedings of the Fourth International Symposium on Glycoconjugates*, Academic, New York, pp. 1011–1014.

Aminoff, D., Bruegge, W. F. V., Bell, W. C., Sarpolis, K., and Williams, R., 1977, Role of sialic acid in survival of erythrocytes in the circulation: Interaction of neuraminidase-treated and untreated erythrocytes with spleen and liver at the cellular level, *Proc. Natl. Acad. Sci. USA* **74:**1521–1524.

Ashwell, G., and Morell, A. G., 1974, The role of surface carbohydrates in the hepatic recognition and transport of circulating glycoproteins, *Adv. Enzymol.* **41:**99–128.

Bartosz, G., Sosynski, M., and Kedziona, J., 1982a, Aging of the erythrocyte. VI. Accelerated red cell membrane aging in Down's syndrome? *Cell Biol. Int. Rep.* **6:**73–77.

Bartosz, G., Sosynski, M., and Wasilewski, A., 1982b, Aging of the erythrocyte XVII. Binding of Autologous immunoglobin, *J. Mech. Aging Dev.* **20:**223–232.

Bennett, G. D., and Kay, M. M. B., 1981, Homeostatic removal of senescent murine erythrocytes by splenic macrophages, *Exp. Hematol.* **9:**297–307.

Bennett, V., and Stenbuck, P. J., 1979, The membrane attachment protein for spectrin is associated with band 3 in human erythrocyte membrane, *Nature (Lond.)* **280:**468–473.

Bosman, G. J. C. G. M., Johnson, G., Beth, A., and Kay, M. M. B. 1988, Band 3 polymers and aggregates, and hemoglobin precipitates in red cell aging, *Blood Cells* **14:**275–289.

Bosman, G. J. C. G. M., and Kay, M. M. B., 1900, Erythrocyte aging: A comparison of model systems for simulating cellula aging in vitro, *Blood Cells* **14:**19–35.

Brown, P. A., Feinstein, M. B., and Shuaki, R. I., 1975, Membrane proteins related to water transport in human erythrocytes, *Nature (Lond.)* **254:**523–525.

Cabantchik, Z. I., and Rothstein, A., 1974, Membrane proteins related to anion permeability of human red blood cells. I. Localization of disulfonic stilben binding sites in proteins involved in permeation, *J. Membr. Biol.* **15:**207–226.

Cheng, S., and Levy, L. D. N., 1980, Characterization of the anion transport system in hepatocyte plasma membranes, *J. Biol. Chem.* **255:**2637–2640.

Cox, J. V., Moon, R. T., and Lazarides, E., 1985, Anion transporter: Highly cell-type-specific expression of distinct polypeptides and transcripts in erythroid and nonerythroid cells, *J. Cell Biol.* **100:**1548–1557.

Dodge, J. T., Cohen, G., Kayden, H. J., and Phillips, G. B., 1967, Peroxidative hemolysis of red blood cells from patients with abetalipoproteinemia, *J. Clin. Invest.* **46:**357–368.

Drenckhan, D., Zinke, K., Schauer, U., Appell, K. C., and Low, P. S., 1984, Identification of immunoreactive forms of human erythrocyte band 3 in nonerythroid cells, *Eur. J. Cell. Biol.* **34:**144–150.

Drenckhahn, D., Schulter, K., Allen, D. P., and Bennett, V., 1985, Colonization of band 3 with ankyrin and spectrin at the basal membrane of intercalated cells in the rat kidney, *Science* **230:**1287–1289.

Elder, J. H., Pickett, R. A. II, Hampton, J., and Lerner, R. A., 1977, Radioiodination of proteins in single polyacylamide gel slices, *J. Biol. Chem.* **252:**6510–6515.

Farrell, P., Bieri, J. G., Fratantoni, J. F., and Wood, R. E., 1977, The occurrence and effects of human Vitamin E deficiency, *J. Clin. Invest.* **60:**233–241.

Furthmayer, H. J., 1978, Glycophorins A, B, and C: A family of sialoglycoproteins: Isolation and preliminary characterization of trypsin derived proteins, *J. Supramol. Struct.* **9:**79–98.

Galili, U., Korkesh, A., Kahane, I., and Rachmilewiltz, A., 1983, Demonstration of a natural antigalactosyl IgG antibody on thalassemic red blood cells, *Blood* **61:**1258–1264.

Galili, U., Rachmilewitz, E. A., Peleg, A., and Flechner, I., 1984, A unique natural human IgG antibody with anti-α-galactosyl specificy, *J. Exp. Med.* **160:**1519–1531.

Galili, U., Flechner, I., and Rachmilewtz, E. A., 1985, A naturally occurring anti-α-galactosyl IgG recognizing senescent human red cells, in: *Cellular and Molecular Aspects of Aging: The Red Cell as a Model* (J. W. Eaton, D. K. Konzen, and J. G. White, eds.), Liss, New York, pp. 263–276.

Galili, U., Clark, M. R., Shohet, S. B., Beuhler, J., and Macher, B. A., 1987, Evolutionary relationship between the natural anti-Gel antibody and the Galαl 3 gel epitope in primates, *Proc. Natl. Acad. Sci. USA* **84:**1369–1373.

Glass, G. A., Gershon, H., and Gershon, D., 1983, The effect of donor and cell age on several characteristics of rat erythrocytes, *Exp. Hematol.* **11:**987–995.

Halhuber, K. T., Stibenz, D., Feuerstein, H., Linss, W., Meyer, H. W., Frober, R., Rumpel, E., and Geyer, G., 1980, *Abstracts of the Ninth International Symposium on Structure and Function of Erythroid Cells, Berlin,* p. 66.

Hebbell, R. P., and Miller, W. J., 1984, Phagocytosis of sickle erythrocytes: Immunologic and oxidative determinants of hemolytic anemia, *Blood* **64:**733–741.

Karadsheh, N. S., Uyeda, K., and Oliver, R. M., 1977, Studies on structure of human erythrocyte phosphofructokinase, *J. Biol. Chem.* **252:**3515–3524.

Kay, M. M. B., 1974, Mechanism of removal of senescent red cells, *Gerontologist* **14:**33.

Kay, M. M. B., 1975, Mechanism of removal of senescent cells by human macrophages *in situ, Proc. Natl. Acad. Sci. USA* **72:**3521–3525.

Kay, M. M. B., 1978, Role of physiologic autoantibody in the removal of senescent human red cells, *J. Supramol. Struct.* **9:**555–567.

Kay, M. M. B., 1981a, Isolation of the phagocytosis inducing IgG-binding antigen on senescent somatic cells, *Nature (Lond.)* **289:**491–494.

Kay, M. M. B., 1981b, The IgG autoantibody binding determinant appearing on senescent cells resides on a 62,000 MW peptide, Presented at the *Ninth International Symposium on Structure and Function of Erythroid Cells, Berlin, Acta. Biol. Med. Geront.* **40:**385–391.

Kay, M. M. B., 1981c, The senescent cell antigen is not a desialylated glycoprotein, *Blood* **58**:90a.

Kay, M. M. B., 1982a, Molecular aging: A termination antigen appears on senescent cells, in: *Protides of the Biological Fluids Molecular*, Vol. 29 (C. Peeters, ed.), Twenty-ninth Annual Colloquium Protides of the Biological Fluids, Brussels, Belgium, 1981, Pergamon Press, Oxford, pp. 325–338.

Kay, M. M. B., 1982b, Accumulation of band 3 breakdown products is a function of cell age, Twenty-third Annual Meeting of the American Society of Hematology, Washington, D. C., *Blood* **60**:21a.

Kay, M. M. B., 1984a, Band 3, the predominant transmembrane polypeptide undergoes proteolytic degradation as cells age, *Monogr. Dev. Biol.* **17**:245–253.

Kay, M. M. B., 1984b, Localization of senescent cell antigen on band 3, *Proc. Natl. Acad. Sci. USA* **81**:5753–5757.

Kay, M. M. B., 1985a, Immune system: Expression and regulation of cellular aging, in: *Thresholds in Aging* (The 1984 Sandoz Lectures in Gerontology), (M. Bergener, M. Ermimi, and H. B. Stahelin, eds.), Academic, London, pp. 59–82.

Kay, M. M. B., 1985b, Aging of cell membrane molecules leads to appearance of an aging antigen and removal of senescent cells, *Gerontology* **31**:215–235.

Kay, M. M. B., 1986, Senescent cell antigen: A red cell aging antigen, in: *Red Cell Antigens and Antibodies* (G. Garratty, ed.), American Association of Blood Banks, Arlington, Virginia, pp. 35–82.

Kay, M. M. B., 1989, in: *Iron, The Lymphomyeloid System, Inflammation and Malignancy* (M. de Sousa and J. Brock, eds.), Wiley, London, pp. 17–33.

Kay, M. M. B., and Bennett, G. D., 1982, Letter to the Editor, *Blood* **59**:1111–1112.

Kay, M. M. B., and Bosman, G. J. C. G. M., 1985, Naturally occurring human "antigalactosyl" IgG antibodies are heterophile antibodies recognizing blood group related substances, *Exp. Hematol.* **13**:1103–1112.

Kay, M. M. B., and Goodman, J. R., 1984, IgG antibodies do not bind to band 3 in intact erythrocytes; enzymatic treatment of cells is required for IgG binding, *Biomed. Biochem. Acta* **43**:841–846.

Kay, M. M. B., Wong, P., and Bolton, P., 1982, Antigenicity, storage and aging: Physiologic autoantibodies to cell membrane and serum proteins, *Mol. Cell. Biochem.* **49**:65–85.

Kay, M. M. B., Goodman, S., Whitfield, C., Wong, P., Zaki, L., and Rudoloff, V., 1983a, The senescent cell antigen is immunologically related to band 3, *Proc. Natl. Acad. Sci. USA* **80**:1631–1635.

Kay, M. M. B., Tracey, C., Goodman, J., Cone, J. C., and Bassel, P. S., 1983b, Polypeptides immunologically related to band 3 are present in nucleated somatic cells, *Proc. Natl. Acad. Sci. USA* **80**:6882–6886.

Kay, M. M. B., Bosman, G. J. C. G. M., Shapiro, S. S., Bendich, A., and Bassell, P. S., 1986, Oxidation as a possible mechanism of cellular aging: Vitamin E deficiency causes premature aging and IgG binding to erythrocytes, *Proc. Natl. Acad. Sci. USA* **83**:2463–2467.

Kay, M. M. B., Lawrence, C., and Bosman, G. J. C. G. M., 1987, Molecular anatomy of an anemia, *Clin. Res.* **35**:599.

Kay, M. M. B., Bosman, G. J. C. G. M., and Lawrence, C., 1988, Functional topography of band 3: A specific structural alteration linked to functional aberrations in human red cells, *Proc. Natl. Acad. Sci. USA* **85**:492–496.

Khansari, N., and Fudenberg, H. H., 1983, Immune elimination of aging platelets by autologous monocytes: Role of membrane-specific autoantibody, *Eur. J. Immunol.* **13**:990–994.

Khansari, N., and Fudenberg, H. H., 1984, Phagocytosis of senescent erythrocytes by autologous monocytes: Requirement of membrane-specific autologous IgG for immune elimination of aging red blood cells, *Cell. Immunol.* **78**:114–121.

Khansari, N., Springer, G. F., Merler, E., and Fudenberg, H. H., 1983, Mechanisms for the removal of senescent human erythrocytes from circulation: Specificity of the membrane-bound immunoglobulin, *J. Mech. Aging Dev.* **21**:49–58.

Kliman, H. J., and Steck, T. L., 1975, Association of glyceraldehyde-phosphate dehydrogenase with the human red cell membrane: A kinetic analysis, *J. Biol. Chem.* **255**:6314–6321.

Lepke, S., Fasold, H., Pring, M., and Passow, H. J., 1976, A study of the relationship between inhibition of anion exchange and binding to the red blood cell membrane of 4,4'-diisothio-cyano-2,2'-disulfonic acid (DIDS) and its dihydro-derivative (H₂DIDS), *J. Membr. Biol.* **29:**147.

Low, P. S., Waugh, S. M., Zinke, K., and Drenckhahn, D., 1985, The role of hemoglobin denaturation and band 3 clustering in red blood cell aging, *Science* **227:**531–533.

Lutz, H. U., 1983, in: *Red Cell Membrane Glycosylates and Related Genetic Markers* (Cartrou, Rayer, and Salumou, eds.), Librairie Aurette, Paris, p. 273.

Lutz, H. U., and Kay, M. M. B., 1981, An age-specific cell antigen is present on senescent human red blood cell membranes, *Mech. Aging Dev.* **15:**65–75.

Lutz, H., and Stringaro-wipf, G., 1984, Identification of a cell-age-specific antigen from human red blood cells, *Biomed. Biochem. Acta* **42:**S117–S121.

Lutz, H. U., Flepp, R., and Stringaro-wipf, G., 1984, Naturally occurring autoantibodies to exoplasmic and cryptic regions of band 3 protein, the major integral membrane protein of human red blood cells, *J. Immunol.* **133:**2610–2618.

McCay, P. B., and King, M. M., 1980, Vitamin E: Its role as a biologic free radical scavenger and its relationship to the microsomal mixed-function oxidase, in: *Vitamin E: A Comprehensive Treatise* (L. Machlin, ed.), Dekker, New York, pp. 289–317.

Menzel, D. B., 1980, Protection against environmental toxicants, in: *Vitamin E: A Comprehensive Treatise* (L. Machlin, ed.), New York, pp. 473–494.

Morrison, M., Mueller, T. J., and Edwards, H. H., 1981, Protein architecture of the erythrocyte membrane, in: *The Function of Red Blood Cells: Erythrocyte Pathobiology* (D. F. M. Wallach, ed.), Liss, New York, pp. 17–34.

Mueckler, M., Caruso, C., Baldwin, S. A., Panico, M., Blench, I., Morris, H. R., Allard, W. J., Lienhard, G. E., and Lodish, H. F., 1985, Sequence and structure of a human glucose transporter, *Science* **229:**941–945.

Mueller, T. J., and Morrison, M., 1977, Detection of a variant of protein 3, the major transmembrane protein of the human erythrocyte, *J. Biol. Chem.* **252:**6573–6576.

Petz, L. D., Yam, P., Wilkinson, L., Garratty, G., Lubin, B., and Mentzer, W., 1984, Proteolytic dissection of band 3, the predominant transmembrane polypeptide of the human erythrocyte membrane, *Blood* **64:**301–304.

Ramjeesingh, M., and Rothstein, A., 1982, The location of a chymotrypsin cleavage site and of other sites in the primary structure of the 17,000-Dalton transmembrane segment of band 3, the anion transport protein of red cell, *Membr. Biochem.* **4:**259–269.

Salhany, J. M., and Shaklai, N., 1979, Functional properties of human hemoglobin bound to the erythrocyte membrane, *Biochemistry* **18:**893–899.

Sayare, M., Fikiet, M., and Paulus, J., 1982, Effect of Vitamin E on the binding of hemoglobin to the red cell membrane, *Ann. NY Acad. Sci.* **393:**251–261.

Shapiro, S. S., Mott, D. J., and Machlin, L. J., 1982a, Altered binding of glyceradehyde-3-phosphate to its binding site Vitamin E deficient red blood cells, *Nutr. Rep. Int.* **25:**507–517.

Shapiro, S. S., Mott, D. J., and Machlin, L. J., 1982b, Alterations of enzymes in red blood cell membranes in Vitamin E deficiency, *Ann. NY Acad. Sci.* **393:**263–276.

Singer, J. A., Jennings, L. K., Jackson, C. W., Dockter, M. E., Morrison, M., and Walker, W. S., 1986, Erythrocyte homeostasis: Antibody-mediated recognition of the senescent state by macrophages, *Proc. Natl. Acad. Sci. USA* **83:**5498–5501.

Smalley, C. E., and Tucker, E. M., 1983, Blood group A antigen site distribution and immunoglobulin binding in relation to red cell age, *Br. J. Haematol.* **54:**209–219.

Steck, T. L., 1974, The organization of proteins in human red blood cell membranes, *J. Cell. Biol.* **62:**1–19.

Steck, T. L., 1978, The band 3 protein of the human red cell membrane: A review, *J. Supramol. Struct.* **8:**311–324.

Steck, T. L., Ramos, B., and Strapazon, E., 1976, Increased IgG molecules bound to the surface of red blood cells of patients with sickle cell anemia, *Biochemistry* **15:**1153–1161.

Strapazon, E., and Steck, T. L., 1977, Interaction of the adolase and membrane of human erythrocytes, *Biochemistry* **16**:2966–2971.

Tannert, C. H., 1978, *Untersuchungen zum altern roter blutzellen*, Ph.D. dissertation, Humbolt University, Berlin.

Vomel, T. H., and Platt, D., 1981, Phagocytic activity of the reticulohistiocyte system in rabbits after splenectomy and activation with ink, *Mech. Aging Dev.* **17**:267–273.

Walker, W. S., Singer, J. A., Morrison, M., and Jackson, C. W., 1984, Preferential phagocytosis of in vivo aged murine red blood cells by a macrophage-like cell line, *Br. J. Haematol.* **58**:259–266.

Waugh, S., Willardson, B. M., Kahan, R., Labotka, R., and Low, P. S., 1986, Heinz bodies induce clustering of band 3, glycophorin, and ankyrin in sickle cell erythrocytes, *J. Clin. Invest.* **78**:155–1160.

Wegner, G., Tannert, C. H., Maretzki, D., Schossler, W., and Strauss, D., 1980, *Abstracts of the Ninth International Symposium on Structure and Function of Erythroid Cells, Berlin,* p. 57.

14

Health Watch: A Longitudinal Prospective Study of Healthy Aging in 2200 Individuals

I. Preliminary Analysis of Biochemical, Hematological, and Physiological Data for Males and Females. Application to the Care of Older Patients

ROBERT M. SCHMIDT, MEIWEN WU, and
GEORGE Z. WILLIAMS

1. INTRODUCTION

Health Watch, a longitudinal, prospective study of healthy aging now in its eighteenth year at Pacific Presbyterian Medical Center, San Francisco, was founded by George Z. Williams in 1970. This study was designed to characterize a healthy population of approximately 2200 individuals, and to follow them annually, with assessment of changes in good or positive health on quantitative laboratory, physiological, and health behavioral tests. The major goal was to provide a solid data base for physicians to undertake meaningful primary care and health promotion and for researchers to quantitate effects of healthy aging, using routine clinical laboratory tests and the information of patients' health behaviors.

The identification, methodology of assessment, evaluation and application of modifiable risk factors affecting the leading causes of disability, morbidity and mortality in older populations have only recently been studied (National Center for Health Services Research and Health Care Technology Assessment, 1986). Comprehensive review of the literature suggests a paucity of existing health risk, health status and functional, quality of life measures as applied to healthy older patients (Omenn, 1987; Office of Disease Prevention, 1986; Rowe and Kahn, 1987; National Center for Health Statistics, 1986; Ward and Tobin, 1987).

ROBERT M. SCHMIDT, MEIWEN WU, and GEORGE Z. WILLIAMS • Health Watch Program, Center for Preventive Medicine and Health Research, Pacific Presbyterian Medical Center and San Francisco State University, San Francisco, California 94132-1789.

Major problems in applying "wellness" and risk reduction knowledge to an older population include difficulties in recruitment, follow-up and compliance, although social marketing techniques have been successfully applied in community intervention programs to facilitate recruitment aims (Farquhar et al., 1984).

Measures of healthy aging evaluated in studies emphasizing individual differences, i.e., physiological age rather than chronological age (Harnly and Williams, 1987; Harris et al., 1980; McDowell and Newell, 1987; Williams, 1981; Williams and Harnly, 1982; Williams, 1987a, 1987b) can be applied to the major chronic diseases that decrease effective function, quality of life, and potential life span (Fries and Crapo, 1981; National Center for Health Services Research and Health Care Technology, 1986; Rowe and Besdine, 1982; Williams and Schmidt, 1989).

Health Watch provides a paradigm of economical, individualized health care for older Americans. Determination of individual health profiles, based on routine biochemical, hematological, physiological, and health behavioral data is readily achieved in the routine practice of medicine. Meaningful primary care includes active intervention advice to assist patients in staying healthy as long as possible. Our rapidly aging society cannot continue to emphasize expensive tertiary, rehabilitative medicine. Rather, primary preventive medicine, the integration of health status and risk factor analysis in the primary care specialties, must replace disease-oriented treatment of signs and symptoms. Johns et al. (1987) summarized these needs with pragmatic application to primary health care. More recently, Callahan (1987) urges all Americans to undertake an active dialogue about the role of society in caring for our elders, if we are to continue with the level of health care to which we have become accustomed.

2. METHODOLOGY

2.1. Participant Selection

2.1.1. Criteria for Selection of Subjects

Health criteria were used to determine whether an individual's values were used in analysis. The criteria of health used in the Health Watch program are defined as (1) no evidence of acute or chronic disease, (2) not under a physician's care, (3) not on any medications, (4) weight within 10% of Metropolitan Life Insurance standards, and (5) blood pressure less than 130/90 mm Hg. Unhealthy criteria are defined as (1) clinical hypertension, (2) on medication for some chronic but nonserious condition, and (3) overweight by 20% or more. The health status of each participant was assessed through a questionnaire and physical examination using the above criteria at the first visit. All participants in the healthy group were accepted as study subjects, and all those in the unhealthy group were excluded. The group between the above classes were also excluded in data analysis.

2.1.2. Age and Sex Distribution of Participants

Recruitment of 2170 individuals from the San Francisco Bay Area was begun in 1970. The age range of persons at entry was 21–80 years. There were 809 subjects in the young age group (18–34 years), 1086 in the middle-age group (35–54 years), and 275 in the old-age group (55 and older). Healthy men and women were actively recruited to the study through the media, speaking engagements at health clubs, professional and business organizations, and through advertisements in newspapers, billboards and magazines. Several feature articles in the Bay Area press also emphasized participation in the study.

2.2. Biochemical, Hematological, and Physiological Data

2.2.1. Laboratories

Laboratories performing tests for the Health Watch Program were also the central laboratories during the 1970s for the National Institutes of Health heart disease prevention program (MRFIT, Multiple Risk Factor Intervention Trials). Williams (1987a,b) used his experience at the Clinical Center laboratory at the National Institutes of Health to design a rigid quality control system in the Health Watch Program.

2.2.2. Laboratory Tests

Laboratory tests used in the study covered a broad spectrum of biochemical, hematological, and physiological variables found useful in the evaluation of healthy aging in pilot studies carried out at the National Institutes of Health (NIH). The initial 13 biochemical tests selected during preliminary studies included glucose, blood urea nitrogen (BUN), creatinine, uric acid, calcium, phosphorus, total protein, cholesterol, lactic dehydrogenase, alkaline phosphotase, aspartate amino transferase (AST, formerly designated SGOT), γ-glutamyl transferase (GGTP) (since 1976), and triglyceride. Eight hematological tests performed included white blood cell (WBC) count, red blood cell (RBC) count, hemoglobin (Hb), hematocrit (Hct), MCV, MCH, MCHC, and platelet count. Six physiological tests performed included height, weight, pulse, systolic blood pressure, diastolic blood pressure, and percent body fat (since 1980). Four additional biochemical test results were added in subsequent years: high-density lipoproteins (HDL) (since 1979), low-density lipoproteins (LDL) (since 1979), thyroxine (T_4) (since 1977), and calculation of the total cholesterol-to-HDL ratio.

2.2.3. Test Schedule

Participants return for annual health evaluations, which usually include, as a minimum, three visits over a 3- to 6-week period, to provide individual means and ranges.

2.2.4. Blood Sample Collection and Physiological Evaluation

In order to facilitate comparability of blood test results from one time to another and to assist subjects in maintaining their physiologically "normal" state for collection of blood samples, the following instructions were given to subjects in reference to rest, food consumption, and physical activity: (1) no alcoholic beverages for 12 hr before the appointment; (2) take your usual vitamins and/or medicines, which reflect your current routine habits; (3) evening meal the night before the Health Watch appointment—exclude foods not typical of your usual diet; (4) drink only water after dinner; (5) get a good night of sleep; (6) breakfast before blood sample—eat at least 1 hr before your appointment (exclude products with caffeine, cream, sugar, fats, or orange juice; and (7) do not exercise the morning of the blood draw.

Participants are requested to return at the same time and day of week during each of the three Health Watch evaluations, preferably at a 3- to 6-week interval, and to begin their annual evaluation in the same month each year.

2.3. Health Behavioral Data

An individual Health Profile Index was developed to evaluate a subject's health based on reported health events and habits. The scores are derived from the subject's responses on the Health Watch Questionnaire. Each of the responses was assigned a weight in proportion to the health benefit of the response. The weights for all of a subject's responses in a given scale were summed to give a raw score. The range for each scale was 0 to 100.

The Health Watch Health Profile Index consists of two areas of health history: Health Status and Health Habits. Health Status is divided into three subscales: (1) Medical Events scale, summarizing a subject's medical history since the last Health Watch update, including medication usage, common clinical conditions, and surgeries; (2) General Well-being scale, ascertaining a subject's energy level and resistance to illness by responses to 13 questions about sleep, physical symptom patterns, and sick days; and (3) Psychological Well-being scale, including two subscales: an adaptation of the index of well-being and a modified version of the social readjustment rating scale (stress scale). Weights on the stress scale are determined according to a subject's own perception of an events stressfulness rather than a fixed value. These two scales and 12 other items determine the subject's scale score.

Health Habits are divided into four subscales: (1) the Nutrition scale evaluates the type and frequency of a subject's food intake according to the American Heart Association List of Preferred Foods for maintaining a healthy heart; (2) the Tobacco and Alcohol scales reflect the presence, amount, and frequency of using these substances; and (3) the Physical Activity scale summarizes the frequency, duration, and potential health benefit of a subject's exercise and sport activities, assessing aspects of aerobic benefit, strength, flexibility, and balance.

An initial questionnaire was prepared for the subject's first visit. Another questionnaire was prepared for subsequent follow-up visits. Every subject completes a questionnaire for each year of evaluation.

2.4. Statistical Analysis

The initial analysis of this huge database places emphasis on establishing a pattern for integrating 26 biochemical, hematological, and physiological variables and determination of the age trends of significantly different tests between two consecutive age groups for males and females. This is a preliminary analysis of the 1974 to 1978 data base, a period showing the least missing data. We focused on 5-year intervals of ages 20 to 74 years. All data from 1974 to 1978 were extracted from the complete data base using the program SUPERSORT.

All subjects included in the data from 1974 to 1978 were selected by the healthy and unhealthy criteria described above by inputting their information from both initial and update questionnaires to a series of computer programs designed to identify the subject's health status. Data from those who were identified as unhealthy were excluded from this analysis.

A subject was represented only once for one test with each 1-year period presented. The one value of a test for 1 year for a subject was the mean value of all the determinations within the year under observation. Since we used a 5-year interval, each subject had five values within the 5-year period. A mean of these five values was calculated for each subject for each test.

For each test, the mean and standard deviation of values for a specific group and the slope based on the mean value of each age group were calculated. For the comparison between male and female sexes, the mean of all values for each year from 1974 to 1978 for a specified test for males in a specified age group was compared with that for females in the same age group, and similarly for all other tests and for all age groups.

3. RESULTS

The trends of biochemical, hematological, and physiological test results by male and female sex for ages 20 to 74 years are shown in Table I. Results are summarized as follows.

TABLE I. Trends in Biochemical,
Hematological, and Physiological Data
by Male and Female Sex, Ages 20
to 74 Years[a]

Male	Female
Increase	
Glucose	Glucose
Blood urea nitrogen	Blood urea nitrogen
Creatinine	Uric acid
Uric acid	Calcium[b]
LDH	Alkaline phosphatase
GGTP	SGOT (AST)
Cholesterol	LDH
Triglyceride	GGTP
WBC	Cholesterol
MCV	Triglyceride
MCH	RBC
Pulse	Hb
Systolic blood pressure	Hct
	Pulse
	Systolic blood pressure
	Diastolic blood pressure
	Weight
Decrease	
Calcium	Platelet count
Phosphorus	Height
Total protein	Calcium[b]
RBC	
HGB	
Hct	
MCHC	
Platelet count	
Height	

[a]Slopes based on mean values of each age group were calculated for each test. Positive slopes with $p < 0.05$ indicate that the rate of change increased. Negative slopes with $p < 0.05$ indicate that the rate of change decreased.
[b]For female sex, calcium decreases with age until age 40, increases after age 40.

(1) For men, test mean values increase with age in glucose, BUN, creatinine, uric acid, LDH, GGTP, cholesterol, triglyceride, WBC, MCV, MCH, pulse, systolic blood pressure; and decrease with age in calcium, phosphorus, total protein, RBC, Hb, Hct, MCHC, platelet count, height. (2) For women, test mean values increase with age in glucose, BUN, uric acid, calcium (after age 40), alkaline phosphatase, SGOT, LDH, GGTP, cholesterol, triglyceride, RBC, Hb, Hct, pulse, systolic blood pressure, diastolic blood pressure, weight; and decrease with age in platelet count, height, and calcium (before age 40).

Most of the clinical tests analyzed indicate that there are obvious trends with age. Some of the trends show linear relationship between age and value; some show curved relationships; some have different trends in different age intervals. Significant gender differences with age are observed.

Generally, results of this pilot data analysis are consistent with those of previous studies (Hodkinson, 1984; Jandl, 1987; Percival and Quinkert, 1987; Rowe and Besdine, 1982).

4. DISCUSSION

A review of the major longitudinal studies that have been or are being conducted on adults indicates that some only involve males, and for those that include both males and females, some only follow subjects during a narrow age range (U.S. Department of Health and Human Services, 1984). The Tecumseh Community Health Study has followed subjects involving both male and female sexes with ages from birth to over 70 years. However, publications from this study have analyzed data only by the cross-sectional method, with special emphasis on the role of physical activity in the maintenance of health. Longitudinal analyses of repeated observations on the same subjects have not been published (Epstein *et al.*, 1986; Montoye, 1975). Review of the gerontology/geriatrics literature suggests that our primary data analysis of the Health Watch Program is the first published longitudinal study showing sex differences with aging based on a broad spectrum of clinical laboratory, physiological, and health behavioral variables.

4.1. Statistical Methodology

The method used for data analysis in this chapter is both longitudinal and cross-sectional (Campbell, 1986). The longitudinal analysis allows us to obtain data for 5 years and calculate the mean value that represents the value at the middle of the period of 5 years, based on the assumption that regression of the variable on age is linear. This is more reasonable than a cross-sectional study, which obtains mean values only by performing tests at a given point in time or several times within a relatively short period of time (Greenhouse, 1986). In addition, our comparison between men and women is also based on the longitudinal data.

Our cross-sectional analysis involves the comparison between two consecutive age groups of the same sex. Although such a cross-sectional study confounds the effects of aging and cohort (Campbell, 1986), it is still useful to define individual health status through an integrated analysis of routinely performed clinical laboratory and physiological test values. If this method is applied to a longitudinal study to determine the age of significant changes for individuals, one can obtain a more detailed understanding of aging changes in each person and a distribution of the frequency of such changes by age and sex for the population. If the healthy population-based patterns and the individual-based patterns are established by such a study, they can be used for assessing health, for making clinical diagnoses, and for determining health risk factors, by combining clinical and behavioral data (Williams, 1987a).

4.2. Gender Differences with Aging

The results of our study provide evidence of sex differences of aging. These are not limited to gender differences in the same age groups but also relate to aspects of variances of test parameters, age change points showing the age of major change and change trends.

Preliminary results of biochemical, hematological, and physiological data comparing healthy men and women over time suggest a trend of sex differences that increase in the age range of 20–29 years, remain stable in the age range of 30–44 years, and subsequently decrease after age 45. This suggests that there is a peak of biomedical differences between the sexes at the age group of 30–44 years. The relationship between this peak and the effect of sex steroids and trophic hormones should be studied in healthy men and women over time. Correlations between this peak and other biomedical and psychosocial/behavioral factors are also high priorities for future research.

4.3. Preventive Medicine in an Aging America: Application to the Care of Older Patients

The Health Watch study presents a paradigm for quantitation of individual rates of aging and provides a solid data base for physicians to undertake meaningful primary care and health promotion using routine clinical laboratory tests. This preventive medicine approach emphasizes traditional clinical medicine in combination with active patient assumption of their own health behavior, an emerging patient–physician preventive medicine paradigm. Routine Health Watch assessments may also provide solutions to some of the questions about health policies for an aging America raised by Callahan (1987).

A review of the current literature (Office of Disease Prevention and Health Promotion, 1986; Farquhar et al., 1984) suggests an urgent need to (1) carry out systematic investigation of processes leading to clinical outcomes rather than investigation of only end points themselves, (2) design health care programs using multifactor interventions with greater potential for successful implementation than single risk-factor interventions, and (3) randomize studies of recruitment and of the effectiveness of behavior change in single versus multiple risk-factor interventions.

The Health Watch study provides a solid data base to apply active multiple intervention techniques without the need to design and carry out additional expensive longitudinal studies of healthy aging. Preliminary results presented here, continuing analysis of the existing data base and research findings from major published longitudinal studies on normal or usual aging (Busse and Maddox, 1985; Greenhouse, 1986; U. S. Department of Health and Human Services, 1984) and behavioral, psychosocial, and economic considerations associated with an aging society (Committee on an Aging Society, 1985; Ward and Tobin, 1987) mandate the application of known risk-reduction techniques to older populations.

Since aging is thought to be the sum of many mechanisms functioning at the molecular to organ level, and the major goal of gerontology should be to increase the quality of life (Schneider et al., 1982), it is likely that further analysis of the enormous Health Watch data base will result in application of a panel of biological markers of physiological aging to serve as intervention guidelines for the health care of older Americans.

5. SUMMARY

Health Watch, a longitudinal prospective study of healthy aging now in its eighteenth year at Pacific Presbyterian Medical Center San Francisco, was founded by George Z. Williams in 1970. The subjects include 2170 men and women, aged 21–80 years at entry, living in the San Francisco Bay Area. The study makes use of well-controlled biochemical, hematological, and physiological tests performed on an annual basis over three weekly visits, combined with a self-administered health events and habits questionnaire. A pilot data analysis of 26 routine biochemical, hematological and physiological tests based on a 5-year window (from 1974–1978) using graphic techniques, with emphasis on trends of change with aging, has been performed. Most of the clinical tests analyzed indicate that there are obvious trends with age. Some of the trends show linear relationships between age and values; some show curved relationships; some have variable trends in different age intervals. These results provide descriptive statistics for further inferential statistical analysis currently underway. Further analysis may also provide a solid data base for physicians to undertake meaningful primary care and health promotion and for researchers to study effects of aging, using routine clinical tests and social/behavioral information.

ACKNOWLEDGMENT. The Health Watch study was carried out at the Institute of Health Research, Medical Research Institute of San Francisco at Pacific Medical Center, until May 1987.

REFERENCES

Benfante, R., Reed, D., and Brody, J., 1985, Biological and social predictors of health in an aging cohort, *J. Chron. Dis.* **38**:385–395.

Busse, E. W., and Maddox, G. L., 1985, *The Duke Longitudinal Studies of Normal Aging. 1955–1980.* Springer, New York.

Callahan, D., 1987, *Setting Limits. Medical Goals in an Aging Society.* Simon & Schuster, New York.

Campbell, R. T., 1986, Longitudinal design and longitudinal analysis. A comparison of three approaches, *Res. Aging* **8**:480–502.

Committee on an Aging Society, 1985, *America's Aging. Health in an Older Society.* Institute of Medicine/National Research Council, National Academy Press, Washington, D. C.

Epstein, F. H., Francis, T., Jr., Hayner, N. S., Johnson, B. C., Kjelsberg, M. O., Napier, J. A., Ostrander, L. D., Jr., Payne, M. W., and Dodge, H. J., 1986, Prevalence of chronic diseases and distribution of selected physiologic variables in a total community, Tecumseh, Michigan, *Am. J. Epidemiol.* **81**:307–322.

Farquhar, J. W., Maccoby, N., and Solomon, D. S., 1984, Community applications of behavioral medicine, in: *Handbook of Behavioral Medicine* (W. D. Gentry, ed.), Guilford Press, New York, pp. 437–478.

Fries, J. F., and Crapo, L. M., 1981, *Vitality and Aging,* W. H. Freeman, San Francisco.

Greenhouse, S. W., 1986, The comparability of longitudinal studies and the role of clinical trails in normal aging research, *Exp. Gerontol.* **21**:341–344.

Harnly, M. E., and Williams, G. Z., 1987, Health status and health habit evaluation, in: *Measurement in Health Promotion and Protection* (T. Abelin, Z. J. Brzezinski, and V. D. L. Carstairs, eds.), European Series No. 22, World Health Organization Regional Publications, Copenhagen, pp. 555–563.

Harris, E. K., Cooil, B. K., Shakarji, G., and Williams, G. Z., 1980, On the use of statistical models of within person variation in long-term studies of healthy individuals, *Clin. Chem.* **26**:383–391.

Hodkinson, M., 1984, *Clinical Biochemistry of the Elderly*, Richard Clay, Singapore.

Jandl, J. L., 1987, *Blood*, Little Brown, Boston.

Johns, M. B., Hovell, M. F., Ganiats, T., Peddlecord, M. K., and Agras, S. W., 1987, Primary care and health promotion: A model for preventive medicine, *Am. J. Prev. Med.* **3**:346–357.

McDowell, I., and Newell, C., 1987, *Measuring Health: A Guide to Rating Scales and Questionnaires*, Oxford University Press, New York.

Montoye, H. J., 1975, *Physical Activity and Health: An Epidemiological Study of an Entire Community*, Prentice-Hall, Englewood Cliffs, New Jersey.

National Center for Health Services Research and Health Care Technology Assessment, 1986, Health risk appraisal: Methods and programs, with annotated bibliography, Publication No. (PHS) 96-3396, U.S. Department of Health and Human Services, Washington, D.C.

National Center for Health Statistics, 1986, Health promotion data for the 1990 objectives. Estimates from the National Health Interview Survey of health promotion and disease prevention, United States, 1985 (O. T. Thornberry, R. W. Wilson, and P. M. Golden, eds.), Advance data from vital and health statistics, No. 126, Publication No. (PHS) 86-1250. Department of Health and Human Services, Hyattsville, Maryland.

Office of Disease Prevention and Health Promotion, 1986, Integration of risk factor interventions, U.S. Government Printing Office No. 116-307, U.S. Department of Health and Human Services, Washington, D.C.

Omenn, G. S. 1987, University of Washington Center for Health Promotion in Older Adults, *Persp. Prev.* **2**:50–55.

Percival, L., and Quinkert, K., 1987, Anthropometric factors, in: *Sex Differences in Human Performance* (M. A. Baker, ed.), Wiley, New York.

Rowe, J. W., and Besdine, R. W. (eds.), 1982, *Health and Disease in Old Age*, Little, Brown, Boston.

Rowe, J. W., and Kahn, R. L., 1987, Human aging: Usual and successful, *Science* **237**:143–149.

Schmidt, R. M., and Kvitash, V. I., 1987, Identification of immunodeficiencies using computer-assisted analysis of hematological, biochemical, immunological, physiological and behavioral data, in: *Proceedings of the Eighth European Immunology Meeting, Zagreb, Yugoslavia, European Society of Immunology.*

Schmidt, R. M., Kvitash, V. I., and Hata, L. E., 1988, Early identification of immunodeficiencies using person-specific data generated in a longitudinal study on healthy aging, in: *Abstracts of Biomedical Advances in Aging 1988*, Washington, D.C., 9–13 May, 1988, p. 78.

Schneider, E. L., Reff, M. E., Finch, C. E., and Meksler, M., 1982, Potential application of biological markers for assessing interventions of physiological aging, in: *Biological Markers of Aging* (M. E. Reff and E. L. Schneider, eds.), *Proceedings of Conference on Nonlethal Biological Markers of Physiological Aging, June 19–20, 1981*, Publication No. (NIH) 82-2221, U. S. Department of Health and Human Services, Bethesda, pp. 237–252.

Sprott, R. L., and Schneider, E. L., 1985, Biomarkers of aging, *Drug–Nutrient Interactions* **4**:43–52.

U.S. Department of Health and Human Services, 1984, Normal human aging: The Baltimore longitudinal study of aging, NIH Publication No. (PHS) 84-2450, National Institute on Aging, Washington, D.C.

Ward, R. A., and Tobin, S. S. (eds.), 1987, *Health in Aging. Sociological Issues and Policy Directions*, Springer, New York.

Williams, G. Z., 1981, Individual-specific normal ranges and identification of trend changes in serum constituents, in: *Progress in Health Monitoring* (T. Yasaka, ed.), Excerpta Medica, New York, pp. 21–34.

Williams, G. Z., and Harnly, M., 1982, Health status and healthy habit evaluation, *Med. Inform.* **7**:193–207.

Williams, G. Z., 1987a, Person-specific health maintenance, in: *Maintaining a Healthy State within the Individual* (E. K. Harris, and T. Yasaka, eds.), Elsevier, Amsterdam, pp. 41–47.

Williams, G. Z., 1987b, Life style and prospects for healthy aging or aging need not be debilitating, in: *Proceedings of the First Linus Pauling Symposium on Nutrition, Health and Peace.* Linus Pauling Institute of Science and Medicine, Stanford, pp. 161–169.

Williams, G. Z., and Schmidt, R. M., 1989, Person specific health assessment and preventive medicine in the 21st century, in: *MEDINFO 89* (B. Barber, D. Cao, D. Qin, and G. Wagner, eds.), North-Holland, Amsterdam, pp. 22–25.

15

Plasma α-Tocopherol Levels in Men and Women of Different Ages

CARLO VERGANI, PATRIZIA STEFANONI, MONICA GRAZIOLI, MARIGRAZIA CLERICI

1. INTRODUCTION

The aging process and age-related changes have been linked to the production of free radicals during normal metabolism (Harman, 1981). α-Tocopherol (AT), the fat-soluble vitamin E, a constituent of biomembranes, plays an important role as a chain-breaking antioxidant in protecting biological molecules against oxidative damage (McCay and King, 1980; Burton and Ingold, 1986).

The transport of AT in the blood seems not to be mediated by a specific carrier, being mainly due to plasma lipoproteins (Bjornson *et al.*, 1976). We determined AT levels in normal subjects of different ages, taking into consideration lipid and lipoprotein parameters.

2. MATERIALS AND METHODS

We examined 240 apparently healthy subjects, 20 men and 20 women, for each decade of life between 20 and 91 years of age. After an overnight fast, 10 ml of blood was drawn from an antecubital vein and collected in heparinized vacutainers. Plasma was isolated immediately and frozen at $-80°C$ until analyzed. The sample analyses were carried out within 3 months of collection. AT was analyzed chromatographically according to the method of Vuilleumier *et al.* (1983) in a Waters high-performance liquid chromatography (HPLC) system (Waters Associates, Milano, Italy) containing a normal phase LiChrosorb Si 60 (5 μm) column, with a mobile phase of *n*-hexane—ethyl acetate (1000:75); detection was performed with a Waters 420-AC fluorescence detector (excitation, 290 nm; emission, 330 nm). This system permits detection and quantitation of as little as 1.0 mg/liter of tocopherol. Quantitation of tocopherol was based on peak height analysis and comparison with known

CARLO VERGANI, PATRIZIA STEFANONI, MONICA GRAZIOLI, and MARIGRAZIA CLERICI
• Institute of Internal Medicine, University of Milan, 20122 Milan, Italy.

amounts of authentic D,L-α-tocopherol (Hoffmann-La Roche, Basel, Switzerland). The co-efficient of variation of concurrently analyzed duplicate assays was 3.2%. Serum total lipids, cholesterol, and triglycerides were determined with the use of the Boehringer–Mannheim methods and for Apo A-I, B, and E, with the use of radioimmunodiffusion (Daiichi Pure Chemicals Co., Ltd, Tokyo, Japan).

High-density lipoprotein (HDL) cholesterol was quantified after precipitation of Apo B-containing lipoproteins by the magnesium chloride–phosphotungstic acid method (Lopes-Virella et al., 1977).

Statistical analysis was performed using the SAS system for personal computers, version 6.03 program. Nonpaired Student's t-test and linear regressions calculated by least-squares method were used.

3. RESULTS

Mean plasma AT, lipid, and lipoprotein levels in men and women of various age groups are presented in Table I. AT increased progressively in men and women with age, up to the sixth decade of life. Thereafter, a decrease of AT levels was observed. Figure 1 shows the plasma AT mean values and the 5th and 95th percentile curves in men and women. In the last two age groups, AT levels were significantly higher in women than in men ($p < 0.001$) (Fig. 2). When correlation coefficients were calculated, a significant positive correlation ($p < 0.001$) was found between AT and total lipids ($r = 0.88$), total cholesterol ($r = 0.61$), triglycerides ($r = 0.27$), HDL cholesterol ($r = 0.19$), Apo B ($r = 0.49$), Apo E ($r = 0.25$), and Apo A-I ($r = 0.12$). The AT–total lipid (mg/g) ratio did not change with advancing age and remained remarkably constant, above 0.6 or 0.8, calculated as the mean ratio of AT to total lipids in adult serum (Farrell et al., 1978) (Fig. 3).

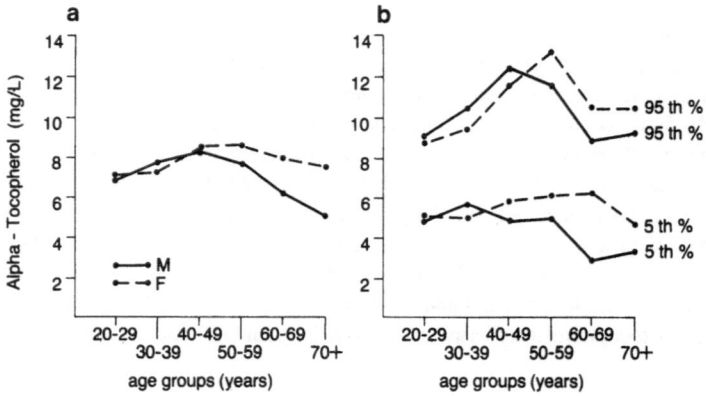

FIGURE 1. Mean levels (a) and 5th and 95th percentiles (b) for plasma α-tocopherol in 20- to 91-year-old men and women.

TABLE I. α-Tocopherol, Lipid, and Lipoprotein Parameters in Different Age Groups[a,b]

Parameters	20–29 M	20–29 F	30–39 M	30–39 F	40–49 M	40–49 F	50–59 M	50–59 F	60–69 M	60–69 F	70+ M	70+ F
α-Tocopherol (mg/liter)	6.8 ±0.1	6.9 ±0.07	7.9 ±0.09	7.1 ±0.09	8.2 ±0.14	8.3 ±0.11	7.9 ±0.12	8.4 ±0.12	6.2 ±0.1	8.0 ±0.08	5.6 ±0.1	7.7 ±0.11
5th percentile	4.8	5.1	5.8	5.0	4.9	5.9	5.1	6.1	3.0	6.2	3.4	4.7
95th percentile	9.4	8.7	10.4	9.7	12.4	11.7	11.7	13.3	9.0	10.6	9.3	10.6
Total cholesterol (mg/liter)	164.4 ±1.9	178.6 ±2.0	192.0 ±1.7	183.7 ±1.6	214.1 ±2.1	205.1 ±1.9	210.9 ±1.8	216.7 ±1.7	198.4 ±2.2	218.2 ±1.9	185.5 ±1.8	197.7 ±1.8
HDL cholesterol (mg/dl)	40.8 ±0.4	56.0 ±0.6	47.3 ±0.8	51.0 ±0.7	49.6 ±0.7	60.1 ±0.8	47.0 ±0.7	60.2 ±0.7	47.9 ±0.8	58.4 ±0.8	48.2 ±0.8	48.8 ±0.9
Triglycerides (mg/dl)	85.8 ±2.1	65.4 ±0.9	99.8 ±2.4	70.0 ±2.1	113.9 ±2.2	88.8 ±2.3	106.6 ±2.0	94.4 ±3.1	111.3 ±2.2	90.9 ±2.1	97.0 ±1.9	90.1 ±1.5
Total lipids (mg/dl)	700.6 ±10.0	721.2 ±7.4	825.7 ±9.2	778.7 ±9.9	858.2 ±11.9	829.4 ±12.2	855.4 ±13.2	856.5 ±10.0	692.4 ±10.2	856.5 ±8.4	647.1 ±8.3	838.4 ±10.4
AT/TL[c] (mg/g)	0.97	0.96	0.96	0.92	0.96	0.99	0.93	0.99	0.91	0.94	0.88	0.93
Apo A-I (mg/dl)	139.4 ±0.9	141.8 ±2.1	152.4 ±1.5	152.4 ±2.0	150.8 ±1.8	161.4 ±1.4	148.3 ±1.6	159.4 ±2.1	140.1 ±2.3	155.0 ±2.0	152.0 ±2.3	143.4 ±1.7
Apo B (mg/dl)	85.6 ±1.0	75.6 ±1.7	86.0 ±1.1	76.4 ±1.4	101.6 ±1.2	90.4 ±2.0	112.3 ±2.1	98.8 ±1.7	109.4 ±1.4	99.9 ±1.6	100.0 ±1.8	96.4 ±2.2
Apo E (mg/dl)	3.5 ±0.06	3.1 ±0.1	3.8 ±0.1	2.9 ±0.04	3.9 ±0.06	3.4 ±0.1	3.9 ±0.1	4.1 ±0.3	4.0 ±0.09	4.4 ±0.1	4.1 ±0.1	4.2 ±0.1

[a]Values are expressed as mean ± SEM.
[b]M, males; F, females.
[c]AT/TL, α-tocopherol/total lipids.

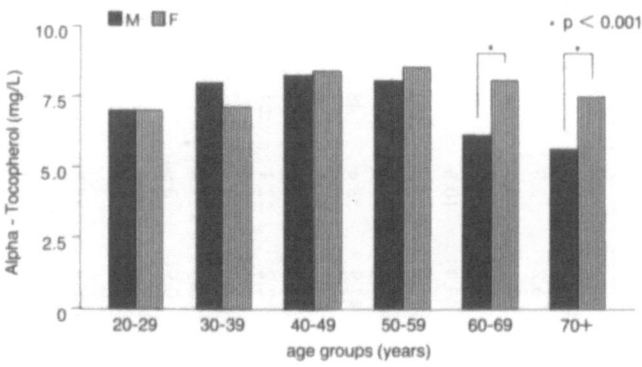

FIGURE 2. Mean plasma α-tocopherol levels in 20- to 91-year-old men and women.

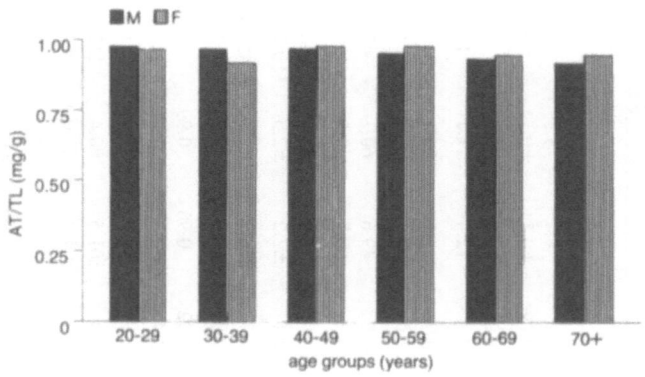

FIGURE 3. Plasma α-tocopherol/total lipid (mg/g) ratios in 20- to 91-year-old men and women.

4. DISCUSSION

Our results on AT plasma concentration in healthy subjects are consistent with those of other studies, which report increasing levels with advancing age (Lewis *et al.*, 1973; Gontzea and Nicolau, 1972). In accordance with Vanderwoude and Vanderwoude (1987), this positive correlation cannot be applied to the elderly. Plasma AT levels depend on the interplay of a number of factors, such as the concentration of triglycerides, phospholipids, cholesterol and lipoprotein carriers, rate of removal from the plasma, and retention rates in individual tissues (Gallo-Torres, 1980).

Different studies show a correlation between lipid and lipoprotein parameters and plasma AT levels (Bjornsen *et al.*, 1976; Behrens *et al.*, 1982). This relationship is particularly close for total lipids (Fig. 4). Horwitt *et al.* (1972) stressed the importance of simultaneous determination of blood lipids and expression of circulating AT as the ratio of AT to total lipid. We obtained highly significant correlations between AT and all lipid and lipoprotein parameters investigated. The correlation with Apo B, a major component of low-density lipoprotein (LDL) (Havel *et al.*, 1980), reflects the importance of this lipoprotein in the

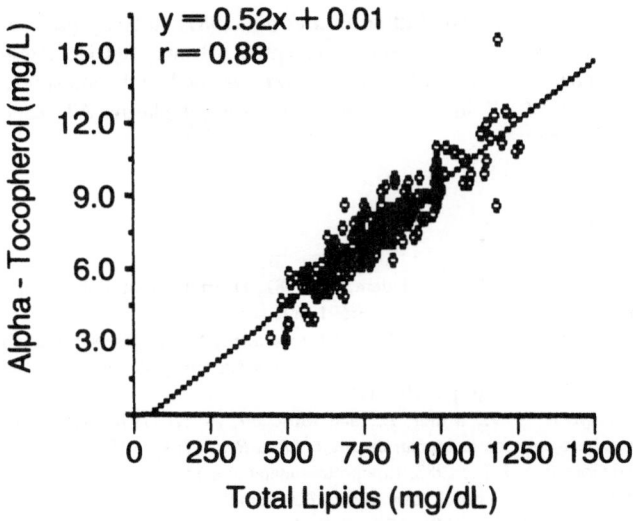

FIGURE 4. Correlation between α-tocopherol and total lipids.

transport of AT delivered to the cell mainly through the LDL receptor (Traber and Kayden, 1984). The absence of Apo B-100 and Apo B-48 in abetalipoproteinemia involves a near absence of AT in blood and tissue (Herbert *et al.*, 1983). Triglyceride-rich lipoproteins ($d <$ 1.006 g/ml) are also carriers of AT, further supported by the positive correlation between AT and Apo E, which is a constituent of very-low-density lipoproteins (VLDL) (Havel *et al.*, 1980). HDL, of which Apo A-I is the main apoprotein component (Havel *et al.*, 1980), also correlate with AT. This is particularly intriguing, taking into consideration the finding of Herman *et al.* (1979) that large doses of tocopherol can increase HDL cholesterol, showing an inverse relationship with the incidence of coronary heart disease (Miller and Miller, 1975; Gordon *et al.*, 1977). However, other studies (Serfontein *et al.*, 1983) do not support this finding. Plasma AT deficiency has been reported in the absence of hypolipidemia (Harding *et al.*, 1985). Some other carriers, different from lipid and lipoproteins, must therefore be proposed.

The behavior of plasma AT levels over different ages parallels that of lipid and lipoprotein parameters, so that the ratio of AT to total lipids is remarkably constant over different age groups. In the normal population, the plasma cholesterol level increases progressively with age in men and women. Not until after the age of 70 does this trend reverse. Above 50 years of age, cholesterol levels are higher for women than for men (Lipid Research Clinics Program Epidemiology Committee, 1979). This finding may explain the sex differences in AT levels observed in our subjects at a late age.

If this is true, AT levels must be considered as an epiphenomenon of plasma lipid levels, not reflecting the real biological tissue activity of vitamin E (Vatassery *et al.*, 1983; Sokol *et al.*, 1984).

However, high levels of circulating AT have been reported as positively modulating the aging process (Schneider and Reed, 1985). The higher levels of plasma AT in elderly women compared with levels in men are also relevant with respect to the difference in longevity between the two sexes. It was recently shown that, after short-term therapy, vitamin E may protect LDL peroxidation *in vivo* (Bittolo-Bon *et al.*, 1987), thereby preventing modified LDL uptake by macrophages via scavenger receptors (Brown and Goldstein, 1983) and atherogenesis (Steinberg, 1983). Further information is needed on the transport, metabolism, and biological activity of AT in order to assess the role of plasma AT, especially in the elderly.

REFERENCES

Behrens, W. A., Thompson, J. N., and Madere, R., 1982, Distribution of alpha tocopherol in human plasma lipoproteins, *Am. J. Clin. Nutr.* **35**:691–696.

Bittolo-Bon, G., Cazzolato, G., Saccardi, M., and Avogaro, P., 1987, Presence of a modified LDL in humans: Effect of vitamin E, in:, *Clinical and Nutrition Aspects of Vitamin E* (O. Hayaishi and M. Mino, eds.), Elsevier, Ireland, pp. 109–120.

Bjornson, L. K., Kayden, H. J., Miller, E., and Moschell, A. N., 1976, The transport of alpha-tocopherol and beta-carotene in human blood, *J. Lipid Res.* **17**:343–352.

Brown, M. S., and Goldstein, J. L., 1983, Lipoprotein metabolism in the macrophage: Implications for cholesterol deposition in atherosclerosis, *Annu. Rev. Biochem.* **52**:223–261.

Burton, G. W., and Ingold, K. U., 1986, Vitamin E: Application of the principles of physical organic chemistry to the exploration of its structure and function, *Acc. Chem. Res.* **19**:194–201.

Farrell, P. M., Levine, S. L., Murphy, D., and Adams, A. J., 1978, Plasma tocopherol levels and tocopherol lipid relationships in a normal population of children as compared to healthy adults, *Am. J. Clin. Nutr.* **31**:1720–1726.

Gallo-Torres, H. E., 1980, Transport and Metabolism, in: *Vitamin E. A Comprehensive Treatise* (L. J. Machlin, ed.), Dekker, New York, pp. 289–347.

Gontzea, I., and Nicolau, N., 1972, Relationship between serum tocopherol level and dyslipidemia, *Nutr. Rep. Int.* **5**:225–230.

Gordon, T., Castelli, W. P., Hjortland, M. C., Kannell, W. B., and Dawber, T. R., 1977, High density lipoprotein as a protective factor against coronary heart disease, The Framingham Study, *Am. J. Med.* **62**:707–714.

Harding, A. E., Matthews, S., Jones, S., Ellis, C. J. K., Booth, I. W., and Muller, D. P. R., 1985, Spinocerebellar degeneration associated with a selective defect of vitamin E absorption, *N. Engl. J. Med.* **313**:32–35.

Harman, D., 1981, The aging process, *Proc. Natl. Acad. Sci. USA* **78**:7124–7128.

Havel, R. J., Goldstein, J. L., and Brown, M. S., 1980, Lipoprotein and lipid transport, in: *Metabolic Control and Disease*, 8th ed. (P. K. Bondy and L. E. Rosenberg, eds.), W. B. Saunders, Philadelphia, pp. 393–494.

Herbert, P. M., Assman, G., Gotto, A. M., Jr., and Fredrickson, D. S., 1983, Familial lipoprotein deficiency: Abetalipoproteinemia, hypobetalipoproteinemia, and Tangier disease, in: *Metabolic Basis of Inherited Disease* (J. B. Stambury, J. B. Wyngaarden, D. S. Fredrickson, J. L. Goldstein, and M. S. Brown, eds.), McGraw-Hill, New York, pp. 589–621.

Herman, W. J., Ward, K., and Faucett, J., 1979, The effect of tocopherol on high-density lipoprotein cholesterol. A clinical observation, *Am. J. Clin. Pathol.* **72**:848–852.

Horwitt, M. K., Harvey, C. C., Dahm, C. H., Searcy, M. T., 1972, Relationship between tocopherol and serum lipid level for determination of nutritional adequacy, *Ann. N.Y. Acad. Sci.* **203**:223–236.

Lewis, J. S., Pian, A. K., Baer, M. T., Acosta, P. B., and Emerson, G. A., 1973, Effect of long-term ingestion of polyunsaturated fat, age, plasma cholesterol, diabetes mellitus and supplemental tocopherol, Am. J. Clin. Nutr., 26: 136–143.

Lipid Research Clinics Program Epidemilogy Committee, 1979, Plasma lipid distribution in selected North American populations: The Lipid Research Clinics Program Prevalence Study, *Circulation* **60**:427–439.

Lopes-Virella, M. F., Stone, P., Ellis, S., and Colwell, J. A., 1977, Cholesterol determination in high-density lipoproteins separated by three different methods, *Clin. Chem.* **23**:882–884.

McCay, P. B., and King, M., 1980, Biochemical function, in: *Vitamin E. A Comprehensive Treatise* (L. J. Machlen, ed.), Marcel Dekker, New York, pp. 289–494.

Miller, G. J., and Miller, N. F., 1975, Plasma high density lipoprotein concentration and development of ischaemic heart disease, *Lancet* **1**:16–19.

Schneider, E. L., and Reed, J. D., 1985, Modulations of aging processes, in: *Handbook of the Biology of Aging,* 2nd ed. (C. E. Finch and E. L. Schneider, eds.), Van Nostrand–Reinhold, New York, pp. 45–76.

Serfontein, W. J., Ubbinink, J. B., and De Villiers, L. S., 1983, Further evidence on the effect of vitamin E on the cholesterol distribution in lipoproteins with special reference to HDL subfractions, *Am. J. Clin. Pathol.* **79**:604–606.

Sokol, R. J., Heubi, J. E., Iannaccone, S. T., Bove, K. E., and Balistrieri, W. F., 1984, Vitamin E deficiency with normal serum vitamin E concentrations in children with chronic cholestasis, *N. Engl. J. Med.* **310**:1209–1212.

Steinberg, D., 1983, Lipoproteins and atheroscloerosis: A look back and a look ahead. *Artheriosclerosis* **3**:283–301.

Traber, M. G., and Kayden, H. J., 1984, Vitamin E is delivered to cells via the high affinity receptor to low-density lipoprotein, *Am. J. Clin. Nutr.* **40**:747–751.

Vanderwoude, M. F. J., and Vanderwoude, M. G., 1987, Vitamin E status in a normal population: The influence of age, *J. Am. College Nutr.* **6**:307–311.

Vatassery, G. T., Krezowski, A. M., and Eckfeldt, J. H., 1983, Vitamin E concentrations in human blood plasma and platelets, *Am. J. Clin. Nutr.* **37**:1020–1024.

Vuilleumier, J. P., Keller, H. E., Gysel, D., and Hunziker, F., 1983, Clinical chemical methods for the routine assessment of the vitamin status in human populations. I. The fat-soluble vitamin A and E and beta carotene, *Int. J. Vitam. Nutr. Res.* **53**:265–272.

16

Polyenoic Fatty Acid Metabolism and Prostaglandin Biosynthesis in Aged Persons

OLAF ADAM

1. INTRODUCTION

The incorporation of polyunsaturated fatty acids (PUFA) in body lipids influences the fluidity of body cells and their capability to form prostaglandins (PG) (Adam and Wolfram, 1984). Recent work has shown that the intake of PUFA has implications on PUFA incorporation (Zöllner *et al.*, 1979), desaturation (Bloj *et al.*, 1973) and PG formation (Adam *et al.*, 1986a,b), which is essential for proper cell function. Aging is a cellular event that may result in impairment of membrane-bound enzymes regulating PUFA metabolism. The objectives of this study were to compare in a group of young adults and in a group of aged persons the incorporation of linoleic acid into plasma lipids. By measuring the elongation product, arachidonic acid, we were able to estimate the activity of the rate-limiting enzyme in this process, the delta-6-desaturase. Finally, we monitored PG formation by measuring the joint urinary metabolite of PGE, PGF, and PGD in 24-hr urine.

2. EXPERIMENTAL SUBJECTS AND DIETS

The group of young adults were six healthy women, judged by clinical examination and laboratory findings, aged 24–32 years. They were given liquid formula diets, in which protein provided 15%, carbohydrates 55%, and fat 30% of total energy intake. The second group consisted of six healthy persons aged 72–84 years, given conventional diets of the same composition. Each of the diets was given to the experimental subject for 2 weeks. To check linoleic acid incorporation and metabolism, a linoleic acid supply of 4% and 20% of total energy intake was provided.

OLAF ADAM • Medical Polyclinic, University of Munich, D-8000 Munich, Federal Republic of Germany.

3. MATERIALS AND METHODS

At the end of the 2-week period, fasting blood samples were drawn from a forearm vein. Lipoprotein fractions were separated by ultracentrifugation and lipid extracts were prepared from plasma, low-density lipoprotein (LDL) and high-density lipoprotein (HDL) (Adam *et al.*, 1985). Cholesterol ester were separated by chromatography on silica gel columns, and lecithin by thin-layer chromatography on silica gel plates, as previously described (Adam *et al.*, 1980). The methyl esters of fatty acids were prepared by transmethylation and analyzed on a capillary column (i.d. 0.3, length 25 m) coated with Silar 10CP. Statistical analyses were done by the unpaired Wilcoxon signed rank test.

Prostaglandin biosynthesis was measured by the determination of tetranorprostanedioic acid in 24-hr urine. This compound is the joint chemical derivative in which 80–90% of the urinary metabolites of PGE, PGF, and PGD with 16 carbon atoms (C_{16}) can be transformed (Nugteren, 1975). This compound is a measure of the overall PG production in the body.

4. RESULTS

In plasma cholesterol esters, linoleic acid was 48 ± 2% of total fatty acids in the younger group and 48 ± 7% in the older group at the end of the diet, providing 4 energy% linoleic acid. With increased intake, linoleic acid augmented to 64 ± 3% in the younger and 62 ± 7% in the older group.

Arachidonic acid decreased with 20 energy% linoleic acid intake by 2% in the younger group, while an increase by 2% was observed in the aged persons. Oleic acid decreased in both groups with augmented linoleic acid intake, while on saturated fatty acids no effect was observed.

In LDL lecithin, the percentage of linoleic acid was 6% lower in the younger group than in the older group at the end of the 2-week period, providing 4 energy% linoleic acid intake and increased in both groups to 80% at the end of the diet providing 20 energy% linoleic acid. The percentage of arachidonic acid in LDL lecithin was not changed with the diet, but in the older group the percentage of arachidonic acid was significantly higher after both diets compared with the values of young adults. The decrease of monounsaturated fatty acids after high linoleic acid intake was the same in both groups, and no change in the percentage of saturated fatty acids was observed. In HDL lecithin (Fig. 1), the increase of linoleic acid at the end of the diet providing 20 energy% linoleic acid was greater in the young adults. Arachidonic acid decreased in this group from 12 ± 4% to 9 ± 1%, while in aged persons an increase from 10 ± 2% to 12 ± 3% was found. For oleic acid, the same decrease was observed in both groups, while the percentage of palmitic acid was not affected by the dietary regimen.

5. PROSTAGLANDIN BIOSYNTHESIS

The excretion of PG metabolites, transformable to tetranorprostanedioic acid was 70% lower in the senior group than in young adults (Fig. 2). Increased linoleic acid intake augmented PG metabolites in 24-hr urines of both groups. In both groups, a fivefold increase of the linoleic acid supply doubled the amount of tetranorprostanedioic acid measured in 24-hr urine.

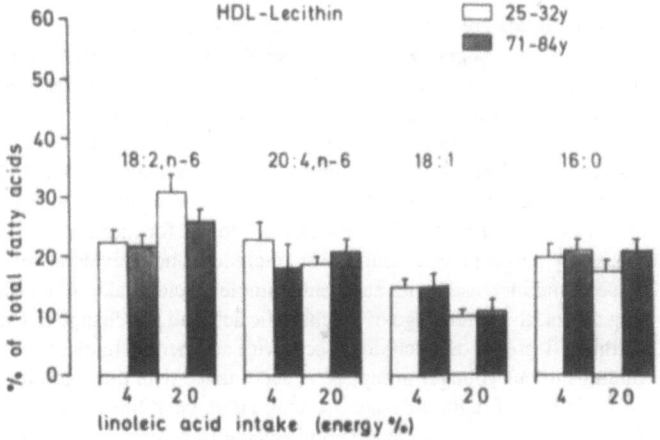

FIGURE 1. Fatty acids of HDL-lecithin in two groups of six healthy women aged 25–32 years (white bars) or six persons aged 71–84 years (dark bars) determined at the end of 2-week periods with diets providing a linoleic acid intake of 4% or 20% of total energy intake.

6. DISCUSSION AND CONCLUSIONS

Linoleic acid levels were very similar in both groups during both dietary regimens, indicating a good adherence of all experimental subjects to the diets. A dietary linoleic acid supply of 20 energy% resulted in a comparable increase of this fatty acid in plasma cholesterol esters. Cholesterol esters are most likely to reflect body lipid composition (Ormsby *et al.*, 1963; Schwartz *et al.*, 1978). From this result, it can be concluded that linoleic acid uptake

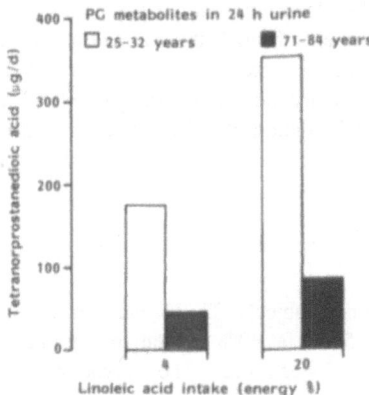

FIGURE 2. Tetranorprostanedioic acid, the joint urinary metabolite of prostaglandin (PG) E, F, and D, determined in 24-hr urine samples of six healthy women aged 25–32 years (white bars) or six healthy seniors aged 71–84 years (dark bars) at the end of diets providing a linoleic acid intake of 4 or 20 energy%.

and transport in plasma lipids are similar in young adults and aged persons. To investigate linoleic acid metabolism, we separated LDL and HDL by ultracentrifugation. Metabolic studies have shown that in LDL, lipids are transported from the intestine to peripheral tissues, while HDL are concerned with the centripedal transport of the lipids to the liver (Bondjers *et al.*, 1980; Green *et al.*, 1979). Therefore, the fatty acid profile of HDL reflects more closely the fatty acid pattern of body lipids than LDL. Phospholipids have been shown to incorporate most of the dietary linoleic acid (Adam *et al.*, 1985); we chose the greatest phospholipid fraction, lecithin, for our analyses. No differences were found for linoleic acid levels in the lipoprotein fractions of young and aged adults. But arachidonic acid levels were significantly higher in aged persons and increased with augmented linoleic acid intake. On the contrary, in the group of young adults, the percentage of arachidonic acid did not change in LDL lecithin, while in HDL lecithin a decrease of arachidonic acid with augmented linoleic acid intake was observed. The findings in our younger group are in accordance with those of other investigators, reporting an inhibition of delta-6-desaturase with augmented linoleic acid intake (Nugteren, 1965; Patil *et al.*, 1979). This enzyme regulates the transformation of linoleic acid to higher unsaturated fatty acids. The downregulation of this enzyme is supposed to enable a high linoleic acid incorporation without an excessive increase in cellular fluidity. Until now, nothing is known about the means by which this enzyme is regulated. It can be assumed that the activity of this enzyme is related to the fluidity of the cell membranes. In fatty acid deficiency, the activity of this enzyme is high, leading to the desaturation of otherwise unprocessed saturated fatty acids, indicating the status of linoleic acid deficiency. With high intake of PUFA, as in our experiment, the activity of delta-6-desaturase obviously decreases only in younger adults, as indicated by the lower percentage of arachidonic acid with high linoleic acid intake. So the availability of the substrate seems to be negatively correlated with enzymatic activity. In aged persons, this regulation obviously is impaired, because an increase of arachidonic acid was found with augmented linoleic intake. The impact of this finding on cellular fluidity or the formation of oxygen radicals, which are also supposed to be triggering substances for other cellular events, e.g., carcinogenesis, is not understood.

Prostaglandin biosynthesis, measured by the determination of tetranorprostanedioic acid in 24-hr urines, was lower in aged persons. PG are effectors of receptor-mediated cell responses, which regulate the electrolyte and energy status of the cell. Reduced PG biosynthesis results in an impairment of renal function and a tendency to gastrointestinal (GI) bleeding, symptoms found with cyclo-oxygenase inhibitors as well. In fact, these side effects of nonsteroidal drugs are commonly found in elderly patients. Whether these side effects can be avoided by the observed stimulation of PG biosynthesis with higher linoleic acid intake must be established.

7. SUMMARY

Two groups of experimental subjects (25–32 years versus 71–84 years) were given diets (protein 15%, carbohydrates 55%, fat 30% of total energy intake) providing a linoleic acid supply of 4 or 20 energie%, for 2 weeks each. The incorporation of linoleic acid was assessed by determination of the fatty acids in plasma cholesterol esters. The activity of the enzyme delta-6-desaturase was estimated by the determination of arachidonic acid in LDL and HDL lecithin. PG biosynthesis was monitored by the determination of tetranorprostanedioic acid, a joint metabolite of PGE, PGF, and PGD in 24-hr urine samples. Incorporation of linoleic acid in plasma cholesterol esters was the same in both groups. The percentage of arachidonic acid in HDL lecithin was higher in aged persons and increased in this group with augmented linoleic acid intake, while a decline of arachidonic acid was found in the younger adults with high linoleic acid intake. PG biosynthesis in the aged persons was only one third that found in young adults. With augmented linoleic acid intake in both groups, the excretion of tetranorprostanedioic acid was stimulated to twofold the control values. From these data, it is concluded that polyunsaturated fatty acid metabolism is affected by aging.

REFERENCES

Adam, O., and Wolfram, G., 1984, Effect of different linoleic acid intake on prostaglandin biosynthesis and kidney function in man, *Am. J. Clin. Nutr.* **40:**763–770.

Adam, O., Wolfram, G., and Zöllner, N., 1980, Phospholipidfraktionen im Plasma des Menschen unter dem Einfluß von Formeldiäten mit modifizierten Fettanteilen. Infusionsther, *Klin. Ernähr. Forsch. Prax.* **6:**176–180.

Adam, O., Wolfram, G., and Zöllner, N., 1985, Wirkung der Linolsäurezufuhr auf die Konzentration der Linolsäure und ihrer Folgeprodukte in einzelnen Plasmalipiden beim Menschen, *Z. Ernährungswiss.* **24:**236–244.

Adam, O., Wolfram, G., and Zöllner, N., 1986a, Vergleich der Wirkung von Linolsäure und Eicosapentaensäure auf die Prostaglandinbiosyntheses beim Menschen, *Klin. Wochenchr.* **64:**274–280.

Adam, O., Wolfram, G., and Zöllner, N., 1986b, Effect of alpha-linolenic acid in human diet on linoleic acid metabolism and prostaglandin biosynthesis, *J. Lipid Res.* **27:**421–426.

Bloj, B., Morero, R. D., Farias, R. N., and Trucco, R. F., 1973, Membrane lipid fatty acids and regulation of membrane-bound enzymes, *Biochem, Biophys. Acta* **311:**67–79.

Bondjers, G., Olsson, G., Nyman, L. L., and Björkerud, S., 1980, High density lipoprotein (HDL) depentend elimination of cholesterol from normal arterial tissue in man, in: *Athersclerosis*, Vol. 4 (G. Schettler, Y. Gotto, G. Kose, and G. Mata, eds.), Springer-Verlag, Berlin, pp. 70–71.

Green, P. H. R., Glickman, R. M., and Saudek, C. D., 1979, Human intestinal lipoproteins, *J. Clin. Invest.* **64:**233–239.

Nugteren, D. H., 1965, The enzymic conversion of gamma-linolenic acid into homo-gamma-linolenic acid, *Biochim. Biophys. Acta* **68:**28–29.

Nugteren, D. H., 1975, The determination of prostaglandin metabolites in human urine, *J. Biol. Chem.* **250:**2808–2812.

Ormsby, J. W., Schnatz, J. D., and Williams, R. H., 1963, The incorporation of linoleic 1-C^{14} acid in human plasma and adipose tissue, *Metabolism* **12:**812–820.

Patil, G. S., Sprecher, H., and Cornwell, D. G., 1979, Correlation between surface area and the rate of enzymatic desaturation with methyl branched 8,11,14-eicosatrieon acid, *Lipids* **14:**826–828.

Schwartz, C. C., Halloran, L. G., Vlahcevic, R., Gregory, D. H., and Swell, L., 1978, Preferential utilization of free cholesterol from high-density lipoproteins for biliary cholesterol secretion in man, *Science* **200:**62–64.

Zöllner, N., Adam, O., and Wolfram, G., 1979, The influence of linoleic acid intake on the excretion of urinary prostaglandin metabolites, *Res. Exp. Med.* **175:**149–153.

17

Altered Phosphatidylinositol Breakdown in Polymorphonuclear Leukocytes with Aging

TAMÀS FÜLÖP, JR., ZSUZSA VARGA, JOZSEF CSONGOR,
MARIE-PAULE JACOB, LADISLAS ROBERT,
ANDRÀS LEOVEY, and GABRIELLA FORIS

1. INTRODUCTION

It is well known that elderly subjects are susceptible to infections, cancer, and autoimmune disorders (Gladstone and Recco, 1976; Doll et al., 1970; Blumenthal and Berns, 1964). The immune functions were studied extensively in aged humans and animals; the results suggest that the B- and T-lymphocyte functions were altered, particularly the T-cell-mediated immune response (Weksler, 1983; Makinodan and Kay, 1980; Antonaci et al., 1987). It is thought that this decline contributes in large part to the increased incidence of the above-mentioned diseases. Most of the effector functions that occur during the immune response necessitate the stimulation of specific receptors. Among these functions, the most important are proliferation, differentiation, secretion, and phagocytosis (Michell, 1987; Snyderman and Pike, 1984; Fülöp et al., 1985). A few studies have been concerned with receptors (Roth, 1986; De Weck et al., 1984) and postreceptor signal-transduction mechanisms (Ito et al., 1982; Fülöp et al., 1987b) in the cells of elderly. The aim of this chapter is to elucidate some aspects of the signal-transduction mechanism in the polymorphonuclear leukocytes (PMNL) of elderly subjects.

TAMÀS FÜLÖP, JR., ZSUZSA VARGA, JOZSEF CSONGOR, ANDRÀS LEOVEY, and GABRIELLA FORIS • First Department of Medicine, University Medical School of Debrecen, 4012 Debrecen, Hungary.   MARIE-PAULE JACOB and LADISLAS ROBERT • Laboratory of the Biochemistry of Connective Tissue, CNRS UA 1174, Faculty of Medicine, University of Paris-Val de Marne, 94010 Créteil, France.

2. THE POSTRECEPTOR SIGNAL-TRANSDUCTION MECHANISM

Currently, it seems to be accepted that three major intracellular signal transduction mechanisms exist coupled with surface receptors. The first, which has long been known, is the receptor–ligand interaction linked to cAMP. The ligand effects are exerted through at least two membrane-associated GTP-binding proteins, referred to as G_s and G_i denoting, respectively, the stimulatory and inhibitory proteins toward adenylate cyclase (Rasenick *et al.*, 1987). The second mechanism, involving the GTP-binding regulatory G_i protein, is the receptor-mediated stimulation of phospholipid turnover, necessitating the initial breakdown of phophatidylinositol bisphosphate (PIP_2) to generate two moieties, each of which is believed to have second messenger characteristics: diacylglycerol (DAG), which activates the protein kinase C (Nishizuka, 1984), and inositol 1,4,5-trisphosphate (IP_3), which mobilizes Ca^{2+} from intracellular stores (Berridge, 1984). The third mechanism, which is still not very well known, is a GTP-binding G protein linked to phospholipase A_2 mediating the release of arachidonic acid (Burch *et al.*, 1986). A huge amount of information is now available on signal transduction mechanisms of various specific receptors, such as chemotactic, cholinergic, α-adrenergic, angiotensin, opioid, and neurotransmitters (Michell, 1987; Abdel-Latif, 1986; Agranoff, 1987), in the cells of young subjects, while the signal-transduction mechanism in the cells of elderly persons has not been completely elucidated.

3. ALTERATIONS IN THE SIGNAL-TRANSDUCTION MECHANISM WITH AGING

3.1. Cyclic Nucleotide Changes

Cyclic nucleotides play an important role as second messengers in signal transduction (Michell, 1987; Roth, 1986; Rasenick *et al.*, 1987; Mepler *et al.*, 1987). Various specific receptors, such as adrenergic (β_1 and β_2), vasopressin (V_2), and histamine (H_2), are coupled to adenylate cyclase, ultimately leading to cAMP production. In various cells of the elderly, the activation of adenylate cyclase is very controversial, as some investigators have found a conserved stimulation (Fülöp *et al.*, 1984, 1985), while other workers have found impaired stimulation (McLaughlin *et al.*, 1986; Tam and Walford, 1978). It seems clear that the basic cAMP level of cells of elderly subjects is lower than that of young subjects (Fülöp *et al.*, 1984; McLaughlin, *et al.*, 1986; Tam and Walford, 1978).

Cyclic guanosine monophosphate (cGMP), another important factor in the signal-transduction mechanism, could not be stimulated by any of the applied stimuli in various cells of elderly subjects (Fülöp *et al.*, 1985, 1987b, 1984; Hauck *et al.*, 1987). Despite the lack of agreement regarding cyclic nucleotide changes with aging, it seems evident that this important second messenger system is altered.

3.2. Alterations of Ca^{2+} Metabolism

The Ca^{2+} concentration in the cytoplasm is held so low (at ~0.1 μmoles) that small ion movements can substantially raise this value: a change in cytoplasmic Ca^{2+} can therefore serve as an effective intracellular signal.

The increased level of intracellular free Ca^{2+} could occur from intracellular stores or from the extracellular medium. When receptors cause a rise in the intracellular concentrations of IP_3, this compound binds to its own "receptors" on the surface of the endoplasmic reticulum, triggering a rapid release of Ca^{2+} into the cytoplasm. Interestingly, the basic intracellular free Ca^{2+} level is much higher in the PMNL of elderly subjects than in the PMNL of young subjects: 332 ± 130 nmoles and 131 ± 30 nmoles, respectively, which correlates with the impaired calmodulin system with aging (Fülöp *et al.*, 1987a). The extrusion of Ca^{2+} through the calmodulin-dependent Ca^{2+} pump is altered, while the influx is conserved (Fülöp *et al.*, 1987a). The net result is an elevation of the intracellular free Ca^{2+} level explaining the alteration of some cellular functions with aging (Varga *et al.*, 1988; Miller *et al.*, 1987). Moreover, this increased intracellular Ca^{2+} level could not be further stimulated by any of the agents known for their Ca^{2+}-increasing effects (Figs. 1 and 2). This can be due to an altered IP_3 formation under receptor stimulation.

3.3. Altered Polyphosphoinositide Metabolism

Recent studies indicate that phospholipase C-induced degradation of the inositol phospholipids leads to the formation of two molecules: 1,2-diacylglycerol, which stimulates protein kinase C, and 1,4,5-inositol trisphosphate, which can mobilize Ca^{2+} from the endoplasmic reticulum to the cytosol. We investigated the phosphatidylinositol breakdown under κ-elastin and FMLP stimulation (Figs. 3 and 4). A decrease was found in all inositol phosphates (IP_1, IP_2, IP_3) in stimulated PMNL of elderly subjects as compared with that of young subjects, but the most marked decrease was observed in IP_3 levels. This could explain the decreased Ca^{2+} stimulation by these same agents (see Figs. 1 and 2).

The basic IP levels in resting PMNL were also studied. It was found that the IP_3 level in

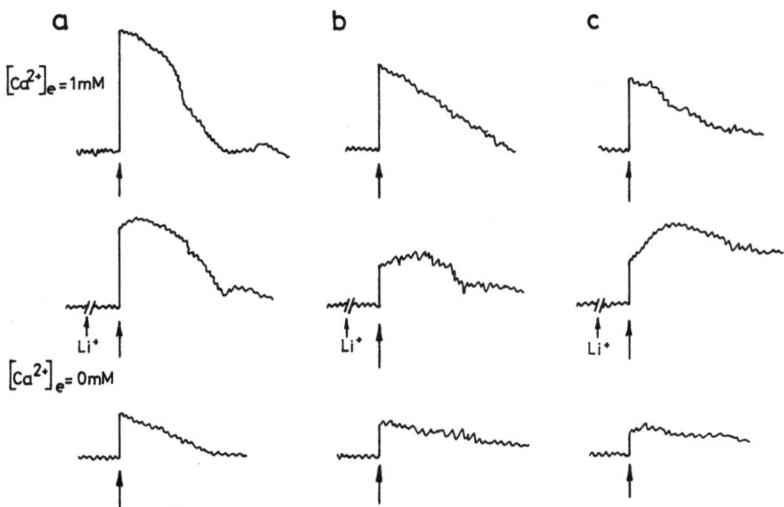

FIGURE 1. FMLP (10^{-8} M)-induced intracellular free Ca^{2+} elevation in the PMNL of young (a) and elderly (b,c) subjects in the presence and absence of 1 mM extracellular Ca^{2+}. Li^+ was applied in 5 mM concentration. The Ca^{2+} free medium contained 2 mM EGTA.

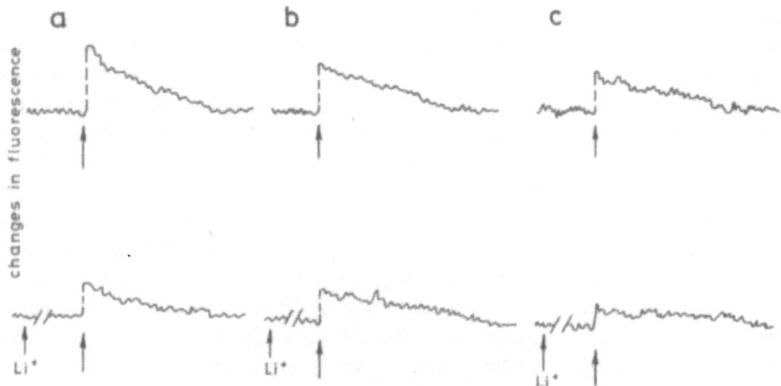

FIGURE 2. κ-Elastin (1.0 μ/ml)-induced intracellular free Ca²⁺ elevation in the PMNL of young (a) and elderly (b,c) subjects in the presence and absence of Li⁺ (5 mM).

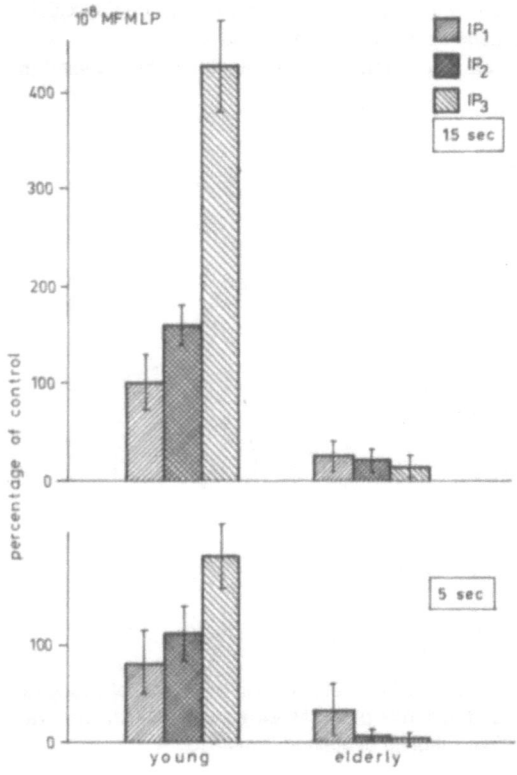

FIGURE 3. Effect of FMLP (10⁻⁸ M) on phosphatidylinositol breakdown in the PMNL of young and elderly subjects. Each value represents the mean ± SD of five independent experiments.

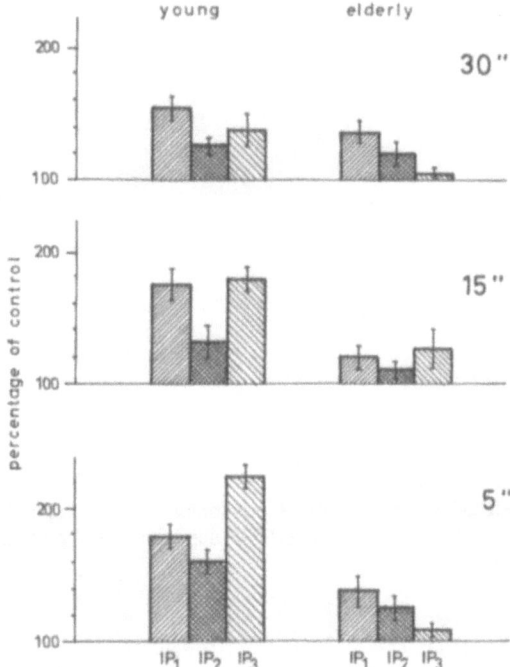

FIGURE 4. Effect of κ-elastin (1.0 μg/ml) on phosphatadylinositol breakdown of young and elderly subjects. Each value represents the mean ± SD of five independent experiments.

resting PMNL of aged subjects was higher than in the PMNL of young subjects. This increased basic IP_3 level could be connected to the enhanced intracellular free Ca^{2+} level in the PMNL of aged subjects. The exact causes of these elevations are unknown, but it can be supposed that a higher metabolism is necessary in an aging cell for the same functional level at rest than in a young cell. As a further consequence of this increased resting metabolism, the stimulation of cells could not be as effective as it should be for an adequate functionment.

The various inhibitors used (Fig. 5), further confirmed that a problem should exist at the level of GTP-binding G protein. Pertussis toxin did not display a significant effect, while neomycin demonstrated an even greater decrease in the IP stimulation in PMNL of elderly subjects. Interestingly, the mepacrin seemed to stimulate IP formation mainly of that of IP_2 and IP_3. In an attempt to investigate the possibility of an alteration in GTP-binding G protein, we tried more direct stimulation of the phosphatidylinositol breakdown in the PMNL of elderly subjects: GTP-γS stimulation.

3.4. Effect of GTP-γS on Phosphoinositide Metabolism

GTP-γS is currently being used to stimulate phosphoinositide metabolism in cell membrane preparations (Lapetina, 1987) as well as in permeabilized cells (Lapetina, 1986). We also tried to investigate its effect on the PMNL of elderly subjects. After our preliminary results, no significant effect could be obtained on phosphatidylinositol breakdown in the PMNL of elderly (Fig. 6). Since it is known that GTP-γS acts on GTP-binding G protein, the

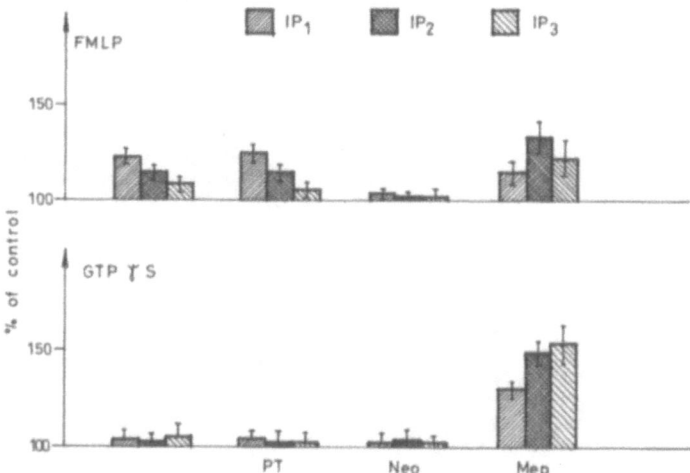

FIGURE 5. Effects of various inhibitors on phosphatidylinositol breakdown in the PMNL of elderly under FMLP and GTP-γS stimulation. PT, pertussis toxin; Neo, neomycin; Mep, mepacrin.

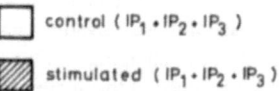

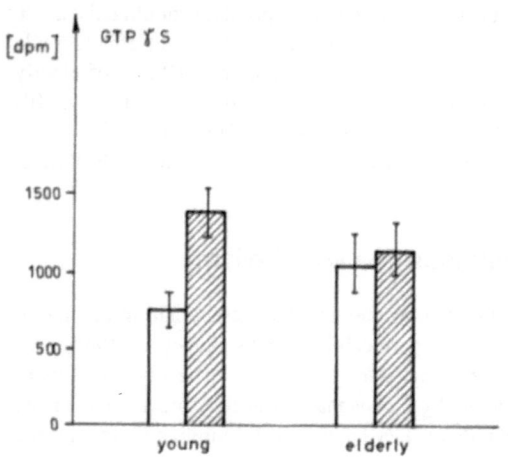

FIGURE 6. Effects of GTP-γS on phosphatidylinositol breakdown in PMNL of young and elderly subjects.

results obtained seem to lend support to our hypothesis that this protein is altered with aging. The direct verification is currently under investigation in our laboratory.

4. CONCLUSION

It seems evident that with aging there exists an alteration of the signal transduction mechanism at various levels of second messenger formation. This is a very complex biochemical process, but one of the basic alteration seems to be the impairment of GTP-binding G protein. Further elucidation of the altered signal-transduction mechanism with aging will help us to better understand the physiological alterations of cell function and to integrate these findings into our present knowledge, in an effort to influence and perhaps prevent, the aging process.

REFERENCES

Abdel-Latif, A. A., 1986, Calcium mobilizing receptors, phosphoinositides and the generation of second messengers, *Pharmacol. Rev.* **38**:227–272.

Agranoff, B. W., 1987, Receptor mediated phosphoinositide metabolism, in: *Molecular Mechanism of Neuronal Responsiveness* (Y. H. Ehrlich, R. H. Lenox, E. Kornecki, and O. W. Berry, eds.), Plenum, New York, pp. 69–79.

Antonaci, S., Jirillo, E., and Bonomo, L., 1987, Immunoregulation in aging, *Diagn. Clin. Immunol.* **5**:55–61.

Berridge, M. J., 1984, Inositol trisphosphate and diacylglycerol as second messengers, *Biochem. J.* **220**:345–360.

Blumenthal, H. T., and Berns, A. W., 1964, Autoimmunity in aging, in: *Recent Advances in Gerontological Research* (B. Strehler, ed.), Academic, New York, pp. 289–304.

Burch, R. M., Luini, A., and Axelrod, J., 1986, Phospholipase A_2 and phospholipase C are activated by distinct GTP-binding proteins in response α-adrenergic stimulation in FRTL5 thyroid cells, *Proc. Natl. Acad. Sci. USA* **83**:7201–7205.

De Weck, A. L., Kristensen, F., Joncourt, F., Bethens, F., Walker, C., and Wang, Y., 1984, Lymphocyte proliferation, lymphokine production and lymphocyte receptors in aging and various clinical conditions, *Springer Semin. Immunopathol.* **7**:273–289.

Doll, R., Muir, C., and Waterhous, J., 1970, *Cancer Incidence in Five Continents,* Vol. 2, IUCC, Springer, Berlin.

Fülöp, T., Jr., Foris, G., and Leovey, A., 1984, Age-related changes in cAMP and cGMP levels during phagocytosis in human PMNLs, *Mech. Aging Dev.* **27**:233–237.

Fülöp, T., Jr., Foris, G., Worum, I., and Leovey, A., 1985, Age dependent alterations of Fc receptor mediated effecter functions in human polymorphonuclear granulocytes, *Clin. Exp. Immunol.* **61**:425–432.

Fülöp, T., Jr., Hauck, M., Worum, I., Foris, G., and Leovey, A., 1987a, Alteration of FMLP induced Ca^{2+} efflux from human monocytes with aging, *Immunol. Lett.* **14**:283–288.

Fülöp, T., Jr., Kekessy, D., and Foris, G., 1987b, Impaired coupling of naloxone sensitive opiate receptors to adenylate cyclase in PMNLs of aged male subjects, *Int. J. Immunopharmacol.* **6**:651–659.

Gladstone, J. L., and Recco, R., 1976, Host factors and infectious diseases in the elderly, *Med. Clin. North Am.* **60**:1225–1240.

Hauck, M., Fülöp, T., Jr., Foris, G., and Leovey, A., 1987, Divergent effects of human lymphokines derived oligopeptides on PMNLs of young and elderly healthy subjects, *Int. J. Immunopharmacol.* **9**:3–9.

Ito, H., Baum, B., Uchida, T., Hoops, M. T., Bodner, L., and Roth, G. S., 1982, Diminished α-adrenergic responsiveness in rat parotid acinar cells with normal receptor characteristics, *J. Biol. Chem.* **246**:9532–9538.

Lapetina, E. G., 1986, Effect of pertussis toxin on the phosphodiesteratic cleavage of the poly-phosphoinositides by guanosine 5'-O-thiotiphosphate and thrombin in permeabilized human platelets, *Biochim. Biophys. Acta.*

Lapetina, E. G., 1987, The role of GTP binding proteins in receptor activation of phospholipase C, in: *Molecular Mechanism of Neuronal Responsiveness* (Y. H. Ehrlich, R. H. Lenox, E. Kornecki, and O. W. Berry, eds.), Plenum, New York, pp. 95–100.

Maede, C. J., Turner, G. A., and Bateman, P., 1986, The role of polyphosphoinositides and their breakdown products in A23187 induced release of arachidonic acid from rabbit polymorphonuclear leukocytes, *Biochem. J.* **238**:425–436.

Makinodan, T., and Kay, M. M. B., 1980, Age influences on the immune system, in: *Advances in Immunology* (C. Kungel, and E. Dixon, eds.), Academic, Orlando, Florida, pp. 287–330.

McLaughlin, B., O'Malley, K., and Cotter, T. G., 1986, Age related differences in granulocyte chemotaxis and degranulation, *Clin. Sci.* **70**:59–62.

Mepler, J. R., Hughes, A. R., and Harden, T. K., 1987, Evidence that muscarinic cholinerg receptors selectively interact with either the cAMP or the inositol phosphate second messenger response system, *Biochem. J.* **247**:793–796.

Michell, R. H., 1987, How do receptors at the cell surface send signals to the cell interior?, *Br. Med. J.* **259**:1320–1323.

Miller, R. A., Jacobson, B., Weil, G., and Simons, E. R., 1987, Diminished calcium influx in lectin-stimulated T cells from old mice, *J. Cell. Physiol.* **132**:337–342.

Nishizuka, Y., 1984, Turnover of inositol phospholipids and signal transduction, *Science* **225**:1365–1370.

Rasenick, M. M., Marcus, M. M., Hatta, Y., DeLeon-Jones, F., and Hatta, S., 1987, Regulation of neuronal adenylate cyclase, in: *Molecular Mechanism of Neuronal Responsiveness* (Y. H. Ehrlich, R. H. Lenox, E. Kornecki, and O. W. Berry, eds.), Plenum, New York, pp. 123–133.

Roth, G. S., 1986, Effects of aging on mechanisms of α-adrenergic and dopaminergic action, *Fed. Proc.* **45**:60–64.

Snyderman, R., and Pike, M. C., 1984, Chemoattractant receptors on phagocytic cells, *Annu. Rev. Immunol.* **2**:257–272.

Tam, C. F., and Walford, R. L., 1978, Cyclic nucleotide levels in resting and mitogen stimulated spleen cell suspensions from young and old mice, *Mech. Aging Dev.* **7**:309–320.

Varga, Zs., Kovàs, E., Paragh, G., Jacob, M. P., Robert, L., and Fülöp, T., Jr., 1988, Effect of kappa-elastin and FMLP on polymorphonuclear leukocytes of healthy middle-aged and aged subjects, κ-elastin induced changes in intracellular free calcium, *Clin. Biochem.* **21**:127–130.

Weksler, M. E., 1983, The senescence of the immune system, *Med. Clin. North Am.* **67**:263–272.

18

Rejoining of X-Ray-Induced DNA Double-Strand Breaks Declines in Unstimulated Human Lymphocytes Aging *in Vivo*

PETER J. MAYER, CHRISTOPHER S. LANGE,
MATTHEWS O. BRADLEY, and WARREN W. NICHOLS

1. INTRODUCTION

If DNA repair plays a major role in aging (Gensler and Bernstein, 1981; Hart *et al.*, 1979; Little, 1976; Yielding, 1974; recently reviewed in Warner *et al.*, 1987), within a species one would expect to see decreased efficacy of repair processes in older animals. Some data support this prediction, whereas others do not (recently reviewed in Tice and Setlow, 1985). In general, as studied in nonhuman animals, *in vivo* age-related DNA repair capacities differ by type of damage, by types of repair, by species, and by strain as well as by organ or tissue (Licastro and Walford, 1985; Niedermuller *et al.*, 1985; Su *et al.*, 1984; Tice and Setlow, 1985; Vijg, 1987).

Data collected from human donors are similarly inconsistent with respect to radiation-induced damage. While the rate of ultraviolet (UV) light-induced unscheduled DNA synthesis (UDS) declines with advancing donor age in human epidermal cells (Nette *et al.*, 1984), no such change is detected in fibroblasts and keratinocytes (reviewed in Tice and Setlow, 1985). Studies of DNA repair in human lymphocytes from donors of different age are also contradictory. Responses to UV irradiation include no change with age in survival (Kutlaca *et al.*, 1982) or in repair synthesis (Kovacs *et al.*, 1984; Madden *et al.*, 1979), decreased repair capacity (Dil'man and Revskoi, 1981; Lambert *et al.*, 1985; Lezhava *et al.*, 1979), and increased repair capacity (Lewensohn *et al.*, 1979; Pero and Ostlund, 1980). Although fewer, studies of the response of human lymphocytes from donors of different ages to ionizing radiation are also inconsistent (Goodwin, 1982; Harris *et al.*, 1986; Kutlaca *et al.*, 1982; Licastro *et al.*, 1982; Turner *et al.*, 1982).

PETER J. MAYER and CHRISTOPHER S. LANGE • Department of Radiation Oncology, SUNY Health Science Center at Brooklyn, Brooklyn, New York 11203.   MATTHEWS O. BRADLEY and WARREN W. NICHOLS • Department of Safety Assessment, Merck Institute for Therapeutic Research, West Point, Pennsylvania 19486.

Rejoining of ionizing radiation-induced DNA single-strand breaks (SSB) in human peripheral blood lymphocytes (HPBL) appears to be complete (Mayer *et al.*, 1986b) and does not alter with age (Turner *et al.*, 1982). By contrast, rejoining of DNA double-strand breaks (DSB) appears to be incomplete (Mayer *et al.*, 1986b) but has not been investigated with respect to human aging. We chose to investigate whether repair of ionizing radiation-induced DSB in HPBL changes with donor age. We examine unstimulated lymphocytes because (1) they "may be a weak link in which the limits of protection and repair processes are most evident" (Doggett *et al.*, 1981, p. 150); (2) they resemble the *in vivo* condition more closely than do stimulated cells; (3) *in vitro* stimulation may introduce artifacts in attempting to distinguish DNA repair from DNA replication; and (4) if activation induces SSB repair (Farzaneh *et al.*, 1982; Johnstone, 1984; cf. Greer and Kaplan, 1986), the use of stimulated lymphocytes may complicate the observation or interpretation of any age effect in DSB repair. The present study demonstrates that the level of incomplete DSB rejoining increases with donor age in unstimulated HPBL (see also Mayer *et al.*, 1989).

2. MATERIALS AND METHODS

As in our earlier study (Mayer *et al.*, 1986b), unstimulated HPBL were separated from anticoagulated whole blood by Ficoll-Paque density centrifugation (Boyum, 1968). Donors giving informed consent were nonsmoking, normotensive Caucasians aged 23–78 years, free from overt pathology and not taking any medication. Lymphocytes were irradiated on ice with 30 Gy X-ray (Philips RT250, 250 kVp, 15 mA, with 2 mm inherent Al filtration, HVL = 0.39 mm Cu, dose rate = 2.5 Gy/min). Cells were kept in medium (RPMI 1640 with L-glutamine, 100 U/liter penicillin, 100 mg/liter streptomycin, 10% fetal calf serum), whether undergoing repair incubation at 37°C or otherwise kept on ice.

DNA DSB were assayed by neutral filter elution (NFE) as previously described (Mayer *et al.*, 1986b). Briefly, $3-8 \times 10^5$ cells are loaded onto 2.0-μm polycarbonate filters under gentle vacuum and then lysed. Eluting solution (nondenaturing pH 9.6) is dripped down the side of Swinnex funnels that hold the filters. The eluate is pumped (at 0.04 ml/min) into six fractions of 90 min each. Loading and lysing cells and eluting DNA occur under subdued lighting in order to avoid inducing strand breaks in DNA (Bradley *et al.*, 1978). The percentage of DNA in each elution fraction and that retained on the filter is quantitated with a fluorometric procedure (see Mayer *et al.*, 1986a, 1989 for details).

Elution profiles (semilog plot of DNA retained on the filter versus elution time) are used to calculate the percentage DSB rejoined by comparing the slope of experimental data to that of DNA from control (unirradiated) cells. Linear profiles indicate first-order elution kinetics (Kohn, 1979) and their slopes can be calculated by

$$[\log (100/F_n)]/(n - 1)$$

where F_n is the nth fraction of DNA retained on the filter and n is the number of elution fractions. The percentage of DSB rejoined is calculated as

$$(1 - [(S_E - S_C)/(S_0 - S_C)]) \times 100$$

where S_E is the slope of DNA from experimental cells, S_C is the slope of DNA from control cells, and S_0 is the slope of DNA from irradiated and unrepaired cells. S_0 (minus S_C) measures DSB induction. In nearly all cases, these slopes are the mean of two replicates.

While neutral filter elution assays DSB as originally discussed (Bradley and Kohn, 1979), the alkaline pH (9.6) of the eluting buffer may induce strand breaks at radiation-induced alkali-labile sites in DNA from irradiated cells (Evans *et al.*, 1986; Flick *et al.*, 1988). Thus, we are measuring induction of "frank" DSB plus any alkali-labile sites which are converted to DSB at pH 9.6 by virtue of their proximity to SSB or to other alkali-labile sites on the opposite strand. Since repair of DNA lesions occurs at physiological pH in our experiments, what we measure as percentage DSB not rejoined could also include unrepaired alkali-labile sites and unrejoined SSB converted to DSB by the pH 9.6 eluting buffer.

3. RESULTS

The completeness of DNA DSB rejoining after various repair incubation times is illustrated in Fig. 1 for unstimulated lymphocytes from young and old donors. Differences between the two groups in the percentage DSB rejoined, as analyzed by Student's *t*-test, are statistically significant for the longer repair times. Mean percentage DSB rejoined for the young group (aged 23–43, mean age = 35.0 ± 7.2, $N = 8$) versus the old group (aged 66–78, mean age = 72.5 ± 4.1, $N = 8$) are as follows: for 15-min repair time, 45.1% versus 40.0% (ns); for 30 min repair time, 59.5% versus 27.8% ($p < 0.01$); for 120-min repair time, 67.8% versus 31.9% ($p < 0.005$). Thus, under the same conditions of 30- or 120-min repair incubation in medium at 37°C, lymphocytes from younger donors rejoin more than twice as many X-ray-induced DSB as lymphocytes from older donors.

The kinetics of DSB repair in the two age groups follow the expected biphasic pattern. As we have observed previously (Mayer *et al.*, 1986b) when data from an age group are pooled, an early rapid component in percent DNA strand breaks rejoined is followed by a level plateau. The level of the "repair plateau" for younger donors (60–70%) (Fig. 1) is essentially identical to that reported previously for similar cells exposed to γ-irradiation

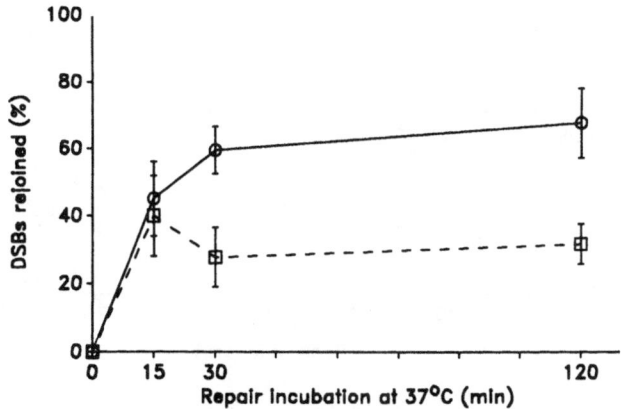

FIGURE 1. Kinetics of DNA double-strand break (DSB) rejoining in unstimulated human lymphocytes from young and old donors. The mean percentage (±SEM) DSB rejoined (calculated as described in Materials and Methods) is plotted for cells X-irradiated (30 Gy) and repair-incubated at 37°C for 15, 30, and 120 min. Lymphocytes from young donors, aged 23–43, mean age: 35.0 ± 7.2, $N = 8$ (○), rejoin twice the percentage of DSB rejoined by lymphocytes from older donors, aged 66–78, mean age: 72.5 ± 4.1, $N = 8$ (□), after 30- and 120-min repair times.

(Mayer *et al.*, 1986b). In the previous study, which examined repair times of 7.5, 15, 30, 60, and 120 min, the repair plateau was attained by 60 min. In the present study, the plateau appears to be attained by 30 min. However one-way analysis of variance within each age group demonstrates no statistically significant differences across the three repair times for percentage DSB rejoined. Thus, based on the present data we cannot conclude when (at what repair time) the plateau is first attained in either age group.

Correlations between donor age and percentage DSB rejoined are negative at all repair times: for 15 min, $r = -0.04$ (ns); for 30 min, $r = -0.62$ ($p < 0.005$); and for 120 min, $r = -0.55$ ($p < 0.05$). Despite small sample sizes and substantial interindividual variability (see Mayer *et al.*, 1989), two out of three of these age-dependent declines are statistically significant.

The correlation between donor age and elution rate (slope) of DNA from unirradiated (control) cells is not statistically significant (Fig. 2). A significant positive correlation would indicate the accumulation of "spontaneous" or "endogenous" DSB with increasing donor age, which has been reported for SSB and/or alkali-labile sites in lectin-stimulated HPBL (Turner *et al.*, 1981).

Induction of DSB by 30-Gy X-irradiation, assessed by the elution rate of DNA from cells irradiated but kept on ice (not repair-incubated), demonstrates a statistically significant correlation with donor age ($r = -0.65$, $p < 0.005$) (see Fig. 2). [The correlation does not change if, for each subject, the elution rate of DNA from unirradiated (control) cells is subtracted from the elution rate of DNA from irradiated but unrepaired cells: $r = -0.68$, $p < 0.001$.] This inverse relationship suggests that X-ray-induction of DSB (radiosensitivity) decreases with increasing donor age.

The correlation between DSB induction and percent DSBs rejoined varies with repair time: after 15 or 30 min repair there is no significant relationship, whereas after 120 min

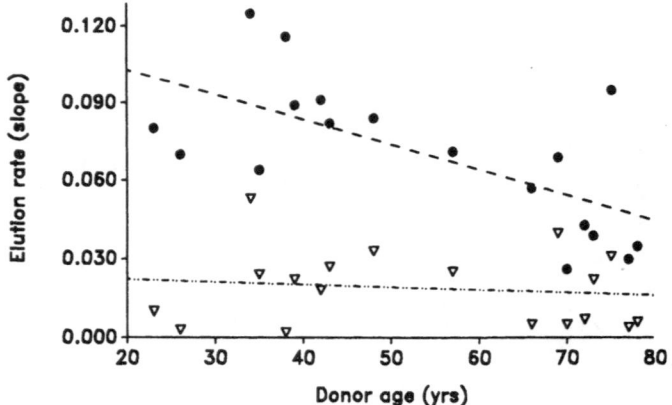

FIGURE 2. Presence of "spontaneous" or "endogenous" DNA double-strand breaks (DSB) and X-ray induction of DSB in unstimulated human lymphocytes from donors of various ages. Low level of "spontaneous" DSB, measured by the elution rate (slope) of DNA from unirradiated cells (∇), does not change with donor age ($r = -0.14$, ns). DSB induction, measured by elution rate (slope) of cells X-irradiated with 30 Gy but kept on ice and not repair-incubated ($\bullet$), decreases with donor age ($r = -0.65$, $p < 0.005$).

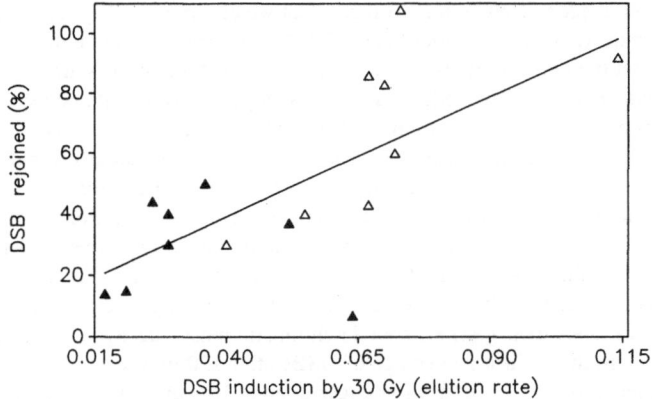

FIGURE 3. Correlation between DNA double-strand break (DSB) induction by 30 Gy X-irradiation and percent DSB rejoined after 120 min repair incubation in unstimulated human lymphocytes. Cells from young [△] and old [▲] donors (same subjects as in Figure 1) which contain more lesions also repair more lesions ($r = 0.69$, $p < 0.01$).

repair the correlation is significant ($r = 0.69$, $p < 0.01$). Moreover, there appears to be an age-related difference in that cells from younger donors tend to have a higher level of damage-induction as well as a higher percentage of DSB rejoined (see Fig. 3). Viability of cells after irradiation and repair incubation, as measured by trypan blue dye exclusion, exceeded 95% in all assays, indicating that there was no immediate cell death.

4. DISCUSSION

This study, the first to examine DSB repair in cells from aging human subjects, demonstrates that unstimulated lymphocytes from older individuals rejoin a lesser percentage of X-ray-induced DSB than unstimulated lymphocytes from younger individuals. The difference between the two groups is statistically significant after 30-min and 120-min repair incubations at 37°C, but not after 15 min. The twofold difference in percentage DSB rejoined is apparent, even though DSB are not completely rejoined in the younger group. Consistent with our previous finding in a similarly aged (young) sample (Mayer et al., 1986b), only 60–70% of ionizing radiation-induced DSB are rejoined (see Fig. 1).

Correlations between percentage DSB rejoined and donor age are negative at all three repair times (15, 30, and 120 min), although the relationships are statistically significant only for the longest incubations. The observed age-dependent decline in percent DSBs rejoined is not due to age-dependent change in the elution rate of DNA from unirradiated (control) cells. Hence, "spontaneous" or "endogenous" DNA DSB do not appear to accumulate with age in unstimulated lymphocytes. This result differs from a study of lectin-stimulated HPBL in which SSB (and/or alkali-labile sites) increased in cells from older individuals (Turner et al., 1981). The physiological state of the cells, the subpopulation of cells studied, the distribution of "spontaneous" SSB along the DNA helix, or a combination of these factors may explain the difference from the present study.

The age-dependent decline in DSB repair that we observe (see Fig. 1) occurs despite an accompanying decrease in the elution rate of DNA from irradiated but unrepaired cells (Fig. 2). We interpret the latter result as indicating that DSB induction by X-irradiation decreases with age. Thus the efficacy of DSB repair processes per se—and not age-related accumulation of lesions or increased susceptibility to DSB induction (radiosensitivity)—is responsible for the observed age-dependent decline in DSB rejoining. The apparently paradoxical finding of *decreased* radiosensitivity with age suggests a possible role for age-related alteration in chromatin conformation. For example, increased chromatin condensation might decrease the accessibility of DNA lesions to repair enzymes (resulting in less complete repair) and simultaneously decrease the exposure of DNA to the indirect action of ionizing radiation (resulting in fewer induced lesions). This idea is supported by the finding that cells which sustain the highest levels of DNA damage (i.e., contain chromatin most "accessible" to radiochemical action) also rejoin the highest percentage of DSBs after 120 min repair-incubation (Fig. 3). Moreover these cells tend to be from younger donors. However, no significant correlation was found at shorter repair times, and in non-aging studies decondensation of chromatin does not affect survival (2.5–15 Gy) or complete rejoining of SSB (10 Gy) in X-irradiated mammalian cells (Yasui et al., 1987). Another possible explanation would be decreased gene expression with aging (see review by Richardson et al., 1985), since unexpressed genomic regions are inefficiently repaired (e.g., Bohr et al., 1986). However, there is no age-related change in SSB rejoining (Turner et al., 1982), which appears to be complete in both unstimulated (Mayer et al., 1986b) and stimulated (Turner et al., 1982) HPBL.

Neutral filter elution assessment of X-ray-induced DNA damage also measures alkali-labile sites, which are converted to DSB at pH 9.6 because of their proximity to either SSB or other alkali-labile sites on the opposite DNA strand (Evans et al., 1986; Flick et al., 1988). In terms of interpreting our data, comparison of pH 9.6 with effects expected at pH 7.0 suggests that we are overestimating the amount of DSB repair. On the one hand, the elution behavior of DNA from cells irradiated and repair-incubated longer than 30 min is probably not affected by the mildly alkaline pH because by 60-min repair incubation HPBL appear to rejoin all their low-dose ionizing radiation-induced SSB and/or alkali-labile sites assayed at pH 12.1 (Mayer et al., 1986b; Turner et al., 1982). On the other hand, if assayed at pH 7.0 the percentage of DSB rejoined would be smaller because of the way this number is calculated. [At pH 7.0, the elution slope of DNA from irradiated but unrepaired cells (S_0) would be smaller, the fraction in which it is the denominator would be larger, so that when this fraction is subtracted from unity, the resulting percentage of DSB rejoined would be smaller.] Put another way, the X-ray-induced DSB rejoining that we observe almost certainly includes repair of alkali-labile sites, sites that would be measured as "DSB" at pH 9.6 in the absence of repair but that would not be detected at pH 7.0.

Along the same lines, the age-related decreased induction of DSB by 30-Gy X-irradiation (see Fig. 2) might be altered if measured at pH 7.0. Specifically, the elution rate of DNA from cells irradiated but unrepaired (from donors of any age) would be flatter at pH 7.0, since the contribution of alkali-labile sites to DSB would be eliminated. However, the age-related decrease in elution rate that we observe at pH 9.6 may underestimate the true extent of decline in X-ray induction of DSB. This would be true if alkali-labile sites were found to increase with age in unstimulated HPBL, as they apparently do in stimulated HPBL (Turner et al., 1981). In the latter case, at older ages the elution rate at pH 7.0 would be flatter than observed at pH 9.6 (due to elimination of alkali-labile sites); thus, the age-related decrease in X-ray induction of (exclusively "frank") DSB would be even greater.

The repair plateau previously observed after 60- to 120-min incubation (Mayer et al.,

1986a,b), meaning that percentage of DSB rejoined does not measurably change during the next 24 hr, occurs at a significantly lower level in cells from older donors. The apparent presence of a plateau plus the rapid half-life ($t\frac{1}{2}$) of less than 30 min for radiation-induced DSB rejoining in HPBL (Mayer et al., 1986b, 1989) suggests that DSB repair enzymes are constitutive and not induced. Thus, any age-related delay in maximal induction of repair enzymes, as seen, for example, in hepatocytes (Adelman, 1970), appears unlikely to bias our results. However, more detailed studies of DSB repair kinetics in HPBL from older subjects are needed to support fully this interpretation. Moreover, such studies would help define the repair time at which the plateau is attained.

The demonstration that lymphocytes from older individuals rejoin a lesser percentage of DSB than do comparable cells from younger individuals (see Fig. 1) is subject to two interpretations: It could mean (1) that all cells from a younger person rejoin more DSB per cell than all cells from an older person (yet no cell completely rejoins all of its DSB), or (2) that the percentage of cells that rejoin all DSB is greater in younger than in older persons (even though a substantial proportion of cells do not rejoin DSB in both age groups). Primarily on the basis of our investigations into the biophysical mechanism of neutral filter elution (Mayer and Lange, 1988), we tentatively support the second interpretation. In other words, we suggest that with age comes a decrease in the proportion of cells that are able to rejoin all their DSB.

Nevertheless, at all adult ages, a significant fraction of ionizing radiation-induced DSB are not rejoined in unstimulated human lymphocytes. This may be attributable to the physiological state of the cells, as cell-cycle-dependent repair has been reported for murine splenocytes (Greer and Kaplan, 1984) and spleen lymphocytes (Licastro and Walford, 1985), for cultured diploid human fibroblasts (Gupta and Sirover, 1981) and for human lymphocytes (Lavin and Kidson, 1977). Mitogen-stimulated lymphocytes are more radioresistant (i.e., have higher survival) (Hashimoto et al., 1975; Kwan and Norman, 1977; Schrek and Stefani, 1964) and demonstrate increased unscheduled DNA (repair) synthesis relative to quiescent cells (Johnstone and Williams, 1982; Lavin and Kidson, 1977; Lewensohn et al., 1979). Data on activation-induced DNA SSB rejoining are contradictory (Farzaneh et al., 1982; Greer and Kaplan, 1986; Johnstone, 1984; Turner et al., 1982).

With regard specifically to response to γ-irradiation of lymphocytes aging in vivo, mitogenic stimulation of murine lymphocytes can increase unscheduled DNA synthesis in old animals, but only at an optimal, and not at a suboptimal, dose of mitogen (Licastro and Walford, 1985). Moreover, even when stimulated, murine lymphocytes from old animals consistently demonstrate less DNA repair activity than do comparable cells from young animals (Licastro and Walford, 1985).

The present results are consistent with other high-dose ionizing radiation studies of aging human lymphocytes: incorporation of tritiated thymidine in the presence of hydroxyurea decreases in unstimulated HPBL irradiated with 26 Gy (Smith et al., 1987) and in stimulated T cells irradiated with 300 Gy (Licastro et al., 1982). Sensitivity to bleomycin, which induces DNA DSB, also increases with donor age (Seshadri et al., 1979).

5. CONCLUSIONS

From our observations, we draw a number of tentative conclusions pertaining to unstimulated HPBL: (1) the age-related decrease in DSB rejoining is caused by a decline in the repair process, and not to accumulation of lesions or increase in radiosensitivity of DNA to strand breakage, (2) this age-related decline involves a step (or steps) in the repair process, which differs between rejoining of radiation-induced SSB and DSB, and (3) there is an age-related decreased induction of DSB by 30-Gy X-irradiation.

As a possible explanation for the latter, unexpected finding, it may be that alterations in chromatin may somehow "sequester" DNA (Williams and Dearfield, 1981) with the effect of "protecting" it from the indirect action of ionizing radiation and simultaneously limiting the access of DNA damage-recognition/repair enzymes. Thus age-related changes in chromatin structure (recently reviewed in Mayer and Baker, 1987), which are unaffected by proteolytic enzymes and detergent but somehow interact with ionizing radiation, may alter elution rate of DNA from lysed lymphocytes. A similar suggestion has been made with respect to cell-cycle variation of DNA neutral filter elution response (Okayasu and Iliakis, 1988). A second possibility, based on the observation that DNA in transcriptionally active chromatin is hypersensitive to ionizing radiation (Chiu et al., 1982), assumes that gene expression in quiescent HPBL decreases with age (reviewed by Richardson et al., 1985).

The heterogeneous nature of density-gradient-separated lymphocytes may account for our observations of decreased DSB rejoining (Mayer et al., 1986b, 1989). Specifically, if subpopulations of HPBL differ in their repair efficacy, e.g., T and B cells (Yew and Johnson, 1978), age-related changes in the distributions of these cell subtypes (e.g., Ligthart et al., 1986; Traill et al., 1985; Yamakido et al., 1985), could explain the present results. The use of monoclonal antibodies to enrich subpopulations of HPBL from differently aged donors, and subsequent assessment of DSB rejoining, represents one method to test this hypothesis.

Immunosenescence, a regular, prominent feature of normal human biological aging (Walford, 1969), manifests age-related increased susceptibility to infection, decreased immune surveillance, and increased autoantibody production (reviewed in Hausman and Weksler, 1985; Nagel et al., 1985; Weksler and Siskind, 1984). The physiological consequences of unrejoined DSB for lymphocyte function are unknown. However, several genetic disorders demonstrate defective DNA repair capability or chromosomal instability and immune system dysfunction (reviewed in Gatti and Walford, 1981; Kraemer, 1977); this suggests a correlation between the efficacy of DNA repair and immune function.

Moreover, a conceptual parallel between rejoining of radiation-induced DSB and genomic rearrangement during activation of T and B cells suggests the possibility of shared enzymatic processes (e.g., ligation) or of common mechanisms such as DNA alteration (Johnson and Wang, 1985). Age-related decline in these processes or mechanisms (as demonstrated by the present study) would diminish cellular response to foreign antigens or alter response to self antigens. Alternatively, cells that cannot rejoin X-ray-induced DSB completely due, for example, to chromatin conformational change, may be unable to proliferate (Dalrymple et al., 1972; Bedford and Cornforth, 1987; Frankenberg-Schwager et al., 1985; Kemp et al., 1984) and under nonirradiated conditions might not clonally expand in response to pathogens (e.g., Staiano-Coico et al., 1984). In the latter case, decline in DSB rejoining would be associated with immune incompetence. If either conjecture (enzymatic or structural) is supported by experimental data, human immunosenescence may involve, in part, decreased efficacy of DNA repair.

6. SUMMARY

In order to test the hypothesis that cellular efficacy of DNA repair declines with age in human beings, we studied peripheral blood lymphocytes from 20 normal, healthy donors (normotensive nonsmokers free from overt pathology and not taking any medications) aged 23–78. Unstimulated lymphocytes were X-irradiated (30 Gy) on ice and incubated at 37°C for repair times of 15, 30, and 120 min. Neutral filter elution was used to assay DNA double-strand break (DSB) induction (including any alkali-labile sites converted to DSB at pH 9.6) as well as kinetics and completeness of DSB rejoining. After 30- or 120-min incubation, cells from older donors rejoin less than one half as many DSB as do cells from younger donors. Correlations between percentage DSB rejoined and donor age are significant for repair times of 30 min ($r = -0.62, p < 0.005$) and 120 min ($r = -0.55, p < 0.05$) but not for 15 min ($r = -0.04$). These age-related declines are observed even though DNA from older donors sustains fewer X-ray-induced strand breaks, as demonstrated by the negative correlation between donor age and DSB induction ($r = -0.68, p < 0.001$). These results suggest that with *in vivo* aging, fewer lymphocytes are capable of responding competently to stress induced by ionizing radiation, most significantly as regards completeness of DSB rejoining. Accessibility to DNA may be one mechanism involved, as suggested by the positive correlation between DSB induction and percent DSB rejoined after 120 min repair-incubation ($r = 0.69, p < 0.01$). Known aspects of immunosenescence (e.g., decreased response to foreign antigens) may be related to diminished DSB rejoining if the latter leads to incomplete genomic rearrangement (during activation of T and B cells) or impaired cell proliferation.

ACKNOWLEDGMENTS. This work was supported, in part, by the Mathers Foundation. We thank Dr. Joan Reibman and Mrs. Marjorie Johnson for help in obtaining blood donations, and the 20 anonymous donors for their contributions.

REFERENCES

Adelman, R. C., 1970, An age-dependent modification of enzyme regulation, *J. Biol. Chem.* **245:**1032–1035.

Bedford, J. S., and Cornforth, M. N., 1987, Relationship between the recovery from sublethal X-ray damage and the rejoining of chromosome breaks in normal human fibroblasts, *Radiat. Res.* **111:**406–423.

Bohr, V. A., Okumoto, D. S., and Hanawalt, P. C., 1986, Survival of UV-irradiated mammalian cells correlates with efficient DNA repair in an essential gene, *Proc. Natl. Acad. Sci. USA* **83:**3830–3833.

Boyum, A., 1968, Isolation of mononuclear cells and granulocytes from human blood, *Scand. J. Clin. Lab. Invest.* **21**(Suppl. 97):77–89.

Bradley, M. O., and Kohn, K. W., 1979, X-ray induced double strand break production and repair in mammalian cells as measured by neutral filter elution, *Nucl. Acids. Res.* **7:**793–804.

Bradley, M. O., Erickson, L. C., and Kohn, K. W., 1978, Nonenzymatic DNA strand breaks induced in mammalian cells by fluorescent light, *Biochim. Biophys. Acta* **150:**11–20.

Chiu, S-M., Oleinick, N. L., Friedman, L. R., and Stambrook, P. J., 1982, Hypersensitivity of DNA in transcriptionally active chromatin to ionizing radiation, *Biochim. Biophys. Acta* **699:**15–21.

Dil'man, V. M., and Revskoi, S. Y., 1981, Correlation between DNA repair and cholesterol concentration in blood serum and lymphocytes, *Fiziol. Cheloveka* **7:**125–129.

Doggett, D. L., Chang, M-P., Makinodan, T., and Strehler, B. L., 1981, Cellular and molecular aspects of immune system aging, *Mol. Cell. Biochem.* **37:**137–156.

Evans, J. W., Limoli, C. L., and Ward, J. F., 1986, Does neutral elution measure intracellular levels of DNA double strand breaks (DSB)? Presented at the *Thirty-fourth Meeting of the Radiation Research Society*, abst., p. 59.

Farzaneh, F., Zalin, R., Brill, D., and Shall, S., 1982, DNA strand-breaks and ADP-ribosyl transferase activation during cell differentiation, *Nature (Lond.)* **300:**362–366.

Flick, M. B., Warters, R. L., and Krisch, R. E., 1988, The number of radiation induced DNA double strand breaks measured by neutral elution or gel electrophoresis depends on pH, presented at the *Thirty-sixth Meeting of the Radiation Research Society*, abst., p. 105.

Frankenberg-Schwager, M., Frankenberg, D., and Harbich, R., 1985, Potentially lethal damage, sublethal damage, and DNA double-strand breaks, *Radiat. Prot. Dosim.* **13:**171–174.

Gatti, R. A., and Walford, R. L., 1981, Immune function and features of aging in chromosomal instability syndromes, in: *Immunological Aspects of Aging* (D. Serge and L. Smith, eds.), Dekker, New York, pp. 449–466.

Gensler, H. L., and Bernstein, H., 1981, DNA damage as the primary cause of aging, *Q. Rev. Biol.* **56:**279–303.

Goodwin, J. S., 1982, Changes in lymphocyte sensitivity to prostaglandin E, histamine, hydrocortisone, and X irradiation with age: Studies in a healthy elderly population, *Clin. Immunol. Immunopathol.* **25:**243–251.

Greer, W. L., and Kaplan, J. G., 1984, Regulation of repair of naturally occurring DNA strand breaks in lymphocytes, *Biochem. Biophys. Res. Commun.* **122:**366–372.

Greer, W. L., and Kaplan, J. G., 1986, Early nuclear events in lymphocyte proliferation, *Exp. Cell Res.* **166:**399–415.

Gupta, P. K., and Sirover, M. A., 1981, Cell cycle regulation of DNA repair in normal and repair deficient human cells, *Chem. Biol. Interact.* **36:**19–31.

Hall, K. Y., Bergmann, K., and Walford, R. L., 1981, DNA repair, H-2, and aging in NZB and CBA mice, *Tissue Antigens* **16:**104–110.

Harris, G., Holmes, A., Sabovljev, S. A., Cramp, W. A., Hedges, M., Hornsey, S., Hornsey, J. M., and Bennett, G. C. J., 1986, Sensitivity to X-irradiation of peripheral blood lymphocytes from aging donors, *Int. J. Radiat. Biol.* **50:**685–694.

Hart, R. W., D'Ambrosio, S. M., and Modak, S. P., 1979, Longevity, stability and DNA repair, *Mech. Aging Dev.* **9:**203–223.

Hashimoto, Y., Ono, T., and Okada, S., 1975, Radiosensitivities of DNA molecules in lymphocytes from the circulating blood of man, *Blood* **45:**503–509.

Hausman, P. B., and Weksler, M. E., 1985, Change in the immune response with age, in: *Handbook of the Biology of Aging* (C. E. Finch and E. L. Schneider, eds.), 2nd ed., Van Nostrand–Reinhold, New York, pp. 414–432.

Johnson, R. C., and Wang, A. A., 1985, DNA repair, antibody diversity, and aging, *Gerontology* **31:**203–214.

Johnstone, A. P., 1984, Rejoining of DNA strand breaks is an early nuclear event during the stimulation of quiescent lymphocytes, *Eur. J. Biochem.* **140:**401–406.

Johnstone, A. P., and Williams, G. T., 1982, Role of DNA breaks and ADP-ribosyl transferase activity in eucaryotic differentiation demonstrated in human lymphocytes, *Nature (Lond.)* **300:**368–370.

Kemp, L. M., Sedgwick, S. G., and Jeggo, P. A., 1984, X-ray sensitive mutants of Chinese hamster ovary cells defective in double-strand break rejoining, *Mutat. Res.* **132:**189–196.

Kohn, K. W., 1979, DNA as a target in cancer chemotherapy: Measurement of macromolecular DNA damage produced in mammalian cells by anti-cancer agents and carcinogens, *Methods Cancer Res.* **16:**291–345.

Kovacs, E., Weber, W., and Muller, Hj., 1984, Age-related variation in the DNA-repair synthesis after UV-C irradiation in unstimulated lymphocytes of healthy blood donors, *Mutat. Res.* **131:**231–237.

Kutlaca, R., Seshadri, R., and Morley, A. A., 1982, Effect of age on sensitivity of human lymphocytes to radiation. A brief note, *Mech. Aging Dev.* **19:**97–101.

Kwan, D. K., and Norman, A., 1977, Radiosensitivity of human lymphocytes and thymocytes, *Radiat. Res.* **69:**143–151.

Lambert, B., Ringborg, U., and Skoog, L., 1985, Age-related decrease of ultraviolet light-induced DNA repair synthesis in human peripheral leukocytes, *Cancer Res.* **39:**2792–2795.

Lavin, M. F., and Kidson, C., 1977, Repair of ionizing radiation induced DNA damage in human lymphocytes, *Nucl. Acids Res.* **4:**4015–4022.

Lewensohn, R., Killander, D., Ringborg, U., and Lambert, B., 1979, Increase of UV-induced DNA repair synthesis during blast transformation of human lymphocytes, *Exp. Cell Res.* **123**:107–110.

Lezhava, R. A., Prokof, V. V., and Mikhel, V. M., 1979, Weakening of the ultraviolet ray-induced unscheduled DNA synthesis in human lymphocytes in extreme old age, *Tsitologilia* **21**:1360–1363.

Licastro, F., and Walford, R. L., 1985, Proliferative potential and DNA repair in lymphocytes from short- and long-lived strains of mice, relation to aging, *Mech. Aging Dev.* **31**:171–186.

Licastro, F., Franceschi, C., Chiricolo, M., Battelli, M. G., Tabacchi, P., Cenci, M., Barboni, F., and Pallenzona, D., 1982, DNA repair after gamma radiation and superoxide dismutase activity in lymphocytes from subjects of far advanced age, *Carcinogenesis* **3**:45–48.

Ligthart, G. J., van Vlokhoven, P. C., Schuit, H. R. E., and Hijmans, W., 1986, The expanded null cell compartment in ageing: Increase in the number of natural killer cells and changes in T-cell and NK-cell subsets in human blood, *Immunology* **59**:353–357.

Little, J. B., 1976, Relationship between DNA repair capacity and cellular aging, *Gerontology* **22**:28–55.

Madden, J. J., Falek, A., Shafer, D. A., and Glick, J. H., 1979, Effects of opiates and demographic factors on DNA repair synthesis in human leukocytes, *Proc. Natl. Acad. Sci. USA* **76**:5769–5773.

Mayer, P. J., and Baker, G. T. III, 1987, Chromatin, in: *Encyclopedia of Aging* (G. L. Maddox, ed.), Springer, New York, pp. 112–115.

Mayer, P. J., Bradley, M. O., and Nichols, W. W., 1986a, No change in DNA damage or repair of single- and double-strand breaks as human fibroblasts age *in vitro*, *Exp. Cell Res.* **166**:497–507.

Mayer, P. J., Bradley, M. O., and Nichols, W. W., 1986b, Incomplete rejoining of DNA double-strand breaks in unstimulated normal human lymphocytes, *Mutat. Res.* **166**:275–285.

Mayer, P. J., Lange, C. S., Bradley, M. O., and Nichols, W. W., 1989, Age-dependent decline in rejoining of X-ray-induced DNA double-strand breaks in normal human lymphocytes, *Mutat. Res.* **219**:95–100.

Mayer, P. J., and Lange, C. S., 1988, Neutral filter elution (pH 9.6) of known molecular weight DNAs demonstrates behavior dependent on pore size, not pore density, *J. Cell Biochem.* **12A** suppl.:270.

Nagel, J. E., Yanagihara, R. H. and Adler, W. H., 1985, Cells of the immune response, in: *Handbook of Cell Biology of Aging* (V. J. Cristofalo, ed.), CRC Press, Boca Raton, Florida, pp. 341–363.

Nette, E. G., Xi, Y-P., Sun, Y-K., Andrews, A. D., and King, D. W., 1984, A correlation between aging and DNA repair in human epidermal cells, *Mech. Aging Dev.* **24**:283–292.

Niedermuller, H., Hofecker, G., and Skalicky, M., 1985, Changes of DNA repair mechanisms during the aging of the rat, *Mech. Aging Dev.* **29**:221–238.

Okayasu, R., and Iliakis, G., 1988, Variation through the cell cycle of DNA neutral filter elution response in synchronous CHO cells, presented at the *Thirty-sixth Meeting of the Radiation Research Society*, abst. p. 87.

Pero, R. W., and Ostlund, C., 1980, Direct comparison, in human resting lymphocytes, of the inter-individual variations in unscheduled DNA synthesis induced by *N*-acetoxy-2-acetylaminofluorene and ultraviolet radiation, *Mutat. Res.* **73**:349–361.

Richardson, A., Roberts, M. S., and Rutherford, M. S., 1985, Aging and gene expression, in: *Review of Biological Research in Aging* Vol. 2 (M. Rothstein, ed.), pp. 395–419.

Schrek, R., and Stefani, S., 1964, Radioresistance of phytohemagglutinin-treated normal and leukemic lymphocytes, *J. Natl. Cancer Inst.* **32**:507–521.

Seshadri, R. S., Morley, A. A., Trainor, K. J., and Sorrell, J., 1979, Sensitivity of human lymphocytes to bleomycin increases with age, *Experientia* **35**:233–234.

Smith, T. A. D., Neary, D., and Itzhaki, R. F., 1987, DNA repair in lymphocytes from young and old individuals and from patients with Alzheimer's disease, *Mutat. Res.* **184**:107–112.

Staiano-Coico, L., Darzynkiewicz, Z., Melamed, M. R., and Weksler, M. E., 1984, Immunological studies of aging. IX. Impaired proliferation of T lymphocytes detected in elderly humans by flow cytometry, *J. Immunol.* **132**:1788–1792.

Su, C. M., Brash, D. E., Turturro, A., and Hart, R. W., 1984, Longevity-dependent organ-specific accumulation of DNA damage in two closely related murine species, *Mech. Aging Dev.* **27**:239–247.

Tice, R. R., and Setlow, R. B., 1985, DNA repair and replication in aging organisms and cells, in: *Handbook of the Biology of Aging* (C. E. Finch and E. L. Schneider, eds.), 2nd ed., Van Nostrand-Reinhold, New York, pp. 173–223.

Traill, K. N., Schonitzer, D., Jurgens, G., Bock, G., Pfeilschifter, R., Hilchenbach, M., Holasek, A., Forster, O., and Wick, G., 1985, Age-related changes in lymphocyte subset proportions, surface differentiation antigen density and plasma membrane fluidity: Application of the EURAGE SENIEUR PROTOCOL admission criteria, *Mech. Aging Dev.* **33**:39–66.

Turner, D. R., Griffith, V. C., and Morley, A. A., 1982, Aging *in vivo* does not alter the kinetics of DNA strand break repair, *Mech. Aging Dev.* **19**:325–331.

Turner, D. R., Morley, A. A., Seshadri, R. S., and Sorrell, J. R., 1981, Age-related variations in human lymphocyte DNA, *Mech. Aging Dev.* **17**:305–309.

Vijg, J., 1987, *DNA Repair and the Aging Process*, TNO Institute for Experimental Gerontology, Rijswijk, The Netherlands.

Walford, R. L., 1969, *The Immunologic Theory of Aging*, Munksgaard, Copenhagen.

Warner, H. R., Butler, R. N., Sprott, R. L., and Schneider, E. L. (eds.), 1987, *Modern Biological Theories of Aging*, Part V: *DNA Damage and Repair*, Raven Press, New York, pp. 173–215.

Weksler, M. E., and Siskind, G. W., 1984, The cellular basis of immune senescence, *Monogr. Dev. Biol.* **17**:110–121.

Williams, J. R., and Dearfield, K. L., 1981, Induction and repair of DNA/chromatin alterations, in: *Biological Mechanisms in Aging* (R. T. Schimke, ed.), U.S. Department of Health and Human Services, Washington, D.C., pp. 245–269.

Yamakido, M., Yanagida, J., Ishioka, S., Matsuzaka, S., Hozawa, S., Akiyama, M., Kobuke, K., Inamizu, T., and Nishimoto, Y., 1985, Detection of lymphocyte subsets by monoclonal antibodies in aged and young humans, *Hiroshima J. Med. Sci.* **34**:87–94.

Yasui, L. S., Higashikubo, R., and Warters, R. L., 1987, The effect of chromatin decondensation on DNA damage and repair, *Radiat. Res.* **112**:331–340.

Yew, F. H., and Johnson, R. T., 1978, Human B and T lymphocytes differ in UV-induced repair capacity, *Exp. Cell Res.* **113**:227–231.

Yielding, E. L., 1974, A model for aging based on differential repair of somatic mutational damage, *Perspect. Biol. Med.* **17**:201–208.

19

Interventive Gerontology, Cloning, and Cryonics
Relevance to Life Extension

HAL STERNBERG, PAUL E. SEGALL, HAROLD WAITZ, and
AVI BEN-ABRAHAM

1. INTRODUCTION

Much of the focus of medical research has been to alleviate age-related diseases. This has led to an increased average life span for humans, and "squaring" of the mortality curve (Schneider and Brody, 1983). However, maximum human life span has not yet been altered by medical intervention.

A number of scientific disciplines are likely to contribute to an increased maximum life span. These include (but are not limited to) (1) interventive gerontology, (2) cloning, (3) cryonics, (4) resuscitation medicine, (5) transplantation, (6) artificial organs, and (7) regeneration. Together they comprise a larger field called the life extension sciences (Kent, 1980; Segall, 1985; Timiras and Segall, 1988).

Considerable work in regeneration (Nylander, 1986), artificial organs (Jarvik, 1981; Nissenson et al., 1986; Pierce, 1986), transplantation (Bjorklund et al., 1987; Bryner et al., 1987), and resuscitation (Safar, 1986) has resulted in important medical advances that are currently being implemented. The rapidly growing areas of interventive gerontology (Regelson and Sinex, 1983; Walker and Cooper, 1983), cryonics (Scholander et al., 1953; Smith, 1956a,b; Hochachka and Guppy, 1987), and cloning (Gurdon, 1968; McKinnel, 1985; Willadsen, 1986; Prather, 1988), which share extensive history, also promise significant medical benefit. Gerontologists are establishing a battery of biomarkers to serve as an index of normal aging, for a more convenient assessment of delayed aging (Reff and Schneider, 1982). Researchers in cloning are developing methods that may permit genetically identical organs to replace damaged or old ones, while cryonics investigators are developing

HAL STERNBERG • Department of Physiology and Anatomy, University of California–Berkeley, Berkeley, California 94720; and Trans Time Inc., Oakland, California 94603.   PAUL E. SEGALL and HAROLD WAITZ • Trans Time Inc., Oakland, California 94603.   AVI BEN-ABRAHAM • American Cryonics Society, San Francisco, California 94102.

technology to preserve terminally ill patients. This chapter describes the scientific progress in interventive gerontology, cryonics, and cloning and discusses the relevance of these disciplines to life extension.

2. INTERVENTIVE GERONTOLOGY

2.1. Aging Theory: A Cascade of Programmed Nerve Cell Death

Programmed nerve cell death is a well-documented phenomenon that takes place throughout life (Hamburger and Oppenheim, 1982; Coleman and Flood, 1987). The nervous system not only can effect endocrine secretions but articulates with almost every tissue of the body. It can potentially influence the cellular composition of various organs and orchestrate metamorphic changes. We propose that a cascade of nerve cell death causes subsequent changes in the peripheral tissues with which the nervous system interacts (Dilman, 1971; Finch, 1978; Segall, 1984; Meites *et al.*, 1987; Segall and Sternberg, 1988). A reduction in either the number of nerve cell processes into tissues or a decrease in trophic excitation by these peripheral neurons may result in the loss of factors necessary to maintain certain cell types, leading to a decline in the capacities of various tissues. While enough cells may be left to enable the organ to maintain homeostasis (Collins and Exton-Smith, 1986), the ability of organs to handle stress (overload) may become impaired because of a lack of functional units (Bellamy, 1986).

A balance of various factors appears to dictate neuronal survival. Neuronal loss can be induced upon binding of certain hormones such as cortisol (Sapolski *et al.*, 1985, 1986) and estrogen (Finch and Mobbs, 1983) or by the depletion of factors such as epidermal growth factor and nerve growth factor (Levi-Montalcini, 1987; Thoenen *et al.*, 1987), which are involved in neuronal regeneration and maintenance.

Nerve cell death may play a key role in aging, as suggested by the following findings:

1. There is an excellent correlation between brain size and life span suggesting a built-in neuronal mechanism to control aging rate (Sacher, 1959, 1965). The greater the number of neurons that have a supportive effect on hypothetical aging-pacemaker regions, the slower the physiological cascade of neuron death and subsequent peripheral age changes (i.e., loss of cells and functional units).
2. Programmed nerve cell death is known to accompany development and metamorphosis (Fahrbach and Truman, 1987).
3. Specific nerve cell death continues throughout life (Agid and Blin, 1987) and may eventually lead to (if allowed to proceed past a threshold) pathologic conditions such as Alzheimer's disease (Coleman and Flood, 1987).
4. Senescence of a physiologic function, female reproductive ability appears to involve the degeneration of hypothalamic neurons (Brawer *et al.*, 1978; Hsu and Peng, 1978; Gottschall *et al.*, 1986).

A cascade of specific nerve cell death may be functional to the aging of the brain as well as peripheral tissues (Segall, 1984). Backtransplantation of lost cells may provide a means of restoring function. The symptoms of Parkinson's disease (where cell death has gone too far and is symptomatic) can be attenuated by backtransplantation of dopamine-secreting neurons (Sladek and Gash, 1988). Thus, it may be possible to replace some neurons that are lost with age and restore the functions that depend on them (Huang *et al.*, 1987). Moreover, transplanted neurons may provide factors that maintain or support other neurons that might otherwise die. If nerve cell death orchestrates aging, slowing the continual cascade of neuron loss may delay aging (the loss of particular cells within peripheral tissues).

2.2. Reproductive Senescence: Role of the Hypothalamus

To understand the mechanisms underlying organismic aging it may be helpful first to focus on the senescence of a specific physiologic function, such as female reproduction (Finch, 1988). An advantage of understanding this function in particular is that it can be assessed easily and unequivocally by monitoring cyclicity, and the ability to reproduce and raise pups. Aging of other physiologic functions is more difficult to assess because these functions may decline more gradually and may also require stress conditions to detect.

Female reproductive ability is one of the best studied examples of how the brain (hypothalamus) is involved in both the development and senescence of a physiologic function (Walker and Cooper, 1983; Finch, 1988). Both sexual maturation (Sherwood and Timiras, 1974) and senescence (Brawer *et al.*, 1978) of reproductive ability in female rats appear to involve the degeneration of particular hypothalamic neurons. With regard to development of reproductive function, the onset of puberty could be accelerated upon lesioning an area between the medial preoptic nucleus and the medial basal hypothalamus (Sherwood and Timiras, 1974). Inhibitory neurons are thought to prevent the onset of puberty. Upon the destruction of these neurons or by naturally occurring programmed neuron death, the hypothalamus may be stimulated to produce the neurohormones needed for maturation (Segall and Sternberg, 1988).

Senescence of the reproductive function appears to be associated with estradiol-induced neuron degeneration (Brawer and Finch, 1983). The involvement of estradiol in hypothalamic neuronal degeneration, hence reproductive senescence, is supported by the observation that high doses of estradiol administered into female rats can cause premature menarchy (Brawer *et al.*, 1978). In addition, removal of the ovaries (of young mice), which produce estrogen/estradiol, prevents aging of the reproductive neuroendocrine axis (Brawer and Finch, 1983); also, old ovariectomized mice can cycle normally after receiving ovaries from young (Nelson *et al.*, 1980). Such studies provide strong evidence for the involvement of the hypothalamus and estrogen/estradiol in reproductive senescence.

In summary, aging of female reproductive function appears to be triggered by a cascade of neuronal degeneration (of estrogen/estradiol-binding neurons) within the arcuate of the hypothalamus. Degeneration of these neurons (which perhaps are involved in maintaining normal cyclicity) may eventually result in the cessation of estrous cycles and reproductive function.

The dynamic continuum of hypothalamic events that may play a role in reproductive function can be studied by serial sectioning of the brain as a cohort of an animal's age. Biochemical and morphologic changes can be characterized in each serial section. Nutritional restriction dramatically delays reproductive aging (Segall *et al.*, 1983). Upon comparing hypothalamic events in the nutritionally restricted animals to normal controls, one may understand the relevance of these events to the development and senescence of reproductive function (Bellport *et al.*, 1987).

Using such an approach we monitored glutamic acid decarboxylase (GAD) activity in discrete hypothalamic regions as a function of maturation in female rats (Sternberg *et al.*,

1987). Although we ultimately wish to examine a variety of cytologic and biochemical parameters, GAD activity was initially chosen because some estrogen-responsive neurons contain this enzyme (Leranth et al., 1985). We found GAD activity to increase significantly in the anterior hypothalamic regions but not the more basal regions. In future studies we hope to determine whether this increase is caused by the release of an inhibition on α-aminobutyric acid (GABA)ergic cells.

2.3. Extending Life Span of Laboratory Animals by Nutritional Restriction

By intervening in the aging process, it may be possible to prolong youth and extend life. Conclusive evidence that the life span of mammals can be dramatically extended comes from studies involving nutritional restriction. Rats maintained on diets low in calories but complete with all the essential nutrients exhibit delayed development and aging (McCay et al., 1935; McCay, 1952; Ross, 1976). Similar observations were made in our laboratory using low tryptophan diets (Segall and Timiras, 1976; Ooka et al., 1988). The more restricted the diet was in tryptophan the greater the enhancement in maximum life span. The maximum life span of rats placed on the diet at 3 weeks of age was 1527 days, using a diet containing 30% of the normal levels of tryptophan (T30%), while those placed on T40% and control diets lived 1347 and 1246 days, respectively (Ooka et al., 1988). It was also noted (using a very small cohort of animals) that the earlier in life the diet is initiated, the greater the effect on maximum life span. Animals started on diets at 3 weeks attained longer life spans than did those started at 3 months. Such work should be repeated with large numbers of experimental animals.

Although severe nutritional restriction is accompanied by a high risk of early mortality, some animals that develop the slowest attain the longest life spans. One Long-Evans rat maintained on a tryptophan-restricted diet (30% that of normal control diets) for 30 months, starting from 3 weeks of age, was able to reproduce at 33 months after being placed back on a normal diet, and lived to be 48 months (Segall et al., 1983). Rats kept on less restricted diets or rats placed on the diet at 3 months instead of 3 weeks cannot reproduce at such late ages and do not obtain such extended life spans as do those rats more severely restricted earlier in life. Control rats cease cyclic estrous activity and stop reproducing at 15–18 months of age (Cooper and Walker, 1979) and die by approximately 24–32 months.

Health and aging are different biological phenomena. Our studies showed that an animal whose aging process is delayed may be unhealthy as determined by a cachetic appearance, convulsions, and a susceptibility to stress (Segall and Timiras, 1976). Maximum life span is the best index for determining whether a particular regimen delays the aging process, not average life span, which reflects more accurately the general health of the treated animals.

Several laboratories have implemented caloric restriction to extend the maximum life span of mice (Weindruch et al., 1986) and rats (Yu et al., 1982). It has been demonstrated that caloric restriction (diets containing all the nutrients for normal development and growth but deficient in calories) can even extend life span if initiated during adult stages (Weindruch and Walford, 1982). However, the effect is not nearly as dramatic as when initiated at younger ages, suggesting that certain developmental events play an important role in aging. Despite this, an experimental nutritional regimen for human adults has been proposed (based on animal studies) that may significantly extend human life span (Walford, 1987).

2.4. Nutritional Restriction: Proposed Mechanism of Delayed Aging

A number of different factors appear to play a role in cell survival. The balance of these factors in a particular environment may dictate cell number, organ size, and thus the functional capabilities of an organ under homeostatic conditions and stress. Nerve cells may secrete factors into both the brain and peripheral tissues that contribute to determining cell number and ratios of various cell types. Under normal physiologic conditions, a cascade of nerve cell death within the brain may affect peripheral nerve cell secretions resulting in specific cell loss within tissues.

Cell death is a well-documented phenomenon that accompanies embryogenesis, development, and aging (Bellamy, 1986). It is possible that nutritional restriction extends maximum life span by preventing programmed cell death, which is fundamental to development and aging. Evidence supporting this hypothesis include the following:

1. Fecal pellets of rats on nutritional restriction are pale compared with controls (Bellport et al., 1987). This may be caused by a decline in red blood cell (RBC) turnover, and thus hemoglobin breakdown, which determines fecal color.
2. DNA synthetic rates in liver, heart, kidney, and abdominal skin (but not thymus or small intestine) are slower in nutritionally restricted animals (Holehan and Merry, 1988).
3. Morphologically intact ovarian follicles have been observed in 3-year-old animals that are nutritionally restricted for 24–30 months, but not in controls of the same age (Ooka et al., 1988).
4. Egg cell number declines more slowly in nutritionally restricted animals (Segall et al., 1983; Nelson et al., 1985). At least some eggs maintain functional viability, in view of the fact that nutritionally restricted female rats can reproduce approaching 3 years of age.
5. Nutritional restriction has also been reported to delay the loss of pinealocytes (Walker et al., 1978) and corneal cells (Nadakavukaren et al., 1986).

With this in mind, it seems plausible that female reproductive maturation and senescence (where hypothalamic neuron loss appears to play a role) is delayed in nutritionally restricted animals due to slowing the physiologic cascade of cell death.

While the mechanism by which nutritional restriction delays aging is highly speculative, it is a very useful tool being used to understand the aging process (Weindruch et al., 1986; Ooka et al., 1988; Segall and Sternberg, 1988). Upon determining what physiologic phenomena are affected by such a regimen we may gain insight as to the underlying mechanisms of aging.

2.5. Products That Potentially Delay Human Aging: Replacement of Lost Factors

Although nutritional restriction is being implemented to delay aging in laboratory animals and to understand the underlying mechanisms of aging, it may have drawbacks when applied clinically. Other areas of interventive gerontology may hold promise for increasing maximum life span.

Perhaps the most profound phenomenon during aging is the involution of the thymus gland and the decline in secretion of thymic hormones (Walford, 1969; Zatz and Goldstein,

1985). With the advent of genetic engineering, protein hormones lost with aging can potentially be replaced. α-Thymosin, an important thymic peptide hormone, is an example of such a factor (Goldstein et al., 1983). This hormone can be manufactured by genetic engineering and is being clinically tested for efficacy. This and other related products not only may help the immune system fight various age-related diseases but may delay aging as well.

A number of other treatments have been shown to reverse age-related changes of the immune system and restore immune function in laboratory animals (Weksler et al., 1978; Fabris et al., 1982; Harrison et al., 1982; Cavagnaro, 1983; Kelley et al., 1986).

Even more interesting to gerontologists, it was reported that some adult rats, mice, and guinea pigs, given serial injections of an early fetal thymic extract over 2½ months, displayed dramatically extended life spans (Czaplicki and Blonska, 1981). Maximal life spans of small cohorts of treated guinea pigs, rats, mice were 12 years and 2 weeks, 4 years and 7 months, and 5 years and 7 months, respectively, while life spans of controls according to the literature are normally 6, 3, and 3, years respectively. This work, although not yet reproduced, demonstrates that it may be possible to extend life span starting from adult stages.

3. CLONING

While genetic engineering can potentially provide protein factors lost with aging, senescent organs might be replaced by isogenic body parts from cloned whole organisms. Clones would also be a source of immunologically compatible tissues that can replace single cells, possibly neurons, that are lost with age.

As early as 1952, investigators successfully formed multiple identical amphibian embryos using nuclear transfer methods (Briggs and King, 1952). Nuclei from early embryonic stages promoted cleavage when transferred into enucleated oocytes. Later, frogs were cloned from intestinal epithelial cell nuclei of tadpoles (Gurdon, 1962, 1968). This was an important accomplishment demonstrating that permanent inactivation of genes does not necessarily accompany animal cell differentiation. The technique involved placement of the intestinal epithelial cell nucleus of a tadpole (using a micropipette) into the unfertilized egg of a frog whose nucleus was destroyed by ultraviolet (UV) light (Gurdon, 1968). Only a very small percentage of nuclei actually developed into fully viable frogs. Most either did not develop at all or displayed limited growth and differentiation. However, the few totipotent transplanted nuclei proved that at least in some cell populations, genes necessary for complete differentiation have not been lost by the tadpole stage.

Nuclear transfer techniques have more recently been reported in mice (McGrath and Solter, 1983, 1984), sheep (Willadsen, 1986), and cows (Robl et al., 1987), using very early-stage embryos. Cows have been cloned by transplanting blastomeres of a 32-cell stage bovine embryo into an enucleated oocyte using micromanipulation and electrofusion (Prather et al., 1987). Even more recent are accounts in the popular press of cloned cows from a 128-cell-stage blastocyst (Kahn, 1988).

Cloning of vertebrates using adult cells has not yet been accomplished. As technology advances with a better understanding of the factors that affect development following nuclear transfer (McKinnell, 1981; Gurdon, 1986; Prather, 1989), cloning from later stages in mammalian development should become possible.

Adult mammalian cloning would extend life and improve the quality of life by providing a source of immunologically compatible organs that could be used to replace functionally impaired ones. This is particularly important to the elderly because of the very limited availability of donor organs and general policy of issuing organs to younger recipients only.

4. CRYONICS

Cryonics can potentially preserve terminally ill patients. It has even been used after clinical death (Kent, 1980). Death is not a moment but a progressive pathophysiologic process that occurs over time (Safar, 1986). Cooling and freezing prevents the normal progression of the dying process. Reversal of death in humans is currently possible 5–20 min after onset (Safar et al., 1987). Advances in resuscitation medicine will permit reversal of clinical death after increasingly longer periods of time.

Currently many mammalian cell types and tissues can be cryopreserved with great success. Examples include corneas (Mueller et al., 1964; Neubauer et al., 1984), blood components (Luff et al., 1985), sperm (Kaden et al., 1985; Serafini and Marrs, 1986), bone marrow (Zhuravlev et al., 1984), erythrocytes (Pyle, 1964), lymphocytes (Pegg, 1970), nasal mucosa (Wulffraat et al., 1985), skin (Lehr et al., 1964), thymus gland (Playfair, 1964), intestine (Hamilton and Lehr, 1967), parathyroid tissue (Russell et al., 1961), kidney tissue (Georgiev and Mateeva, 1967), spleen (Barner and Schenk, 1966), and teeth (Schwartz and Andreasen, 1983). Although a great variety of cell types and tissues can be cryopreserved, it has not yet been possible to achieve reversible freezing of entire vertebrates or even whole organs of appreciable size. However, there is strong evidence to suggest such technology is feasible. Many species of insects can tolerate deep subzero (°C) temperatures (Asahina, 1959; Baust and Rojas, 1985; Hochachka and Guppy, 1987). Insects are highly complex organisms composed of many cell types in an organized array. Thus, nature demonstrates that freezing of highly complex tissues is possible.

Perhaps of greater relevance to humans, it is known that some species of frogs such as *Hyla versicolor* and *Rana sylvatica* can tolerate partial freezing during winter months in the northern United States (Schmid, 1982; Storey, 1985). These frogs produce cryoprotective polyols (such as glucose or glycerol) that allow them to survive temperatures of −9°C where 35–50% of their body water turns to ice. Likewise, the golden Syrian hamster (*Mesocricetus auratus*) can survive temperatures between 0 and −2°C after their body water reaches up to 50% ice, but only for periods of up to 1 hr (Lovelock and Smith, 1956; Smith, 1956a,b). The hamster can tolerate this extent of freezing without cryoprotectants. The investigators suggested that hamsters, and perhaps other mammalian species as well, might be able to tolerate long-term storage in the partially frozen state if cryoprotectants could be administered and distributed throughout their bodies as occurs naturally in frogs.

Almost any cell suspension can be reversibly cyropreserved using many different regimens and cryoprotectants. Freeze-tolerant species use a variety of substances and mechanisms to avoid freeze damage. Therefore, the technology to freeze mammalian organs and whole mammals may be accomplished by a number of approaches.

4.1. Technical Approach, Recent Progress, and Immediate Medical Applications

To develop technology in low-temperature medicine and cryonics we continued Smith's (1961) work using hamsters. To partially freeze hamsters for long durations without significant damage, cryoprotectants must be distributed throughout the hamsters tissues (Lovelock and Smith, 1956). The technique that we developed over the past decade to accomplish this is as follows. The hamsters are anesthetized, body temperature is lowered by surface cooling with ice, and respiration is continued with 100% O_2. The hamsters are then placed on a custom-made surgical platform below a dissecting microscope. The carotid artery and vena cava are exposed for the insertion of microcannulas. The arterial cannula is connected to a peristaltic pump and the venous cannula is connected to a collecting duct. The venous effluent is analyzed periodically. An ice-cold non-blood-based flush solution containing oncotic polymer, electrolytes, buffer, and sugar is perfused into the carotid artery and through the circulatory system replacing the blood (Waitz et al., 1984; Gan et al., 1985). After various periods of ice-cold blood substitution, blood is placed back and they are rewarmed. Hamsters have been revived after up to 2 hr of bloodless cold.

The revival of ice-cold bloodless hamsters (which are not cryoprotected or frozen) is important for low-temperature medicine. A number of surgical and experimental procedures can potentially be performed in an ice-cold bloodless condition without certain risk factors that accompany such operations performed at normothermia (Klebanoff et al., 1972; Haff et al., 1974).

Even of greater relevance to cryonics, hamsters have been revived after levels of cryoprotectants up to 1.0 M were administered into the circulatory system. The hamsters that revived after such treatment were never frozen. However, in partially frozen (below −3°C for 1 hr) similarly cryoprotected hamsters, steady electrocardiographic (EKG) signals were monitored for 1 hr, following rewarming and reperfusion. Also, some electrical activity was recorded in vivo from the hearts of thawed hamsters, which were frozen to −20°C overnight. Interestingly, it was reported that a dog placed in a freezer at −20°C for 6 hr was able to resume heartbeat and breathing upon rewarming (Dogliotti, 1960). Although the higher brain centers did not recover, a substantial amount of physiologic function did. The extent of ice formation (if any) was not monitored, but the experiment demonstrates the tolerance of mammalian tissues to very cold temperatures.

Technology developed in hamsters is quickly upscaled to dogs (Segall et al., 1987). A series of 10 dogs were kept bloodless and cold for varying times using different protocols. Five of the dogs in this series at least partially revived. The two animals (beagles) that were allowed to survive long-term recovered to unimpaired health after being kept bloodless and below 10°C for more than 70 min. This indicates that methodology obtained using hamsters is applicable to larger, more humanlike mammals. Moreover, it shows that at least part of the cryonics suspension procedure (i.e., replacement of blood with a substitute and lowering of body temperature to the ice point) is potentially reversible. One Newfoundland was exsanguinated and chilled for 8 hr before reinfusion with blood and rewarming. This was planned as an acute experiment and for ethical reasons was terminated before full revival. Restoration of rhythmic heartbeats, breathing, and mean arterial pressure consistent with recovery were observed. A previous study by Air Force physicians included survival of a dog after 8 hr of bloodless cold (Haff et al., 1974).

The blood substitutes and protocols developed to advance cryonics technology have immediate applications in low-temperature medicine. Such applications include multiorgan preservation, bloodless surgery, therapy for ridding blood-borne symptomatic infections that accompany acquired immune deficiency syndrome (AIDS), and specific organ-directed high-dose cancer chemotherapy (Segall et al., 1988).

4.2. Cryonics Suspension Procedure

The technique currently used to place an individual into cryonic suspension upon legal death involves administration of an anticoagulant to prevent blood aggregation, continued oxygen delivery, and blood circulation. Concomitantly, body temperature is lowered by surface cooling. A major artery and vein is exposed, cannulated, and attached to a bypass apparatus equipped with roller pumps, extracorporeal oxygenation, and temperature regulation for core cooling. The blood is replaced with a substitute solution; increasing levels of cryoprotectants are then perfused, circulated, and distributed to body tissues. The individual is placed in a dry ice chest and body temperature is lowered gradually to −79°C. Finally, the individual is placed in a capsule containing liquid nitrogen, and body temperature is gradually reduced to −196°C.

Cryonics is used to preserve biologic information. Current evidence suggests that upon lowering body temperature to −196°C, there is freeze damage. As stated above, no vertebrate has ever been, or can currently be, revived after deep freezing and thawing. However, the extent of freeze damage is unpredictable, as its measurement currently requires thawing. Improved thawing techniques may be available in the future. Progress in repair and resuscitation can also be expected.

5. CONCLUSION

Interventive gerontology along with cloning and cryonics provide a powerful combination of technologies to extend life. Cloning would make available youthful, immunologically compatible organs. Cryonics would provide a means of storing organs and terminally ill patients. Moreover, cryonics is the one technology that can potentially prevent death caused by almost any illness, whether it be cancer, heart disease, Alzheimer's disease, or a disease of unknown etiology. This chapter outlines the current knowledge in these rapidly growing disciplines. Advances in these areas would be of great medical value and may not be more difficult to achieve than cures for biologically complex age-related illnesses.

REFERENCES

Agid, Y., and Blin, J., 1987, Nerve cell death in degenerative diseases of the central nervous system: Clinical aspects, *Selective Neuronal Death,* Ciba Foundation Symposium 126 (G. Bock and M. O'Conner, eds.), Wiley, Chichester, pp. 3–29.

Asahina, E., 1959, Prefreezing as a method enabling animals to survive freezing at an extremely low temperature, *Nature (Lond.)* **184:**1003–1004.

Barner, H. B., and Schenk, E. A., 1966, Autotransplantation of the frozen-thawed spleen, *Arch. Pathol. Lab. Med.* **82:**267–271.

Baust, J. G., and Rojas, R. R., 1985, Review insect cold hardiness: Facts and fancy, *J. Insect Physiol.* **31:**755–759.

Bellamy, D., 1986, Cell death and the loss of structural units of organs, in: *The Biology of Human Aging* (A. H. Bittles and K. J. Collins, eds.), Cambridge University Press, New York, pp. 119–132.

Bellport, V., Steinberg, R., Young, G. W., Ranganatham, S., Sternberg, H., Segall, P. E., and Timiras, P. S., 1987, Maturational changes in regional hypothalamic neurochemistry of tryptophan-restricted rats, presented at the *Seventy-first Annual Meeting of the Federation of the American Society of Experimental Biology, Washington, D.C.*

Bjorklund, A., Lindvall, O., Isacson, O., Brundin, P., Wictorin, K., Strecker, R. E., Clarke, D. J., and Dannett, S. B., 1987, Mechanisms of action of intracerebral neural implants: Studies on nigral and striatal grafts to the lesioned striatum, *Trends Neurosci.* **12:**509–516.

Brawer, J. R., and Finch, C. E., 1983, Normal and experimentally altered aging processes in the rodent hypothalamus and pituitary, in: *Experimental and Clinical Interventions in Aging* (R. F. Walker and R. L. Cooper, eds.), Dekker, New York, pp. 45–65.

Brawer, J. R., Naftolin, F., Martin, J., and Sonnenschein, C., 1978, Effects of a single injection of estradiol valerate on the hypothalamic arcuate nucleus and on reproductive function in the female rat, *Endocrinology* **103:**501–512.

Briggs, R., and King, T. J., 1952, Transplantation of living nuclei from blastula cells into enucleated frogs' eggs, *Zoology* **38**:455–463.

Bryner, H., Blohme, I., and Karlberg, I., 1987, Third Congress of the European Society for Organ Transplantation, June 11–13, Gothenburg, Sweden, *Transplant. Proc.* **19**:3531–4396.

Cavagnaro, J., 1983, Treatments that retard or reverse immunological losses due to aging, in: *Experimental and Clinical Interventions in Aging* (R. F. Walker and R. L. Cooper, eds.), Dekker, New York, pp. 133–162.

Coleman, P. D., and Flood, D. G., 1987, Neuron numbers and dendritic extent in normal aging and Alzheimer's disease, *Neurobiol. Aging,* **8**:521–545.

Collins, K. J., and Exton-Smith, A. N., 1986, Effects of aging on homeostasis, in: *The Biology of Human Aging* (A. H. Bittles and K. J. Collins, eds.), Cambridge University Press, New York, pp. 261–275.

Cooper, R. L., and Walker, R. F., 1979, Potential therapeutic consequences of age-dependent changes in brain physiology, *Interdiscipl. Topics Gerontol.* **15**:54–76.

Czaplicki, J., and Blonska, B., 1981, Some cases of animal longevity following treatment with early fetal thymic extracts, *Thymus* **3**:185–186.

Dilman, V. M., 1971, Age-associated elevation of hypothalamic threshold to feedback control, and its role in development, aging and disease, *Lancet* **1**:1211–1219.

Dogliotti, A. M., 1960, Hypothermia in surgery, *J. Cardiovasc. Surg.* **1**(2):120–132.

Fabris, N., Muzzioli, M., and Mocchegiani, E., 1982, Recovery of age-dependent immunological deterioration in Balb/c mice by short-term treatment with L-thyroxine, *Mech. Aging Dev.* **18**:327–338.

Fahrbach, S. E., and Truman, J. W., 1987, Mechanisms for programmed cell death in the nervous system of a moth, in: *Selective Neuronal Death* (G. Bock and M. O'Conner, eds.), Ciba Foundation Symposium 126, Wiley, Chichester, pp. 65–76.

Finch, C. E., 1978, The brain and aging, in: *The Biology of Aging* (J. A. Behnke, C. E. Finch, and G. B. Moment, eds.), Plenum, New York, pp. 301–310.

Finch, C. E., 1988, Aging in the female reproductive system: A model system for analysis of complex interactions during aging, in: *Emergent Theories of Aging* (J. E. Birren and V. L. Bengtson, eds.), Springer, New York, pp. 128–150.

Finch, C. E., and Mobbs, C. B., 1983, Hormonal influences on hypothalamic sensitivity during aging in female rodents, in: *Neuroendocrinology of Aging* (J. Meites, ed.), Plenum, New York, pp. 143–171.

Gan, S. C., Segall, P. E., Waitz, H. D., and Sternberg, H., 1985, Ice-cold blood-substituted hamsters revive, *Fed. Proc.* **44**:623.

Georgiev, I., and Mateeva, G., 1967, Survival and growth of kidney tissues in culture *in vitro* after freezing and preservation at low temperatures, *C. R. Acad. Bulg. Sci.* **20**:261–262.

Goldstein, A. L., Low, T. L. K., Hall, N., Naylor, P. H., and Zatz, M. M., 1983, Thymosin: Can it retard aging by boosting immune capacity? in: *Intervention in the Aging Process. Part A: Quantitation, Epidemiology and Clinical Research* (W. Regelson and F. M. Sinex, eds.), Liss, New York, pp. 169–197.

Gottschall, P. E., Sarkar, D. K., and Meites, J., 1986, Persistence of low hypothalamic dopaminergic activity after removal of chronic estrogen treatment, *Proc. Soc. Exp. Biol. Med.* **181**:78–86.

Gurdon, J. B., 1962, The developmental capacity of nuclei taken from intestinal epithelium cells of feeding tadpoles, *J. Embryol. Exp. Morphol.* **10**:622–640.

Gurdon, J. B., 1968, Transplanted nuclei and cell differentiation, *Sci. Am.* **219**(6):24–35.

Gurdon, J. B., 1986, Nuclear transplantation in eggs and oocytes, *J. Cell Sci.* **4**(suppl.):287–318.

Haff, R. C., Klebanoff, G., Brown, B. G., and Koreski, W. R., 1975, Asanguinous hypothermic perfusion as a means of total organism preservation, *J. Surg. Res.* **19**:13–19.

Hamburger, V., and Oppenheim, R. W., 1982, Naturally occurring neuronal death in vertebrates, *Neurosci. Comment,* **1**:39–55.

Hamilton, R., and Lehr, H. B., 1967, Survival of small intestine after storage for 7 days at −196°C, *Cryobiology* **3**:375.

Harrison, D. E., Archer, J., and Astle, C. M., 1982, The effect of hypophysectomy on thymic aging in mice, *J. Immunol.* **129**:2673–2677.

Hochachka, P. W., and Guppy, M. 1987, *Metabolic Arrest and the Control of Biological Time*, Harvard University Press, London.

Holehan, A. M., and Merry, B. J., 1988, Experimental manipulation of aging by diet, in: *Physiological Basis of Geriatrics* (P. S. Timiras, ed.), Macmillan, New York, pp. 232–240.

Hsu, H. K., and Peng, M. T., 1978, Hypothalamic neuron number of old female rats, *Gerontology* **124**:434–440.

Huang, H. H., Kissane, J. Q., and Hawrylewicz, E. J., 1987, Restoration of sexual function and fertility by fetal hypothalamic transplant in impotent aged male rats, *Neurobiol. Aging* **8**:465–472.

Jarvik, R. K., 1981, The total artificial heart, *Sci. Am.* **244**:74–80.

Kaden, R., Klippel, F. F., Katzorke, T., Propping, D., and Schone, D., 1985, A new instant cryoprotectant for human sperm, *Arch. Androl.* **14**(2–3):133–137.

Kahn, C., October 1988, *Omni* **II**(1):58.

Kelley, K. W., Brief, S., Westly, H. J., Novakofski, J., Bechtel, P. J., Simon, J., and Walker, E. B., 1986, GH₃ pituitary adenoma cells can reverse thymic aging in rats, *Proc. Natl. Acad. Sci. USA* **83**:5663–5667.

Kent, S., 1980, *The Life-Extension Revolution*, William Morrow, New York.

Klebanoff, G., Armstrong, R. G., Cline, R. E., Powell, J. R., and Bedingfield, J. R., 1972, Resuscitation of a patient in stage IV hepatic coma using total body washout, *J. Surg. Res.* **13**:159–165.

Lehr, H. B., Berggren, R. B., Lotke, P. A., and Coriell, L. L., 1964, Permanent survival of preserved skin autografts, *Surgery* **56**:742–746.

Leranth, C., Sakamoto, H., Maclosky, J. J., Shanabrough, M., and Naftolin, F., 1985, Estrogen responsive cells in the arcuate nucleus of the rat contain glutamic acid decarboxylase (GAD): An electron microscopic immunocytochemical study, *Brain Res.* **331**:376–381.

Levi, Montalcine, R., 1987, The nerve growth factor 35 years later, *Science* **237**:1154–1162.

Lovelock, J. E., and Smith, A. V., 1956, Studies on golden hamsters during cooling to and rewarming from body temperatures below 0°C. III. Biophysical aspects and general discussion, *Proc. R. Soc. Lond. [Biol.]* **145**:427–442.

Luff, R. D., Kessler, C. M., and Bell, W. R., 1985, Microwave technology for the rapid thawing of frozen blood components, *Am. J. Clin. Pathol.* **83**(1):59–64.

McCay, C. M., 1952, Chemical aspects of ageing and the effect of diet upon ageing, in: *Cowdry's Problems of Ageing* (A. F. Lansing, ed.), Williams & Wilkins, Baltimore, pp. 139–202.

McCay, C. M., Crowell, M. F., and Maynard, L. A., 1935, The effect of retarded growth upon length of lifespan and upon ultimate body size, *J. Nutr.* **10**:63–69.

McGrath, J., and Solter, D., 1983, Nuclear transplantation in the mouse embryo by microsurgery and cell fusion, *Science* **220**:1300–1302.

McGrath, J., and Solter, D., 1984, Inability of mouse blastomere nuclei transferred to enucleated zygotes to support development *in vitro*, *Science* **226**:1317–1319.

McKinnell, R. G., 1981, Amphibian nuclear transplantation: State of the art, in: *New Technologies in Animal Breeding* (B. G. Brackett, G. E. Seidel, and S. M. Seidel, eds.), Academic, New York, pp. 163–180.

McKinnel, R. G., 1985, *Cloning of Frogs, Mice and Other Animals*, University of Minnesota Press, Minneapolis.

Meites, J., Goya, R., and Takahashi, S., 1987, Review article: Why the neuroendocrine system is important in aging processes, *Exp. Gerontol.* **22**:1–15.

Mueller, F. O., Casey, T. A., and Trevor-Roper, P. D., 1964, Use of deep frozen human cornea in full-thickness grafts, *Br. Med. J.* **2**:473–475.

Nadakavukaren, M. J., Fitch, K. L., and Richardson, A., 1986, Rat corneal epithelial cells as markers of physiological age: Dietary restriction retards age-related increase in cell area, *Gerontologist* **26**:157A.

Nelson, J. F., Felicio, L. S., and Finch, C. E., 1980, Ovarian hormones and the etiology of reproductive aging in mice, in: *Aging, Its Chemistry* (A. Dietz, ed.), American Association of Clinical Chemistry, Washington, D.C., pp. 64–81.

Nelson, J., Goschen, R., and Felicio, L., 1985, Effect of dietary restriction on estrous cyclicity and follicular reserves in aging C57BL/6J mice, *Biol. Reprod.* **32**:515–522.

Neubauer, L., Smith, R. S., Leibowitz, H. M., and Laing, R. A., 1984, Endothelial findings in cryopreserved corneal transplants, *Ann. Ophthalmol.* **16**:980–984.

Nissenson, A. R., Gentile, D. E., Soderblom, R. E., Brak, C., and the Medical Review Board, NCC#4, Los Angeles, 1986, Long-term outcome of continuous ambulatory peritoneal dialysis. The Southern California/Southern Nevada experience, *Trans. Am. Soc. Artif. Intern. Organs* **32**:560–563.

Nylander, G., 1986, Tissue ischemia and hyperbaric oxygen treatment: An experimental study, *Acta Chir. Scand.* **533**:1–109.

Ooka, H., Segall, P. E., and Timiras, P. S., 1988, Histology and survival in age-delayed low-tryptophan fed rats, *Mech. Aging Dev.* **43**:79–98.

Pegg, D. E., 1970, Banking of cells, tissues and organs at low temperatures, in: *Current Trends in Cryobiology* (A. Smith, ed.), Plenum, New York, pp. 153–180.

Pierce, W. S., 1986, The artificial heart, *Trans. Am. Soc. Artif. Intern. Organs* **32**:5–10.

Playfair, J. H. L., and Davies, A. J. S., 1964, Successful preservation of mouse thymuses by freezing, *Transplantation*, **2**:271–273.

Prather, R. S., 1988, Nuclear transfer in mammals and amphibians: Nuclear equivalence, species specificity?, in: *The Molecular Biology of Fertilization* (H. Schatten and G. Schatten, eds.), Academic, Orlando, Florida, pp. 323–340.

Prather, R. S., Barnes, F. L., Sims, M. M., Robl, J. M., Eyestone, W. H., and First, N. L., 1987, Nuclear transplantation in the bovine embryo: Assessment of donor nuclei and recipient oocyte, *Biol. Reprod.* **37**:859–566.

Pyle, H. M., 1964, Glycerol preservation of red blood cells, *Cryobiology* **1**:57–60.

Reff, M. E., and Schneider, E. L. (eds.), 1982, *Biological Markers of Aging*, U.S. NIH Publication no. 82-2221, Bethesda, Maryland.

Regelson, W., and Sinex, M. F. (eds.), 1983, *International Symposium on Intervention in the Aging Process, 1982, Boston, Mass. Vol. A*, Alan Liss, New York, pp. 3–323; *Vol. B*, pp. 3–375.

Robl, J. M., Prather, R., Barnes, F., Eyestone, W., Northey, D., Gilligan, B., and First, N., 1987, Nuclear transplantation in bovine embryos, *J. Anim. Sci.* **64**:642–647.

Ross, M. H., 1976, Nutrition and longevity in experimental animals, in: *Nutrition and Aging* (M. D. Winick, ed.), Wiley, New York, pp. 43–57.

Russell, P. S., Wood, M. L., and Gittes, R. F., 1961, Preservation of living systems in the frozen state: A study using parathyroid tissue, *J. Surg. Res.* **1**:23–31.

Sacher, G. A., 1959, Relation of lifespan to brain weight in mammals, in: *Colloquium on Aging*, Vol. 5 (G. E. W. Wolstenholme and M. O'Conner, eds.), Ciba Foundation Symposium, Little, Brown, Boston, pp. 115–141.

Sacher, G. A., 1965, The role of physiological fluctuations in the aging process and the relation of longevity to the size of the central nervous system, in: *Aging and Levels of Biological Organization* (A. M. Brues and G. A. Sacher, eds.), University of Chicago Press, Chicago, pp. 226–331.

Safar, P., 1986, Cerebral resuscitation after cardiac arrest: A review, *Circulation* **74**(suppl. IV):138–153.

Safar, P., Breivik, H., Abramson, N., and Detre, K., 1987, Reversibility of clinical death in patients: The myth of the 5 minute limit, *Ann. Emerg. Med.* **16**:495.

Sapolsky, R. M., Kery, L. L., and McEwen, B. S., 1985, Prolonged glucocorticoid exposure reduces hippocampal neuron number: Implications for aging, *J. Neurosci.* **5**:1221–1227.

Sapolsky, R. M., Kery, L. L., and McEwen, B. S., 1986, The neuroendocrinology of stress and aging: The glucocorticoid cascade hypothesis, *Endocrine Rev.* **7**:284–301.

Schmid, W. D., 1982, Survival of frogs in low temperature, *Science* **215**:697–698.

Schneider, E. L., and Brody, J. A., 1983, Aging, natural death, and compression of morbidity: Another view, *N. Engl. J. Med.* **309**: 854–856.

Scholander, P. F., Flagg, W., Hock, R. J., and Irving, L., 1953, Studies on the physiology of frozen plants and animals in the arctic, *J. Cell. Comp. Physiol.* **42**(1):1–56.

Schwartz, O., and Andreasen, J. O., 1983, Cryopreservation of mature teeth before replantation in monkeys. I. Effect of different cryoprotective agents and freezing devices, *Int. J. Oral. Surg.* **12**:425–536.

Segall, P. E., 1984, Aging as a programmed cascade of specific cell death, *Age* **7**:149.

Segall, P. E., 1985, The life extension sciences: A non-traditional approach to gerontology, in: *First International Congress of Biomedical Gerontology, American Aging Association, New York, July 10–11.*

Segall, P. E., and Sternberg, H., 1988, Aging: A CNS–endocrine perspective, in: *Regulation of Age Changes Along the Hypothalamic–Pituitary Axis* (A. V. Everitt and J. D. Walton, eds.), S. Karger, Basel, pp. 9–20.

Segall, P. E., and Timiras, P. S., 1976, Pathophysiologic findings after chronic tryptophan deficiency in rats: A model for delayed growth and aging, *Mech. Aging Dev.* **5**:109–124.

Segall, P. E., Timiras, P. S., and Walton, J. R., 1983, Low-tryptophan diets delay reproductive aging, *Mech. Aging Dev.* **23**:245–252.

Segall, P. E., Waitz, H. D., Sternberg, H., Steinberg, R., Young, G. W., Bellport, V., Strack, D., Cain, C. R., Schertel, E. R., Breznock, A. L., and Breznock, E. M., 1987, Ice-cold bloodless dogs revived using protocol developed in hamsters, *Fed. Proc.* **46**:1338.

Segall, P. E., Sternberg, H., and Waitz, H., 1988, Blood substitute, U.S. Patent Pending.

Serafini, P., and Marrs, R. P., 1986, Computerized staged-freezing technique improves sperm survival and preserves penetration of zona-free hamster ova, *Fertil. Steril.* **45**:854–858.

Sherwood, N. M., and Timiras, P. S., 1974, Comparison of direct current and radio-frequency lesions in the rostral hypothalamus with respect to sexual maturation in the female rat, *Endocrinology* **9**:1275–1286.

Sladek, J. R., and Gash, D. M., 1988, Nerve cell grafting in Parkinson's disease, *J. Neurosurg.* **68**:337–351.

Smith, A. V., 1956a, Studies on golden hamsters during cooling to and rewarming from body temperatures below 0°C. I. Observations during chilling, freezing and supercooling, *Proc. R. Soc. Lond. [Biol.]* **145**:391–407.

Smith, A. V., 1956b, Studies on golden hamsters during cooling to and rewarming from body temperatures below 0°C. II. Observations during and after resuscitation, *Proc. R. Soc. Lond. [Biol.]* **145**:407–426.

Smith, A. V., 1961, *Biological Effects of Freezing and Supercooling,* Edward Arnold, London.

Sternberg, H., Segall, P. E., Bellport, V., and Timiras, P. S., 1987, Glutamic acid decarboxylase activity in discrete hypothalamic nuclei during the development of rats, *Dev. Brain Res.* **34**:316–317.

Storey, K. B., 1985, Freeze tolerance in terrestrial frogs, *Cryo-Letters* **6**:115–134.

Thoenen, H., Barde, Y., Daview, A. M., and Johnson, J. E., 1987, Neurotrophic factors and neuronal death, in: *Selective Neuronal Death* (G. Bock and M. O'Conner, eds.), Ciba Foundation Symposium 126, Wiley, Chichester, pp. 82–95.

Timiras, P. S., and Segall, P. E., 1988, An agenda for healthful aging: Life extension sciences, Chapter 27, in: *Physiological Basis of Geriatrics* (P. S. Timiras, ed.), Macmillan, New York, pp. 449–455.

Waitz, H. D., Yee, H., Gan, S., and Segall, P. E., 1984, Reviving hamsters after asanguinous hypothermic perfusion, *Cryobiology* **21**:699 (abst.).

Walford, R. L., 1969, *The Immunological Theory of Aging,* Williams & Wilkins, Baltimore.

Walford, R. L., 1987, *The 120-Year Diet: How to Double Your Vital Years,* Simon & Schuster, New York.

Walker, R. F., and Cooper, R. L. (eds.), 1983, *Experimental and Clinical Interventions in Aging,* Dekker, New York.

Walker, R. F., McMahon, K. M., and Pivorun, E. B., 1978, Pineal gland structure and respiration as affected by age and hypocaloric diet, *Exp. Gerontol.* **13:**91–99.

Weindruch, R. H., and Walford, R. L., 1982, Dietary restriction in mice beginning at 1 year of age: Effect on life-span and spontaneous cancer incidence, *Science* **215:**1415–1418.

Weindruch, R. H., Walford, R. L., Fligiel, S., and Guthrie, D., 1986, The retardation of aging in mice by dietary restriction: Longevity, cancer, immunity and lifetime energy intake, *J. Nutr.* **116:**641–654.

Weksler, M. E., Innes, J. B., and Goldstein, G. J., 1978, Immunological studies of aging. IV. The contribution of thymic involution to the immune deficiencies of aging mice and reversal with thymopoietin, *Exp. Med.* **148:**996–1006.

Willadsen, S. M., 1986, Nuclear transplantation in sheep embryos, *Nature (Lond.)* **320:**63–65.

Wulffraat, N. M., Veerman, A. J., and Stalmhuis, I. H., 1985, Frequency and coordination of ciliary beat after cryopreservation of respiratory epithelium, *Cryobiology* **22**(2):105–110.

Yu, B. P., Masoro, E. J., Murata, F., Bertand, H. A., and Lynd, F. T., 1982, Life-span study of SPF Fischer 344 male rats fed *ad libitum* or restricted diets: Longevity, growth, lean body mass and disease, *J. Gerontol.* **37:**130–141.

Zatz, M. M., and Goldstein, A. L., 1985, Thymosins, lymphokines, and the immunology of aging, *Gerontology* **31:**263–277.

Zhuravlev, V. A., Svedentsov, E. P., Kriazhev, L. N., Simkin, D. S., and Kokoulin, B. E., 1984, New aspects of obtaining and cryopreserving cadaveric bond marrow with "hemegel" solution, *Gematol. Transfuziol.* **29**(9):27–30.

20

Effects of Various Stimulators and Inhibitors on the Respiratory Burst of PMNL with Aging

ZSUZSA VARGA, GABRIELLA FORIS, SÀNDOR SZUCS,
TAMÀS FÜLÖP, JR., and ANDRÀS LEOVEY

1. INTRODUCTION

It is well known that the incidence of certain diseases such as infections (Gardner, 1980), atherosclerosis (Stout, 1987), diabetes mellitus (DeFronzo, 1981), and tumors (Doll *et al.*, 1970) is increased with aging. It can be assumed that the cause of this increased incidence is multifactorial, but the decrease of the immune response certainly plays an important role (Makinodan and Kay, 1980; Corberand *et al.*, 1981). It was established that the oxidative burst plays an essential role in the host defense against pathogens and other microorganisms (Johnston *et al.*, 1976; Babior and Crowley, 1983); therefore, an alteration of the respiratory burst could contribute to the increased incidence of infectious diseases with aging.

The basic oxidative processes were found to be increased in resting cells, i.e., polymorphonuclear leukocytes (PMNL), of healthy elderly subjects (Harman *et al.*, 1977, 1978; Fülöp *et al.*, 1985); the detoxification processes were also altered (Thompson *et al.*, 1977; Abraham *et al.*, 1978). This increased oxidative process could be rendered further responsible for cell membrane changes, e.g., increased rigidity, decreased fluidity, and degradation of membrane lipids and proteins with aging (Tappel, 1973; Halliwell *et al.*, 1978). Nagel *et al.* (1982), in agreement with our studies, (Fülöp *et al.*, 1988), found a diminished O_2^- production after phagocytic stimulation in PMNL of elderly patients. The question arises as to what is the basic alteration underlying this decreased oxidative response. Several possibilities seem to emerge: either decreased NADPH oxidase activity, or altered signal transduction mechanism, or both.

The aim of the present study was to investigate NADPH oxidase activity, measured by O_2^- production, with both specific stimulation, e.g., κ-elastin (KE), FMLP, opsonized

ZSUZSA VARGA, GABRIELLA FORIS, SÀNDOR SZUCS, TAMÀS FÜLÖP, JR., and ANDRÀS LEOVEY • First Department of Medicine, University Medical School of Debrecen, 4012 Debrecen, Hungary.

zymosan (OZ), and carbachol, and nonspecific stimulation, e.g., A23187 and PMA, in the presence and absence of various inhibitors, e.g., pertussis toxin (PT), for GTP-binding G_i protein; neomycin for phospholipase C (PLC); and chloroquin for phospholipase A_2 (PLA_2).

2. PHYSIOLOGICAL CELL FUNCTION ALTERATIONS WITH AGING

Aging of human cells has been demonstrated to involve structural and functional changes in cell membrane proteins as well as alterations of various cell functions. McLaughlin et al. (1986) demonstrated that the granulocytes of elderly subjects exhibit reduced chemotaxis and degranulation in response to stimulation with a chemotactic peptide such as FMLP. Negoro et al. (1987) studied the T-cell functions with aging. The proliferative response was markedly decreased and was more pronounced for CD8-positive cells than for CD4-positive cells, compared with young subjects. It is worthwhile to note that the proportion of CD8 cells in the peripheral blood as well as the erythrocyte–antibody–complement (EAC)-rosette-forming cells from elderly subjects were significantly reduced compared with that in young subjects. Furthermore, an alteration in the Ca^{2+} metabolism in the monocytes of healthy elderly patients under stimulation was also demonstrated (Fülöp et al., 1987).

It is now well accepted that all these cell functions are mediated by various agents, such as chemotactic peptides, opsonized micro-organisms, or interleukin-2 (IL-2), acting through their specific receptors. Roth (1986) showed an altered mechanism of α-adrenergic and dopaminergic receptors in mammalian parotid glands with aging. The signal transduction of various ligands (KE, FMLP, OZ) has also been investigated in aging; a marked alteration in the mechanism of transduction of these Ca^{2+}-mobilizing receptors was found (Varga et al., 1988). These ligands, stimulating the cells through the phosphatidylinositol (PIP_2) breakdown, can mobilize the inositol phosphate much less intensively than in young subjects. As a consequence of this altered PIP_2 breakdown with aging, the most important second messengers, such as cyclic adenosine monophosphate (cAMP), cyclic guanosine monophosphate (cGMP), or intracellular free Ca^{2+}, are also impaired.

3. INTRACELLULAR FREE CALCIUM AND RESPIRATORY BURST IN PMNL OF ELDERLY SUBJECTS

3.1. Changes in Intracellular Free Ca^{2+} Levels

The important role of Ca^{2+} as an intracellular second messenger in many cell types is well known (Berridge, 1986; Abdel-Latif, 1986). The elevation of intracellular free Ca^{2+} after stimulation could occur through the formation of inositol 1,4,5-trisphosphate (IP_3) from intracellular pools and from extracellular medium stimulated by 1,3,4,5-tetrakisphosphate (IP_4) (Berridge, 1986).

We have studied $[Ca^{2+}]_i$ in the PMNL of elderly subjects and found a marked elevation in the resting cells of aged compared with that of young subjects (Table I). After stimulation, a decreased elevation was found in the PMNL of elderly patients (Table II) compared with that of young subjects. Thus a decreased reactivity of intracellular free Ca^{2+} was demonstrated with aging concomitant with a high basic level.

TABLE I. Intracellular Free Ca^{2+} Level
in the Resting PMNL of Young
and Elderly Subjects[a]

Subjects (N = 20)	Intracellular free Ca^{2+} (nmoles)
Young	
25–30 years	131 ± 30
Elderly	
65–80 years	332 ± 130
90 years	270 ± 80

[a]Each value represents the mean ± SD of 20 independent experiments.

3.2. Study of NADPH Oxidase Activation

NADPH oxidase, which is responsible for the O_2^- production, can be activated in different ways. Sakata et al. (1987) demonstrated that arachidonic acid (AA) is able to stimulate NADPH oxidase, because it can be partly generated during the PIP_2 breakdown from diacylglycerol (DAG). Parini et al. (1986) found that activation of NADPH oxidase by AA can involve the PLA_2 in human neutrophils. Activation of PLA_2 can occur either through specific receptors, e.g., α_1-adrenergic receptors in FRTL5 cells (Burch et al., 1986), or through PIP_2 breakdown by DAG formation, activating the DAG kinase (Westwick and Poll, 1986). PLA_2 can be activated directly by a Ca ionophore such as A23187 (McPhail et al., 1981). Protein kinase C (PKC) is another intracellular agent that can activate NADPH oxidase during receptor-mediated stimulation (McPhail et al., 1981). PKC can also be directly activated by phorbol esters (Castagne et al., 1982) such as PMA.

TABLE II. Elevation of Intracellular Free
Ca^{2+} after κ-elastin (KE) and FMLP
Stimulation in Percentage of Saturation in
the PMNL of Young and Elderly Subjects[a]

Subjects (N = 20)	Intracellular free Ca^{2+} (% of saturation)	
	KE	FMLP
Young		
25–30 years	59 ± 17	78 ± 4
Elderly		
65–80 years	40 ± 10	56 ± 10
90 years	32 ± 20	47 ± 20

[a]Each value represents the mean ± SD of 20 independent experiments.

Taking into consideration these experimental results, we were interested to study the basic alteration underlying the decreased O_2^- production in the PMNL of elderly subjects (Fig. 1). Pertussis toxin, an inhibitor of the GTP-binding G_i protein, was found unable to inhibit receptor-stimulated O_2^- production in the elderly in the same manner as in young persons (Fig. 2), while the effect of neomycin, an inhibitor of PLC, was similar in all age groups (Fig. 3). The effect of chloroquin, an inhibitor of PLA_2, was very surprising (Fig. 4) because it could inhibit the KE, OZ, and carbachol-induced O_2^- production in young subjects, while in the PMNL of the elderly it could restore the O_2^- production in the presence of OZ and carbachol.

The effects of nonspecific agents (A23187 and PMA) on O_2^- production as well as the effect of various inhibitors were similar in both young and elderly subjects (Figs. 1–4). In view of these results, it can be concluded that NADPH oxidase could function equally well in the PMNL of young and elderly subjects and the decreased O_2^- production found in the PMNL of the elderly could be due to an altered signal transduction mechanism.

4. CONCLUSION

The oxidative burst plays an important role in host defense. Decreased oxidative metabolism was demonstrated in the PMNL of elderly subjects after various types of stimulations (Fülöp *et al.*, 1985; Abraham *et al.*, 1978; Nagel *et al.*, 1982). According to our results, it can be assumed that this altered respiratory burst is not due to altered NADPH oxidase activity because the nonspecific stimulating agents (A23187 and PMA) can activate the enzyme similarly in the PMNL of both young and elderly subjects. The altered signal-

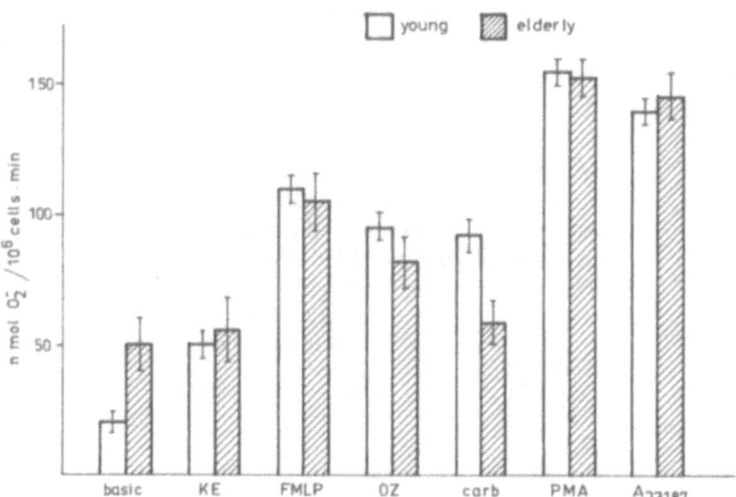

FIGURE 1. Effect of specific and nonspecifi stimulants on O_2^- prodution in the PMNL of young and elderly subjects. Specific stimulants: ×-elastin (KE), FMLP; opsonized zymozan (OZ), carbachol. Nonspecific stimulants: A23187; PMA. Each value represents the mean + SD of 10 experiments.

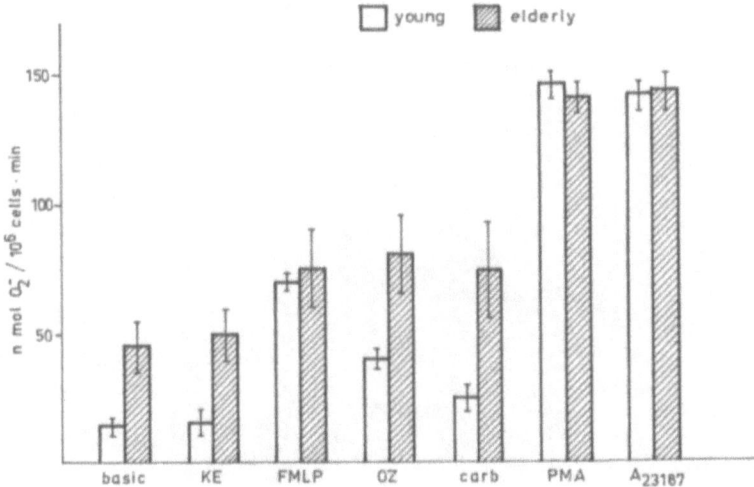

FIGURE 2. Effect of pertussis toxin on specific and nonspecific stimulants inducing O_2^- production in the PMNL of young and elderly subjects. See Fig. 1 for stimulants used.

transduction mechanism, as demonstrated in elderly subjects (Fülöp *et al.*, 1988; Varga *et al.*, 1988), can explain the decreased O_2^- production under specific stimulation. The precise alteration in the signal transduction mechanism is actually unknown, but it can be assumed to be a very complex problem. Nevertheless, based on a recent data, we can say that (1) GTP-binding G_i protein might be altered; (2) PIP_2 breakdown is decreased; (3) $[Ca^{2+}]_i$ in resting

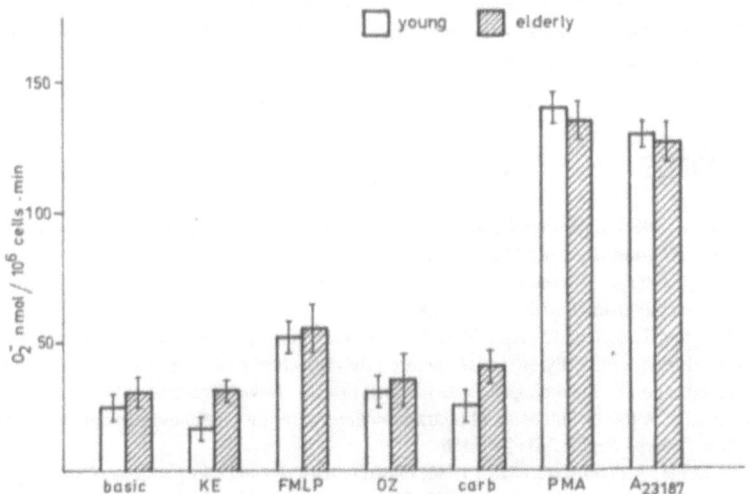

FIGURE 3. Effect of neomycin on specific and nonspecific stimulants inducing O_2^- production in the PMNL of young and elderly subjects. See Fig. 1 for stimulants used.

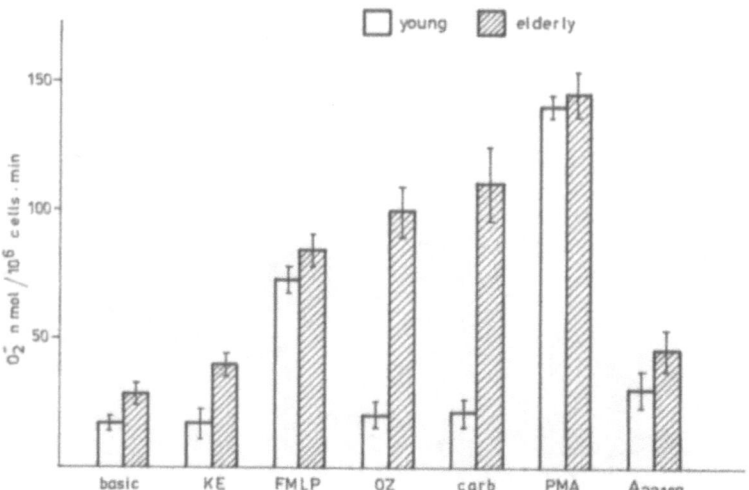

FIGURE 4. Effect of chloroquin on specific and nonspecific stimulants inducing O_2^- production in the PMNL of young and elderly subjects. See Fig. 1 for stimulants used.

cells is increased, while Ca^{2+} enhancement is decreased after stimulation; and (4) the NADPH oxidase activity is conserved with aging.

Drazmin *et al.* (1987) showed that there exists an optimal cytosolic free Ca^{2+} range for insulin-stimulated glucose transport in rat adipocytes. Thus, the role of increased basic $[Ca^{2+}]_i$ in resting PMNL with aging should be further investigated in the altered signal-transduction mechanism. In our case, it can be supposed that the fact that chloroquin markedly decreased the intracellular free Ca^{2+} (unpublished data) in resting cells might explain its O_2^- production restoring effect in presence of OZ and carbachol in the PMNL of elderly subjects. The alterations found in cell functions with aging could be attributable in part to the altered signal-transduction mechanism found at various levels.

REFERENCES

Abdel-Latif, A. A., 1986, Calcium mobilizing receptors, phosphoinositides and the generation of second messengers, *Pharmacol. Rev.* **38**:227–272.
Abraham, E. C., Taylor, J. F., and Lang, C. A., 1978, Influence of mouse age and erythrocyte age on glutathione metabolism, *Biochem. J.* **174**:819–825.
Babior, B. M., and Crowley, C. A., 1983, Chronic granulomatous disease and other disorders of oxidative killing by phagocytes, in: *Metabolic Basis of Inherited Diseases* (J. B. Stanburg, J. B. Wyngaarden, and D. S. Fredickson, eds.), McGraw-Hill, New York, pp. 1956–1985.
Berridge, M. J., 1986, Intracellular signalling transductions of inositol trisphosphate and diacylglycerol, *Biol. Chem. Hoppe-Seyler* **367**:447–456.
Burch, R. M., Luine, A., and Axelrod, J., 1986, Phospholipase A_2 and phospholipase C are activated by distinguished GTP-binding protein in FRTL5 thyroid cells, *Proc. Natl. Acad. Sci. USA* **83**:7201–7205.

Castagne, M., Tokai, Y., Kaibuchi, K., Kikkawa, U., and Nishizuka, Y., 1982, Direct activation of calcium activated phospholipid dependent protein kinase by tumor promoting phorbol esters, *J. Biol. Chem.* **257**:7847–7853.

Corberand, G., Ngyen, F., Laharrague, P., Fontanilles, A. N., Gleyzes, B., Gyrard, E., and Senegas, C., 1981, Polymorphonuclear functions and aging in humans, *J. Am. Geriatr. Soc.* **29**:391–397.

DeFronzo, R. A., 1981, Glucose intolerance and aging, *Diabetes Care* **4**:493–501.

Doll, R., Muir, C., and Waterhous, J., 1970, *Cancer Incidence in Five Continents*, Vol. 2, IUCC, Springer, Berlin.

Drazmin, B., Sussman, K., Kao, M., Lewis, D., and Sherman, N., 1987, The existence of an optimal range of cytosolic free calcium for insulin stimulated glucose transport in rat adipocytes, *J. Biol. Chem.* **262**:14385–14388.

Fülöp, T., Jr., Foris, G., Worum, I., Paragh, G., and Leovey, A., 1985, Age-related variations of some polymorphonuclear leukocyte functions, *Mech. Aging Dev.* **29**:1–8.

Fülöp, T., Jr., Hauck, M., Worum, I., Foris, G., and Leovey, A., 1987, Alterations of the FMLP-induced Ca^{2+} efflux from human monocytes with aging, *Immunol. Lett.* **14**:283–286.

Fülöp, T., Jr., Foris, G., Nagy, T. J., Varga, Z., and Leovey, A., 1988, Respiratory burst and aging, in: *Respiratory Burst and Its Physiologic Significance in Medicine* (A. J. Sbarra and R. R. Strauss, eds.), Plenum, New York, pp. 419–435.

Gardner, I. D., 1980, The effect of aging on susceptibility to infections, *Rev. Infect. Dis.* **2**:801–810.

Halliwell, B., 1978, Biochemical mechanisms accounting for the toxic action of oxygen in living organisms: The key role of superoxide dismutase, *Cell. Biol. Int. Rep.* **2**:113–128.

Harman, D., 1978, Free radical theory of aging: Nutritional implications, *Age* **1**:143–150.

Harman, D., Heidrick, M. L., and Eddy, D. E., 1977, Free radical theory of aging. Effect of free-radical-reaction inhibitors on the immune response, *J. Am. Geriatr. Soc.* **25**:400–407.

Johnston, R. B., Lehmeyer, J. E., and Guthrie, L. A., 1976, Generation of superoxide anion and chemiluminescence by human monocytes during phagocytosis and on contact with surface-bound immunoglobulin G, *J. Exp. Med.* **143**:1551–1563.

Makinodan, T., and Kay, M. M. B., 1980, Age-influences on the immune system, in: *Advances in Immunology* (E. Kungel and B. C. Dixon, eds.), Academic, New York, pp. 287–300.

McLaughlin, B., O'Malley, K., and Cotter, T. G., 1986, Age-related differences in granulocyte chemotaxis and degranulation, *Clin. Sci.* **70**:59–62.

McPhail, L. C., Henson, P. M., and Johnston, R. B., 1981, Respiratory burst enzyme in human neutrophils. Evidence for multiple mechanisms of action, *J. Clin. Invest.* **67**:710–716.

Nagel, J. E., Pyle, R. S., Chrest, F. J., and Adler, W., 1982, Oxidative metabolism and bactericidal capacity of polymorphonuclear leukocytes from normal young and aged adults, *J. Gerontol.* **37**:529–534.

Negoro, S., Hara, H., Miyata, S., Saiki, O., Tanaka, T., Yoshizaki, K., Nishimoto, N., and Kishimoto, S., 1987, Age-related changes of the function of T cell subsets predominant defect of the proliferative response in CD8 positive T cell subsets in aged persons, *Mech. Aging Dev.* **39**:263–279.

Parini, I. M., and Tauber, A. I., 1986, Activation of NADPH oxidase by arachidonic acid involves phospholipase A_2 in intact human neutrophils but not in the cell free system, *Biochem. Biophys. Res. Commun.* **138**:1099–1105.

Roth, G. S., 1986, Effect of aging on mechanisms of α-adrenergic and dopaminergic action, *Fed. Proc.* **45**:60–64.

Sakata, A., Ida, E., Tominaga, M., and Onone, K., 1987, Arachidonic acid acts as an intracellular activator of NADPH oxidase in Fc receptor-mediated superoxide generation in macrophages, *J. Immunol.* **138**:4353–4359.

Stout, R. W., 1987, Aging and atherosclerosis, *Age Aging* **26**:65–72.

Tappel, A. L., 1973, Lipid peroxidation damage to cell components, *Fed. Proc.* **32**:1870–1875.

Thompson, C. D., Rea, H. M., and Robinson, M. F., 1977, Low blood selenium levels and glutathione peroxidase activity in elderly people, *Proc. Univ. Otego Med. Sch.* **55**:19–26.

Varga, Z. S., Kovàcs, E. M., Paragh, G., Fülöp, T., Jr., Jacob, M. P., Robert, L., 1988, Effect of K-elastin (KE) and N-Formyl-methionyl-leucyl-phanylalanine (FMLP) on PMNLs of healthy middle-aged and aged subjects, *Clin. Biochem.* **21**:127–130.

Westwick, J., and Poll, C., 1986, Mechanism of calcium homeostasis in the polymorphonuclear leukocytes, *Agents Actions* **19**:80–86.

21

Quantitative Approaches to Pathogenesis of Age-Related Metabolic Conditions

RICHARD N. BERGMAN

1. INTRODUCTION

Accompanying the subtle but unrelenting increment in the fasting blood sugar with aging, at a rate of about 1 mg/dl per decade (Davidson, 1979), is a more profound impairment of glucose tolerance. The 2-hr blood sugar increases at least 5 mg/dl each decade of life. Thus, it is clear that with aging the tissues of the body are exposed to a steadily increasing glycemic environment. From the Whitehall study in 1980 (Fuller *et al.*, 1980), we know that glucose intolerance is associated with increased mortality: death rate per 1000 individuals increased from 59 to 94, comparing normal with impaired intolerant individuals; in newly diagnosed diabetics (preidentified overt diabetics were eliminated from their 7.5-year observational study), mortality was 175 per 1000. The close association among hyperglycemia, glucose intolerance, and mortality justifies obtaining a deeper understanding of the pathogenesis of glucose intolerance with aging, with the hope of intervention to reduce risk.

That the association of intolerance with mortality may be more than associative, and possibly causal, is supported by the important studies of the glycosylation of proteins by Cerami and Brownlee and colleagues (1987). These investigators have championed the hypothesis that irreversible binding of carbohydrate moieties to peptides may be important in many aspects of the aging process. Because these reactions are glucose concentration dependent, one may suppose that improvement of glucose control could reduce the integrated glycemic environment and stem, if not reverse, at least some aspects of the normal aging process. Thus, it is a justifiable goal to understand the individual factors that determine the ability of the young individual to closely regulate glycemia and to ask which of these physiologic processes degenerates with time. In addition, it is of interest to consider whether environmental factors are involved in the hyperglycemia of aging and whether the progression can be reversed with appropriate life-style and/or therapeutic approaches.

RICHARD N. BERGMAN • Department of Physiology and Biophysics, University of Southern California Medical School, Los Angeles, California 90033.

2. FACTORS REGULATING GLUCOSE TOLERANCE

Regulation of the blood glucose *in vivo* can be described using the hydraulic analogue shown in Fig. 1. Blood glucose in the fasting state is determined by an exquisite balance between the rate of endogenous glucose production (predominantly by the liver) and the rate of glucose utilization by it and other tissues of the body, of which muscle is quantitatively most important.

Carbohydrate intake transiently elevates the blood glucose level. Renormalization occurs due first, to the effects of glucose per se, and also to the effects of insulin and other hormones. Glucose self-normalizes (1) by augmenting its own uptake due to mass action, as well as glucose control of rate-limiting enzymes, and (2) by inhibiting hepatic glucose output (glucose autoregulation) (Sacca *et al.*, 1978). We have termed the overall effect of glucose to self-normalize, *glucose effectiveness*. These insulin-independent effects to renormalize glycemia are quantitatively important (Ader *et al.*, 1985; Baron *et al.*, 1985) and allow the blood sugar to be regulated even without an increment in plasma insulin (Fig. 2).

While glucose effectiveness is important, insulin generally does increase after glucose ingestion and, under such conditions, in normal individuals, glucose tolerance is determined primarily by insulin. The influence of insulin is determined first by the magnitude of the plasma insulin response to the carbohydrate intake, and second by the efficacy of the responding insulin to suppress endogenous glucose production and enhance its uptake. The magnitude of the hormonal response is established as a balance between insulin secretion and clearance (coalesced as insulin kinetics) (Fig. 1); the ability of the secreted insulin to enhance glucose renormalization is determined by the sensitivity of the individual tissues to insulin.

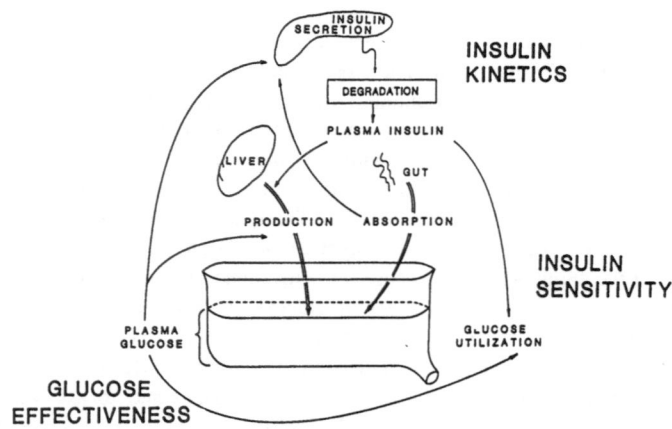

FIGURE 1. Hydraulic analogue of the regulation of the blood glucose concentration. The height of water in the tank represents the blood glucose. An increase in level from the fasting value is self-regulating in that it will increase glucose disappearance; a lowering of the level will decrease disappearance. The self-regulating effect of glucose (at basal insulin) is glucose effectiveness. Insulin augments glucose regulation by virtue of the hormone's portal and peripheral levels, determined by a balance between secretion and insulin metabolism (insulin kinetics). The final factor determining glucose tolerance is insulin's ability to enhance glucose utilization and restrain production (insulin sensitivity). (From Bergman, 1988.)

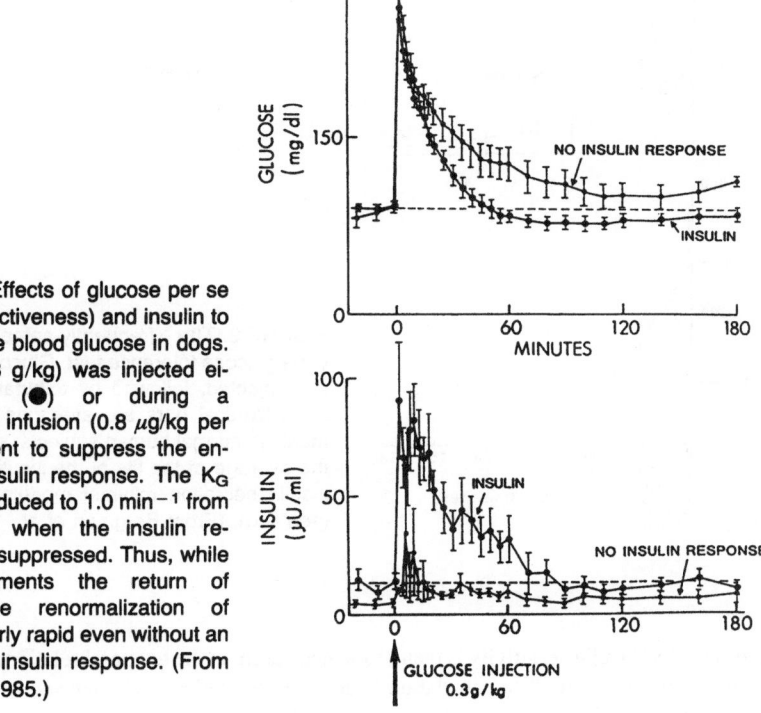

FIGURE 2. Effects of glucose per se (glucose effectiveness) and insulin to normalize the blood glucose in dogs. Glucose (0.3 g/kg) was injected either alone (●) or during a somatostatin infusion (0.8 μg/kg per min), sufficient to suppress the endogenous insulin response. The K_G value was reduced to 1.0 min^{-1} from 2.65 min^{-1} when the insulin response was suppressed. Thus, while insulin augments the return of glucose, the renormalization of glucose is fairly rapid even without an endogenous insulin response. (From Ader et al., 1985.)

2.1. Insulin Resistance

It is clear that insulin resistance is an important component of impaired glucose tolerance in a variety of conditions, including obesity (Olefsky et al., 1974), type 2 diabetes (Ginsburg et al., 1975), and aging (Kimmerling et al., 1977). However, assessment of the degree of this defect is problematic (Bergman et al., 1985; Ader and Bergman, 1987). Insulin sensitivity is a distributed parameter, as the overall ability of the body to dispose of glucose in response to insulin may not reflect the sensitivity of any single insulin-dependent tissue, but may well be an overall average of the functions of individual tissues. Also, because of the closed-loop nature of the feedback relationship between glucose and insulin (Fig. 1), any imposed change in insulin will affect the blood glucose, which in turn will cause compensatory changes in insulin, and so on, rendering it difficult to perceive changes in insulin sensitivity separate from changes in insulin secretion.

2.2. Minimal Model Approach

We introduced the minimal model approach to measuring insulin sensitivity (Bergman et al., 1979, 1981, 1987; Bergman, 1988). The concept underlying this approach is that glucose is administered systemically (Fig. 3), the time courses of plasma glucose and insulin are

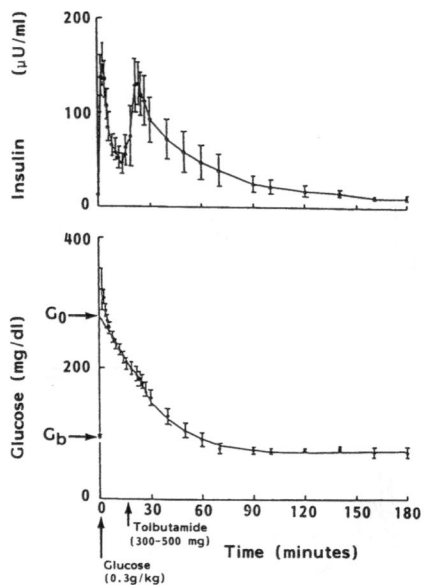

FIGURE 3. The frequently-sampled intravenous glucose tolerance test. Glucose (0.3 g/kg) was injected, followed by tolbutamide 20 min later. Vertical bars are averages of 8 experiments in normal human subjects; solid lines are the average of the fits of the insulin action and insulin secretion minimal models to the data (see text). (From Bergman et al., 1987.)

recorded, and insulin sensitivity is then calculated based on the temporal relationship between hormone and substrate. The calculation is done on the digital computer and uses a specific mathematical model of insulin action based on known glucose and insulin physiology. In brief (Fig. 4) (cf. Bergman et al., 1979; Bergman, 1988), what is implemented in the model of glucose regulation are the concepts that (1) it is not plasma insulin per se, but insulin at a site remote from plasma (interstitial compartment?) that alters glucose utilization; and (2) remote insulin acts to suppress net endogenous glucose production and augment glucose uptake, which occurs at any given plasma glucose concentration.

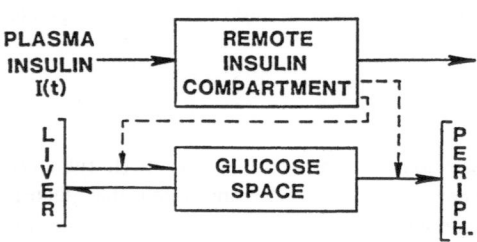

FIGURE 4. Representation of the minimal model of insulin action. Plasma insulin is envisioned as being transported into a remote compartment (interstitial fluid?); remote insulin acts to accelerate glucose utilization and retard endogenous glucose production. Frequently sampled intravenous glucose tolerance test (FSIGT) data (Fig. 3) are submitted to the computer program in which this model is implemented, and the insulin sensitivity index (S_I) is calculated. (Equations for the model can be found in Bergman et al., 1979.)

2.3. Frequently Sampled Intravenous Glucose Tolerance Test

The question arose as to the best diagnostic protocol to use for calculation of insulin sensitivity exploiting the minimal model. We were able to demonstrate that a combined glucose/tolbutamide injection protocol (see Fig. 3) yielded the most accurate results (Yang *et al.*, 1987). The extra secretagogue was required because in some cases (e.g., in aging subjects) glucose did not elicit an insulin response that was at the best time, and of sufficient magnitude, to allow for an accurate calculation. The protocol can be described thus: after a basal sample is taken, a moderate dose of glucose is injected intravenously (IV) (300 mg/kg) followed by tolbutamide (200 mg) 20 min later. Thirty-one blood samples are taken over 3 hr, glucose and insulin are measured, and the results are submitted to the computer. The computer uses the program MINMOD (Pacini and Bergman, 1986) to calculate the insulin sensitivity index (S_I). Values of S_I in normal subjects average between 5 and 6 $\times$ 10^{-4} min$^{-1}/\mu$U per ml.

The units of the insulin sensitivity index S_I seem daunting; however, when carefully considered, they make good sense. Glucose clearance is the ratio of the disappearance of glucose from the blood to the prevailing glucose concentration. Thus, glucose clearance is an index of the ability of glucose to enhance its own utilization. It is related to the total number of pathways in the body for glucose uptake (i.e., the number of glucose transporters on cell membranes). S_I represents the degree to which insulin increases glucose clearance, hence the extent to which insulin can increase the available pathways for glucose utilization. Since this is the primary mechanism by which insulin acts, we can interpret S_I as the ability of insulin, in a given individual, to access pathways for glucose uptake in all the tissues of the body. Clearly, when insulin resistance is present (as in the aging individual), it is this action of insulin that is impaired.

2.4. Glucose Resistance

An additional index that emerges from minimal model analysis is the glucose sensitivity index, S_G. This parameter is analogous to glucose clearance at basal insulin; i.e., it reflects the ability of glucose to enhance its own utilization independent of any increment in insulin. It should be thought of both as a measure of the pathways of glucose uptake of the insulin-independent tissues, e.g., brain, red blood cells, liver, gut, as well as glucose uptake by insulin-dependent tissues (muscle, adipose tissue, fat), at basal plasma insulin levels.

3. RESISTANCE IN AGING

Older subjects are insulin resistant (Kimmerling *et al.*, 1977); however, they also demonstrate increased adiposity (Novak, 1972). In collaboration with Dr. Mei Chen and Dr. Daniel Porte, Jr., in Seattle, we considered whether resistance in aging occurs independent of adiposity. The value of factor K_G, which is a measure of glucose tolerance, was diminished in these subjects from the value in young controls of 2.21 $\pm$ 0.22 to 1.32 $\pm$ 0.10 min^{-1} in the older subjects, despite no evidence of increased adiposity in the elderly group (Fig. 5). These lean elderly subjects were substantially insulin resistant, with S_I diminished 73% from normal (Fig. 6). By contrast, there was no impairment in the insulin-independent glucose utilization in these subjects. This latter observation further demonstrates that the insulin

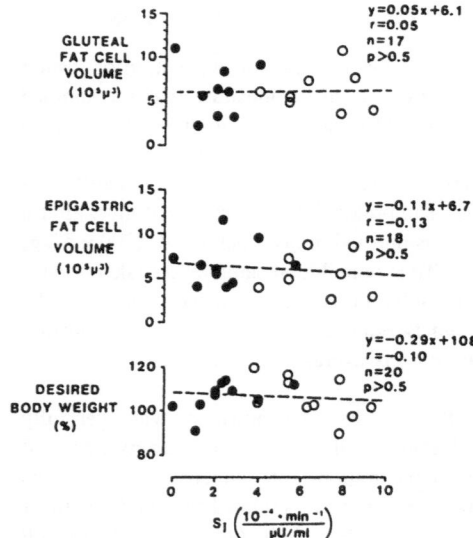

FIGURE 5. Independence of insulin sensitivity from adiposity among young (○) and older (●) patients. Insulin resistance of older subjects could not be explained on the basis of adiposity. (From Chen *et al.*, 1985.)

resistance shown in older subjects is independent of adiposity, since glucose resistance has been reported in the obese, young subject (Bergman *et al.*, 1981).

4. PANCREATIC B-CELL FUNCTION

While insulin resistance is clearly characteristic of elderly subjects, even if nonobese, it is not necessarily fully responsible for the glucose intolerance of such subjects. Thus, it is important to consider whether changes in insulin kinetics—secretion and/or clearance from blood—can also be implicated in the intolerance of the aging subject. This question is of great significance because it is now recognized by many investigators that insulin resistance

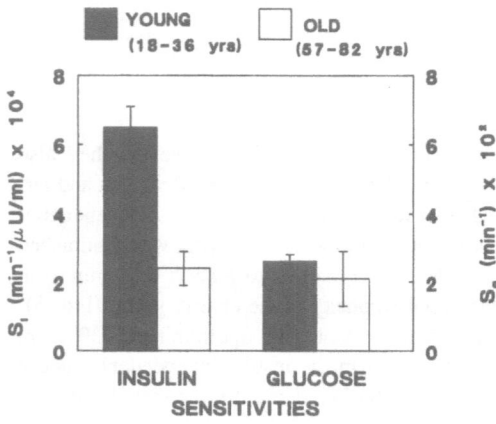

FIGURE 6. Effect of aging on insulin sensitivity (S_I) and glucose (S_G) effectiveness. Insulin resistance of the older patients was highly significant ($p < 0.01$); no difference was seen in S_G.

alone is not sufficient to cause overt diabetes mellitus, but that B-cell dysfunction is a requisite component. Because type 2 diabetes mellitus is an age-related disorder, it would be important if diminished B-cell function were also age related, because the pancreatic locus could then be implicated in the increased risk of type 2 with advancing age.

4.1. Assessment of Insulin Kinetics

As with insulin sensitivity, adequate methodology is important for assessment of B-cell function and insulin clearance *in vivo*. It is possible simply to observe plasma insulin following glucose injection (cf. Fig. 3), as such an approach is sufficient to distinguish total B-cell dysfunction. However, it is particularly difficult to identify subtle changes in B-cell response from plasma observations for several reasons: (1) changes in plasma insulin after glucose administration can be due to alterations in secretion and/or clearance, and it is difficult to distinguish them; and (2) as glucose intolerance develops, the stimulus to the pancreas increases (i.e., glucose stays elevated longer after injection), and what may seem like an adequate insulin response may simply reflect a greater stimulus to B cells rather than a healthy B-cell response. Finally, secreted insulin must pass through the liver before reaching the systemic circulation, and changes in first-pass hepatic insulin extraction may occur with age.

4.2. Exploitation of C-Peptide

A discovery that has greatly influenced assessment of insulin kinetics is the equimolar secretion of insulin and C-peptide (Rubenstein *et al.*, 1969). (The latter peptide is broken off during biosynthesis when proinsulin is converted to insulin in the B cells.) Eaton and colleagues (1980), and later Polonsky *et al.* (1984, 1986), calculated the C-peptide secretion rate by measuring kinetics of the peptide in each subject on one day, and stimulating endogenous secretion on a second day. Using compartmental modeling to combine these results, the pattern of prehepatic insulin secretion could be calculated.

We have recently simplified the Eaton approach (Volund *et al.*, 1987). Our method exploits insulin and C-peptide concentrations following glucose administration simultaneously to calculate the pattern of insulin secretion. The patterns of plasma insulin and C-peptide after glucose injection (Fig. 7) are fitted using a combined compartmental model of insulin and C-peptide kinetics (Fig. 8); from this, the pattern of insulin secretion as well as the fractional insulin clearance rate can be determined (Fig. 9).

It has long been known that insulin secretion is a biphasic phenomenon; application of the combined insulin/C-peptide model confirms the importance *in vivo* of the two phases (Fig. 9). R. Watanabe in our laboratory has studied the two phases in a group of normal lean young women (Watanabe *et al.*, 1988). He has demonstrated that the initial phase represents most (67%) of the incremental insulin secretion elicited by glucose in normal individuals.

4.3. Secretion Model

We have expressed the two phases of insulin secretion in terms of a secretory model (Fig. 10) based on the concepts that (1) when an IV glucose tolerance test is performed, the sum total of the potential first-phase contribution is released by the B cells into the portal vein; and (2) the rate of second-phase secretion is a function of the plasma glucose concentra-

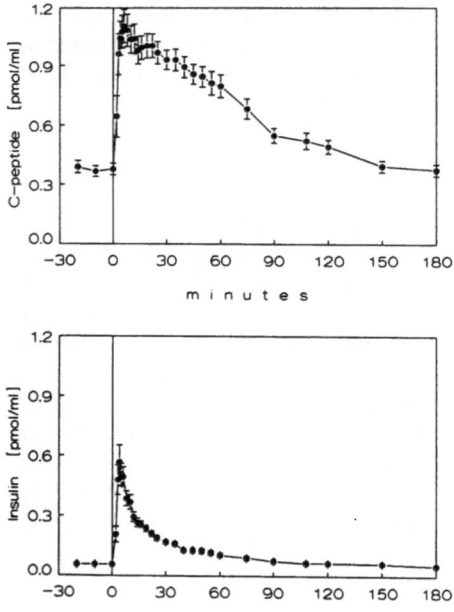

FIGURE 7. Plasma levels of insulin and C-peptide in human subjects (N = 26) following injection of glucose alone (300 mg/kg) at t = 0.

tion in excess of a threshold value. Application of the model to the biphasic secretory patterns calculated from the combined insulin/C-peptide model results in two specific parameters of B-cell function: ϕ_1 and ϕ_2, which explicitly represent the sensitivity of first- and second-phase insulin release to glucose, following glucose injection. First-phase insulin secretion and insulin clearance were clearly not reduced in the aging subjects (Fig. 11, $p > 0.50$ for

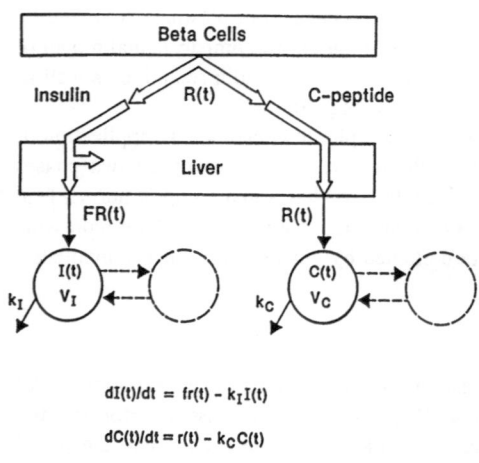

$$dI(t)/dt = fr(t) - k_I I(t)$$

$$dC(t)/dt = r(t) - k_C C(t)$$

$$r(t) = R(t)/V_C; \quad f = FV_C/V_I$$

FIGURE 8. Model used to calculate the temporal pattern of insulin secretion during the intravenous glucose tolerance test. Insulin and C-peptide are secreted at equimolar rate, R(t), from the B cells; secreted C-peptide survives passage through the liver while insulin is partially degraded. It is assumed that insulin and C-peptide have first-order metabolic kinetics; however the clearance rate for insulin (k_I) exceeds substantially that for C-peptide (k_C). From plasma insulin and C-peptide measurements, I(t) and C(t), pattern R(t) is calculated. (From Volund et al., 1987.)

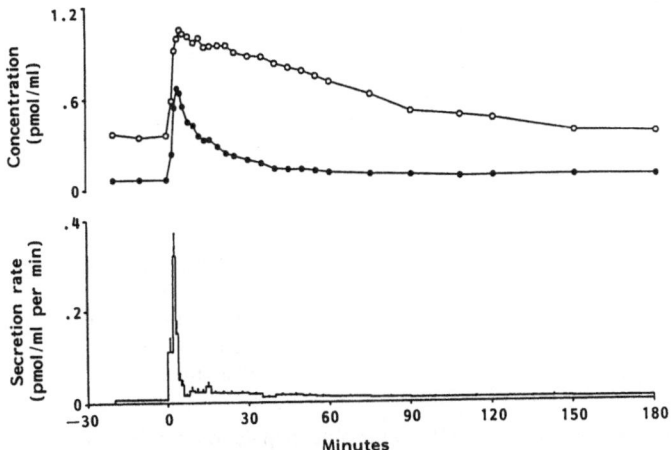

FIGURE 9. Plasma concentrations of insulin (●) and C-peptide (○) in a single normal individual (top) and the calculated insulin secretory pattern (bottom). Glucose was injected at time 0. Note that first-phase insulin release is twice as great as total second-phase increment.

both). However, there was a tendency for second-phase pancreatic responsivity (ϕ_2) to be reduced, with the mean of the aging subjects equal to 13 ± 3 μU/ml min^{-2}/mg/dl, compared with a value of 19 ± 3 in the young. The age dependence of second-phase B-cell responsiveness was marginally significant when we examined the correlation between ϕ_2 and age ($r = -0.47$, $p < 0.05$).

5. INSULIN SECRETION/INSULIN ACTION RELATIONSHIP

Taken at face value, the above results would lead to the conclusion that glucose intolerance of aging is due primarily to insulin resistance and is independent of a pancreatic

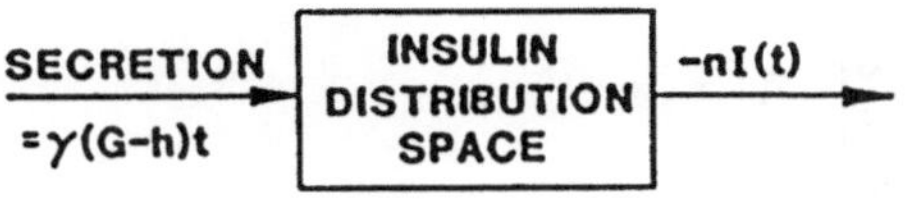

FIGURE 10. Model of insulin kinetics *in vivo*. Instantaneous appearance in plasma of first-phase insulin release after glucose injection is assumed; first-phase secretion is considered an initial condition ($I(0)^+$) = I_O. Second-phase secretion is proportional by parameter γ to the rate of increase of glucose, above a threshold in plasma [(G-h)t]. First- and second-phase sensitivities to glucose are expressed as ϕ_1 and ϕ_2, defined as here. For further details, see Bergman (1988). (From Toffolo *et al.*, 1980.)

$$\text{SECRETION} \xrightarrow{=\gamma(G-h)t} \boxed{\begin{array}{c}\text{INSULIN}\\\text{DISTRIBUTION}\\\text{SPACE}\end{array}} \xrightarrow{-nI(t)}$$

$$\frac{dI}{dt} = \gamma(G-h)t - nI$$

$$I(o) = I_O \text{ (apex of 1st peak)}$$

$$\Phi_1 = \frac{I_O}{n\,\Delta G}$$

$$\Phi_2 = \gamma$$

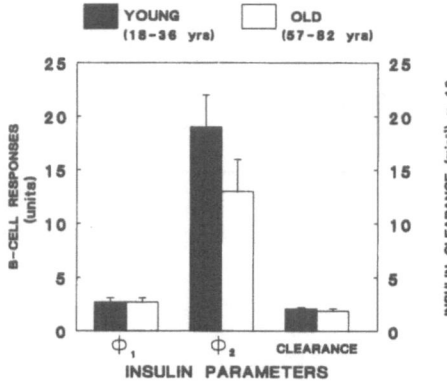

FIGURE 11. Effect of aging on secretory parameters and fractional insulin clearance. The latter is expressed as the fraction of the insulin pool disappearing per unit time.

defect, because S_I was reduced 73% in the older population, while ϕ_1 was normal and ϕ_2 was reduced only 31%. However, the flaw in such reasoning is that, even in the normal individual, there is an important interaction between insulin secretion and insulin action, such that we expect that normally, insulin resistance should be offset by a compensatory increase in B-cell responsiveness. If we can demonstrate that this putative compensatory B-cell mechanism did not occur with the aging subjects, this may reveal a latent B-cell defect that is not obvious simply by observing the islet cell response to glucose stimulation.

In the obese, but not aged, individual with normal glucose tolerance, there is an apparent B-cell compensation for insulin resistance (Perley and Kipnis, 1966; Bergman et al., 1981). The result is that parameters ϕ_1 and ϕ_2 are elevated in the obese individual. This relationship may be envisioned in terms of a plot between S_I and ϕ_2 (Fig. 12), showing a tendency for the B-cell parameter to be elevated in the more resistant subjects, and vice-versa. This can be expressed quantitatively by stating that the $S_I \times \phi_2$ product was overall equal to 75 (units omitted). This value of 75 can be considered the closed-loop gain of the glucose regulating system; it reflects the ability of the individual to renormalize elevated glycemia by a combination of B-cell response and the action of insulin to accelerate glucose disposition.

Evidence from other studied populations supports the concept of a strong interaction between pancreatic islets and insulin-sensitive cells. Dr. Thomas Buchanan and colleagues,

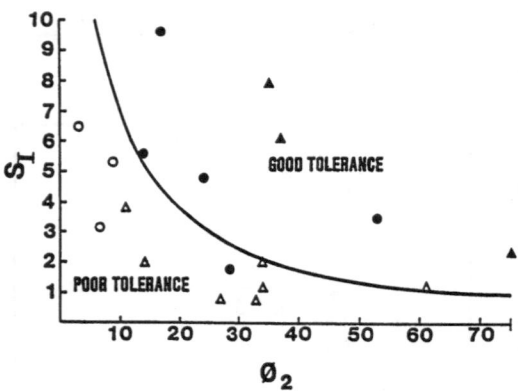

FIGURE 12. Relationship between insulin sensitivity and second-phase B-cell responsiveness in a group of normal-weight subjects with good glucose tolerance (●) $K_G > 1.5$ min^{-1}) or poor tolerance (○) $K_G < 1.5$ min^{-1}), and obese subjects with good (▲) or poor (△) tolerance. Solid line represents the expression $\phi_2 \times S_I = 75$. Note that the $\phi_2 \times S_I$ product usually exceeds 75 for subjects with $K_G > 1.5$ min^{-1}. (From Bergman et al., 1981.)

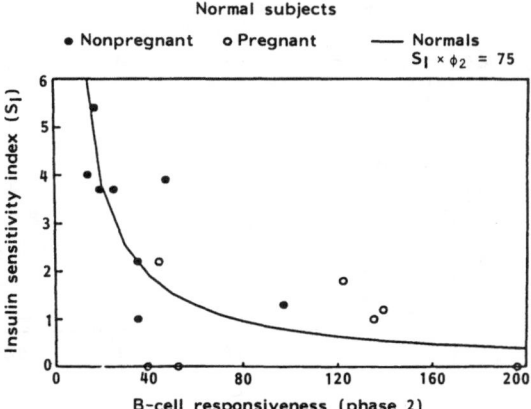

FIGURE 13. Insulin sensitivity/insulin action relationship for a group of normal women (●) and a group of normal, pregnant women of matched nonpregnant body weight (○). Note that pregnancy decreases S_I overall, but there is a compensatory increase in ϕ_2 such that the $\phi_2 \times S_I$ relationship is obeyed during the course of pregnancy. (From T. Buchanan et al., 1987.)

when he was at Northwestern, examined this relationship in normal women and compared the results with a second group of normal but pregnant subjects. In preliminary data, shown in Fig. 13, the pregnant subjects were, as expected, more resistant (Ryan et al., 1985; Buchanan et al., 1987); however, their islet cell responses increased so as to maintain the $S_I \times \phi_2$ product exactly. Thus, pregnancy represents a natural experiment that demonstrates the concept of the normalcy of the islet cell/insulin action relationship.

The converse is demonstrated by a group of high-risk siblings of type 1 diabetic subjects, studied in Seattle by Johnston, Raghu, Palmer, and colleagues (1987) (Fig. 14). These siblings had normal glucose tolerance; however, all the patients fell below the $S_I \times \phi_2$ curve (actually, a different method was used in this case to measure islet cell function). In this group, therefore, a latent B-cell defect was uncovered only by simultaneous consideration of the islet cell/insulin action relationship.

What, then, of the aged population? Clearly, although it was problematic to demonstrate

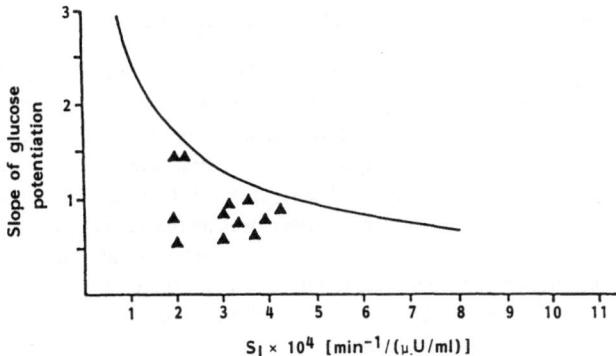

FIGURE 14. Insulin sensitivity/insulin action relationship for a group of high-risk but nondiabetic siblings of type 1 diabetics. Note that all siblings fall below the $\phi_2 \times S_I$ hyperbola. (From Johnston et al., 1987.)

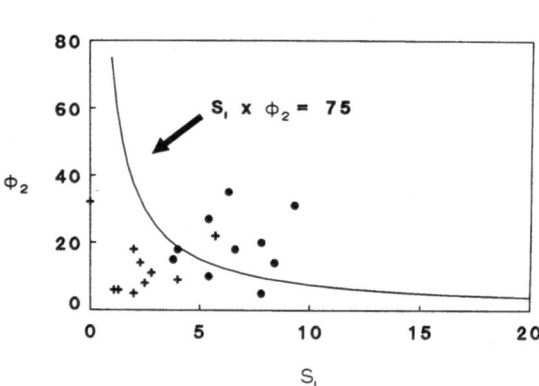

FIGURE 15. Insulin sensitivity/ insulin action relationship for a group of young and elderly male nonobese subjects. As in earlier examples, ϕ_2 is inappropriately low for the degree of insulin resistance in these subjects, revealing a latent B-cell defect. (From Chen *et al.*, 1985.)

a decrease in B-cell function (see Fig. 11), the aging group (with a single exception) was entirely located below the normal $S_I \times \phi_2$ relationship (Fig. 15). The B-cell response of the older subjects is clearly inappropriately low for the degree of insulin resistance in that population. Therefore, insulin resistance alone cannot explain the glucose intolerance in the elderly population, and islet cell deficiency is clearly implicated by the data of Fig. 15. Both the HLA-identical siblings of type 1 diabetics and the elderly population are at greater risk of diabetes than is the general population; it remains a clear possibility that the latent and virtually identical B-cell defects exposed in Fig. 14 and 15 may be causative for the increased risk.

It is of interest to consider whether the insulin resistance or the latent B-cell deficiency of the older population may be a "primary" defect. Reaven and colleagues (1977) showed that alloxan diabetes in dogs is associated with substantial insulin resistance; we may therefore propose that it is the latent B-cell defect that results in insulin resistance in older subjects, independent of adiposity. Longitudinal studies are needed to test the hypothesis of the primacy of the B-cell defect in age-related glucose intolerance.

Lability of Glucose Tolerance in Aging Subjects

If we presume that glucose intolerance in older subjects may be detrimental, it is reasonable to consider therapeutic approaches to improve tolerance and reduce the risk associated with persistent elevated post-meal glycemia. It has been known for some time that glucose intolerance of aging can be improved with a high carbohydrate diet. We have recently confirmed this finding (Chen *et al.*, 1988); after a 3- to 5-day regimen of high (85%) carbohydrate intake, the K_G value in elderly subjects was increased from 1.5 ± 0.2 min^{-1} to 2.0 ± 0.3 min^{-1}. It is interesting that while glucose tolerance was normalized by this dietary regimen, the diet did not totally ameliorate the metabolic profile of the elderly subjects (Fig. 16). The increase in tolerance was caused by the well-known effect of high carbohydrate on pancreatic responsiveness; ϕ_2 was increased from 9 ± 3 to 22 ± 1 μU/ml min^{-2}/mg per dl, even in excess of ϕ_2 in young normal subjects. This overcompensation of pancreatic responsiveness was necessary because insulin sensitivity was not totally normalized by the high carbohydrate diet. However, as demonstrated in Fig. 16, B-cell overcompensation in the face of moderate insulin resistance was sufficient in the elderly subjects to return the insulin

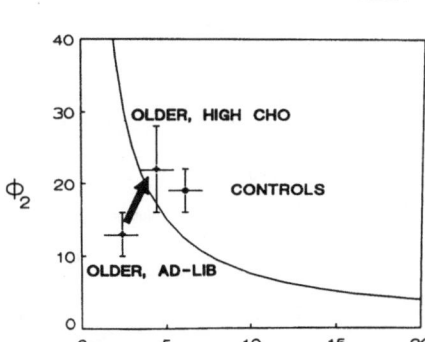

FIGURE 16. Corrective effects of high carbohydrate diet on intolerance of aging. (From Chen
et al., 1988.)

secretion–insulin action relationship to the hyperbola of good tolerance; i.e., for these
subjects, $\phi_2 \times S_I$ was greater than 75 because of pancreatic overcompensation in the face of
moderate insulin resistance. The resultant hyperinsulinemia seems to have improved the
insulin sensitivity of the peripheral tissues (Kahn *et al.*, 1987).

6. OVERVIEW: EVENTS LEADING TO GLUCOSE INTOLERANCE IN THE ELDERLY

The arguments presented here are consistent with the hypothesis that glucose intolerance
in aging results from a combination of insulin resistance and a subtle B-cell defect. The islet
cell defect can only be identified if the relationship between B-cell responsiveness and insulin
sensitivity is considered. An important question arises: Which is primary with glucose
intolerance of aging, the B-cell defect or the insulin resistance? Because of the evidence that
the insulin environment influences insulin sensitivity, such that hypoinsulinemia will lead to
insulin resistance (Reaven *et al.*, 1977), we propose that it is the B-cell defect that is primary,
and the insulin resistance is secondary for the glucose intolerance of the elderly individual.

The hypothesis may be understood by consideration of Fig. 17a–d. Let us assume that
the B cell develops insensitivity to glucose with age. This insensitivity will be expressed as a
rightward shift of the curve relating plasma glucose level and insulin secretory rate (Fig.
17a). This rightward shift will lead initially to a subtle lowering of plasma insulin at the
fasting glycemia level. Lowered insulin will invoke a modest insulin resistance, resulting in
diminished glucose uptake by peripheral tissues (cf. Fig. 17b) and increased glucose production by the liver (Fig. 17c). Concomitant elevated production and inhibited utilization of
glucose will conspire to elevate plasma glucose modestly. Because the "gain" of the pancreatic B cell depends on the ambient glucose to which the pancreas responds, we expect that
there will be a renormalization of plasma glucose, which is accomplished by a glucose-
mediated increase in the slope of the insulin secretory curve (Fig. 17d).

According to the hypothesis expressed in Fig. 17a–d, then, a subtle age-related rightward shift of the insulin secretory curve results in a slight hyperglycemia. Thus, we may
explain the modest (1 mg/dl per decade) hyperglycemia of aging. The hyperglycemia is due

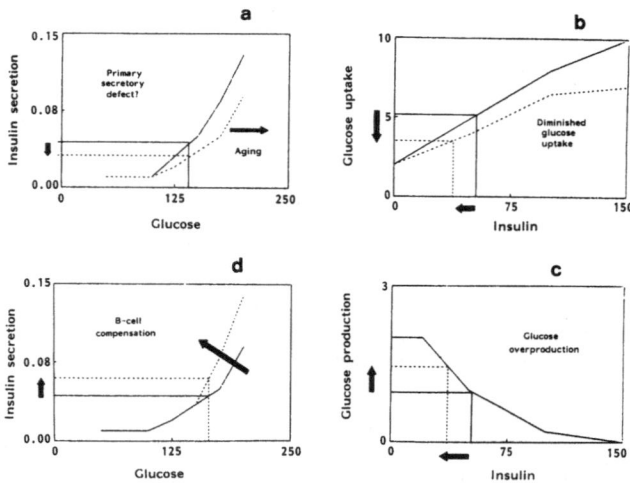

FIGURE 17. Hypothetical course of events in the development of glucose intolerance of aging. (a) Aging-related rightward shift in B-cell responsiveness to glucose. (b) Steady-state relationship between plasma insulin and peripheral glucose utilization; modest hypoinsulinemia is proposed to reduce sensitivity. (c) Lower insulin also increases hepatic glucose output. (d) Compensation is increased slope of the relationship between B-cell function and plasma glucose, possibly representing B-cell stress.

to subtle increases in glucose production and decrease in glucose uptake. Thus, this hypothesis accounts for the glucose intolerance of aging, since glucose tolerance is determined by the balance between glucose production and utilization. Finally, the renormalization of the plasma glucose level occurs at the expense of a glucose-potentiated B-cell "gain" (i.e., the slope of the relationship between glucose and insulin secretion will be increased) in the face of a rightward shift in the insulin secretory relationship. We may envision that this renormalization of the insulin/glucose relationship puts a moderate "stress" on the B cells which may themselves ultimately fail in those individuals who have a lesser pancreatic reserve. It is those subjects who may be envisioned to be at greatest risk of age-related diabetes mellitus.

7. CONCLUSION

We have attempted to describe the factors determining the glucose tolerance *in vivo* and how they may be altered in the aging state. We believe that there is a subtle (even latent) B-cell defect that is exacerbated with age (for unknown reasons), but that is hidden because of the ability of the closed-loop insulin glucose control system to reregulate the plasma glucose level, albeit at a greater B-cell "gain." While a high carbohydrate diet can ameliorate the glucose intolerance of aging, it does this at the cost of an even greater increase in B-cell gain, and possibly a greater stress to the pancreas. We suggest that it is in those individuals who are, for genetic or environmental reasons, least able to increase their islet cell responsiveness that aging-related glucose intolerance may develop into full-blown diabetes mellitus. This process is exacerbated by other factors, such as obesity, which will add to insulin resistance and further stress the B cells. We also suggest that approaches must be found to uncover the subtle B-cell defects outlined here to begin to consider early interventions in those patients most susceptible to age-related frank metabolic disease.

8. SUMMARY

Inappropriately elevated plasma glucose is implicated in pathogenesis of tissue changes in aging per se, as well as in aging-related diseases including diabetes, diabetes-related complications and atherosclerosis. The pathogeneses of the steady increase in the fasting blood glucose level, as well as the more precipitous increment in the transient meal-related hyperglycemia with age remain to be determined. While reduced glucose intolerance is characteristic of obesity, and relative adiposity increases even in "thin" aging subjects, it is clear that glucose tolerance declines even independent of the increased adiposity. Glucose tolerance may deteriorate because of insulin resistance, impaired function of the pancreatic islets (which secrete insulin), or both. Overproduction of glucose by liver is implicated in fasting hyperglycemia. We have described new approaches to quantification of the importance of these various factors. One approach, the "minimal model" method, measures the degree of insulin resistance, as well as B-cell function from a noninvasive method, allowing for longitudinal studies in aging subjects. Normally, tissue sensitivity to insulin and islet cell function interact to optimize glucose tolerance, and return the blood sugar to its "non-pathologic" value with great efficiency. Thus, B-cell response normally increases in exact proportion to compensate for insulin resistance, stabilizing glucose tolerance. Such a compensation is seen in obesity of the young, who exhibit insulin resistance and markedly increased B-cell response. Characteristic of aging is the inability of the B cell to compensate adequately for the resistance to insulin of peripheral tissues, leading to a decline in glucose tolerance, with the associated increase in the 24-hr glucose pattern that is believed to be pathogenic. Ability to quantify the pathogenic factors promises approaches to stem the rate of decline of tolerance and increase in fasting blood sugar. One promising approach is diet. A high-carbohydrate diet increases B-cell function relative to insulin resistance in the older population and can act to normalize glucose tolerance in aging. The possibility exists that this will slow the pathogenicities of aging.

ACKNOWLEDGMENTS. This work was supported by grants DK-29867 and DK-27619 from the National Institute of Health. I am grateful to Dr. Marilyn Ader for her commentary on the text as well as help in production of the manuscript. I also am indebted to Dr. Daniel Porte, Jr., for arousing my interest in aging research.

REFERENCES

Ader, M., and Bergman, R. N., 1987, Insulin sensitivity in the intact organism, in:*Bailliere's Clinics in Endocrinology and Metabolism. Techniques for Metabolic Investigation in Man,* Vol. 1(4) (K. G. M. M. Alberti, P. D Home, and R. Taylor, eds.), Bailliere Tindall, London, pp. 879–910.
Ader, M., Yang, Y., Pacini, G., and Bergman, R. N., 1985, Importance of glucose per se to intravenous glucose tolerance: comparison of the minimal model prediction with direct measurements, *Diabetes* **34:**1092–1103.

Baron, A. D., Kolterman, O. G., Bell, J., Mandarino, L. J., and Olefsky, J. M., 1985, Rates of noninsulin-mediated glucose uptake are elevated in Type II diabetic subjects, *J. Clin. Invest.* **76:**1782–1788.

Bergman, R. N., 1988, Integration of pathogenic factors in impaired glucose tolerance and NIDDM, in: *Pathogenesis of Noninsulin-Dependent Diabetes Mellitus* (V. Grill and S. Efendic, eds.), Raven, New York, pp. 241–269.

Bergman, R. N., Finegood, D. T., and Ader, M., 1985, Assessment of insulin sensitivity in vivo, *Endocr. Rev.* **6:**45–86.

Bergman, R. N., Ider, Y., Bowden, C. R., and Cobelli, C., 1979, Quantitative estimation of insulin sensitivity, *Am. J. Physiol.* **236:**E667–E677.

Bergman, R. N., Phillips, L. S., and Cobelli, C., 1981, Physiologic evaluation of factors controlling glucose tolerance in man: Measurement of insulin sensitivity and B-cell glucose sensitivity from the response to intravenous glucose, *J. Clin. Invest.* **68:**1456–1467.

Bergman, R. N., Prager, R., Volund, A., and Olefsky, J. M., 1987, Equivalence of the insulin sensitivity index in man derived by the minimal model method and the euglycemic glucose clamp, *J. Clin. Invest.* **79:**790–800.

Buchanan, T., Metzger, B., and Freinkel, N., 1987, Impaired B-cell function rather than exaggerated insulin resistance distinguishes gestational diabetes from normal pregnancy, *Diabetes,* **36:**5A.

Cerami, A., Vlassara, H., and Brownlee, M., 1987, Glucose and aging, *Sci. Am.* **256:**91–96.

Chen, M., Bergman, R. N., Pacini, G., and Porte, D., Jr., 1985, Pathogenesis of age-related glucose intolerance in man: Insulin resistance and decreased B-cell function, *J. Clin. Endocrinol. Metab.* **60:**13–20.

Chen, M., Bergman, R. N., and Porte, D., Jr., 1988, Insulin resistance and beta-cell dysfunction in aging: The importance of dietary carbohydrate, *J. Clin. Endocrinol. Metab.* **67:**951–957.

Davidson, M. B., 1979, The effect of aging on carbohydrate metabolism: A review of the English literature and a practical approach to the diagnosis of diabetes mellitus in the elderly, *Metabolism* **28:**688–705.

Eaton, R. P., Allen, R. C., Schade, D. S., Erickson, K. M., and Standefer, J., 1980, Prehepatic insulin production in man: Kinetic analysis using peripheral connecting peptide behavior, *J. Clin. Endocrinol. Metab.* **51:**520–528.

Fuller, J. H., Shipley, M. J., Rose, G., Jarrett, R. J., and Keen, H., 1980, Coronary–heart-disease risk and impaired glucose tolerance: The Whitehall study, *Lancet* **1:**1373–1376.

Ginsburg, H., Kimmerling, G., Olefsky, J. M., and Reaven, G. M., 1975, Demonstration of insulin resistance in untreated adult onset diabetic subjects with fasting hyperglycemia, *J. Clin. Invest.* **55:**454–461.

Johnston, C., Raghu, P., McCulloch, D. K., Beard, J. C., Ward, W. K., Klaff, L. J., McKnight, B., Bergman, R. N., and Palmer, J. P., 1987, B-cell function and insulin sensitivity in nondiabetic HLA-identical siblings of insulin-dependent diabetics, *Diabetes* **36:**829–837.

Kahn, B. B., Horton, E. S., and Cushman, S. W., 1987, Mechanism for enhanced glucose transport response to insulin in adipose cells from chronically hyperinsulinemic rats. Increased translocation of glucose transporters from an enlarged intracellular pool, *J. Clin. Invest.* **79:**853–858.

Kimmerling, G., Jovorski, W. C., and Reaven, G. M., 1977, Aging and insulin resistance in a group of non-obese male volunteers, *J. Am. Geriatr. Soc.* **25:**349–353.

Novak, L. P., 1972, Aging, total body potassium, fat-free mass, and cell mass in males and females between ages 18 and 85 years, *J. Gerontol.* **27:**438–443.

Olefsky, J., Reaven, G. M., and Farquhar, J. W., 1974, Effects of weight reduction on obesity: Studies of lipid and carbohydrate metabolism in normal and hyperlipoproteinemic subjects, *J. Clin. Invest.* **53:**64–76.

Pacini, G., and Bergman, R. N., 1986, MINMOD: A computer program to calculate insulin sensitivity and pancreatic responsivity from the frequently sampled intravenous glucose tolerance test, *Comp. Meth. Progr. Biomed.* **23:**113–122.

Perley, M., and Kipnis, D. M., 1966, Plasma insulin responses to glucose and tolbutamide of normal weight and obese diabetic and nondiabetic subjects, *Diabetes* **15**:867–874.

Polonsky, K., Lucinio-Paixao, J., Given, B. D., Pugh, W., Rue, P., Galloway, J., Karrison, T., and Frank, B., 1986, Use of biosynthetic human C-peptide in the measurement of insulin secretion rates in normal volunteers and type 1 diabetic patients, *J. Clin. Invest.* **77**:98–105.

Polonsky, K. S., Pugh, W., Jaspan, S. J., Cohen, D. M., Karrison, T., Tager, H. S., and Rubenstein, A. H., 1984, C-peptide and insulin secretion: Relationship between peripheral concentrations of C-peptide and insulin and insulin secretion rates in the dog, *J. Clin. Invest.* **74**:1821–1829.

Reaven, G. M., Sageman, W. S., and Swenson, R. S., 1977, Development of insulin resistance in normal dogs following alloxan-induced insulin deficiency, *Diabetologia* **13**:459–462.

Rubenstein, A. H., Clark, J. L., Melani, F., and Steiner, D. F., 1969, Secretion of proinsulin C-peptide by pancreatic beta cells and its circulation in blood, *Nature (Lond.)* **224**:697–699.

Ryan, E. A., O'Sullivan, M. J., and Skyler, J. S., 1985, Insulin action during pregnancy. Studies with the euglycemic clamp technique, *Diabetes* **34**:380–389.

Sacca, L., Hendler, R., and Sherwin, R. S., 1978, Hyperglycemia inhibits glucose production in man independent of changes in glucoregulatory hormones, *J. Clin. Endocrinol. Metab.* **47**:1160–1163.

Toffolo, G., Bergman, R. N., Finegood, D. T., Bowden, C. R., and Cobelli, C., 1980, Quantitative estimation of beta-cell sensitivity to glucose in the intact organism, *Diabetes* **29**:979–990.

Volund, A., Polonsky, K. S., and Bergman, R. N., 1987, Calculated pattern of intraportal insulin appearance without independent assessment of C-peptide kinetics, *Diabetes* **36**:1195–1202.

Watanabe, R., Roy, S., and Bergman, R. N., 1988, Estimation of prehepatic B-cell secretion from the IVGTT in humans, *Diabetes* **37**:100A.

Yang, Y. J., Youn, J. H., and Bergman, R. N., 1987, Modified protocols improve insulin sensitivity estimation using the minimal model, *Am. J. Physiol.* **253**:E595–E602.

III

Role of Nutritional, Dietary, and Immune Factors in the Pathogenesis of Aging

22

Nutritional Requirements in Aging

DAVID KRITCHEVSKY

1. INTRODUCTION

The number of Americans living to 65 years (an arbitrary, and possibly obsolete, cutoff) is increasing. Katz *et al.* (1983) estimated that men and women aged 65–69 years in Massachusetts had 13.1 and 19.5 years of life remaining, respectively. At age 85, remaining years of life were 6.5 for men and 7.7 for women. As the life span has continued to increase, the recognition has come that attention needs to be paid to the nutritional requirements of the elderly. These requirements are influenced by the physiological realities of aging as well as by sociological and psychological factors which do not play an important role in younger persons. All these problems must be addressed in order to provide the elderly with a diet replete in macro- and micronutrients.

Albanese (1980) listed degrees of change in physiological function that occur between the ages of 30–80 (Table I). Bidlack *et al.* (1986) summarized some of the chronic conditions associated with aging (Table II). Increases in occurrence with aging between the ages of 45–64 to 65+ years include 88% for arthritis, 46% for diabetes, 75% for diseases of the urinary tract, and 125% for heart conditions. There is a 15% drop in asthma. Recognition of these changes requires adjustment of nutrient quantity and spectrum. In addition, malnutrition in old age may be caused by physical disability, social isolation, poverty, ignorance, dental problems, and dental status, among other factors, all of which must be integrated into nutrition programs for the elderly. Clearly, it is not possible to address these questions adequately in a short essay, so the ensuing discussion will be incomplete. Fortunately, there are several excellent monographs relating to nutrition and the elderly (Albanese, 1980; Munro, 1988; Watkin, 1983; Young, 1986).

The most recently published Recommended Dietary Allowances (RDA) (Food and Nutrition Board, 1980) are recommended for everyone 51 years and older. Current estimates are being made for groups aged 51–75 years and 75+ years. The FAO/WHO (1973) recommended a 5% per decade decrease in calories for ages 40–59, a 10% decrease in caloric consumption for persons aged 60–69, and a further 10% decrease beyond age 70. In other words, a 30% decrease in caloric intake between the ages of 40 and 70 years. The National

DAVID KRITCHEVSKY • Wistar Institute of Anatomy and Biology, Philadelphia, Pennsylvania 19104.

TABLE I. Changes in Physiologic
Function with Aging[a,b]

Function	Reduction (%)
Basal metabolic rate	8
Hemoglobin	23
Glucose tolerance	30
Bone density	39
Protein synthesis	48
Total body water	55
Renal capacity	70

[a]From Albanese (1980).
[b]Functions at age 80 as percentage of functions at age 30.

TABLE II. Selected Chronic Conditions
Associated with Aging

Condition	Occurrence per 1000	
	45–64 years	65+ years
Arthritis	247	465
Hypertension	244	379
Heart conditions	123	277
Diabetes	57	83
Disease of urinary tract	32	56
Asthma	34	29

[a]From Bidlack et al. (1986).

Health and Nutrition Examination Surveys (NHANES) are beginning to present a picture of nutrient intake in the elderly. Lowenstein and Stanton (1988) compared the results of NHANES I (1971–1974) and NHANES II (1976–1980). Table III summarizes differences in subjects aged 65–74 (1811 women and 1655 men) observed between the first and second surveys. There were no significant differences in total calories, fat, of calcium. Women were found to ingest significantly less protein and cholesterol. Iron and vitamin intakes were increased significantly in both women and men. Diets for the elderly need to provide high nutrient density and contain required amounts of protein, fat, vitamins, and minerals. Some of the major dietary sources of vitamins and minerals are listed in Tables IV and V.

The recommended intake of 0.8 g of protein/kg per day may be low for some individuals. Kohrs and Czajka-Narins (1986) find this level generally adequate, but several studies (Albanese, 1980; Munro, 1981; Gersovitz et al., 1982) find this level of protein inadequate for maintenance of nitrogen balance in subjects aged 70–99. Albanese (1980) and Young et al. (1982) suggested that an adequate protein intake for the elderly might be 12–14% of total calories. There appears to be a need for further studies in this area.

Energy requirements of healthy individuals decrease by about 30% between the ages of

TABLE III. Differences in Mean Values for Daily Intake
of Selected Nutrients between NHANES I (1971–1974)
and NHANES II (1976–1980) in Men and Women Aged 65–74[a]

	Group			
	Men		Women	
	I	II	I	II
kcal	1794	1829	1308	1295
Protein, g	72	73	54	51[b]
Fat, g	73	75	52	50
Cholesterol, mg	410	387	276	240[b]
Calcium, mg	711	698	564	542
Iron, mg	12.0	14.1[c]	9.2	10.2[c]
Vitamin C, mg	88	100[b]	89	105[c]
Vitamin A, mg	5492	6579[b]	5214	5481

[a]From Lowenstein and Stanton (1988).
[b]$p < 0.05$.
[c]$p < 0.001$.

30–80. Since fat is the most concentrated source of energy, a reduction in fat might be indicated. The requirement for essential fatty acids amounts to about 3% of total calories. However, fat is also a vehicle for the fat-soluble vitamins and enhances the palatability of food. The latter is an important consideration in feeding individuals who, for various reasons, eat poorly.

A number of scientific bodies have recommended that the contribution of fat to our daily caloric intake be reduced from 40% to 30% of calories. This change seems to be taking place. Suggestions regarding the type of dietary fat are in flux, and earlier recommendations for a high ratio of polyunsaturated to saturated fat have been modified to equal levels of polyunsaturated to monounsaturated to saturated fatty acids, with saturated fatty acids representing

TABLE IV. Some Dietary Sources of Vitamins

Vitamin	Sources
B_1 (thiamin)	Pork, organ meats, legumes, whole grains
B_2 (riboflavin)	Liver, yeast, wheat germ
Niacin	Liver, meats, grains, legumes
B_6 (pyridoxine)	Meats, whole grains
B_{12}	Meats, eggs, dairy products
A	Green vegetables, milk
C	Fruits, vegetables
D	Cod liver oil, eggs, dairy products
E	Seeds, vegetable oils, vegetables
K	Leafy green vegetables

TABLE V. Some Dietary Sources
of Minerals

Mineral	Source
Calcium	Milk, cheese, dried legumes
Phosphorus	Milk, cheese, meat, grains
Sulfur	Protein foods
Potassium	Fruit, meat, milk
Magnesium	Whole grains, nuts
Iron	Meat, eggs, whole grains
Zinc	Animal sources
Copper	Liver, seafood
Iodine	Fish, shellfish
Chromium	Meat, grains, yeast

no more than 10% of calories. The roles of specific fatty acids (e.g., oleic and stearic) are still being delineated, and suggestions in this area should be regarded as interim.

Plasma cholesterol elevation is one of the major risk factors for development of coronary disease (along with hypertension, diabetes, and cigarette smoking). The strength of plasma cholesterol as a predictor of heart disease risk declines beyond age 60 but is still considered significant at older ages. The ratio of low- to high-density lipoprotein cholesterol is an important prognosticator of heart disease in people aged 70 or older (Castelli *et al.*, 1977). Although dietary cholesterol may affect plasma cholesterol levels in man, the effect of fat saturation is much greater (McNamara *et al.*, 1987). There are also differences in response to dietary cholesterol and genetic disposition to lipidemia and heart disease which must be considered.

Gertler *et al.* (1950) found that subjects with coronary disease exhibited significantly higher levels of serum cholesterol than did controls regardless of comparable cholesterol intake; these workers also found that men who ingested 7.0 g of cholesterol weekly had cholesterol levels similar to those of men who ingested 1.4 g/wk (213 ± 11 mg/dl compared with 222 ± 16 mg/dl). Comparison of diets in men with and without overt heart disease in large studies in Puerto Rico, Honolulu, and Framingham showed no differences in fat and cholesterol intake (Gordon *et al.*, 1981).

It should also be noted that between 1968 and 1978 there was a 27% reduction in coronary heart disease mortality. There is evidence that the actual severity of atherosclerosis has also declined (Strong and Guzman, 1980). The reason for the decline in coronary mortality has been attributed to many factors but no clear explanation has emerged. The decline in cigarette smoking and pharmacologic control of hypertension have resulted in reduction in two of the major risk factors and have undoubtedly been major contributors to the decline (Stern, 1979). Bearing special requirements in mind, a diet for the elderly that reflects general suggestions for moderation of fat intake would be prudent.

The elderly suffer from increasing incidence of digestive diseases (Young and Urban, 1986). As can be seen in Table VI, as we go from 45 to 65 years of age, ulcers increase by 44%, constipation by 428%, gallbladder disease by 147%, gastritis by 107% and diverticular disease by more than 1800%. Many of these conditions can be ameliorated by dietary fiber.

TABLE VI. Chronic Digestive Diseases (per 1000)
in the United States[a]

Disease	45–64 years	65+ years
Ulcer	37.7	30.8
Constipation	23.6	67.1
Hiatal hernia	34.3	62.2
Gallbladder disease	4.4	3.7
Diverticular disease	13.2	31.0
Gastroenteritis, colitis	9.7	13.5
Intestinal disorders	8.7	10.7

[a]From Young and Urban (1986).

Fiber is a generic term that covers a number of substances of varying chemical composition and diverse physiological function. Their commonality lies in the fact that they are not digested by enzymes of the human alimentary tract.

Constipation is probably the most common gastrointestinal (GI) complaint among the elderly, one half of whom take laxatives. Wheat bran, soy polysaccharide, or ispaghula increase the frequency of defecation and stool weight and eliminate the need for laxatives (Clark and Scott, 1976; Smith et al., 1980; Graham et al., 1982; Fischer et al., 1985; Hope and Down, 1986). Cummings (1986) reviewed the effect of dietary fibers on fecal weight (Table VII). The most effective substance appears to be wheat bran.

Gastric ulcer is a common complaint of the elderly (Grossman, 1981). Moderate (8.9 g/day) and high (22.6 g/day) levels of dietary fiber seem to promote similar levels of healing (Harju and Larmi, 1985; Rydning et al., 1986). Recurrence of healed ulcers is higher on a low-fiber diet (Rydning et al., 1982). More work is needed in this area.

Diverticular disease increases with advancing age (Parks, 1975). A decade ago, Rogers (1975) estimated that 15 million people aged 70 years or older had diverticular disease. Diets high in fiber generally relieve symptoms of diverticular disease (Mitchell and Eastwood, 1976; Brodribb, 1980). Originally Painter et al. (1972) achieved relief of diverticular symp-

TABLE VII. Increase in Fecal Output per Gram
of Ingested Fiber[a,b]

Fiber source	No studies	Increase in fecal weight (g/g fiber ±SEM)
Wheat bran	31	5.7 ± 0.5
Fruits and vegetables	20	4.9 ± 0.9
Gums, mucilages	16	3.5 ± 0.7
Pectins	10	1.3 ± 0.3

[a]From Cummings (1986).
[b]Only data from >10 studies are shown.

toms with diets high in bran, but since then other types of fiber have proved equally effective (Eastwood *et al.*, 1978).

There is a marked increase in the incidence of gallstones as individuals age (Glen, 1981). About 10% of people under 30 years of age exhibit gallbladder problems; at 50–60 years of age, the incidence goes up to about 30%, and 55% of subjects aged 80 or older have gallstones. There are no reported studies in which dietary fiber treatment affected gallbladder disease, but influences of fiber on bile saturation or on the lithogenic index (calculated from biliary concentrations of bile acids, phospholipids, and cholesterol) have been observed. Bran (Watts *et al.*, 1978) or guar gum (Hansen *et al.*, 1983) reduce bile saturation in normal subjects. Wheat bran and pectin reduce the lithogenic index, but cellulose and lignin have no effect (Pomare *et al.*, 1976; Wechsler *et al.*, 1984; Hillman *et al.*, 1986). The use of dietary fiber to treat irritable bowel syndrome or Crohn's disease has produced equivocal results (Soltoft *et al.*, 1976; Manning *et al.* 1977; Brandes and Lorenz-Meyer, 1981; Levenstein *et al.*, 1985).

Horwitz (1982) estimated that almost 17% of Americans older than 65 years have diabetes in some form, and the incidence in those 85 years or older may be more than 25%. Blood glucose was reduced in more than 90% of studies in which diet was supplemented with fiber in the form of wheat bran, guar gum, apple fiber, psyllium, glucomannan, or cellulose. A similar level of blood glucose reduction was seen in studies in which fiber-rich foods were used, in contrast to addition of specific fibers (Anderson, 1986).

Colon cancer contributes significantly to morbidity and mortality among the elderly. The role of diet in this disease has been the subject of numerous reviews. Although colon cancer appears later in life, the influence of diet must extend over the entire life span. Several surveys of the literature conclude that the role of dietary fiber in colon cancer is moot (Cummings, 1985; Committee on Diet, Nutrition and Cancer, 1982).

Dietary levels of calcium (Lowenstein, 1986) and zinc (Greger, 1984) are low in older Americans. The effects of specific fibers on mineral balance vary. Sandstead *et al.* (1978) found wheat or corn bran to exert no effect on iron, zinc, or copper balance. Cummings *et al.* (1979a,b) found negative calcium balance to be induced by wheat bran, but not by pectin. Cellulose was shown to affect calcium but not magnesium balance (Slavin and Marlett, 1980). In studies using fiber-rich foods rather than specific fibers, no effects on calcium, magnesium, iron, or zinc balance were observed (Kelsay *et al.*, 1981; Andersson *et al.*, 1983).

There may be deleterious effects of excess fiber intake, and high intake of fiber may be a problem in a population whose overall food intake is low, such as the elderly. A review of the health consequences of fiber has prompted an expert committee to conclude that the optimum intake of fiber should be viewed as a function of total caloric intake and has recommended 10–13 g of fiber per 1000 kcal/day, with the distribution being 3 parts insoluble fiber to 1 part soluble fiber (Pilch, 1987).

More data are needed to establish nutritional needs for healthy, active people aged 70–90. An ideal diet would provide low-cost items having high nutrient density, with sufficient protein, minerals, and vitamins. Vitamin and mineral fortification may be necessary. Attention must also be paid to texture, palatability, and ease of preparation. Fluid intake is frequently overlooked, but it should be encouraged.

ACKNOWLEDGMENTS. This work was supported, in part, by a Research Career Award (HL-00734) from the National Institutes of Health and by funds from the Commonwealth of Pennsylvania.

REFERENCES

Albanese, A. A., 1980, *Nutrition for the Elderly*, Liss, New York.

Anderson, J. W., 1986, Dietary fiber in nutrition management of diabetes, in: *Dietary fiber: Basic and Clinical Aspects* (G. V. Vahouny and D. Kritchevsky, eds.), Plenum, New York, pp. 343–360.

Andersson, H., Nävert, B. Bingham, S. A., Englyst, H. N., and Cummings, J. H., 1983, The effects of breads containing similar amounts of phytate but different amounts of wheat bran on calcium, zinc and iron balance in man, *Br. J. Nutr.* **50:**503–510.

Bidlack, W. R., Smith, C. H., Clemens, R. A., and Omaye, S. T., 1986, Nutrition and the elderly, *Food Technol.* **40:**81–88.

Brandes, J. W., and Lorenz-Meyer, H., 1981, Zuckerfreie Diät: eine neue Perspektive zur Behandlung des Morbus Crohn: Eine randomisierte, kontrollierte Studie, *Z. Gastroenterol.* **19:**1–12.

Brodribb, A. J. M., 1980, Dietary fiber in diverticular disease of the colon, in: *Medical Aspects of Dietary Fiber* (G. A. Spiller and R. M. Kay, eds.), Plenum, New York, pp. 43–66.

Castelli, W. P., Doyle, J. T., Gordon, T., Hames, C. G., Hjortland, M. C., Hulley, S. B., Kagan, A., and Zukel, W. J., 1977, HDL cholesterol and other lipids in coronary heart disease. The Cooperative Lipoprotein Phenotyping Study, *Circulation* **55:**767–772.

Clark, A. N. G., and Scott, J. F., 1976, Wheat bran in dyschezia in the aged, *Age Aging* **5:**149–154.

Committee on Diet, Nutrition and Cancer, 1982, *Diet, Nutrition and Cancer*, National Academy of Sciences, Washington, D.C.

Cummings, J., 1985, Cancer of the large bowel in: *Dietary Fibre, Fibre-Depleted Foods and Disease* (H. Trowell, D. Burkitt, and K. Heaton, eds.), Academic, London, pp. 161–189.

Cummings, J. H., 1986, The effect of dietary fiber on fecal weight and composition, in: *CRC Handbook of Dietary Fiber in Human Nutrition* (G. A. Spiller, ed.), CRC Press, Boca Raton, Florida, pp. 211–280.

Cummings, J. H., Southgate, D. A. T., Branch, W. J., Wiggins, H. S., Houston, H., Jenkins, D. J. A., Jivraj, T., and Hill, M. J., 1979a, The digestion of pectin in the human gut and its effect on calcium absorption and large bowel function, *Br. J. Nutr.* **41:**477–485.

Cummings, J. H., Hill, M. J., Jivraj, T., Houston, H., Branch, W. J., and Jenkins, D. J. A., 1979b, The effect of meat protein and dietary fiber on colonic function and metabolism. I. Changes in bowel habit, bile acid excretion, and calcium absorption, *Am. J. Clin. Nutr.* **32:**2086–2093.

Eastwood, M. A., Smith, A. N., Brydon, W. G., and Pritchard, J., 1978, Comparison of bran, ispaghula and lactulose on colon function in diverticular disease, *Gut* **19:**1144–1147.

FAO/WHO, 1973, *Energy and Protein Requirements*, WHO Technical Reports, Series No. 522, World Health Organization, Geneva.

Fischer, M., Adkins, W., Hall, L., Scaman, P., Hsi, S., and Marlett, J., 1985, The effects of dietary fibre in a liquid diet on bowel function of mentally retarded individuals, *J. Ment. Defic. Res.* **29:**373—381.

Food and Nutrition Board, 1980, *Recommended Dietary Allowances*, 9th ed., National Academy of Sciences, National Research Council, Washington, D.C.

Glen, F., 1981, Surgical management of acute cholecystis in patients 65 years of age and older, *Ann. Surg.* **193:**56–59.

Gersovitz, M., Motil, K., Munro, H. N., Scrimshaw, N. S., and Young, V. R., 1982, Human protein requirements: Assessment of the adequacy of the current recommended dietary allowance for dietary protein in elderly men and women, *Am. J. Clin. Nutr.* **35:**6–14.

Gertler, M. M., Garn, S. M., and White, P. D., 1950, Diet serum cholesterol and coronary artery disease, *Circulation* **2:**696–702.

Gordon, T., Kagan, A., Garcia-Palmieri, M., Kannel, W. B., Zukel, W. J., Tillotson, J., Sorlie, P., and Hjortland, M., 1981, Diet and its relation to coronary heart disease and death in three populations, *Circulation* **63:**500–515.

Graham, D. Y., Moser, S. E., and Estes, M. K., 1982, The effect of bran on bowel function in constipation, *Am. J. Gastroenterol.* **77:**599–603.

Greger, J. L., 1984, Zinc and copper requirements of the elderly, in: *Annual Conference on Trace Substances in Environmental Health,* Vol. 13 (D. Hemphill, ed.), University of Missouri, Columbia, Missouri, pp. 463–475.

Grossman, M. I., 1981, *Peptic Ulcer: Guide for the Practicing Physician,* Yearbook, Chicago, pp. 10–11.

Hansen, W. E., Maurer, H., Vollmer, J., and Bräuning, C., 1983, Guar gum and bile: effects on postprandial gallbladder contraction and on serum bile acids in man, *Hepatogastroenterology* **30:**131–133.

Harju, E. J., and Larmi, T. K., 1985, Effect of guar gum added to the diet of patient with duodenal ulcer, *J. Parenter. Enter. Nutr.* **9:**496–500.

Hillman, L. C., Peters, S. G., Fisher, C. A., and Pomare, E. W., 1986, Effects of the fibre components pectin, cellulose, and lignin on bile salt metabolism and biliary lipid composition in man, *Gut* **27:**29–36.

Hope, A. K., and Down, E. C., 1986, Dietary fibre and fluid in the control of constipation in a nursing home population, *Med. J. Aust.* **144:**306–307.

Horwitz, D. L., 1982, Diabetes and aging, *Am. J. Clin. Nutr.* **36:**803–808.

Katz, S., Branch, L. G., Branson, M. H., Papsidero, J. H., Beck, J. C., and Greer, D. S., 1983, Active life expectancy, *N. Engl. J. Med.* **309:**1218–1224.

Kelsay, J. L., Clark, W. M., Herbst, B. J., and Prather, E. S., 1981, Nutrient utilization by human subjects consuming fruits and vegetables as sources of fiber, *J. Agric. Food Chem.* **29:**461–465.

Kohrs, M. B., and Czajka-Narins, D. M., 1986, Assessing the Nutritional Status of the Elderly, in: *Nutrition, Aging and Health* (E. A. Young, ed.), Liss, New York, pp. 61–89.

Levenstein, S., Prantera, C., Luzi, C., and D'Ubaldi, A., 1985, Low residue or normal diet in Crohn's disease: A prospective controlled study in Italian patients, *Gut* **26:**989–993.

Lowenstein, F. W., 1986, Nutritional requirements of the elderly, in: *Nutrition, Aging and Health* (E. A. Young, ed.), Liss, New York, pp. 61–89.

Lowenstein, F. W., and Stanton, M. F., 1988, Comparison of some results from two National Nutrition Surveys in the United States of America, *Front. Gastrointest. Res.* **14:**24–40.

Manning, A. P., Heaton, K. W., Harvey, R. F., and Uglow, P., 1977, Wheat fibre and irritable bowel syndrome: A controlled trial, *Lancet* **2:**417–418.

McNamara, D. J., Kolb, R., Parker, T. S., Batwin, H., Samuel, P., Brown, C. D., and Ahrens, E. H., Jr., 1987, Heterogeneity of cholesterol homeostasis in man. Response to changes in dietary fat quality and cholesterol quantity, *J. Clin. Invest.* **79:**1729–1739.

Mitchell, W. D., and Eastwood, M. A., 1976, Dietary fiber and colon function, in: *Fiber in Human Nutrition* (G. A. Spiller and R. J. Amen, eds.), Plenum, New York, pp. 185–206.

Munro, H. N., 1981, Nutrition and Aging, *Br. Med. Bull.* **37:**83–88.

Munro, H. N. (ed.), 1988, *Human Nutrition,* Vol. 6: *Nutrition, Aging and the Elderly,* Plenum, New York.

Painter, N. S., Almeida, A. Z., and Colebourne, K. W., 1972, Unprocessed bran in treatment of diverticular disease of the colon, *Br. Med. J.* **2:**137–140.

Parks, T. G., 1975, Natural history of diverticular disease of the colon, *Clin. Gastroenterol.* **4:**53–69.

Pilch, S. M. (ed.), 1987, *Physiological Effects and Health Consequences of Dietary Fiber,* FASEB, Bethesda, Maryland.

Pomare, E. W., Heaton, K. W., Low-Beer, T. S., and Espiner, H. J., 1976, The effect of wheat bran upon bile salt metabolism and upon the lipid composition of bile in gallstone patients, *Am. J. Dig. Dis.* **21:**521–536.

Rogers, A. I., 1975, *Colonic Diverticular Disease,* Hoechst-Roussel Pharmaceuticals, Somerville, New York, pp. 1–20.

Rydning, A., Berstad, A., Aadland, E., and Odegaard, B., 1982, Prophylactic effect of dietary fibre in duodenal ulcer disease, *Lancet* **2:**736–739.

Rydning, A., Weberg, R., Lange, O., and Berstad, A., 1986, Healing of benign gastric ulcer with low-dose antacids and fiber diet, *Gastroenterology* **91:**56–61.

Sandstead, H. H., Munoz, J. M., Jacob, R. A., Klevay, L. M., Reck, S. J., Logan, G. M., Jr., Dintzis, F. R., Inglett, G. E., and Shuey, W. C., 1978, Influence of dietary fiber on trace element balance, *Am. J. Clin. Nutr.* **31**:S180–S184.

Slavin, J. L., and Marlett, J. A., 1980, Influence of refined cellulose on human bowel function and calcium and magnesium balance, *Am. J. Clin. Nutr.* **33**:1932–1939.

Smith, R. G., Rowe, M. J., Smith, A. N., Eastwood, M. A., Drummond, E., and Brydon, W. G., 1980, A study of bulking agents in elderly patients, *Age Aging* **9**:267–271.

Soltoft, J., Gudmand-Hoyer, E., Krag, B., Kristensen, E., and Wulff, H. R., 1976, A double-blind trial of the effect of wheat bran on symptoms of irritable bowel syndrome, *Lancet* **1**:270–272.

Stern, M. P., 1979, The recent decline in ischemic heart disease mortality, *Ann. Intern. Med.* **91**:630–640.

Strong, T. P., and Guzman, M. A., 1980, Decrease in coronary atherosclerosis in New Orleans, *Lab. Invest.* **18**:509–526.

Watkin, D. M., 1983, *Handbook of Nutrition, Health and Aging,* Noyes, Park Ridge, New Jersey.

Watts, J. M., Jablonski, P., and Toouli, J., 1978, The effect of added bran to the diet in the saturation of bile in people without gallstones, *Am. J. Surg.* **135**:321–324.

Wechsler, J. G., Swobodnik, W., Wenzel, H., Heuchemer, T., Nebelung, W., Hutt, V., and Ditschuneit, H., 1984, Ballaststoffe vom Typ Weizenkleie senken Lithogenität der Galle, *Dtsch. Med. Wochenschr.* **109**:1284–1288.

Young, E. A. (ed.), 1986, *Nutrition, Aging and Health,* Liss, New York.

Young, E. A., and Urban, E., 1986, Aging, the aged and the gastrointestinal tract, in: *Nutrition, Aging and Health* (E. A. Young, ed.), Liss, New York, pp. 91–131.

Young, V. R., Gersovitz, M., and Munro, H. N., 1982, Human aging: Protein and amino acid metabolism and implications for protein and amino acid requirements, in: *Nutritional Approaches to Aging Research* (G. B. Moment, ed.), CRC Press, Boca Raton, Florida, pp. 47–81.

23

Influence of Dietary Restriction and Aging on Gene Expression in the Immune System of Rats

MOHAMMAD A. PAHLAVANI, H. TAK CHEUNG, NIAN-SHENG CAI, and ARLAN RICHARDSON

1. INTRODUCTION

Gene expression is a fundamental process for all cells, and alterations in the expression of a gene(s) can have a dramatic effect on cell structure and function. During the past two decades, there has been a large number of studies on the effect of aging on various aspects of gene expression. The area that has been most extensively studied has been protein synthesis. Most studies in this area have shown that the protein synthetic activity of tissues from a variety of organisms declines with increasing age (Richardson, 1981; Richardson and Birchenall-Sparks, 1983; Richardson and Semsei, 1987). Because this decrease has been observed in organisms ranging from fungi to humans, it has been proposed that the age-related decline in protein synthesis is a universal phenomenon (Richardson, 1981). The effect of aging on transcription has been studied to a lesser extent than protein synthesis, and, in general, a related decline in transcription is usually observed in tissues (Richardson et al., 1983; Richardson and Semsei, 1987). Currently, investigators are beginning to use complementary DNA (cDNA) probes to measure the effect of aging on the expression of specific genes at the level of transcription (Richardson et al., 1985; Richardson and Semsei, 1987).

The immune system offers one an excellent system to study the effect of aging on gene expression because it is well established that a variety of immunological functions decline with age (Walford, 1974; Makinodan and Kay, 1980). This decline is associated with an increase in the incidence of infectious diseases and malignancies. The age-related decline in the responsiveness of the immune system to foreign substances is shown by the ability of mitogens to stimulate lymphocytes to proliferate. The induction of lymphocyte proliferation by mitogens involves dramatic changes in gene expression at the level of both translation and

MOHAMMAD A. PAHLAVANI, H. TAK CHEUNG, NIAN-SHENG CAI, and ARLAN RICHARDSON • Departments of Biological Sciences and Chemistry, Illinois State University, Normal, Illinois 61761.

transcription (Varesiol and Holden, 1980; Varesiol *et al.*, 1980). Thus, it is possible that changes at the level of gene expression are responsible for the decline in mitogenesis in lymphocytes.

Our laboratory was the first group to show that changes in gene expression occurred in lymphocytes isolated from old rats (Cheung *et al.*, 1983). Mitogen induction of protein synthesis in spleen lymphocytes declined with increasing age; this decline paralleled the decline in lymphocyte proliferation. Subsequently, Tollefsbol and Cohen (1986) showed that mitogen-induced protein synthesis decreased with age in lymphocytes isolated from human subjects.

The importance of gene expression in the response of the immune system has become more evident with the discovery that lymphocytes synthesize and secrete small polypeptides, lymphokines, in response to mitogens or infectious agents. The lymphokines are important in the regulation of the complex cellular interactions that occur during the immune process. One of these lymphokines, which has been studied extensively, is interleukin-2 (IL-2). IL-2 is produced by a subpopulation of helper T cells, and its interaction with IL-2 receptors on other T cells drives the cells to proliferate (Gillis *et al.*, 1978; Robb *et al.*, 1981). Several laboratories have shown that IL-2 production by mitogen-stimulated lymphocytes from rodents (Thoman and Weigle, 1981; Chang *et al.*, 1982; Cheung *et al.*, 1983) and human subjects (Gillis *et al.*, 1981) declines with increasing age. Recently, our laboratory showed that the age-related decrease in IL-2 production was due to a decline in the induction of IL-2 mRNA (Wu *et al.*, 1986). Thus, it appears that the expression of this particular gene is altered with increasing age in lymphocytes.

In the following experiments, the effect of dietary restriction on the age-related decline in gene expression in lymphocytes has been studied. Dietary restriction, i.e., underfeeding, and not malnutrition, is the only experimental method known to increase the life span of mammals (Masaro, 1984; Yu *et al.*, 1984), and it has been shown to have a beneficial effect on several immune functions (Weindruch *et al.*, 1986). In this study, we have measured the effect of aging and dietary restriction on the protein synthetic activity of mitogen-stimulated lymphocytes as well as the expression of the lymphokines IL-2 and interleukin-3 (IL-3).

2. MATERIALS AND METHODS

2.1. Animals and Diets

Male specific pathogen-free (SPF) Fischer 344 rats were obtained from Harlan Industries (Indianapolis, Indiana). The rats were caged individually in a barrier facility at the V.A. Medical Center in St. Louis, Missouri. The rats were maintained on two diets on a 12-hr light–dark cycle as described by Birchenall-Sparks *et al.* (1985) and Armbrecht *et al.* (1988). Briefly, rats were caged individually and fed a semisynthetic casein diet. The dietary restriction was initiated when the rats were 6 weeks old. One group (control) was fed the diet *ad libitum*, and the second group (restricted) was fed daily 60% of the diet consumed by the control rats.

2.2. Measurement of Proliferation and Interleukin Expression

Rats were killed by decapitation, and the spleens were removed aseptically. The preparation of single-cell suspensions of lymphocytes from the spleen and the measurement of lymphocyte proliferation were accomplished as described by Cheung *et al.* (1981). Lymphocytes (5×10^5 cells per 0.2 ml) were incubated with either 5 μg/ml of Concanavalin A (Con A) or 20 μg/ml of lipopolysaccharide (LPS), which give maximum proliferation. Proliferation was quantified by the amount of [^{3}H]thymidine incorporated into DNA after 48 hr of incubation with the mitogens.

IL-2 and IL-3 expression were determined in lymphocytes incubated with Con A (5 μg/ml) for 24 hr. Previous studies have shown that maximum expression of IL-2 and IL-3 is obtained at this time (Wu *et al.*, 1986; Li *et al.*, 1988). The activities of IL-2 and IL-3 were determined by the ability of culture supernatants from Con A-stimulated lymphocytes to support the growth of the IL-2- and IL-3-dependent cell lines CTLL-20 and FDC-P1, respectively (Li *et al.*, 1988). The unit activity of IL-2 or IL-3 was determined using IL-2 and IL-3 standards obtained from Collaborative Research (Lexington, Massachusetts). The levels of IL-2 messenger RNA (mRNA) were determined by cytoplasmic dot blot hybridization as described by Wu *et al.* (1986). Cytoplasmic extracts were prepared from 1×10^8 lymphocytes incubated with Con A (5 μg/ml) for 20 hr and the level of IL-2 mRNA in the extracts determined using a cDNA probe to IL-2 (p3-16), obtained from Dr. Tadasugu Taniguchi (Japanese Foundation for Cancer Research, Tokyo, Japan). The quantification of the IL-2 mRNA in the cytoplasmic extracts following hybridization was determined by exposing the nitrocellulose filters to X-ray film and measuring the relative spot intensities on the autoradiograms with a scanning densitometer.

2.3. Measurement of Lymphocyte Protein Synthesis

Five-ml cultures of lymphocytes (1×10^7 cells /ml) were resuspended in RPMI-1640 culture medium. After incubation for 15 min at 37°C, 10 μCi/ml of [^{3}H]valine (57 Cimmole) were added to the cultures together with 5 μg/ml of Con A. After incubating for 3 hr, 50 μl of 20% trichloroacetic acid (TCA) was added to the cultures to stop protein synthesis. The resulting suspensions were incubated at 90°C for 10 min, and the acid-insoluble material was collected on glass fiber filters. The radioactivity in the acid-insoluble material was determined using a liquid scintillation counter.

2.4. Statistical Analysis of Data

Analysis of variance was used to determine whether mitogenesis, protein synthesis, and IL-2 expression by lymphocytes isolated from restricted and control animals changed significantly with age. Student's T-test was used to determine when values from restricted and age-matched controls were significantly different.

3. RESULTS

3.1. Effect of Dietary Restriction on Survival and Lymphocyte Proliferation

The survival of the rats maintained on the two diets is shown in Fig. 1. Both the median and 10% survival was 30% greater for the restricted rats. In this study, the various immunological parameters were determined with lymphocytes isolated from 5-, 12-, 21-, and 28-

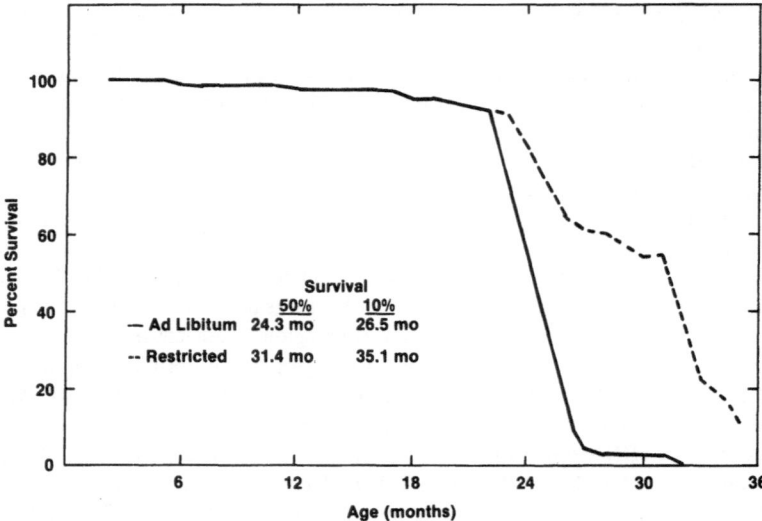

FIGURE 1. Survival curve of male Fischer F344 rats fed *ad libitum* or 60% of the diet consumed by the rats fed *ad libitum* (restricted).

month-old rats. The survival of the rats fed *ad libitum* was only 3% at 28 months of age, while the survival of the restricted rats was more than 60% at this age.

Mitogen-induced proliferation of spleen lymphocytes isolated from restricted and control rat is shown in Tables I and II. In the absence of mitogen, lymphocyte proliferation was similar for control and restricted rats at all ages studied. In the presence of either LPS or Con

TABLE I. LPS-Induced Lymphocyte Proliferation by Spleen Lymphocytes
Isolated from Restricted and Control Rats

Age (months)	Group	*N*	Lymphocyte proliferation (dpm)[a]		
			No mitogen	+LPS	SI
5	Control	6	2,429 ± 172	44,946 ± 3,429[c]	18.3 ± 0.8[c]
	Restricted	7	2,394 ± 104	38,037 ± 1,061	15.8 ± 0.6
12	Control	6	2,341 ± 113	36,442 ± 1,498	15.6 ± 1.6
	Restricted	6	2,504 ± 118	34,537 ± 3,544	13.8 ± 1.3
21	Control	9	2,178 ± 48	13,914 ± 1,438	6.4 ± 0.6
	Restricted	8	2,294 ± 54	16,374 ± 1,375	7.1 ± 0.6
28	Control	3	1,901 ± 78	6,093 ± 479[b]	3.2 ± 0.3[b]
	Restricted	5	2,021 ± 72	9,490 ± 697	5.4 ± 0.4

[a]Each value represents the mean ± SEM for the number of animals (*N*) shown. The stimulation index (SI) was calculated by dividing the incorporation of [³H]thymidine by stimulated lymphocytes by the [³H]thymidine incorporation of unstimulated lymphocytes.
[b]These values are significantly different from those for the restricted rats at the $p < 0.01$ level.
[c]These values are significantly different from those for the restricted rats at $p < 0.05$ level.

TABLE II. Con A-Induced Lymphocyte Proliferation by Spleen Lymphocytes
Isolated from Restricted and Control Rats

Age (months)	Group	N	Lymphocyte proliferation (dpm)[a]		
			No mitogen	+Con A	SI
5	Control	6	2,429 ± 122	59,427 ± 3,776	24.5 ± 1.1
	Restricted	7	2,394 ± 104	56,247 ± 3,932	23.4 ± 1.1
12	Control	6	2,341 ± 113	38,551 ± 3,467	16.3 ± 0.8
	Restricted	6	2,504 ± 118	41,126 ± 3,280	17.1 ± 0.8
21	Control	9	2,178 ± 48	20,121 ± 1,237[b]	9.2 ± 0.5[b]
	Restricted	8	2,294 ± 54	28,953 ± 2,701	12.6 ± 1.1
28	Control	3	1,901 ± 78	10,788 ± 865[c]	5.6 ± 0.9[c]
	Restricted	5	2,021 ± 72	16,815 ± 1,735	8.4 ± 0.9

[a]Each value represents the mean ± SEM for the number of animals (N) shown. The stimulation index (SI) was calculated by dividing the incorporation of [^{3}H]thymidine by stimulated lymphocytes by the [^{3}H]thymidine incorporation of unstimulated lymphocytes.
[b]These values are significantly different from those of the restricted rats at the $p < 0.01$ level.
[c]These values are significantly different from those of the restricted rats at $p < 0.05$ level.

A, lymphocyte proliferation was increased 10- to 30-fold. Lymphocytes from both restricted and control rats showed a significant ($p < 0.001$) decline in proliferation with increasing age. When the data are expressed as stimulation index, it was found that LPS-induced lymphocyte proliferation decreased 66% and 82% in restricted and control rats, respectively, between 5 and 28 months of age. A 64% and a 77% decrease in Con A-induced lymphocyte proliferation was observed in restricted and control rats, respectively. Thus, the age-related decrease in mitogen-induced lymphocyte proliferation was less for the restricted rats than for the control rats.

When mitogen-induced lymphocyte proliferation from restricted and control rats was compared, the stimulation index in the presence of LPS at 5 months of age was significantly lower (15%) for the restricted rats compared with the control rats (see Table I). No significant difference in LPS-induced lymphocyte proliferation was observed at 12 and 21 months of age. However, at 28 months of age, LPS-induced lymphocyte proliferation was significantly greater (41%) for lymphocytes isolated from restricted rats compared with control rats. The stimulation index observed in the presence of Con A was similar for the lymphocytes isolated from restricted and control rats at 5 and 12 months of age (see Table II). However, at 21 and 28 months of age, Con A-induced lymphocyte proliferation for restricted rats was significantly greater than that of control rats, e.g., Con A-induced lymphocyte proliferation was 30% and 35% higher at 21 and 28 months of age, respectively.

3.2. Effect of Age and Dietary Restriction on IL-2 and IL-3 Expression

The induction of IL-2 expression was measured in culture supernatants obtained from lymphocytes that had been incubated with Con A for 24 hr. IL-2 activity was determined by the ability of the culture supernatants to sustain the growth of an IL-2-dependent cell line. Table III shows the levels of IL-2 activity in culture supernatants obtained from lymphocytes

TABLE III. Effect of Age and Diet on IL-2 Expression

Age (months)	Group	N	IL-2 Expression[a] Activity (U/ml)	IL-2 Expression[a] mRNA levels (area)
5	Control	6	28.1 ± 1.3	4.2
	Restricted	7	26.8 ± 0.7	4.0
12	Control	6	17.1 ± 1.1	3.0
	Restricted	6	18.3 ± 0.9	2.9
21	Control	9	11.3 ± 0.8[b]	1.8
	Restricted	8	14.5 ± 1.0	2.3
28	Control	3	4.4 ± 0.9[b]	0.6
	Restricted	5	6.5 ± 0.8	0.9

[a]The IL-2 activity in supernatants of cultured lymphocytes is expressed as the mean ±SEM of the number of animals (*N*) shown. mRNA levels were determined on cytoplasmic extracts prepared from lymphocytes pooled from the number of animals (*N*) shown.
[b]These values are significantly different from restricted rats at $p < 0.05$ level.

isolated from 5-, 12-, 21-, and 28-month-old restricted and control rats. No IL-2 activity was detectable in the culture supernatants from unstimulated lymphocytes. In the presence of Con A, maximum IL-2 activity was found in the culture supernatants of lymphocytes isolated from 5-month-old rats. Con A-induced IL-2 production by lymphocytes isolated from restricted and control rats decreased 75% and 84%, respectively, between 5 and 28 months of age. Thus, the age-related decline in IL-2 production by lymphocytes is less for the restricted rats than for control rats. A comparison of IL-2 production by lymphocytes from restricted and control rats showed no significant difference in IL-2 activity at 5 and 12 months of age. However, at 21 and 28 months of age, Con A-induced IL-2 activity was significantly greater for lymphocytes isolated from restricted rats, e.g., the IL-2 activity was 22% and 32% higher at 21 and 28 months of age, respectively.

The induction of IL-2 mRNA expression was also measured in the cytoplasmic extracts of Con A-induced lymphocytes. Figure 2 presents the autoradiogram showing the hybridization of the IL-2 containing cDNA probe to cytoplasmic extracts obtained from 5- to 28-month-old rats fed *ad libitum* or the restricted diet. The induction of IL-2 mRNA decreased

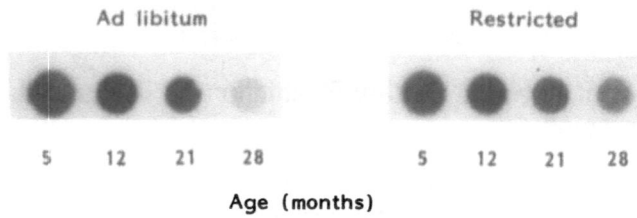

FIGURE 2. Autoradiograph of dot blot analysis of cytoplasmic RNA obtained from Con A-stimulated lymphocytes isolated from rats fed *ad libitum* or a restricted diet.

TABLE IV. Effect of Age and Diet
on IL-3 Activity

Age (months)	Group	N	IL-3 activity[a] (U/ml)
5	Control	6	165.5 ± 4.7
	Restricted	7	132.2 ± 8.2
12	Control	6	118.3 ± 11.5
	Restricted	6	118.6 ± 9.7
21	Control	9	80.8 ± 4.5
	Restricted	8	134.7 ± 10.7
28	Control	3	76.0 ± 3.7
	Restricted	5	152.8 ± 14.3

[a]IL-3 activity was measured in culture supernatants obtained from lymphocytes pooled from the number of animals (N) shown. IL-3 activities are expressed as the mean ±SEM of triplicate measurements.

with age in both restricted and control rats. When autoradiographs were quantified with a scanning densitometer (Table III), it was found that the induction of IL-2 mRNA for both restricted and control rats decreased 78% and 85%, respectively, between 5 and 28 months of age. The levels of IL-2 mRNA were similar for restricted and control rats at 5 and 12 months of age. However, at 21 and 28 months of age, the induction of IL-2 mRNA was 28% and 50% higher, respectively, for restricted rats. Thus, similar changes were observed in Con A induction of IL-2 activity or IL-2 mRNA level with age or dietary restriction.

We also studied the effect of age and diet on Con A stimulation of IL-3. Because of the limited amount of supernatant available, it was necessary to conduct these experiments on samples pooled from all the animals for each age and diet. Table IV shows that the activity of IL-3 in culture supernatants from Con A-stimulated lymphocytes isolated from control rats decreased more than 50% between 5 and 28 months of age. This observation is in agreement with our recent study, in which a decrease in Con A-induction of IL-3 production was observed with spleen lymphocytes from mice (Li *et al.*, 1988). By contrast, there was very little change in the induction of IL-3 activity with age in lymphocytes isolated from the rats fed the restricted diet.

3.3. Effect of Dietary Restriction on Protein Synthesis

The level of protein synthesis in lymphocyte cultures was measured by the incorporation of [3H]valine into protein after 3 hr of incubation in the presence and absence of Con A. Table V shows that the age-related decrease in protein synthesis by lymphocytes from control and restricted rats in the absence of Con A was similar. At 5 and 12 months of age, protein synthesis in the absence of Con A was the same for lymphocytes isolated from restricted and control rats. Although protein synthesis for unstimulated lymphocytes from restricted rats was higher than the control rats at 21 and 28 months of age, only at 21 months of age was this difference statistically significant. In the presence of Con A, protein synthesis was induced two- to fivefold. In lymphocytes isolated from control rats, protein synthesis decreased 85%

TABLE V. Comparison of Protein Synthesis by Spleen
Lymphocytes Isolated from Restricted and Control Rats

Age (months)	Group	N	Protein synthesis (dpm)[a]	
			No mitogen	+Con A
5	Control	6	5,493 ± 120	26,073 ± 1,492[b]
	Restricted	7	4,902 ± 403	17,605 ± 1,507
12	Control	6	4,156 ± 84	17,682 ± 919
	Restricted	6	4,294 ± 65	16,746 ± 612
21	Control	9	3,393 ± 110[c]	9,429 ± 627[b]
	Restricted	8	3,759 ± 140	13,312 ± 855
28	Control	3	1,695 ± 197	3,808 ± 344[c]
	Restricted	5	1,957 ± 162	5,481 ± 514

[a]Each value represents the mean ±SEM for the number of animals (N) shown.
[b]These values are significantly different from those of the dietary restricted rats at the $p < 0.01$ level.
[c]These values are significantly different from those of the dietary restricted rats at $p < 0.05$ level.

between 5 and 28 months of age. Protein synthesis decreased less than 70% in the restricted rats. When Con A induction of protein synthesis from restricted and control rats was compared, it was found that [³H]valine incorporation was significantly lower (32%) for lymphocytes isolated from restricted than from control rats at 5 months of age. Protein synthesis was similar for restricted and control rats at 12 months of age; however, at 21 and 28 months of age, [³H]valine incorporation was more than 40% higher for lymphocytes isolated from restricted rats compared with control rats. Thus, the data in Table V show that dietary restriction has a marked effect on the age-related decline in Con A-induced protein synthesis.

4. DISCUSSION

McCay *et al.* (1935) reported that the severe reduction of calories increased the life span of rats dramatically. During the past two decades, numerous laboratories have confirmed this observation and have shown that dietary restriction not only increases the survival of rodents but also retards/reduces the incidence of a variety of age-related diseases, e.g., cancer and renal disease (Weindruch *et al.*, 1982; Masaro, 1984; Yu *et al.*, 1984). Because the immune system plays an important role in protecting an organism from disease processes and because it is well documented that the immunological status of an organism declines with increasing age, it has been suggested that dietary restriction increases the survival of rodents through its action on the immune system (Walford, 1974). The initial study in this area was conducted by Walford (1974), who showed that lymphocyte proliferation in response to phytohemagglutinin (PHA) and pokeweed mitogen (PWM) was similar for control and restricted mice at 18 weeks of age. However, at 52 and 118 weeks of age, lymphocytes from restricted mice showed a higher proliferation to these two mitogens. Several other studies by Walford's laboratory with other strains of mice confirmed the initial observation that mitogen-induced lymphocyte proliferation was greater in rodents fed a restricted diet (Gerbase-Delima *et al.*,

1975; Weindruch *et al.*, 1982, 1986). In addition, Fernandes *et al.* (1976) showed that dietary restriction improved PHA- and Con A-induced proliferation in lymphocytes isolated from a short-lived autoimmune-prone strain of mice (NZB).

The dietary restriction procedure used in this study increased the survival of male Fischer F344 rats 30%. The immunological status of these rats was determined at 5, 12, 21, and 28 months of age by measuring lymphocyte proliferation in response to LPS and Con A. Dietary restriction altered the age-related decline in mitogenesis after midlife (e.g., at 21 and 28 months of age). Lymphocytes isolated from old rats fed the restricted diet had a significantly higher response to LPS and Con A than did lymphocytes isolated from rats fed *ad libitum*.

Although the effect of dietary restriction on survival and the immunological status of rodents is well established, the biochemical mechanism underlying the effect of dietary restriction on these two parameters is unknown. Recent studies suggest that dietary restriction can affect gene expression in various tissues (Richardson, 1985; Richardson *et al.*, 1988). Because changes in gene expression can have a profound effect on cellular function, it is possible that the mechanism underlying the effect of dietary restriction on the immune system could occur at the level of gene expression.

Research over the past two decades has shown that the protein synthetic activity of most tissues decreases with increasing age (Richardson, 1981; Richardson and Semsei, 1987). Recently, several investigators have shown that dietary restriction delays the age-related decline in protein synthesis in liver (Birchenall-Sparks *et al.*, 1985; Ward, 1988), kidney (Ricketts *et al.*, 1985) and whole body (Lewis *et al.*, 1985) of rats. Protein synthesis by mitogen-stimulated lymphocytes from rats and humans has been shown to decrease with age (Cheung *et al.*, 1983; Tollefsbol and Cohen, 1986). In this study, we also observed a dramatic age-related decrease (over 85%) in protein synthesis by Con A-stimulated lymphocytes from rats fed *ad libitum*. More importantly, we found that dietary restriction had a marked effect on the level of protein synthesis in the Con A-stimulated lymphocytes. In young adult rats (5 months), protein synthesis was significantly lower for lymphocytes from restricted rats than for control rats. However, the level of protein synthesis remained constant between 5 and 21 months of age in the restricted rats, while protein synthesis in the rats fed *ad libitum* decreased over 60%. Only between 21 and 28 months of age was a significant decrease in protein synthesis observed in the Con A-stimulated lymphocytes obtained from the restricted rats. At 21 and 28 months of age, the level of protein synthesis was significantly greater for the lymphocytes isolated from the restricted rats. Thus, dietary restriction significantly alters gene expression at the level of protein synthesis in spleen lymphocytes.

The effect of dietary restriction on the expression of two specific proteins (IL-2 and IL-3) produced by mitogen-stimulated lymphocytes was also studied. We chose to study these two proteins because they play a critical role in the immune system and because previous studies have shown that their expression declines with increasing age (Wu *et al.*, 1986; Li *et al.*, 1988). IL-2 is required for the proliferation of activated T lymphocytes, particularly cytotoxic (Wagner *et al.*, 1980) and helper T lymphocytes (Robb *et al.*, 1981). IL-3 plays an important role in the formation and maturation of erythrocytes, granulocytes, monocytes, and lymphocytes (Ihle *et al.*, 1982). The induction of IL-2 activity or mRNA levels declined with age in lymphocytes isolated from rats fed *ad libitum* or the restricted diet. At 5 and 12 months of age, there was no difference in the induction of IL-2 expression; however, at 21 and 28 months of age, IL-2 expression, i.e., activity and mRNA level, was higher in the lymphocytes isolated from restricted rats. Previous studies with autoimmune-prone mice indicated that the induction of IL-2 activity by mitogens was higher in restricted mice (Jung et al., 1982; Kubo et al., 1984). We also observed an excellent correlation between Con A-induced lymphocyte proliferation and IL-2 expression. Both parameters decreased with age and were higher in restricted rats at 21 and 28 months of age. These data support the suggestion that changes in IL-2 expression play an important role in the age-related decline in mitogen-induced proliferation.

In a preliminary experiment, we compared the induction of IL-3 expression in lympho-cytes isolated from rats fed ad libitum and the restricted diet. An age-related decline in IL-3 activity was observed in rats fed ad libitum. This observation is in agreement with our recent study in which the expression of IL-3, i.e., activity and mRNA levels, was found to decrease with age in spleen lymphocytes from mice (Li et al., 1988). Interestingly, the activities of IL-3 did not decrease with age in the restricted rats. Thus, our preliminary experiments suggest that dietary restriction has a very dramatic effect on the age-related change in IL-3. Additional studies are necessary to establish that dietary restriction can prevent the age-related decline in IL-3 expression.

5. SUMMARY

We have shown that dietary restriction alters gene expression at several levels in spleen lymphocytes isolated from rats. The age-related decline in mitogen-induced protein synthesis is dramatically retarded and the expression of two specific genes, IL-2 and IL-3, are en-hanced in spleen lymphocytes from restricted rats. Thus, it is possible that the ability of dietary restriction to improve the immune system might be at least in part due to its effect on the process of gene expression.

ACKNOWLEDGMENTS. This work was supported by grant AG 01548 from the National In-stitutes of Health. The authors thank the following investigators for generously supplying the following cell lines and cDNA probe: FDC-P1 cells from Dr. Sandra K. Ruscetti (National Cancer Institute, Bethesda, Maryland), CTLL-20 cells from Dr. Charles Orosz (Therapeutic Immunology Laboratories, Ohio; State University, Columbus, Ohio), and the human IL-2 cDNA probe from Dr. Tadasugu Taniguchi (Japanese Foundation for Cancer Research, Tokyo, Japan).

REFERENCES

Armbrecht, J. H., Strong, R., Boltx, M., Rocco, D., Wood, W. G., and Richardson, A., 1988, Modulation of age-related changes in serum 1,25-dihyroxyvitamin D and parathyroid hormone by dietary restriction, J. Nutr. 118:1360–1365.
Birchenall-Aarks, M. C., Roberts, M. S., Staecker, J., Hardwick, J. P., and Richardson, A., 1985, Effect of dietary restriction on liver protein synthesis in rats, J. Nutr. 115:944–950.
Chang, M. P., Makinodan, T., Peterson, W. J., and Strechler, B. L., 1982, Role of T-cells and adherent cells in age-related decline in murine Interleukin-2 production, J. Immunol. 129:2426–2430.
Cheung, H. T., Twu, J. S., and Richardson, A., 1983, Mechanism of age-related decline in lymphocyte proliferation: Role of IL-2 production and protein synthesis, Exp. Gerontol. 18:620–629.
Cheung, H. T., Volvoka, J. D., and Terry, D. S., 1981, Age- and maturation-dependent changes in the immune system of Fischer F344 rats, J. Reticuloendothelial Soc. 30:563–572.
Fernandes, G., Yunis, E. J., and Good, R. A., 1976, Influence of protein restriction on immune function in NZB mice, J. Immunol. 116:782–790.

Gerbase-Delima, M., Liu, R. K., Cheney, K. E., Mickey, R., and Walford, R. L., 1975, Immune function and survival in the long-lived mouse strain subjected to undernutrition, *Gerontologia* **21**:184–202.

Gillis, S., Ferm, M. M., Ou, W., and Smith, K. A., 1978, T cell growth factor: Parameters of production and a quantitative microassay for activity, *J. Immunol.* **120**:2027–2037.

Gillis, S., Kozak, R., Durante, M., and Weksler, M. E., 1981, Immunological studies of aging. Decreased production of and response to T-cell growth factor by lymphocytes from aged human, *J. Clin. Invest.* **67**:937–942.

Ihle, J., Keller, J., Henderson, L., Klein, F., and Palaszynski, E., 1982, Procedures for the purification of interleukin 3 to homogeneity, *J. Immunol.* **129**:2431–2436.

Jung, L. K., Palladino, M. A., Calvano, S., Mark, D. A., Good, R. A., and Fernandes, G., 1982, Effect of calorie restriction on the production and responsiveness to interleukin 2 in (NZB × NZW)F1 mice, *Clin. Immunol. Immunopathol.* **25**:295–301.

Kubo, C., Johnson, C. B., Day, N. K., and Good, R. A., 1984, Calorie source, calorie restriction, immunity and aging of (NZB/NZW)F1 mice, *J. Nutr.* **114**:1884–1899.

Lewis, S. E., Goldspink, D. F., Philips, J. G., Merry, B. J., and Holehan, A. M., 1985, The effect of aging and chronic dietary restriction on whole body growth and protein turnover in the rat, *Exp. Gerontol.* **20**:253–263.

Li, D. D., Chien, Y. K., Gu, M. Z., Richardson, A., and Cheung, H. T., 1988, The age-related decline in interleukin 3 expression in mice, *Life Sci.* **43**:1215–1222.

Makinodan, T., and Kay, M. M. B., 1980, Age influence on the immune system, *Adv. Immunol.* **29**:287–330.

Masoro, E. J., 1984, Nutrition as a modulator of the aging process, *Physiologist* **27**:98–101.

McCay, C. M., Crowell, M. F., and Maynard, L. M., 1935, The effect of retarded growth upon the length of life span and upon the ultimate body size, *J. Nutr.* **10**:63–68.

Richardson, A., 1981, The relationship between aging and protein synthesis, in: *Handbook of Biochemistry in Aging* (J. R. Florini, ed.), CRC Press, Boca Raton, Florida, pp. 79–101.

Richardson, A., 1985, The effect of age and nutrition on protein synthesis by cells and tissues from mammals, in: *Handbook of Nutrition in the Aged* (R. R. Watson, ed.), CRC Press, Boca Raton, Florida, pp. 31–47.

Richardson, A., and Birchenall-Sparks, M. C., 1983, Age-related changes in protein synthesis, in: *Review of Biological Research in Aging*, Vol. 1 (M. Rothstein, ed.), Liss, New York, pp. 255–275.

Richardson, A., Birchenall-Sparks, M. C., and Staecker, J. L., 1983, Aging and transcription, in: *Review of Biological Research in Aging*, Vol. 1 (M. Rothstein, ed.), Liss, New York, pp. 275–294.

Richardson, A., Butler, J. A., Rutherford, M. S., Semsei, I., Gu, M. Z., Fernandes, G., and Chiang, W. H., 1988, Effect of age and dietary restriction on the expression of α2u-globulin, *J. Biol. Chem.* **262**:12821–12825.

Richardson, A., Rutherford, M. S., Birchenall-Sparks, M. C., Roberts, M. S., Wu, W. T., and Cheung, H. T., 1985, Levels of specific messenger RNA species as a function of age, in: *Molecular Biology of Aging: Gene Stability and Gene Expression* (R. S. Sohal, L. S. Birnbaum, and R. G. Cutler, eds.), Raven, New York, pp. 229–241.

Richardson, A., and Semsei, T., 1987, Effect of aging on translation and transcription, in: *Review of Biological Research in Aging*, Vol. 3 (M. Rothstein, ed.), Liss, New York, pp. 467–483.

Ricketts, W. G., Spark, M. C., Hardwick, J. P., and Richardson, A., 1985, Effect of age and dietary restriction on protein synthesis by isolated kidney cells, *J. Cell Physiol.* **125**:492–498.

Robb, R., Munck, A., and Smith, K. A., 1981, T-cell growth factor receptors: Quantitation, specificity, and biological relevance, *J. Exp. Med.* **154**:1455–1474.

Thoman, M., and Weigle, W., 1981, Lymphokines and aging: Interleukin-2 production and activity in aged animals, *J. Immunol.* **127**:2102–2105.

Tollefsbol, T. O., and Cohen, H. J., 1986, Decreased protein synthesis of transforming lymphocytes from aged humans. *Mech. Aging Dev.* **30**:53–62.

Varesio, L., and Holden, H. T., 1980, Mechanisms of lymphocyte activation. I. Linkage between early protein synthesis and late lymphocyte proliferation, *J. Immunol.* **124**:2288–2294.

Varesio, L., Holden, H. T., and Taramelli, D., 1980, Mechanisms of lymphocyte activation. II. Requirements for macromolecular synthesis in the production of lymphokines, *J. Immunol.* **125**:2810–2817.

Wagner, H., Hardt, C., Heeg, K., Rollinghoff, M., and Pfizenmaier, K., 1980, T-cell-drived helper factor allows in vitro induction of cytotoxic T cells in nu/nu mice, *Nature (Lond.)* **284**:278–280.

Walford, R. L., 1974, Immunological theory of aging: Current status, *Fed. Proc. Fed. Am. Soc. Exp. Biol.* **33**:2020–2027.

Ward, W. F., 1988, Enhancement by food restriction of liver protein synthesis in aging Fischer 344 rat, *J. Gerontol.* **43**:B50–B53.

Weindruch, R., Gottesman, S. R., and Walford, R. L., 1982, Modification of age-related immune decline in mice dietary restricted from or after midadulthood, *Proc. Natl. Acad. Sci. USA* **79**:898–902.

Weindruch, R., Walford, R. L., Fligiel, S., and Guthrie, D., 1986, The retardation of aging in mice by dietary restriction: Longevity, cancer, immunity and lifetime energy intake, *J. Nutr.* **116**:641–654.

Wu, W., Pahlavani, M. A., Cheung, H. T., and Richardson, A., 1986, The effect of aging on the expression of interleukin-2 messenger ribonucleic acid, *Cell. Immunol.* **100**:224–231.

Yu, B. P., Maeda, H., Murata, I., and Masoro, E. J., 1984, Nutritional modulation of longevity and age-related diseases, *Fed. Proc. Fed. Am. Soc. Exp. Biol.* **43**:858–863.

24

Zinc, Immunity, and Aging

NICOLA FABRIS, EUGENIO MOCCHEGIANI, MARIO MUZZIOLI, and MAURO PROVINCIALI

1. INTRODUCTION

A good body of experimental and clinical evidence supports the idea that, with advancing age, the immune system undergoes a progressive deterioration of efficiency and that such a decline largely depends on the involution of the thymus, this phenomenon being considered one of the earliest and irreversible age-related events (Walford, 1969). With advancing age, the thymus shows a progressive decline in function, as demonstrated by the reduced size of the organ, by hystological evidence of hypotrophy of the cortex with frequent corticomedullary inversion (G. Goldstein and Mackay, 1969) and by the reduced plasma level of thymic hormones such as thymosin α_1 (McClure *et al.*, 1982), thymopoietin (Lewis *et al.*, 1978), and the *facteur timique sérique* (FTS), more recently called thymulin in its zinc-bound active form (J. F. Bach *et al.*, 1972; Fabris *et al.*, 1984).

All these humoral factors are produced by the epithelial component of the thymus (Savino and Dardenne, 1984) and are required for proliferation and differentiation of thymocytes toward mature T cells (A. L. Goldstein, 1984). The causes of such an age-dependent thymic deterioration are undefined; the progressive decline of thymic endocrine activity with advancing age may be due to alterations of either epithelial cells that become unable to synthesize and/or release thymic factors or occurring in those extrinsic mechanisms that seem to control the function of the endocrine epithelium (Fabris and Piantanelli, 1982).

Experiments in mice have demonstrated that both intrinsic and extrinsic factors can play a role. In fact, thymuses from old mice, when grafted into young adult thymectomized recipients, can at least partially restore the plasma thymulin level of the recipients, whereas newborn thymuses are less efficient in restoring the plasma level of thymulin when transplanted into old recipients than in young adult thymectomized mice (M. A. Bach and Beaurain, 1979).

Among the microenvironmental factors that may be responsible for these findings,

NICOLA FABRIS, EUGENIO MOCCHEGIANI, MARIO MUZZIOLI, and MAURO PROVINCIALI
• Gerontology Research Department, Italian National Research Center on Aging, 60100 Ancona, Italy.

neuroendocrine factors are certainly of primary relevance (Fabris and Piantanelli, 1982; Fabris et al., 1988a), either because some of them have been proven to act on thymus endocrine activity (Fabris et al., 1988b), or because a progressive deterioration of the neuroendocrine balance is among the detrimental processes more frequently encountered in old age (Meites et al., 1987).

It has, in fact, been demonstrated that the age-dependent thymic involution may be reversed by some endocrine manipulations known to influence thymus growth during development (Fabris, 1981); exogenous administration of thyroxine (T4) (Fabris and Mocchegiani, 1985) or growth hormone (Kelley et al., 1986) or of inhibitors of luteinizing hormone releasing hormone (LH-RH) (Greenstein et al., 1987) is able to induce regrowth of the thymus, even when applied in old age.

While it is clear that these observations necessarily point to a need to consider the age-dependent involution of the thymus as a reversible phenomenon, it is still unclear as to whether the physiological causes of such an involution are restricted to neuroendocrine imbalances, (which, by the way, do not occur in all species) or whether other microenvironmental mechanisms must be invoked.

The question has been raised as to the possible role, within this context, of the altered turnover of zinc, since (1) marginal zinc deficiency is a common finding with advanced age (Hsu, 1979), (2) it is involved in regulation of immune functioning (Chandra, 1985), or (3) one, at least, of the known thymic peptides, i.e., thymulin, is certainly zinc dependent (Dardenne et al., 1982).

This chapter reviews some of the major features of zinc metabolism, their implications for the immune system, and the possible role of alterations in zinc turnover in age-related immune deterioration.

2. BIOLOGICAL ROLE OF ZINC

The biological relevance of zinc has been initially suggested by the observation of high incidence of growth retardation with sexual underdevelopment and mental retardation in children living in zinc-deficient ecological system (Prasad, 1982). Studies performed in those ecosystems or experimentally in animals fed a zinc-deprived diet have demonstrated that zinc has a widespread action on various biological functions. Enzymatic efficiency as well as neuroendocrine balance are both affected by zinc deficiency.

During the past 15 years, more than 200 zinc metalloenzymes have been recorded, including dehydrogenase, peptidases, polymerases, and phosphatase (Sandstead, 1982) (Table I). Zinc enzymes are known to participate in many metabolic processes, including carbohydrate, lipid, protein, and nucleic acid synthesis or degradation. Zinc is therefore required for both DNA and RNA synthesis and, owing to its involvement in ATPase and phospholypase A_2, for the structure and function of the plasma membranes as well (Chvapil, 1976).

The role played by zinc in various endocrinological functions is clearly evidenced by the observation that in zinc-deprived animals, the blood level of some hormones and neurotransmitters, such as insulin, growth hormone, thyrotropic hormone, thyroid hormones, gonadotropins, testosterone, and vasointestinal peptide (VIP), are reduced, whereas other hormones, such as prolactin (PRL), cortisol, corticosterone, and catecholamines, are found at increased levels (Prasad, 1985) (Table II). Some of these alterations, such as the reduced

TABLE I. Primary Zinc-Requiring Enzymes

Phosphotransferases
  Thymidine kinase
  Pyruvate kinase
  Adenylate kinase
  Deoxynucleotide transferase
	Polymerases
	  RNA polymerases
	  DNA polymerases

Hydrolases
  Diadenosine tetraphosphate ($A_{P_4}A$)
    hydrolase
  Peptidyldipeptide hydrolase (angiotensin
    I converting enzyme)
  5'-Ribonucleotide phosphohydrolase
  3'-Ribonucleotide phosphohydrolase
	Phosphatases
	  Alkaline phosphatase
	  Creatine phosphatase
	  ATPase
	  Phospholipase A_2

Dehydrogenases
  Alcohol dehydrogenase
  Superoxide dismutase
  "Malic" enzyme
  Isocitrate dehydrogenase
  Lactate dehydrogenase
	Peptidases
	  Carboxypeptidase A
	  Carboxypeptidase B
	  Arginine carboxypeptidase
	  Carboxypeptidase N

TABLE II. Neurohormonal Variation in Zinc Deficiency

Diminished	Augmented
Thyroid-releasing hormone (TRH)	PRL
Thyroid-stimulating hormone (TSH)	Cortisol
Triiodothyronine (T3) and thyroxine	Corticosterone
(T4)	DOPA (brain)
Insulin	Norepinephrine (brain)
Growth hormone (GH)	Epinephrine (brain)
Gonadotropins	
Testosterone	
Progesterone	
Gastric Inhibitory peptide (GIP)	
Vasoactive intestinal polypeptide	
(VIP)	
Enkephalin	
Endorphin	
Prostaglandin E_1 (PGE_1)	
Prostaglandin E_2 (PGE_2)	

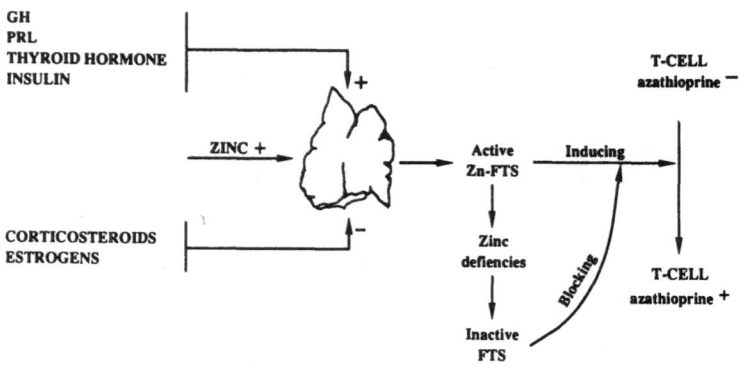

FIGURE 1. Role of hormones and zinc on thymulin production and activation.

testosterone and the increased PRL blood level, have been demonstrated also in zinc-deficient humans.

It has been shown that some hormones, such as nerve growth factor (NGF) and one of the thymic peptides (i.e., thymulin), are strictly zinc dependent (Dardenne et al., 1982; Pattison and Dunn, 1975). With regard to thymulin, it has been demonstrated that zinc is bound to the peptide in an equimolar ratio and that biological activity resides in the zinc-bound form (Dardenne et al., 1982), whereas the zinc-unbound peptide is able to bind to target sites but is inactive and probably prevents the active form from exerting its action (Fabris et al., 1984) (Fig. 1). The presence of inactive hormone molecules in biological fluids may be demonstrated by measurement of their capacity to inhibit known amounts of synthetic active thymulin (Fabris et al., 1984; Bach and Beaurain, 1979), and indirectly by measuring thymulin activity in biological samples before and after in vitro addition of zinc ions, which may unmask the presence of inactive hormone (Fabris et al., 1986).

3. ROLE OF ZINC IN THE IMMUNE SYSTEM

During recent years, zinc has been demonstrated to be essential for the immunocompetence in man (Chandra, 1985) and animals (Iwata et al., 1979). Zinc deficiency in animals causes thymic and lymphe node atrophy and impaired cell-mediated cutaneous hypersensitivity reactions. Lymphocytes isolated from zinc-deficient animals show impaired response to phytohemagglutinin (PHA) and depression of T-cell-dependent antibody production. Furthermore, a zinc-deficient diet in experimental animals causes impaired T-helper and T-suppressor function and decreased T-killer and natural killer (NK) activity (Iwata et al., 1979) (Table III). Assessment of the role of zinc in the development and function of different lymphoid cell populations indicates that this element has an effect predominantly on T lymphocytes (Iwata et al., 1979). In humans, the effect of zinc deficiency on immune function has been studied in congenital diseases, such as acrodermatitis enteropathica, sickle cell anemia (Prasad, 1985), and Down's syndrome (Fabris et al., 1984), and in conditions characterized by acquired altered zinc turnover, such as uremia (Travaglini et al., 1988), or during total parenteral nutrition (TNP). Depending on the severity and duration, zinc defi-

TABLE III. Immunological Consequences
of Zinc Deprivation

Function	Consequences
Histological	Thymic atrophy
	Structural abnormalities of T-dependent areas
Thymus	Reduced thymic hormone production
	Reduced peripheral activation of thymulin (Zn-FTS)
	Reduced proliferation and differentiation of T lymphocytes
T cell	Impaired T-helper activity
	Impaired T-suppressor activity
	Reduced mitogen responsiveness
	Reduced T-killer activity
	Depressed Ab response to T-dependent antigens
B cell	Normal response to B-dependent antigens
Natural killer (NK)	Decreased NK activity

ciency produces hypoplasia of the thymus, spleen, lymphe nodes, and Peyer's paches (Mac-Clain, 1985). Alterations in the lymphocyte population, including reduced T-helper lymphocyte function, reduced NK activity, decreased number of total T lymphocytes, and increased B lymphocytes, are a common and constant aspect in zinc-deficiency diseases (Chandra, 1985; Allen et al., 1981).

The mechanism by which zinc may affect the immune system is certainly multifaceted, due to the widespread action on zinc on different enzymes and hormones involved in various physiological steps of immune development and response. A direct effect of zinc on immune cells is supported by evidence that zinc is a potent in vitro T-lymphocyte mitogen for both humans and animals over a narrow range of concentrations (Fraker et al., 1977) and that zinc is required for the nucleoside phosphorylase, a purine enzyme that is required also by T cells for its functioning (Underwood, 1977).

In addition to a direct effect on lymphoid cells, zinc may influence the immune system through its action on the biological activity of thymulin. In fact, it has been demonstrated that in conditions characterized by more or less profound zinc deficiencies, such as those associated with physiological aging (Fabris et al., 1984), or with congenital diseases, such as acrodermatitis enteropathica, cystic fibrosis, Down's syndrome (Fabris et al., 1984), and Duchenne's dystrophy (Fabris et al., 1988c), or with infectious diseases such as acquired immune deficiency syndrome (AIDS) (Fabris et al., 1988a), a reduction in the circulating level of active thymulin is observed with a concomitant appearance of inactive zinc-unbound FTS molecules (Table IV). The in vitro addition to plasma samples of zinc ions is able to unmask the inactive circulating FTS molecule, showing that the total amount of the thymic hormone (zinc bound plus zinc unbound FTS) is frequently much higher than the active fraction in all the above-reported zinc marginal deficiencies.

TABLE IV. Zinc Serum Level and Plasma Level of Active (Zn-FTS), Inactive (FTS), and Total Thymulin (ZnFTS + FTS) in Various Human Pathologies

Group	Zinc[a] (μg/dl)	Active An-FTS[b] (log-2)	Inactive FTS[c] (pg/ml)	Total FTS[d] (log-2)
Normal	113 ± 2.4	5.3 ± 0.4	0.3 ± 0.1	5.8 ± 0.5
Acroderm. ENT.	58 ± 1.3	1.4 ± 0.3	65 ± 4.3	5.4 ± 0.4
Cystic fibrosis	71 ± 3.0	1.7 ± 0.3	64 ± 3.2	4.7 ± 0.5
Down's syndrome	86 ± 3.9	1.0 ± 0.2	45 ± 4.6	4.8 ± 0.4
Duchenne dystrophy	67 ± 9.4	1.2 ± 0.2	40 ± 3.5	3.5 ± 0.5
AIDS	57 ± 5.0	1.0 ± 0.3	not done	5.7 ± 0.4

[a]Measured by atomic absorption spectroscopy.
[b]Measured by conventional rosette inhibition assay (J. F. Bach et al., 1972).
[c]Measured by inhibitory activity on synthetic thymulin (M. A. Bach and Beaurain, 1979).
[d]Measured by modified rosette inhibition assay (Fabris et al., 1986).

4. ZINC AND AGING

The possibility that trace elements may play a role in physiological aging processes was originally hypothesized following the observation that, with advancing age, at least in humans, alimentary habits vary consistently and defective intake of various micronutrients is almost unavoidable.

With regard to zinc intake and turnover in old individuals, data are incomplete. According to a major survey, performed by the U.S. Department of Agriculture (USDA), zinc intake appears to be reduced in old age (USDA, 1980). Plasma level of zinc is reduced, but no definite data are available on intracellular zinc content. It has been shown, however, that zinc absorption is also affected by age (i.e., reduced). Also, zinc levels are reduced through urine and feces; this phenomenon has been considered compensatory in nature, although not sufficient to prevent progressive reduction of zinc plasma levels (Turnlund et al., 1986) (Table V).

TABLE V. Zinc Turnover in Young and Old Humans and Rate of Absorption of [67]Zn after Single Administration[a]

Factors	Young	Old
Serum Zn μg/dl	105 ± 4	78 ± 3
Urinary Zn mg/day	0.92 ± 0.11	0.67 ± 0.13
Fecal Zn mg/day	15.3 ± 0.7	14.2 ± 0.9
% [67]Zn absorption[b]	29.9 ± 3.4	17.3 ± 4.1

[a]Redrawn from Turnland et al., (1986).
[b]Rate of absorption of [67]Zn, orally administered (10 mg/day), evaluated 12 weeks later.

The relevance of this age-dependent decline of plasma zinc level is unknown. It does not seem to be a pure temporal coincidence, however, that some of the known zinc-dependent functions, such as wound healing, skin cell turnover, taste acuity, and immune efficiency, are all found to be depressed in older individuals and that in some instances the age-dependent deterioration can be reversed by zinc supplementation (Chandra, 1986).

The hypothesis that alterations of zinc turnover are common in old age requires confirmation in species other than humans, as very few data are available. Recent findings from our laboratory have demonstrated that in mice and rats, plasma zinc levels are significantly reduced even though food intake is not changed as compared with that in young individuals. These observations would suggest that alteration in zinc turnover is a common finding in old age and that such a defect may be relevant for various age-related processes.

5. EFFECT OF ZINC SUPPLEMENTATION IN OLD AGE

The observation of age-associated alterations in zinc turnover, together with the knowledge of its role in immune efficiency, has prompted investigation of the effect that a zinc supplementation may have on age-related decline of immune functions. Experiments performed in rodents, involving dietary zinc supplementation during the animal's whole life span, have demonstrated that in these conditions many of the known age-related immune modifications, including decreased thymic hormone production, reduced T-helper and T-suppressor activity, and depressed NK cytotoxicity, could be prevented by such treatment (Iwata et al., 1979).

Furthermore, when applied to autoimmune susceptible NZB mice, zinc supplementation succeeded in delaying the time of appearance of autoaggressive reactions (Beach et al., 1981). These findings have been interpreted in terms of a possible prevention of age-related alterations. A major question raised by these data has been whether age-related immune deterioration could be corrected, even after immune alterations have occurred.

Trials performed in elderly humans have shown that, in fact, zinc supplementation might be able to increase the cutaneous sensitivity to various antigens and the antibody response to tetanus toxoid (Ducheateu et al., 1981) and to recover thymic endocrine activity (Chandra, 1988).

Recent experiments in our laboratory have been conducted in an attempt to elucidate the mechanism of such an action; it has been demonstrated that oral zinc supplementation, even when applied to elderly mice, is able to induce regrowth of the thymus (Fig. 2) with increased thymic hormone production and augmented percentage of thymulin-producing cells, complete recovery of the reduced number of Thy 1.2^+ cells in the spleen, and partial reconstitution of PHA response and NK cytotoxic activity of spleen cells (Muzzioli et al., 1988; Mocchegiani and Fabris, 1988a).

The increased thymulin plasma level depends not only on the peripheral reactivation of zinc-unbound FTS, but on a control effect on the rate of production of thymic hormones. In fact, after oral zinc supplementation, the total thymulin (Zn-FTS + FTS) results increased over the values observed in age-matched controls.

Administration of zinc salts in vitro to spleen cells from old mice failed to recover peripheral immune efficiency, whereas zinc-bound thymulin was succeeded. This last observation suggests that one of the major effects of zinc supplementation in old age is to recover thymic endocrine activity and that such a restoration is responsible for the recovery of peripheral immune efficiency.

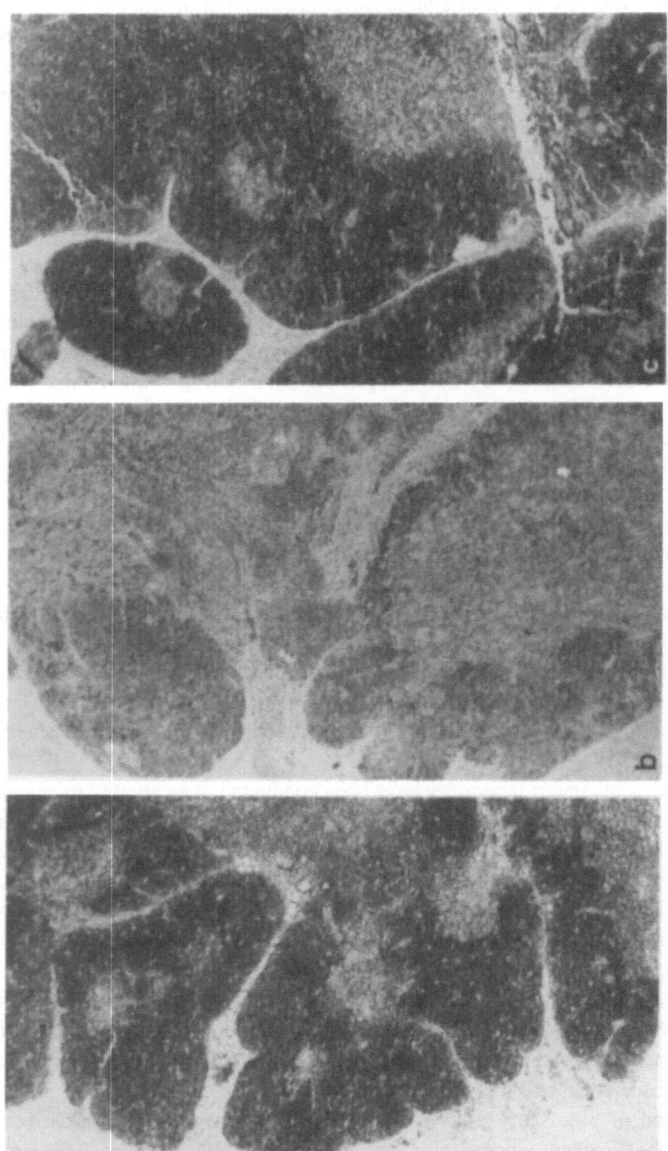

FIGURE 2. Reconstitution of thymic histology in a 22-month-old BALB/c mouse. (a) Oral administration of zinc sulfate (0.1 mg zinc sulfate/mouse/days). (b) Untreated old mouse. (c) Untreated young mouse.

That zinc supplementation may recover thymic endocrine activity has been recently supported by observations in old uremic patients, treated with oral zinc for 6 months. In these conditions, patients showed, after 2-week treatment, an increase in the circulating level of thymulin, which reached values in young individuals by the fourth week of treatment (Travaglini *et al.*, 1989).

With regard to the mechanism by which zinc can exert its action on the thymus, the available data do not provide substantial information. Because of the widespread action on zinc ions, it can be hypothesized that zinc supplementation may reactivate the enzyme cascade (Prasad, 1982) necessary for thymic peptide synthesis or that it may correct the turnover of some hormones, such as growth hormone (GH), thyroid-stimulating hormone (TSH), and thyroid hormones (Prasad, 1985) which are of great relevance for thymus functioning (Fabris and Mocchegiani, 1985). Preliminary data from our laboratory have shown that zinc supplementation in old mice recovers the abnormally low serum level of triiodothyronine (T3), a hormone that can directly modulate the thymic peptide synthesis by the thymic epithelial cells (Mocchegiani and Fabris, 1988b).

6. CONCLUSION

The present data together with other investigators' findings stress the following points:

1. The age-related involution of the thymus does not seem to be attributable to an intrinsic failure of the organ, but to a functional alteration, probably related to age-associated modifications of microenvironmental factors relevant to immune functioning, such as neuroendocrine factors and bioavailability of trace elements.
2. With regard to the neuroendocrine system, experimental support to this assumption has been offered by the demonstration of the possibility of restoring thymic histology and thymic endocrine activity in old animals by different hormonal interventions and particularly by treatment with thyroxine (T4) or with inhibitors of LH-RH or by transplanting a GH-producing GH_3 tumor cell line.
3. Among nutritional factors, zinc plays a relevant role in the maintenance of thymic efficiency. Age-associated marginal zinc deficiency is responsible for low thymic endocrine activity. Zinc supplementation, at physiological doses, can completely restore crippled thymic function, even when applied in old age, and can recover various peripheral immune functions, thus representing an interesting and rather physiological approach to immunological potentiation in the elderly.
4. It is difficult to reconcile the restoration of thymic function achieved by zinc supplementation with the similar effect obtained by hormonal manipulation. The knowledge that zinc is required to ensure functional efficiency of different endocrine glands and the observation that during zinc supplementation, at least in mice, increased thyroid function is recorded, may offer a tool for future work.

ACKNOWLEDGMENTS. This work was supported in part by grant 86.01763.04 from the Italian National Research Council (N.F.) and from the Italian Health Ministry, Italian National Research Center on Aging (INRCA), targeted program on Nutrition in the Elderly. We thank Marzio Marcellini, Mrs. Nazzarena Gasparini, and Mrs. Clara Chesi for their excellent technical assistance.

REFERENCES

Allen, J. I., Kay, E. N., and MacClain, C. S., 1981, Severe zinc deficiency in humans. Association with a reversible T-lymphocyte dysfunction, *Ann. Intern Med.* **95**:154–157.

Bach, J. F., Dardenne, M., Papiernik, M., Barois, A., Levasseur, P., and Le Brigant, H., 1972, Evidence for a serum thymic factor produced by the human thymus, *Lancet* **2**:1056–1058.

Bach, M. A., and Beaurain, G., 1979, Respective influence of extrinsic and intrinsic factors on the age-related decrease of thymic secretion, *J. Immunol.* **122**:2505–2507.

Beach, R. S., Gershwin, M. E., and Hurley, L. S., 1981, Nutritional factors and autoimmunity. I. Immunopathology of zinc deprivation in New England mice, *J. Immunol.* **126**:1999–2006.

Chandra, R. K., 1985, Trace element regulation of immunity and infection, *J. Am. Coll. Nutr.* **4**:5–16.

Chandra, R. K., 1989, Nutritional regulation of immunity and risk of infection in old age, *Immunology* **67**:141–147.

Chvapil, M., 1976, Effect of zinc on cells and biomembranes, *Med. Clin. North Am.* **60**:799–812.

Dardenne, M., Pleau, J. M., Nabama, B., Lefancier, P., Denien, M., Choay, J., and Bach, J. F., 1982, Contribution of zinc and other metals to the biological activity of the serum thymic factor, *Proc. Natl. Acad. Sci. USA* **79**:5370–5373.

Ducheateu, J., Delespesse, G., Vrijen, R., and Coolet, H., 1981, Beneficial effects of oral zinc supplementation on the immune response of old people, *Am. J. Med.* **70**:1001–1004

Fabris, N., 1981, Ontogenetic and phylogenetic aspects of neuroendocrine–immune network, *Dev. Comp. Immunol.* **5**(1):46–53.

Fabris, N., and Piantanelli, L., 1982, Thymus–neuroendocrine interactions during development and aging, in: *Hormones and Aging* (R. C. Adelman and G. S. Roth, eds.), CRC Press, Boca Raton, Florida, pp. 167–171.

Fabris, N., and Mocchegiani, E., 1985, Endocrine control of thymic serum factor production in young-adult and old mice, *Cell Immunol.* **91**:325–385.

Fabris, N., Mocchegiani, E., Amadio, L., Zannotti, M. Licastro, F., and Franceschi, C., 1984, Thymic hormone deficiency in normal aging and Down's syndrome: Is there a primary failure of the thymus?, *Lancet* **1**:983–986.

Fabris, N., Mocchegiani, E., Mariotti, S., Pancini, F., and Pinchera, A., 1986, Thyroid function modulates thymus endocrine activity, *J. Clin. Endocrinol. Metab.* **62**:474–478.

Fabris, N., Mocchegiani, E., Galli, M., Irato, L., Lazzarin, A., and Moroni, M., 1988a, AIDS, zinc deficiency, and thymic hormone failure, *JAMA* **259**:839–840.

Fabris, N., Mocchegiani, E., Muzzioli, M., and Provinciali, M., 1988b, Neuroendocrine–thymus interaction: Perspectives for intervention in aging, in: *Neuroimmunomodulation: Interventions in Aging and Cancer* (W. Pierpaoli and H. Spector, eds.), Annals of the New York Academy of Science, New York, pp. 145–149.

Fabris, N., Mocchegiani, E., and Palloni, R., 1988c, Zinc-dependent failure of thymic hormones in human pathologies, in: *Trace Elements in Man and Animals* (L. S. Hurtley, ed.), Plenum, New York, pp. 315–317.

Fraker, P. J., Haas, S., and Luecke, R. W., 1977, Effect of zinc deficiency on the immune response of the young adult A/Jax mouse, *J. Nutr.* **107**:1889–1895.

Goldstein, A. L. (ed.), 1984, *Thymic Hormones and Lymphokines*, Plenum, New York, pp. 1–669.

Goldstein, G., and Mackay, I. R., 1969, *The Human Thymus*, Heinemann, London, p. 1–168.

Greenstein, B. D., Fitzpatrick, F. T., Kendall, M. D., and Wheeler, M. J., 1987, Regeneration of the thymus in old male rats treated with a stable analogue of LHRH, *J. Endocr.* **112**:345–350.

Hsu, J. M., 1979, Current Knowledge on zinc, copper and chromium in ageing, *World Rev. Nutr. Diet* **33**:42–69.

Iwata, T., Incefy, G. S., Tanaka, T., Fernandes, G., Menendez-Botet, C. I., Pih, K., and Good, R. A., 1979, Circulating thymic hormone levels in zinc deficiency, *Cell Immunol.* **47**:100–105.

Kelley, K. W., Brief, S., Westly, H. J., Novakofski, J., Bechtel, P. J., Simon, J., and Walker, E. B.,

1986, GH3 pituitary adenoma cells can reverse thymic aging in rats, *Proc Natl Acad Sci. USA* **83:**5663–5667.

Lewis, V. M., Twomey, J. J., Bealmear, P., Goldstein, G., and Good, R. A., 1978, Age, thymic involution, and circulating thymic hormone activity, *J. Clin. Endocrinol. Metab.* **47:**145–150.

McClain, C. S., 1985, Zinc metabolism in malabsorption syndromes, *J. Am. Coll. Nutr.* **4:**49–64.

McClure, J. E., Lameris, N., Wara, D. W., and Goldstein, A. L., 1982, Immunochemical studies on thymosin: Radioimmunoassay of thymosin alpha 1, *J. Immunol.* **128:**368–372.

Meites, J., Goya, R., and Takahashi, S., 1987, Why the neuroendocrine system is important in aging processes, a review, *Exp. Gerontol.* **22:**1–15.

Mocchegiani, E., and Fabris, N., 1989a, Trace elements, immunity and aging. II. Recovery of thymic endocrine activity by zinc supplementation in old mice, submitted.

Mocchegiani, E., and Fabris, N., 1989b, Neuroendocrine–thymus interactions. I. "In vitro" modulation of thymic factor secretion by thyroid hormones, *J. End. Invest.* (in press).

Muzzioli, M., Mocchegiani, E., Provinciali, M., Zaia, A. M., and Fabris, N., 1989, Trace elements immunity and aging. I. Recovery of mitogen responsiveness and natural cytotoxicity by zinc supplementation in old mice, submitted.

Pattison, S. E., and Dunn, M. F., 1975, On the relationship of zinc ion to the structure and function of the 7S nerve growth factor protein, *Biochemistry* **14:**2373–2377.

Prasad, A. S., 1982, *History of Zinc in Human Nutrition in Clinical Applications of Recent Advances in Zinc Metabolism*, Liss, New York, pp. 1–17.

Prasad, A. S., 1985, Clinical, endocrinological and biochemical effects of zinc-deficiency, *Clin. Endocrinol. Metab.* **14:**567–589.

Sandstead, H. H., 1982, Availability of zinc and its requirements in human subjects, in: *Clinical, Biochemical and Nutritional Aspects of Trace Elements* (A. S. Prasad, ed.), Liss, New York, pp. 83–102.

Savino, W., and Dardenne, M., 1984, Thymic hormone-containing cells. VI. Immunohistologic evidence for the simultaneous presence of thymulin, thymopoietin and thymosin alpha 1 in normal and pathological human thymuses, *Eur. J. Immunol.* **14:**987–991.

Travaglini, P., Moriondo, P., Togni, E., Venegoni, P., Bocchicchio, D., Faglia, G., Ambroso, G., Ponticelli, C., Mocchegiani, E., and Fabris, N., 1989, Effect of oral zinc administration on prolactin and thymulin circulating levels in uremic patients, *J. Clin. Endocrinol. Metab.* **68:**186–190.

Turnlund, J. R., Durvin, N., Costa, F., and Margen, S., 1986, Stable isotope studies of zinc absorption and retention in young and elderly men, *J. Nutr.* **116:**1239–1247.

Underwood, E. J., 1977, *Trace elements in human and animal nutrition*, 4th ed., Academic, New York, pp. 1–302.

USDA, 1980, Science and Education Administration, Food and Nutrient Intakes of Individuals in 1 day in the United States, Spring 1977, Preliminary Report No. 2, U.S. Department of Agriculture, Washington, D. C., 1980, Vol. 40, p. 45.

Walford, R. L., 1969, *The Immunologic Theory of Aging*, Munksgaard, Copenhagen, pp. 1–248.

25

Neuroendocrine Effects of Lifelong Dietary Restriction by Intermittent Feeding in Mice

BARBARA J. DAVIS, ROBERT W. HAMILL,
THOMAS H. McNEILL, ELAINE BRESNAHAN,
and DONALD K. INGRAM

1. INTRODUCTION

Lifelong dietary restriction has been shown to increase mean and maximum life span and to delay the onset of pathophysiologic changes associated with aging in rodents (Barrows and Kokkonen, 1978). The mechanisms underlying the modulation of aging by dietary restriction remain unknown. Based on studies using several levels of dietary restriction in mice, Weindruch et al. (1986) suggested that increased metabolic efficiency may be related to longevity, since the longest-lived mice at each level of dietary restriction studies also were the heaviest. Although a number of studies support the hypothesis that increased body weight is associated with increased longevity in dietarily restricted rodents, (reviewed by Ingram and Reynolds, 1987), the relationship between body weight and life span is complex, and it is difficult to make generalized statements relating longevity to body weight.

Studies specifically aimed at defining metabolic consequences of lifelong dietary restriction have shown that lifelong dietary restriction in rats is accompanied by marked alterations in hepatocyte and adipocyte metabolism (Bertrand et al., 1983; Yu et al., 1984). Insulin and glucagon are two of the major hormones that regulate overall body fuel metabolism (Unger et al., 1978). Despite growing evidence that antiaging effects of lifelong dietary restriction may be fundamentally related to metabolic changes (Masoro et al., 1984), very few data are available with respect to the effects of lifelong dietary restriction on circulating

BARBARA J. DAVIS, ROBERT W. HAMILL, and THOMAS H. McNEILL • Department of Neurology, University of Rochester School of Medicine and Dentistry, Rochester, New York 14642.   ELAINE BRESNAHAN • Gerontology Research Center, National Institute on Aging, National Institutes of Health, Francis Scott Key Medical Center, Baltimore, Maryland 21224.   DONALD K. INGRAM • Molecular Physiology and Genetics Section, Laboratory of Cellular and Molecular Biology, Gerontology Research Center, National Institute on Aging, National Institutes of Health, Francis Scott Key Medical Center, Baltimore, Maryland 21224.   Present address of T. H. M: Andrus Gerontology Center, University of Southern California, Los Angeles, California 90089.

levels of insulin or glucagon. Moreover, although the sympathoadrenal system is significantly involved in neuroendocrine regulation of metabolism (Smith and Davis, 1983), no data are available with respect to the effects of lifelong dietary restriction on sympathoadrenal activity. In the present study, we assessed the effects of lifelong dietary restriction on plasma glucose, insulin, and glucagon levels and on adrenal tyrosine hydroxylase (TH) activity in C57B1/6J mice. TH is the rate-limiting enzyme in catecholamine biosynthesis (Levitt *et al.*, 1965) and may be used as a marker of sympathetic and sympathoadrenal activity (Cooper *et al.*, 1986).

2. METHODS

Male C57B1/6J mice were obtained from the Jackson Laboratories (Bar Harbor, Maine) at 6 weeks of age. Mice were housed in groups of four in polycarbonate cages (28 × 18 × 13 cm) equipped with removable food hoppers and water spouts. Wood shavings were provided for bedding. Mice were housed in a specially designated room (standard temperature and humidity, lights on from 6:30 AM to 5:30 PM daily, and low background noise) in the vivarium facility at the National Institute on Aging, Gerontology Research Center, Baltimore, Maryland. All mice were provided NIH-07 diet, a pelleted diet containing 24% protein and 10% fat. Mice were randomly assigned to one of two experimental groups: (1) *ad libitum* (AL) mice were allowed *ad libitum* access to the diet throughout the entire experiment, and (2) dietary-restricted (DR) mice were allowed *ad libitum* access to the diet on Mondays, Wednesdays, and Fridays only. Food was removed from the cages and was not available on Tuesdays, Thursdays, Saturdays, or Sundays. All mice had *ad libitum* access to water throughout the experiment. Mice were allowed to survive until they reached 20 months of age. All mice were killed between the hours of 11:00 AM and 2:00 PM, after 24 hr of access to food. Mice were killed by decapitation following cervical dislocation. Trunk blood was collected into chilled, heparinized microhematocrit centrifuge tubes containing aprotinin (Trasylol, Sigma, 500K IU/ml) to inhibit proteolytic degradation of hormones. Tubes containing blood were kept on ice until centrifuged (within 6 hr of blood collection). Plasma was separated and stored at −20°C until assay. No more than 1 week had elapsed between the time of blood collection and assay. Samples of liver were fixed in Bouin's fluid for 8 hr, then dehydrated in graded alcohols, cleared in xylene, and embedded in paraffin. Tissue blocks were cut at 5 μm. Sections were stained using periodic acid-Schiff (PAS) and hematoxylin.

Plasma glucose was determined using a Beckman Glucose Analyzer (glucose oxidase method). Plasma insulin (Morgan and Lazarow, 1963) and glucagon (Hazzard *et al.*, 1968) were determined by double-antibody radioimmunoassays (RIA) using commercially prepared RIA kits (Cambridge Medical Diagnostics, Billerica, Massachusetts). Adrenal TH activity was determined on alumina-absorbed extracts of adrenal medullae using a modification (Melvin and Hamill, 1986) of the radiochemical assay of Black (1975). Student's *t*-tests were used to determine significant differences between AL and DR groups for each parameter measured.

3. RESULTS

The effects of dietary manipulation on survival and life span are presented in Fig. 1. AL mice showed a marked increase in mortality at 96 weeks (24 months) of age. A similar increase in mortality rate was seen at 132 weeks (33.3 months) of age in DR mice (Fig. 1A).

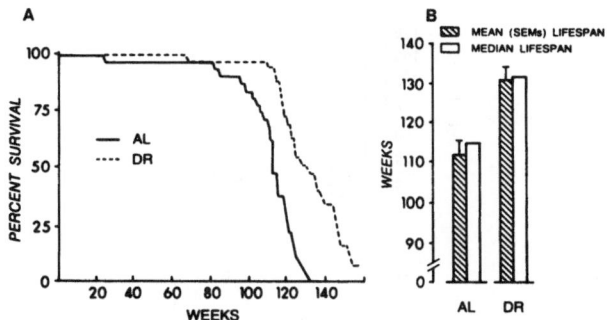

FIGURE 1. (A) Survival curves and (B) lifespan data (mean +SEM) from cohort groups of AL and DR mice housed and fed according to protocols described in the Methods section.

The dietary restriction regimen of intermittent feeding used in the present study increased mean and median lifespan by approximately 18% (Fig. 1B). Figure 2 illustrates the effects of dietary manipulation on weekly food intake and on final body weight. Dietary restriction by intermittent feeding resulted in a small (10%) but significant ($p < 0.01$) reduction of food intake (Fig. 2a). However, final body weights of the AL and DR mice did not differ significantly at 20 months of age (Fig. 2b). Plasma glucose, insulin, and glucagon levels of AL and DR mice are presented in Fig. 3. Glucose levels of AL and DR mice were comparable (Fig. 3a). However, DR mice showed a significant increase of plasma insulin ($p < 0.01$) (Fig. 3b) and a significant decrease of plasma glucagon ($p < 0.05$) (Fig. 3c) when compared with AL mice. The effect of dietary manipulation on adrenal TH activity is presented in Fig. 4. Dietary restriction by intermittent feeding resulted in a significant increase of adrenal TH activity ($p < 0.025$). Moreover, there was a significant positive correlation between plasma insulin level and adrenal TH activity ($p < 0.001$) (Fig. 4b).

Typical patterns of glycogen distribution in the livers of AL and DR mice are illustrated in Fig. 5. Compared with AL mice, DR mice showed histochemical evidence of increased glycogen and lipid deposition in hepatocytes. Differences in glycogen deposition between AL and DR mice were most pronounced in periportal regions of the liver. However, evidence of increased lipid deposition in DR livers occurred uniformly in periportal and centrolobular hepatocytes.

FIGURE 2. (a) Average daily food intake (total weekly food intake /7) for 32 mice (8 cages containing 4 mice/cage) on AL or DR feeding regimens. Data were obtained when mice were 7 months of age. Asterisk (*) $p < 0.01$ difference between groups. (b) Final body weights (mean +SEM) of AL ($N = 16$) and DR ($N = 17$) mice studied at 20 months of age.

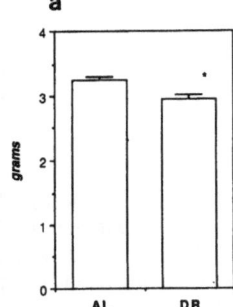

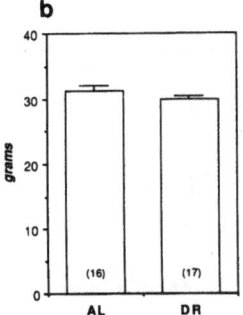

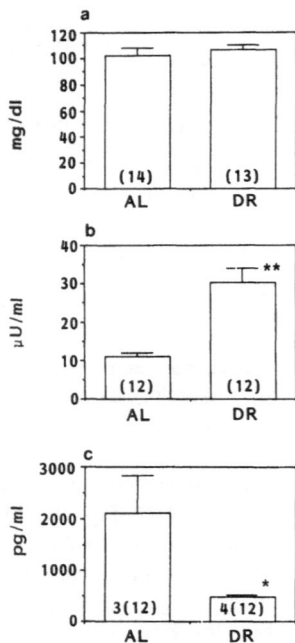

FIGURE 3. Plasma levels of glucose (a), insulin (b) and glucagon (c) of 20-month-old AL and DR mice. Gulcagon values are for pooled plasma samples. Bar height = mean +SEM. Asterisk (*) $p < 0.05$ difference; double asterisk (**) $p < 0.01$ difference.

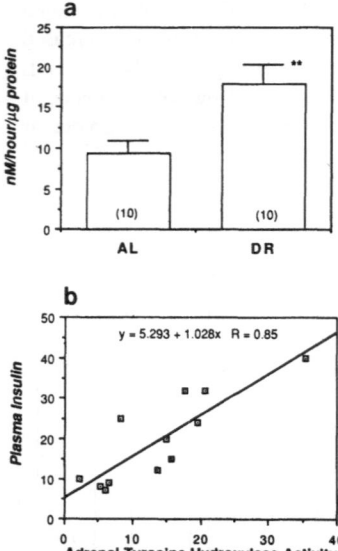

FIGURE 4. (a) Adrenal tyrosine hydroxylase (TH) activity of 20-month-old AL and DR mice. Bar height = mean +SEM. Double asterisk (**) $p < 0.025$ difference. (b) Correlation between plasma insulin and adrenal TH activity.

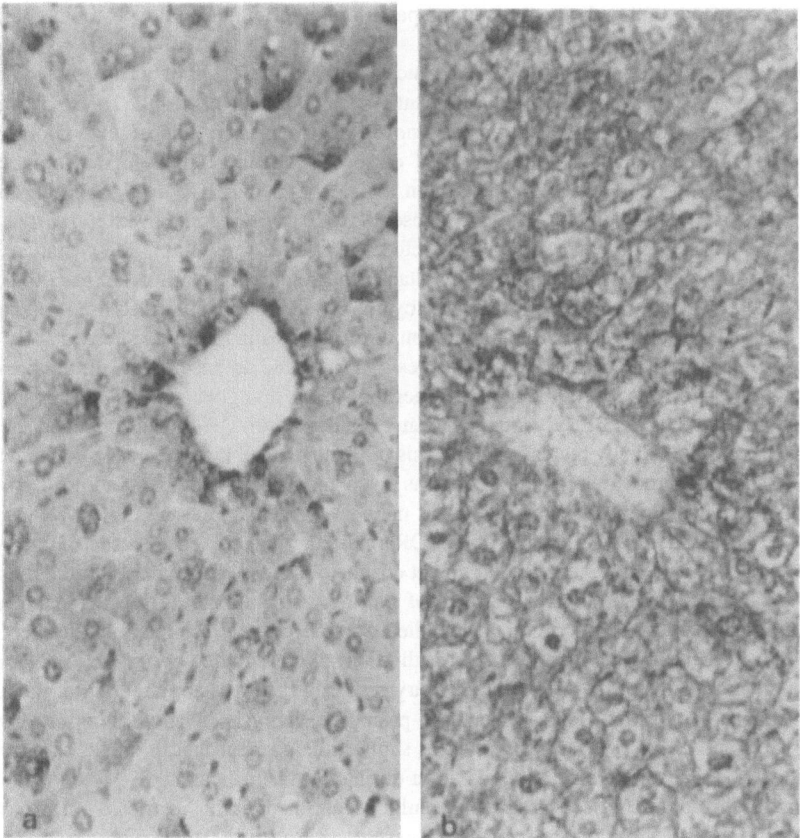

FIGURE 5. Periportal region of the liver from a typical 20-month-old AL (a) and DR (b) mouse. Sections were stained with PAS and hematoxylin. Note evidence of increased glycogen (more intense staining) and lipid deposition (vacuolization) in hepatocytes of the DR mouse. (×200)

4. DISCUSSION

The restriction of daily intake to specified levels in dietary restriction studies usually involves presentation of a measured amount of food that the animals consume over a short period of time. Thus, most dietary restriction studies inadvertently involve a regimen of intermittent feeding. In the present study, dietary-restricted animals were given free access to food (i.e., the amount consumed was not restricted) but only were allowed access to food on 3 nonconsecutive days during the week. Thus, the dietary restriction imposed in the present study was by intermittent feeding, with the amount consumed determined by the animals themselves. Analysis of total weekly caloric consumption revealed that intakes of DR mice were approximately 90% that of AL mice. Despite this relatively mild level of dietary restriction, DR mice showed a significant (18%) increase in mean life span. These data support the concept that both the amount and pattern of caloric intake may profoundly affect life span.

Our results show that when AL and DR mice are killed after 24 hr of access to food (i.e., in the fed state), DR mice show a significant increase of plasma insulin, evidence of a significant decrease of plasma glucagon but no change of plasma glucose. This hormonal profile is similar to what has been reported during the feeding phase in rats trained to consume their total daily allotment of food in a single 2-hr meal (Ip *et al.*, 1977). These investigators, as well as others (Cohn and Joseph, 1970; Wiley and Leveille, 1970) have reported that chronic regimens of fasting and refeeding, such as those imposed by an intermittent feeding regimen, are accompanied by metabolic adaptations that allow animals to store nutrients in a short period of time (favored by increased insulin and decreased glucagon during the feeding phase) for rapid mobilization during the fasting period. These adaptations include increases in lipogenesis and glycogenesis in liver and adipose tissue. In the present study, histochemical evidence of adaptive hyperlipogenesis and glycogenesis was present in livers of DR mice. These results suggest that hepatocytes of DR mice responded to the increased level of insulin by increasing synthesis of glycogen and lipid. However, despite the increased levels of circulating insulin, there was no apparent gross increase of adiposity in the DR animals. Thus, adipocytes of DR mice may have been expressing selective insulin resistance. Alternatively, adipocytes of the DR mice may have been exposed to lipolytic hormones on the fasted day, resulting in no net change of adipose depot mass. In the present study, we did not assess hormonal effects of our DR regimen during the fasting phase. However, studies by Masoro's group using a dietary-restricted regimen in which Fischer 344 rats consumed their daily allotment of food within 3 hr of presentation (Yu *et al.*, 1984), rats that had undergone a regimen of lifelong dietary restriction showed a retardation of the age-related decline in glucagon and epinephrine-promoted lipolysis in adipose tissue during fasting (Bertrand *et al.*, 1987). Those studies support the concept that regimens of chronic intermittent feeding improve fuel mobilization during the fasting phase.

Our finding of increased circulating insulin levels in dietarily restricted mice would appear to be in conflict with the results of Reaven and Reaven (1981), who reported that dietary restriction beginning at 1.5 months of age in Sprague-Dawley rats was associated with decreased basal insulin levels when animals were studied at 3–4, 6–8, or 10–12 months of age. However, it should be noted that, unlike C57B1/6J mice, Sprague-Dawley rats exhibit obesity and hyperinsulinemia early in adulthood (Reaven and Reaven, 1981). Thus, direct comparisons of insulin responses between these two metabolically different rodent models may not be appropriate.

A striking finding of the present study was the elevation of TH activity in adrenals of DR mice. Hypoglycemia is known to be a powerful stimulus for adrenal epinephrine secretion. The lipolytic and glycogenolytic actions of epinephrine result in mobilization of fuels to counteract the hypoglycemia (reviewed by Tepperman and Tepperman, 1987). Adrenal TH activity is increased in response to systemic insulin injections (Ulus and Wurtman, 1979; Fluharty *et al.*, 1983), presumably in response to the concomitant hypoglycemia. Thus, the increase in adrenal TH activity observed in the present study might be expected to result in increased adipose tissue lipolysis through the action of epinephrine. This would counteract the lipogenic effects of the increased circulating insulin resulting in no net change in adipose tissue mass. While acute increases of adrenal TH activity might be expected on the fasting day of an intermittent fasting–refeeding regimen, our results suggest that dietary restriction by intermittent feeding results in chronic upregulation of adrenal TH, since increased TH activity was observed in the fed state, presumably when there is no shortage in the supply of nutrients. Adrenal TH activity may be increased by two fundamental mechanisms: enzyme activation and enzyme induction (Fluharty *et al.*, 1983). Enzyme activation results in a rapid increase in the affinity of TH for its cofactor (Roth *et al.*, 1974) while enzyme induction results in synthesis of new enzyme protein (Mueller *et al.*, 1969). Since the assay used to assess TH activity in the present study measures total enzymatic activity (induction), rather than acute activation of existing enzyme, we hypothesize that the regimen of lifelong dietary restriction by intermittent feeding used in the present study led to persistent upregulation of TH enzyme protein synthesis.

Although there was a strong positive correlation between adrenal TH activity and plasma insulin levels, it is not known whether there is a causal relationship between these two phenomena. Epinephrine infusions result in increased levels of circulating insulin through a β-adrenergic receptor-mediated mechanism, but this is usually observed in the presence of α-adrenergic blockade (Porte and Woods, 1983). On the other hand, insulin increased adrenal TH activity (Ulus and Wurtman, 1979; Fluharty *et al.*, 1983), but this presumably was in response to hypoglycemia, rather than a direct action of insulin on expression of TH activity in adrenal chromaffin cells. In order to investigate the relationship between changes in plasma insulin levels and adrenal TH activity in mice subjected to lifelong regimens of intermittent feeding, it will be necessary to assess insulin and TH activity responses to fasting and refeeding and to assess the time course of changes in these parameters across the life span.

5. SUMMARY

Lifelong dietary restriction by intermittent feeding in C57B1/6J mice results in increased circulating levels of insulin, increased activity of adrenal TH, and histochemical evidence of increased glycogen and lipid deposition in liver when mice are studied after 24 hr of access to food. These findings suggest that lifelong regimens of intermittent feeding are associated with neuroendocrine changes that promote both the production and utilization of glucose.

ACKNOWLEDGMENTS. This work was supported by grants AG07194, AG05445, and NS22103 from the National Institutes of Health. The authors with to express their appreciation for the expert technical assistance of Sally Brown, Jeff Davis, Stephen Hawes, Barbara Schroeder, and Ed Spangler.

REFERENCES

Barrows, C. H., and Kokkonen, G. C., 1978, Diet and life extension in animal model systems, *Age* **1**:131–143.

Bertrand, H. A., 1983, Nutrition–aging interaction: Life-prolonging action of food restriction, in: *Review of Biological Research in Aging* (M. Rothstein, ed.), Liss, New York, pp. 359–378.

Bertrand, H. A., Anderson, W. R., Masoro, E. J., and Yu, B. P., 1987, Action of food restriction on age-related changes in adipocyte lipolysis, *J. Gerontol.* **42**:666–673.

Black, I. B., 1975, Increased tyrosine hydroxylase activity in frontal cortex and cerebellum after reserpine, *Brain Res.* **95**:170–176.

Cohn, C., and Joseph, D., 1970, Effects of caloric intake and feeding frequency on carbohydrate metabolism of the rat, *J. Nutr.* **100**:78–84.

Cooper, J. R., Bloom, F. E., and Roth, R. H., 1986, *The Biochemical Basis of Neuropharmacology*, 5th ed., Oxford University Press, New York.

Fluharty, S. J., Snyder, G. L., Stricker, E. M., and Zigmond, M. J., 1983, Short- and long-term changes in adrenal tyrosine hydroxylase activity during insulin-induced hypoglycemia and cold stress, *Brain Res.* **267**:384–387.

Hazzard, W. R., Crockford, P. M., Buchanan, K. D., Vance, J. E., and Williams, R. H., 1968, A double antibody immunoassay for glucagon, *Diabetes* **17**:179–186.

Ingram, D. K., and Reynolds, M. A., 1987, The relationship of body weight to longevity within laboratory rodent species, in: *Evolution of Longevity in Animals* (A. D. Woodhead and K. H. Thompson, eds.), Plenum, New York, pp. 247–282.

Ip, M., Ip, C., Tepperman, H. M., and Tepperman, J., 1977, Effect of adaptation to meal feeding on insulin, glucagon and the cyclic nucleotide–protein kinase system in rats, *J. Nutr.* **107**:746–757.

Levitt, M., Spector, S., Sjoersdma, A., and Udenfriend, S., 1965, Elucidation of the rate-limiting step in norepinephrine biosynthesis in the perfused guinea-pig heart, *J. Pharmacol. Exp. Ther.* **148**:1–8.

Masoro, E. J., 1984, Nutrition as a modulator of the aging process, *Physiologist* **27**:98–101.

Melvin, J., and Hamill, R. W., 1986, Gonadal hormonal regulation of neurotransmitter synthesizing enzymes in developing hypogastric ganglia, *Brain Res.* **383**:38–46.

Morgan, C. R., and Lazarow, A., 1963, Immunoassay of insulin: two antibody system. Plasma levels of normal, subdiabetic and diabetic rats, *Diabetes* **12**:115–126.

Mueller, R. A., Thoenen, H., and Axelrod, J., 1969, Inhibition of transsynaptically increased tyrosine hydroxylase activity by cycloheximide and actinomycin D, *Mol. Pharmacol.* **5**:463–469.

Porte, D., Jr., and Woods, S. C., 1983, Neural regulation of islet hormones and its role in energy balance and stress hyperglycemia, in: *Diabetes Mellitus, Theory and Practice*, 3rd ed. (M. Ellenburg and N. Rifkin, eds.), Medical Examination Publishing Co., New York, pp. 267–294.

Reaven, E. P., and Reaven, G. M., 1981, Structural and functional changes in the endocrine pancreas of aging rats with reference to the modulating effects of exercise and caloric restriction, *J. Clin. Invest.* **68**:75–84.

Roth, R. H., Salzman, P. M., and Morganroth, V. H., 1974, Noradrenergic neurons: Allosteric activation of hippocampal tyrosine hydroxylase by stimulation of the locus coeruleus, *Biochem. Pharmacol.* **23**:2779–2784.

Smith, P. H., and Davis, B. J., 1983, Morphological and functional aspects of pancreatic islet innervation, *J. Autonomic Nerv. Syst.* **9**:53–56.

Tepperman, J., and Tepperman, H. M., 1987, *Metabolic and Endocrine Physiology*, 5th ed., Yearbook, Chicago.

Ulus, I. H., and Wurtman, R. J., 1979, Selective response of rat sympathetic nervous system to various stimuli, *J. Physiol.* **293**:513–523.

Unger, R. H., Dobbs, R. E., and Orci, L., 1978, Insulin glucagon and somatostatin secretion in the regulation of metabolism, *Annu. Rev. Physiol.* **40**:307–343.

Weindruch, R., Walford, R. L., Fligiel, S., Guthrie, D., 1986, The retardation of aging in mice by dietary restriction: Longevity, cancer, immunity and lifetime energy intake, 1986, *J. Nutr.* **116**:641–654.

Wiley, J. H., and Leveille, G. A., 1970, Influence of periodicity of eating on the activity of adipose tissue and muscle glycogen synthesizing enzymes in the rat, *J. Nutr.* **100**:85–93.

Yu, B. P., Wong, G., Lee, H-C., Bertrand, H. A., and Masoro, E. J., 1984, Age changes in hepatic metabolic characteristics and their modulation by dietary manipulation, *Mech. Aging Dev.* **24**:67–81.

26

Age-Associated Decline in Renal Response to Vasopressin

Diminished Adenylate Cyclase Activation in Collecting Ducts

PATRICIA D. WILSON, MARK A. DILLINGHAM, and
ROBERT J. ANDERSON

1. INTRODUCTION

It has long been known that the ability of the kidney to conserve water can decline quite dramatically in old age (Epstein, 1979). Renal water reabsorption is dependent on the action of arginine vasopressin (AVP) to increase the permeability to water of the apical surface of collecting tubule cells and on the presence of an osmotic gradient to provide the force to facilitate the movement of water out of the tubule into the interstitium. An age-associated renal concentrating defect could be caused by a decline in pituitary release of the hormone, diminished renal interstitial osmolality, or a reduced sensitivity of renal tubule cells of the collecting duct to the action of AVP. Since circulating levels of AVP have been reported unchanged or increased with age (Rowe *et al.*, 1976; Helderman *et al.*, 1978; Miller, 1987), and renal interstitial osmolality has also been reported to increase (Bengele *et al.*, 1981), the present studies were designed to study target tubule cell sensitivity. The effects of age on renal cortical collecting duct sensitivity to AVP were determined by measuring AVP-induced water conductivity and adenylate cyclase activation in isolated rabbit tubules and monolayer cultures of collecting duct epithelia.

PATRICIA D. WILSON • Department of Physiology and Biophysics, UMDNJ-Robert Wood Johnson (formerly Rutgers) Medical School, Piscataway, New Jersey 08854.   MARK A. DILLINGHAM and ROBERT J. ANDERSON • Department of Medicine, University of Colorado Health Science Center and VA Hospital, Denver, Colorado 80220.

2. METHODS

Individual cortical collecting tubules were microdissected, without the use of collagenase or dissociative enzymes, from kidney slices from six young adult (3 months); six "middle-aged" (2.5 years), and six old (4.5 years) New Zealand white rabbits. From each animal, 50 cortical collecting ducts from one kidney were used for tissue culture and four cortical collecting ducts from the contralateral kidney were used for microperfusion studies. For culture, individual collecting ducts were explanted into depressions on glass slides coated with type I collagen (Ethicon, Sommerville, New Jersey) and grown to confluence in fully defined serum-free growth factor-supplemented media according to our previously reported techniques (Wilson and Horster, 1983; Wilson *et al.*, 1987). Monolayer cultures were subjected to hypo-osmotic shock and membrane adenylate cyclase activity, determined using a highly sensitive microassay and [^{32}P]-ATP as substrate (Wilson *et al.*, 1985). Basal activity was compared with activity after incubation in the presence of arginine vasopressin (AVP, 10–250 μU, 10^{-9}–10^{-6} M), cholera toxin (5–1 μg/ml), forskolin (1–25 μM), and after preincubation in media containing pertussis toxin (1 ng–1 μg/ml, 1–24 hr). In addition, binding studies were carried out in which permeabilized cultures from young and old donors were exposed to [^{3}H]-AVP (100 μCi/ml, 66.7 Ci/mM, New England Nuclear) in the presence of 10^{-9} and 10^{-6} M AVP and specific binding determined in the presence of 1000-fold molar excess cold AVP (Cornet and Dorsa, 1986). Cultures were washed extensively with phosphate-buffered saline, extracted with 1 N NaOH, and radioactivity counted by scintillation techniques. Protein was measured according to the method of Lowry *et al.*, (1951). Collecting ducts for microperfusion studies were mounted between micropipets in a lucite perfusion chamber and hydraulic water conductivity determined by measuring the rate of appearance of the impermeant marker [^{14}C]inulin in the collection pipet (Dillingham *et al.*, 1986). Osmotic water flux was determined under basal unstimulated conditions and after incubation in the presence of the agonist AVP (10–250 μU, 10^{-9}–10^{-6} M), cholera toxin (1 μg/ml), forskolin (1–25 μM), and *p*-chlorophenylthio- cyclic adenosine monophosphate (cAMP) (0.2 mM).

3. RESULTS

Figure 1 shows the normal dose response of adenylate cyclase to AVP in confluent cultures of collecting duct epithelia derived from normal young adult rabbit kidneys. Stimulation of activity was seen at 10^{-9} M and was maximal at 10^{-6} M. Similar increases in hydraulic water conductivity (Lp) were seen over this concentration range of AVP with maximal, 6- to 10-fold increases at 250 μU AVP. The effects of age on collecting duct hydraulic conductivity (Lp) and adenylate cyclase activity are shown in Table I. No significant alterations in basal responses were seen, but the response of both hydraulic conductivity and adenylate cyclase to AVP activation was significantly decreased with age. This was most marked in the collecting ducts isolated from old animals, in which adenylate cyclase and hydraulic conductivity responses to AVP were reduced by 76% and 63%, respectively, as compared with the response seen in young adults. In old animals, stimulation above basal levels was only 2.9-fold and 2.5-fold. Intermediate values were seen in the middle-aged group.

Incubation of microperfused tubules in *p*-chlorophenylthio-cAMP stimulated a signifi-

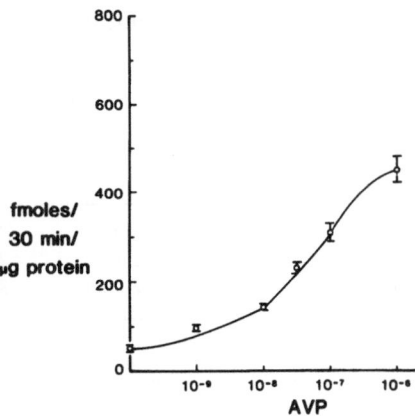

FIGURE 1. Dose response of adenylate cyclase to AVP 10^{-9}–10^{-6} M in confluent cultures of collecting duct epithelia from young rabbits (3 months). Eight cultures were used at each concentration, and six different rabbit preparations were examined. Enzymatic activity was measured on permeabilized cells and expressed as fmoles cAMP generated in a 30-min assay per μg total cell protein.

cant increase in water conductivity in collecting ducts from old rabbits, which was 78% that seen in tubules isolated from young rabbits (Table II).

Figure 2 shows the specific binding of [^{3}H]-AVP to permeabilized collecting duct epithelial cultures in response to low and high doses of AVP. No significant difference in binding was seen in cultures derived from young adult and old rabbits. Incubation of collecting tubules from both young and old rabbits in media containing pertussis toxin, caused a 2.5-fold increase in the basal level of adenylate cyclase activity in cultures derived from young rabbits and a 1.7-fold increase in cultures from old kidneys (Table II). The effects of the potent agonists of adenylate cyclase activity, cholera toxin, and forskolin were much more pronounced in magnitude and with respect to age. Both the degree of adenylate cyclase activity stimulation and hydraulic water conductivity were significantly diminished in collecting tubules from old rabbits (Table II).

4. DISCUSSION

The action of AVP in mammalian renal collecting ducts has been shown to be mediated via cAMP (Imbert *et al.*, 1975). In the studies reported here, a direct correlation was seen

TABLE I. Effects of Age on Collecting Duct Sensitivity to AVP

	Hydraulic conductivity (Lp)[a]		Adenylate cyclase activity[b]	
	Basal	+AVP (250 μU)	Basal	+AVP (10^{-6} M)
Young	21 ± 8	162 ± 10	44 ± 4	462 ± 12
Middle-aged	29 ± 10	119 ± 14	51 ± 14	298 ± 14
Old	15 ± 7	29 ± 8	39 ± 7	101 ± 15

[a]Lp is cm/atm 0.5×10^{-7}.
[b]fmoles cAMP/30 min per μg protein.

TABLE II. Effects of Age on Sensitivity
to AVP Modulators

	% Change vs. basal levels		
	Young	Old	Old/Young (%)
cAMP	757	591	78[a]
Forskolin	5227	679	12[b]
Cholera toxin	843	259	29[a,b]
Pertussis toxin	250	169	68[b]

[a]Hydraulic conductivity (Lp).
[b]Adenylate cyclase activity (fmoles/30 min per μg protein).

between hydraulic water conductivity and adenylate cyclase levels in the absence and presence of varying doses of AVP. Using this combined physiological and biochemical approach, it has also been shown that an increase in age was accompanied by a dramatic decrease in the sensitivity of collecting tubule epithelia to the actions of AVP, as manifested by a significant decline in hydraulic water conductivity and adenylate cyclase activation. Somewhat surprisingly, this decline was already marked before senescence, at 4.5 years, since the maximum life span of these rabbits was approximately 8 years. Presumably, this decline in epithelial sensitivity would be compensated for by increased osmoreceptor sensitivity, vasopressin release, or interstitial osmolality, since these animals did not normally exhibit a significant concentrating defect at this age.

AVP is known to exert its effects on collecting tubules by binding to specific receptors located on the basolateral membranes of principal cells (Campbell et al., 1972), thereby signalling stimulation of the catalytic activity of adenylate cyclase, via G–protein (G_s) interaction, with the net result of elevated levels of cellular cAMP. The resulting phosphorylation of, as yet, ill-determined protein substrates is thought to trigger the insertion of

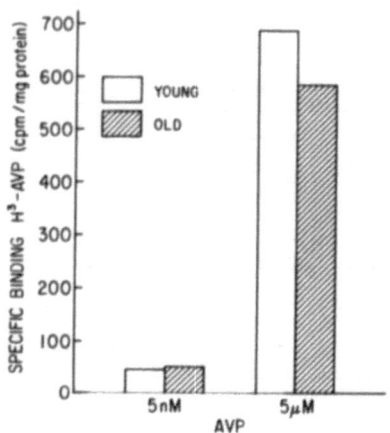

FIGURE 2. Specific binding of 5-nM and 5-μM [³H]-AVP to permeabilized collecting duct epithelial cultures from three young (3 months) and three old (4–4.5 years) rabbits. Specific binding was expressed as cpm above that measured in the presence of excess unlabeled AVP, per mg protein.

water conducting channels into the apical cell membranes (Hays *et al.*, 1987). The age-associated decline in cellular response to AVP was apparently not caused by reduction in receptor density, since no change in specific binding of labeled AVP was demonstrable. However, the age-associated defect was apparently predominantly a pre-cAMP phenomenon since stimulation of water conductivity by a permeable cAMP derivative was >70% of that seen in tubules derived from young rabbits. Since normal regulation of cAMP levels is controlled by receptor–G protein–adenylate cyclase catalytic unit interactions, the age defect might reside at any one or more of these sites. Inhibitory G protein (G_i) interactions were little changed with age, since pertussis toxin, which inactivates G_i by ADP-ribosylation, caused a derepression of adenylate cyclase in old kidney epithelia which was 68% of that seen in the young. However, major differences were seen in the effects of both cholera toxin, which activates G_s, and forskolin, which activates the catalytic subunit of adenylate cyclase (Stryer and Bourne for review; Seaman and Daly, 1981). The actions of both agonists were significantly diminished in renal collecting duct epithelia from old animals.

This suggested that the age-associated decline in AVP sensitivity was caused by a defect in Gs interactions in the membrane receptor–G protein–adenylate cyclase complex.

ACKNOWLEDGMENTS. This work was supported by grant AG06533 from the National Institutes of Health. We wish to thank Ms. Ruth Breckon and Mr. David Hreniuk for their excellent technical assistance.

REFERENCES

Bengele, H. H., 1981, Urinary concentrating defect in the aged rat, *Am. J. Physiol.* **240**:F147–F150.

Campbell, B. J., Woodward, G., and Borberg, V., 1972, Calcium-mediated interactions between the antidiuretic hormone and renal plasma membranes, *J. Biol. Chem.* **247**:6167–6175.

Cornett, L. E., and Dorsa, D. M., 1986, Regulation of [3H]arginine vasopressin binding to the rat renal medulla by guanine nucleotides, *J. Receptor Res.* **6**:127–140.

Dillingham, M. A., Dixon, B. S., Kim, J. K., Wilson, P. D., 1986, Effect of trifluoperazine on rabbit cortical collecting tubular response to vasopressin, *J. Physiol. (Lond.)* **372**:41–50.

Epstein, M., 1979, Effects of aging on the kidney, *Fed. Proc.* **38**:168–172.

Helderman, J. H., Vestal, R. E., Rowe, J. W., Tobin, J. D., Andres, R., Robertson, G. L., 1978, The response of arginine vasopressin to intravenous ethonol and hypertonic saline in man: the impact of aging, *J. Gerontol.* **33**:39–47.

Hays, R., Franki, N., and Ding, G., 1987, Effects of antidiuretic hormone on the collecting duct, *Kidney Int.* **31**:530–537.

Imbert, M., Chabardes, D., Montegut, M., Clique, A., and Morel, F., 1975, Vasopressin dependent adenylate cyclase in single segments of rabbit kidney tubule, *Pfluegers Arch.* **357**:173–186.

Lowry, O. H., Rosenbrough, N. J., Farr, A. L., and Randall, R. J., 1951, Protein measurement with Folin phenol reagent, *J. Biol. Chem.* **193**:265–275.

Miller, M., 1987, Increased vasopressin secretion: An early manifestation of aging in the rat, *J. Gerontol.* **42**:3–7.

Rowe, J., Shock, N., and DeFronzo, R., 1976, Influence of age on the renal response to water deprivation in man, *Nephron* **17**:270–278.

Seamon, K., and Daly, J. W., 1981, Activation of adenylate cyclase by the diterpene forskolin does not require the guanine nucleotide regulatory protein, *J. Biol. Chem.* **256**:9799–9801.

Stryer, L. and Bourne, H. R., 1986, G Proteins: A family of signal transducers, *Annu. Rev. Cell Biol.* **2**:391–419.

Wilson, P. D. and Horster, M. N., 1983, Differential response to hormones of defined distal nephron epithelia in culture, *Am. J. Physiol.* **244**:C166–C174.

Wilson, P. D., Anderson, R. J., Breckon, R. D., Nathrath, W., and Schrier, R. W., 1987, Retention of differentiated characteristics by cultures of defined rabbit kidney epithelia, *J. Cell Physiol.* **130**:245–254.

Wilson, P. D., Dillingham, M. A., Breckon, R., and Anderson, R. J., 1985, Defined human tubular epithelia in culture: Growth, characterization and hormonal response, *Am. J. Physiol.* **248**:F436–F443.

27

Obesity and Lipoproteins

Influence of Weight Reduction in Postmenopausal Women

PETER WEISWEILER

1. INTRODUCTION

Excess body fat adversely affects plasma lipoproteins in humans (Brunzell, 1984). Specifically, obesity results in increased levels of very-low-density lipoproteins (VLDL) and low-density lipoproteins (LDL), which are considered atherogenic, and decreased levels of high-density lipoproteins (HDL), which are considered antiatherogenic (Wolf and Grundy, 1983). Turnover studies of apolipoprotein B, the main constituent of VLDL and LDL, have demonstrated overproduction of hepatic VLDL in obese subjects (Kesäniemi *et al.*, 1985). Furthermore, increased plasma postheparin hepatic triglyceride lipase (HTGL) (Reitmann *et al.*, 1982) and lecithin–cholesterol acyltransferase (LCAT) (Akanuma *et al.*, 1973) activities have been reported. The inverse relationship between HTGL activity and HDL cholesterol levels substantiates the role of this enzyme in the metabolism of HDL (Kuuisi *et al.*, 1980). LCAT contributes to the mobilization of cholesterol from peripheral cells by esterifying free cholesterol contained in HDL (Glomset, 1968). Since VLDL are preferred acceptors for cholesteryl ester (Eisenberg, 1985), one consequence of VLDL overproduction in obesity is thought to be the impairment of cholesterol mobilization (Wallentin and Angelin, 1978).

It is commonly assumed that the metabolic effects of obesity can be reversed by weight loss (Reitmann *et al.*, 1982; Wolf and Grundy, 1983). This study was carried out to determine the patterns of change in plasma lipoprotein lipid and apolipoprotein concentrations, postheparin lipases, and LCAT in obese postmenopausal women during a supervised program of hypocaloric diet and exercise.

2. MATERIALS AND METHODS

2.1. Study Design

Ten women were studied. Their body weights varied from 79.1 to 121.5 kg (105.7 ± 31.1 kg); these weights corresponded to a range of 33.1–42.9 kg/m² (37.6 + 3.3 kg/m²)

PETER WEISWEILER • Metabolic Research Munich, 8000 Munich 5, Federal Republic of Germany.

body mass index (BMI). The program included three dietary periods. Period I lasted 3 weeks, during which time the patients ate a weight-maintenance diet. During period II, total calories were restricted to 600 kcal/day for 3 weeks. A diet calculated to maintain the lower weight then was given for another 6 weeks (period III). The diets were prepared by a dietitian and were given to subjects under supervision. The diets contained 25% of calories as protein, 25% as fat, and 50% as carbohydrate. The polyunsaturated-to-saturated fat ratio was approximately 0.8, and cholesterol intake ranged from 0.15 to 0.25 g/day. Patients were weighed daily; during periods I and III, caloric intakes were adjusted to keep weight to within 2 kg of the weight at the beginning of the periods.

2.2. Analyses

After an overnight fast at the end of each period, blood was drawn into tubes containing 1 g/liter EDTA. The plasma was separated immediately by low-speed centrifugation. VLDL were isolated from plasma by ultracentrifugation (Havel et al., 1955). HDL in the infranate were separated from LDL by precipitation of LDL with heparin manganese chloride (Warnick et al., 1985). Free and total cholesterol and triglycerides were measured enzymatically, using commercially available kits. Plasma apolipoproteins A-I and B were determined by end-point immunonephelometry (Weisweiler et al., 1984).

For the enzyme measurements, the subjects were injected with 100 U/kg porcine heparin. Blood samples were collected before and 20 min after heparin injection. LPL and HTGL activities were quantified using a nonradioisotopic method, as described by Nozaki et al. (1984). In this method, HTGL activity was inactivated by sodium dodecyl sulfate (SDS) before assay of LPL activity. HTGL activity was measured in the presence of 750 mmoles/liter sodium chloride to inactivate LPL activity in the samples. The rate of LCAT activity was determined by a self-substrate method, in which the decrease in free cholesterol is measured enzymatically after incubation of the plasma itself with synthetic dipalmitoyl lecithin sol (Nagasaki and Akanuma, 1977). All analyses were performed in duplicate. Statistical evaluation was performed using the paired Wilcoxon rank test for comparisons between periods.

3. RESULTS

After 3 weeks of caloric restriction (period II), obese subjects had an average weight loss of 8.9 ± 1.5 kg (range: 6.0–10.7 kg), leading to a significant fall in BMI (from 37.6 ± 3.3 to 34.4 ± 3.0 kg/m²; $p < 0.01$). Since individual plasma lipoprotein responses to the diets were similar, the results from all subjects were pooled for analysis. Mean values for all parameters (except the ratio of LDL to HDL cholesterol) were significantly lower after period II than after period I (Table I). At the end of period III, the apolipoprotein B concentration remained lowered, while the HDL cholesterol and apolipoprotein A-I levels increased. The mean HDL cholesterol level significantly exceeded the level of period I (+26.6%). After period III, the mean LDL-to-HDL cholesterol ratio was therefore significantly reduced by 32.5%. In all subjects, mean values for postheparin LPL and HTGL activities and for the molar esterification rate of the LCAT enzyme were significantly lower after period II than after period I (Table II). However, the percentage conversion of free to esterified cholesterol (fractional esterification rate of the LCAT enzyme) did not change significantly after weight loss. At the end of period III, the mean LPL and LCAT activities had increased. The fractional esterifica-

TABLE I. Effects of Weight Reduction in Plasma and Lipoprotein Lipid and Apolipoprotein Concentrations[a]

Parameters	After period I	After period II	After period III
Plasma total cholesterol (mmol/L)	5.51 ± 1.32	4.58 ± 1.16[b]	5.38 ± 1.16
Plasma triglycerides (mmol/L)	2.18 ± 0.90	1.61 ± 0.71[c]	1.66 ± 0.66
VLDL cholesterol (mmol/L)	0.60 ± 0.41	0.36 ± 0.26[c]	0.42 ± 0.23
LDL cholesterol (mmol/L)	4.03 ± 1.11	3.49 ± 1.19[c]	3.84 ± 1.11
HDL cholesterol (mmol/L)	0.88 ± 0.31	0.73 ± 0.18[c]	1.12 ± 0.23[b]
LDL/HDL cholesterol	5.4 ± 3.3	5.1 ± 2.0	3.6 ± 0.5[b]
Apolipoprotein A-I (g/L)	1.20 ± 0.31	0.64 ± 0.19[b]	1.18 ± 0.38
Apolipoprotein B (g/L)	1.28 ± 0.42	1.10 ± 0.32[c]	1.15 ± 0.32[c]

[a]Data are expressed as the mean ± SD (n = 10).
[b]$p < 0.01$ versus period I.
[c]$p < 0.05$ versus period I.

tion rate of the LCAT enzyme was higher after period III than after period I (+38.2%), providing for a significantly elevated mean ratio of esterified cholesterol to free cholesterol in plasma (+21.4%).

4. DISCUSSION

This study examined the effects of weight reduction on plasma lipoprotein concentrations and postheparin lipase and LCAT activities in postmenopausal obese women. All studies were done under metabolic ward conditions, so that the caloric intakes and the composition of the diet could be kept constant.

The fall in plasma lipids during caloric restriction was probably due to a reduction in VLDL synthesis (Olefsky et al., 1974; Grundy et al., 1979). The causes could have been decreased availability of substrate for triglyceride synthesis and/or reduced insulin concentra-

TABLE II. Effects of Weight Reduction on Plasma Postheparin Lipase and LCAT Activities[a]

Parameters	After period I	After period II	After period III
LPL (mmol/L·h)	9.3 ± 4.3	7.4 ± 3.9[b]	10.4 ± 5.9
HTGL (mmol/L·h)	26.3 ± 15.3	16.3 ± 8.3[c]	19.9 ± 15.2[b]
LCAT$_{MER}$ (μmol/L·h)	104.6 ± 62.2	67.2 ± 28.4[b]	132.5 ± 75.5
LCAT$_{FER}$ (%/h)	7.1 ± 4.4	6.1 ± 2.7	10.5 ± 4.0[b]
EC/FC	2.8 ± 0.7	3.0 ± 1.0	3.4 ± 0.8

[a]Data are expressed as the mean ± SD (n = 10). LCAT$_{MER}$ and LCAT$_{FER}$, molar and fractional esterification rates of LCAT, respectively; EC/FC, ratio of esterified cholesterol to free cholesterol in plasma.
[b]$p < 0.05$ versus period I.
[c]$p < 0.01$ versus period I.

tions (Grundy *et al.*, 1979; Wolf and Grundy, 1983; Bosello *et al.*, 1984). Immediately after weight loss, a decline in LDL and HDL cholesterol reportedly occurs (Thompson *et al.*, 1979; Wechsler *et al.*, 1981). Indeed, caloric restriction decreases the input of VLDL into LDL (Kesäniemi and Grundy, 1983). The accompanying fall in plasma apolipoprotein B confirms the reduced turnover rate of these lipoproteins (Ginsberg *et al.*, 1985). However, while the lowered apolipoprotein B levels persisted after stable weight reduction, the possibly adverse alterations in HDL, i.e., the falls in plasma HDL cholesterol and apolipoprotein A-I after the low calorie diet, were temporary (Tokunaga *et al.*, 1982; Wolf and Grundy, 1983; our study). The rise in HDL cholesterol above the initial values and the increase in apolipoprotein A-I to the baseline value after weight stabilization can be explained by a net increase in HDL_2 particles (Albers *et al.*, 1978), accounting to a major extent for the negative correlation between HDL levels and coronary heart disease (Pilger *et al.*, 1983). Together with the reduced ratio of LDL to HDL cholesterol, our results therefore confirm previous data that successful weight loss improve adverse plasma lipoprotein profiles in obese subjects (Wolf and Grundy, 1983).

Further insight into the mechanisms of plasma lipoprotein changes is provided by analysis of the key enzymes of lipoprotein metabolism. The fall in postheparin lipase and LCAT activity after the low-calorie diet resulted from the decline of VLDL overproduction in obesity (Reitmann *et al.*, 1982; Ginsberg *et al.*, 1985; Dieplinger *et al.*, 1985). However, the lowered HTGL activity in most subjects after weight stabilization must be emphasized. The negative relationship to HDL cholesterol levels underlines the major role of this enzyme in HDL metabolism (Applebaum-Bowden *et al.*, 1985). In contrast to LPL activity, HTGL activity does not appear to have regulatory functions in the catabolism of lipoproteins (Reardon *et al.*, 1982). Thus, it is possible that lowering the HTGL enzyme by successful weight reduction positively affects HDL metabolism. The net increase in the percentage conversion of free to esterified cholesterol by the LCAT enzyme must be further emphasized. One abnormality of obesity is the increased transfer of cholesteryl ester from HDL to VLDL, leading to cholesteryl ester-depleted HDL (Eisenberg *et al.*, 1984). After caloric restriction, HDL with normal composition seems to be more capable of transporting cholesterol, together with the LCAT enzyme, from peripheral cells to the liver (Fielding *et al.*, 1983).

5. SUMMARY

The results in obese subjects demonstrate decreased concentrations of the apolipoprotein B-containing plasma lipoproteins and of HTGL activity after stable weight loss. The resulting increase in HDL and in the fractional esterification rate of the LCAT enzyme may be responsible for the antiatherogenic properties of hypocaloric diets in obesity.

REFERENCES

Akanuma, J., Kuzuya, T., Hayashi, M., Ide, T., and Kuzya, N., 1973, Positive correlation of serum lecithin : cholesterol acyltransferase activity with relative body weight, *Eur. J. Clin. Invest.* 3:136–141.

Albers, J. J., Warnick, G. R., and Cheung, M. C., 1978, Quantitation of high density lipoproteins, *Lipids* 13:926–932.

Applebaum-Bowden, D., Haffner, S. M., Wahl, P. W., Hoover, J. J., and Warnick, G. R., 1985,

Postheparin plasma triglyceride lipases. Relationships with very low density lipoprotein triglyceride and high density lipoprotein$_2$ cholesterol, *Arteriosclerosis* **5**:273–282.

Bosello, O., Cigolini, M., Battaggia, A., Ferrari, F., Micciolo, R., Corsato, M., and Olivetti, R., 1984, Interrelationship between serum insulin levels and adipose tissue lipoprotein lipase activity in obesity, in: *Recent Advances in Obesity and Diabetes Research* (N. Melchionda, ed.), Raven, New York, pp. 395–400.

Brunzell, J. D., 1984, Obesity and coronary heart disease. A targeted approach, *Arteriosclerosis* **4**:180–182.

Dieplinger, H., Zechner, R., and Kostner, G. M., 1985, The in vitro formation of HDL$_2$ during the action of LCAT: The role of triglyceride-rich lipoproteins, *J. Lipid. Res.* **26**:273–282.

Eisenberg, S., 1985, Preferential enrichment of large-sized very low density lipoprotein populations with transferred cholesteryl esters, *J. Lipid. Res.* **26**:487–494.

Eisenberg, S., Gavish, D., Oschry, Y., Fainaru, M., and Deckelbaum, R. J., 1984, Abnormalities in very low, low, and high density lipoproteins in hypertriglyceridemia. Reversal toward normal with bezafibrate treatment, *J. Clin. Invest.* **74**:470–482.

Fielding, P. E., Fielding, C. J., Havel, R. J., Kane, J. P., and Tun P., 1983, Cholesterol net transport, esterification, and transfer in human hyperlipidemic plasma, *J. Clin. Invest.* **71**:449–460.

Ginsberg, H. N., Le, N. A., and Gibson, J. C., 1985, Regulation of the production and catabolism of plasma low density lipoproteins in hypertriglyceridemic subjects. Effects of weight loss, *J. Clin. Invest.* **76**:614–623.

Glomset, J. A., 1968, The plasma lecithin: Cholesterol acyltransferase reaction, *J. Lipid. Res.* **9**:155–167.

Grundy, S. M., Mok, H. Y. I., Zech, L., Steinberg, D., and Berman, M., 1979, Transport of very low density lipoprotein triglycerides in varying degrees of obesity and hypertriglyceridemia, *J. Clin. Invest.* **63**:1274–1283.

Havel, R. J., Eder, H. A., and Bragdon, J. H., 1955, The distribution and chemical composition of ultracentrifugally separated lipoproteins in human serum, *J. Clin. Invest.* **34**:1345–1353.

Kesäniemi, Y. A., and Grundy, S. M, 1983, Increased low density lipoprotein production associated with obesity, *Arteriosclerosis* **3**:170–177.

Kesäniemi, J. A., Beitz, W. F., and Grundy, S. M., 1985, Comparisons of metabolism of apolipoprotein B in normal subjects, obese patients, and patients with coronary heart disease, *J. Clin. Invest.* **76**:586–595.

Kuuisi, T., Saarinen, P., and Nikkilä, E. A., 1980, Evidence for the role of hepatic endothelial lipase in the metabolism of plasma high density lipoprotein$_2$ in man, *Atherosclerosis* **36**:589–593.

Nagasaki, T., and Akanuma, G., 1977, A new colorimetric method for the determination of plasma lecithin: cholesterol acyltransferase activity, *Clin. Chim. Acta* **75**:371–375.

Nozaki, S., Kubo, M., Matsuzawa, Y., and Tarni, S., 1984, Sensitive nonradioisotopic method for measuring lipoprotein lipase and hepatic triglyceride lipase in post-heparin plasma, *Clin. Chem.* **30**:749–751.

Olefsky, J., Reaven, G. M., and Farquhar, J. W., 1974, Effects of weight reduction on obesity. Studies of lipid and carbohydrate metabolism in normal and hyperlipoproteinemic subjects, *J. Clin. Invest.* **53**:64–76.

Pilger, E., Pristantz, H., Pfeiffer, K. H., and Kostner, G. M., 1983, Retrospective evaluation of risk factors for peripheral atherosclerosis by stepwise discriminant analysis, *Arteriosclerosis* **3**:57–63.

Reardon, M. F., Sakai, H., and Steiner, G., 1982, Roles of lipoprotein lipase and hepatic triglyceride lipase in the catabolism in vivo of triglyceride-rich lipoproteins, *Arteriosclerosis* **2**:396–402.

Reitmann, J. S., Kosmakos, F. C., Howard, B. V., Taskinen, M. R., Kuusi, T., and Nikkilä, E. A., 1982, Characterization of lipase activities in obese Pima Indians. Decreases with weight reduction, *J. Clin. Invest.* **70**:791–797.

Thompson, P. D., Jeffery, R. W., Wing, R. R., and Wood, P. D., 1979, Unexpected decrease in plasma high density lipoprotein cholesterol with weight loss, *Am. J. Clin. Nutr.* **32**:2016–2021.

Tokunaga, K., Ishikawa, K., and Matsuzawa, Y., 1982, Lipids and lipoproteins during a very-low-calorie diet, *Int. J. Obesity,* **6**:416–418.

Wallentin, L., and Angelin, B., 1978, LCAT in plasma and its relation to lipoprotein concentrations and to kinetics of bile acids and triglycerides in hyperlipoproteinemic subjects, *Scand. J. Clin. Lab. Invest.* **38**:103–110.

Warnick, G. R., Ngyuen, T., and Albers, A. A., 1985, Comparison of improved precipitation methods for quantification of high density lipoprotein cholesterol, *Clin. Chem.* **31**:217–222.

Wechsler, J. G., Hutt, V., Wenzel, H., Klör, H. U., and Ditschuneit, H., 1981, Lipids and lipoproteins during a very-low-calorie diet, *Int. J. Obesity* **5**:325–331.

Weisweiler, P., Schwandt, P., and Friedl, C., 1984, Determination of human apolipoproteins A-I, B and E by laser nephelometry, *J. Clin. Chem. Clin. Biochem.* **22**:113–118.

Wolf, R. N., and Grundy, S. M., 1983, Influence of weight reduction on plasma lipoproteins in obese patients, *Arteriosclerosis* **3**:160–169.

28

Phenotype and Function of Lymphocyte Clones from Old and Young Subjects

ERMINIA MARIANI, PATRIZIA RODA,
ADRIANA RITA MARIANI, MARCO VITALE,
ALBERTO DEGRASSI, STEFANO PAPA,
FRANCESCO ANTONIO MANZOLI, RENÉ VAN DE GRIEND,
and ANDREA FACCHINI

1. INTRODUCTION

Alterations of the immune system during human aging affect different lymphocyte functions. A progressive modification in the distribution of lymphocyte subpopulations in peripheral blood has been described, the major finding being a decrease in circulating T cells after adulthood (Kay and Makinodan, 1981).

These changes have been associated with impaired lymphocyte proliferation after mitogen stimulation *in vitro* (Facchini *et al.*, 1986b). The functional basis of this decline can be explained by a T-cell failure to expand into a pool of proliferating clones and/or the reduced number of mitogen responsive cells (Inkeles *et al.*, 1977).

These data are in agreement with the finding that mitogen-stimulated lymphocyte cultures in the elderly produce a lower amount of interleukin-2 (IL-2) and incorporate less [³H]thymidine than do cultures from young subjects (Mariani *et al.*, 1986a,b; Mariani *et al.*, 1987; Schwab and Weksler, 1987).

In addition, a reduced response in some cytotoxic T lymphocyte (CTL)-dependent reactions has been demonstrated during human aging (Kay and Makinodan, 1981). Lytic activity and the binding capacity of natural killer (NK) cells are also decreased (Herberman *et al.*, 1975; Kiessling *et al.*, 1975), suggesting that in elderly people only a reduced proportion of NK cells is functionally active (Facchini *et al.*, 1986a, 1987). Most studies conducted on

ERMINIA MARIANI, PATRIZIA RODA, ALBERTO DEGRASSI, and ANDREA FACCHINI • Institute Rizzoli, University of Bologna, 40136 Bologna, Italy.   ADRIANA RITA MARIANI, MARCO VITALE, STEFANO PAPA, and FRANCESCO ANTONIO MANZOLI • Institute of Normal Human Anatomy, University of Bologna, 40138 Bologna, Italy.   RENÉ VAN DE GRIEND • Radiobiological Institute, TNO, 2280 HV Rijswijk, The Netherlands.

lymphocyte function during human aging have used bulk cultures that prevent cellular modification being investigated at the single-cell level.

Clonal expansion of human T and NK cells with well-defined functional activity has become an important tool in the study of cells involved in immune response; a limiting dilution assay has been developed to clone human lymphocytes at very high efficiency (Van de Griend *et al.*, 1984).

In this technique, the interaction between cellular and humoral factors is sustained by the addition of irradiated feeder cells and exogenous IL-2. As a consequence, the frequency of clone formation is entirely dependent on a single population of clone-forming cells; selected clones must be multiplied to permit further characterizations, as proliferative capacity and differentiation patterns of cloned cells descendants.

In this study, we used a cloning technique to estimate the frequency of proliferating T-lymphocyte precursors (PTL-p) in peripheral blood lymphocytes (PBL). This procedure is well suited for determination of the effect of age on PTL-p because the deficiency in IL-2 production can be overcome. The frequency of PTL-p, the proliferative ability of clone-forming cells, and the functional activity of grown clones were analyzed in young and old subjects. A decreased number of proliferating precursors, associated with a reduced functional activity, was demonstrated in CD8+ and CD16+ clones derived from old subjects.

2. MATERIAL AND METHODS

2.1. Subjects

Old and young healthy subjects were selected according to the SENIEUR protocol (Lightart *et al.*, 1984). All subjects were outpatients, considered healthy on the basis of clinical and biochemical findings; none was taking any drugs known to affect the immune system.

2.2. Lymphocyte Separation

Peripheral blood lymphocytes were isolated from the blood of healthy donors by centrifugation on Ficoll–Hypaque density gradient.

2.3. Tumor Cell Lines

Two Epstein–Barr virus (EBV) transformed B cell (B-LCL) lines (APD and BSM) were maintained in culture with RPMI 1640 (pH 7.4), buffered with bicarbonate and 10% supplemented heat-inactivated fetal calf serum (FCS), 2 mM glutamine, and 100 IU/ml penicillin-streptomycin.

K562 (myeloid cell line) and P815 (mastocytoma cell line) were cultured in RPMI 1640 buffered with HEPES (25 mM) and supplemented with 10% FCS, 2 mM glutamine, and 100 IU/ml penicillin-streptomycin.

2.4. Cloning and Expansion Technique

Lymphocytes were plated after separation in 96-well round-bottomed microtiter plates in limiting dilution at concentrations of 3000, 1000, 300, 100, 30, 10, 3, and 1 cell/well in presence of feeder cells. As a feeder source, 2×10^4 PBL and 10^4 allogenic EBV-transformed B-LCL (APD and BSM) were added to each well after 3000-rad irradiation.

Culture medium RPMI 1640, buffered with HEPES (25 mM), was supplemented with 10% fresh pooled human serum, 4 mM glutamine, 1 μg/ml leukoagglutinin, 1 μg/ml indomethacin, penicillin-streptomycin, and 5% IL-2 from supernatant cultures of mitogen-stimulated mononuclear cells.

After about 11 days, wells with growing cells were transferred to new wells in fresh medium with new feeder cells; about 1 week later, the clones were selected and expanded for further investigation by subculturing them each week in microtiter wells, starting with 1000–2000 responder cells/well and a mixture of fresh feeder cells as described above (Van de Griend et al., 1984).

The frequency of proliferating cells per well was calculated from the proportion of negative wells, using the chi-square minimization method suggested by Taswell (1981).

The number of viable cells in positive wells was measured by a hemocytometer. Cells were only enumerated in positive wells with more than an 80% probability of having originated from a single cell, as calculated from the proportion of negative wells by Poisson statistics (Lefkovits and Waldmann, 1979).

2.5. Cryopreservation of Clones in Liquid Nitrogen

Cells were frozen at several time intervals in 1-ml samples using a computer-controlled freezing program with a freezing rate of 1°C/min to −30°C and 5°C/min to −120°C. $1–5 \times 10^6$ cells were resuspended in FCS and dropwise diluted on ice with an equal volume of RPMI with 20% of dimethylsulfoxide (DMSO). After freezing, the vials were maintained in liquid nitrogen for different periods.

2.6. Proliferative Capacity

The mean growing rate of the clones was evaluated by two methods: (1) by calculating the multiplication factor per week of each clone on the basis of the cells seeded/well on the starting culture day; (2) by evaluating [³H]thymidine uptake after 18-hr incubation of a constant number of cells (9000 cells/well in triplicate) after 1 week's culture.

2.7. Phenotype Characterization

Each clone phenotype was determined using a panel of monoclonal antibodies (MoAb): Leu1 (CD5), Leu2a (CD8), Leu3a (CD4), Leu7, and Leu11c (CD16) (Becton Dickinson, Mountain View, California); 50,000–100,000 cells were incubated in a V-bottom microtiter plate with a MoAb for 30 min at 4°C; the percentage of positive cells was analyzed by means of a flow cytometer (FACS IV Becton Dickinson, Mountain View, California) (Mariani et al., 1984).

2.8. Functional Analysis

Cytolytic clone activity was tested against different cell lines as targets: K562, NK-susceptible line; P815 pretreated with immunoglobulin (IgG)-specific fraction for antibody-dependent cellular cytotoxicity (ADCC); and nontreated P815 cells for specific lysis. The cytotoxicity assay was performed in V-bottom microtiter plates. Varying numbers of effector cells in 100-μl RPMI-HEPES with 10% FCS, and 50 μl of ^{51}Cr-labeled target cells (5 × 10^3/well) were seeded in triplicate. After centrifugation at 4°C, the plates were incubated for 3 hr at 37°C in 5% CO_2. Thereafter, plates were centrifuged again, 75 μl of supernatant was harvested, and ^{51}Cr release was determined with a gamma counter.

The results were expressed as follows: (test counts − spontaneous counts)/(maximum counts − spontaneous counts) × 100% (Ortaldo *et al.*, 1977).

3. RESULTS

The frequency of proliferating T-lymphocyte percursors was estimated in the peripheral blood from old and young donors. All points were determined from a minimum of 32 to a maximum of 288 cultures at each density of responder cells/culture for each subject examined. The mean frequency of proliferating precursors in young peripheral lymphocytes was 1/142 (range: 1/112–1/186) compared with 1/416 (range: 1/154–1/627) for cells from the elderly.

The effect of adding of leukoagglutinin to the culture medium only slightly influenced the frequency of precursors in old subjects. By contrast, precursor frequency from the young dropped by about 25% (data not shown) when the medium was depleted of leukoagglutinin.

Most of the microcultures studied had a high probability of being clonal (mean $p = 0.93$ ± 0.06 standard error (SE), according to Poisson statistics) and were therefore assumed to be clonal proliferations. To evaluate the proliferative capacity of clones with different phenotype, we cultured 6 CD8$^+$, 4 CD4$^+$, and 1 CD16$^+$ clones from the old group and 4 CD8$^+$, 9 CD4$^+$, and 1 CD16$^+$ clones from the young group, for a maximum of 4 weeks.

Clones with CD4$^+$ phenotype showed the highest multiplication factor per week, while CD8$^+$ clones presented the lowest growing rate. When these data on proliferative capacity were expressed considering the growing rate of clones from young people as 100% (Fig. 1a), CD4$^+$ and CD16$^+$ clones presented similar values in the two groups, while CD8$^+$ clones derived from old subjects presented a growing rate of about 50%. The results obtained from [^{3}H]thymidine uptake (Fig. 1b), confirmed a lower growing rate of CD8$^+$ clones derived from aged lymphocytes.

A total of 62 clones were also examined by phenotypical and functional analysis: 35 CD5$^+$ CD4$^+$ CD8$^-$ clones (12 from elderly, 23 from young people), 11 CD5$^+$ CD4$^-$ CD8$^+$ clones (6 from old, 5 from young), 16 CD5$^+$ CD4$^-$ CD8$^-$ CD16$^+$ clones (8 from old and 8 from young).

CD4$^+$ clones from both groups did not show any functional activity against any cell line used as target (K562, P815-IgG), while CD8$^+$ and CD16$^+$ were cytolytic.

CD8$^+$ clones from old people presented a decreased cytotoxic activity against K562 and IgG-coated P815 cell lines compared with CD8$^+$ clones from young people and this was particularly evident in some target–effector ratios (Fig. 2a,b). Similar results were also obtained analyzing the functional activity of CD16$^+$ clones (Fig. 3a,b). No cytotoxicity was observed against P815 cells uncoated with specific IgG (data not shown).

4. DISCUSSION

In this study, we have investigated the proliferative capacity and cytolytic activity of T and NK lymphocytes derived from the peripheral blood of young and old subjects. Cells were

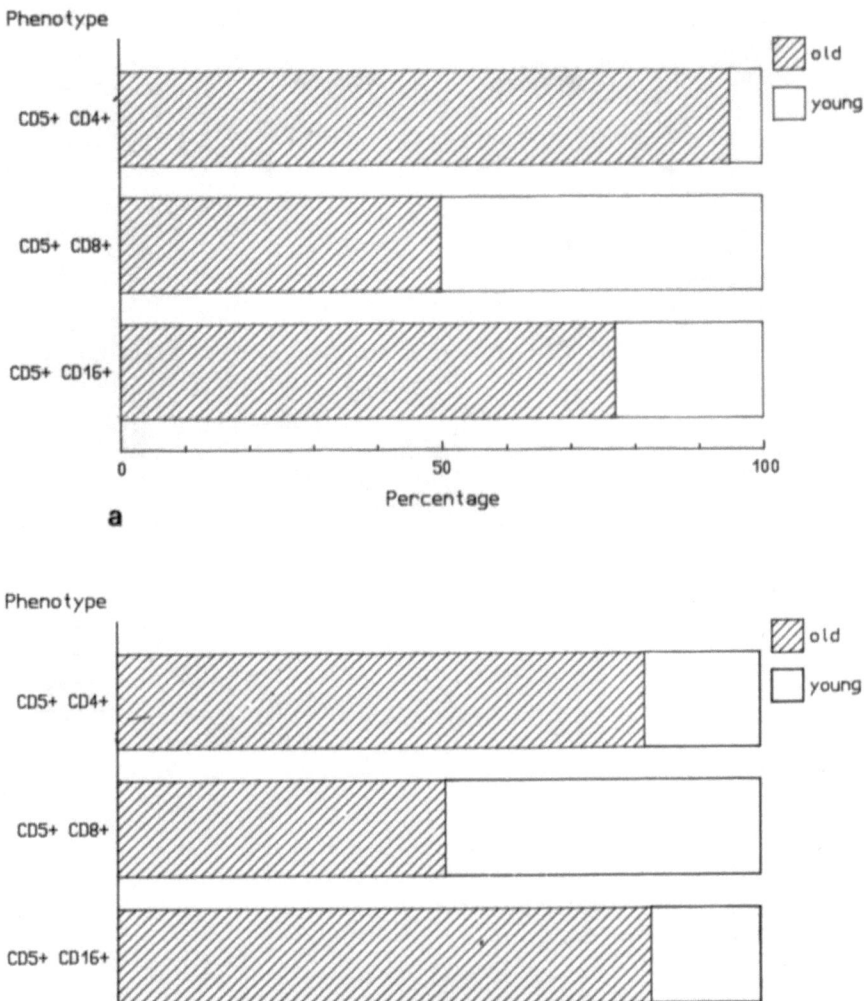

FIGURE 1. Proliferative capacity of clones with different phenotype. (a) Multiplication factor per week. (b) [³H]thymidine uptake. All young subjects are considered 100%.

cultured in a limiting dilution assay that permits quantitative estimation of proliferating and functional precursors in the cloned populations. T and NK cell clones were also tested for their ability to lyse K562 cells and P815 cells in the ADCC assay.

Some investigators have examined age-associated changes in precursor frequencies of old mice, finding a diminished number of precursor cells, but no impairment of functional activity in each precursor cell (Miller and Harrison, 1987).

These data on the mouse partially agree with our results and those of other groups

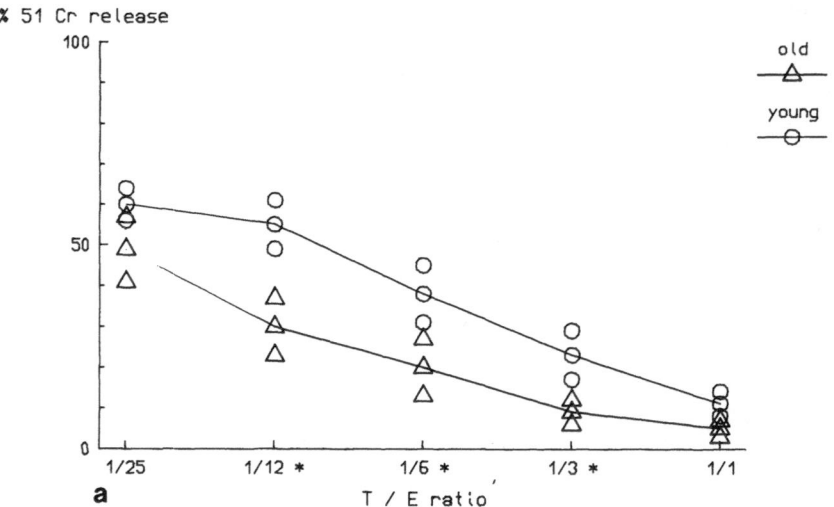

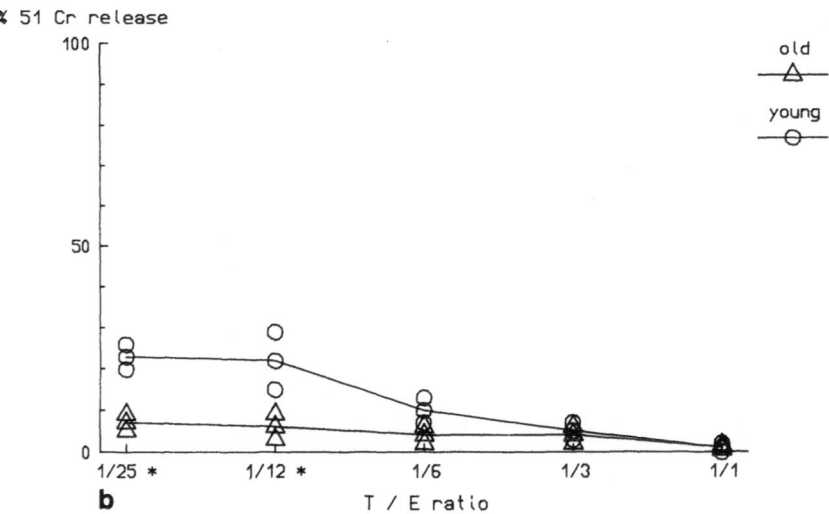

FIGURE 2. Cytolytic activity of CD5+ CD4− CD8+ clones against (a) K562 and (b) P815-IgG (ADCC) cell lines. Asterisk (*) $p < 0.05$.

showing diminished clone formation in the elderly due to a defective number of precursors, both when cells were cultured in soft agar and in limiting dilution assay (Adler *et al.*, 1982; Chrysostomou *et al.*, 1984).

Despite the decreased frequencies of proliferating T-lymphocyte precursors in all our preparations derived from elderly cells compared with those of young subjects, many of the microcultures that proliferated displayed cytolytic activity either against the K562 target or in the ADCC assay.

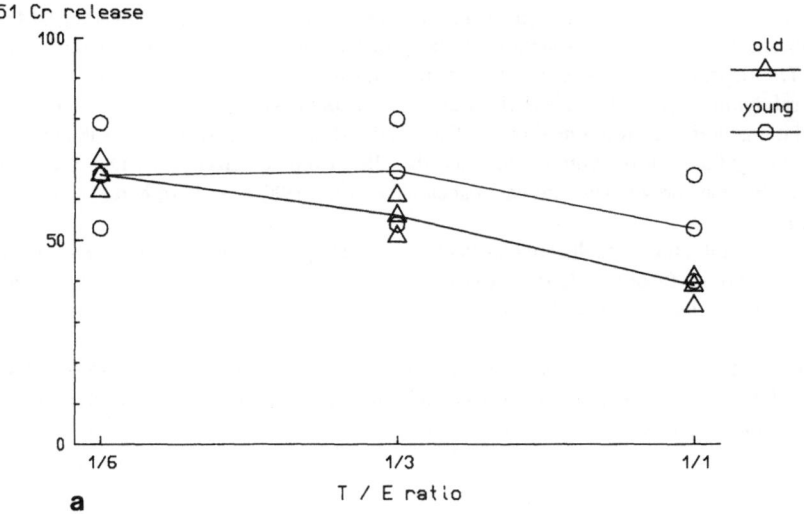

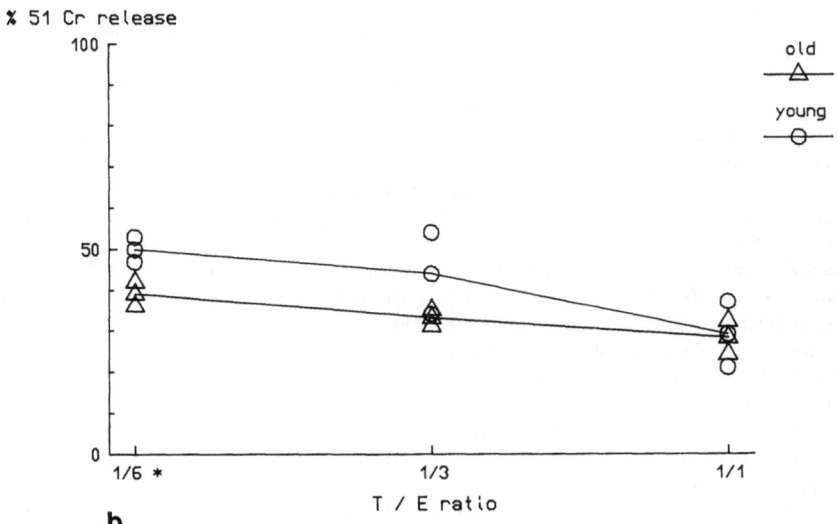

FIGURE 3. Cytolytic activity of CD5+ CD4- CD8- CD16+ clones against (a) K562 and (b) P815- IgG (ADCC) cell lines. Asterisk (*) $p < 0.05$.

The PTL-p frequency of old lymphocytes is markedly decreased as compared with young PBL and was less influenced by the presence of leukoagglutinin in the medium. This finding confirms the reduced capacity of T cells from elderly subjects to respond to mitogens and a drop in cell division after activation in culture.

Clones derived from young subjects seem to be more sensitive to the absence of lectin in their proliferation, although the number of membrane receptors for PHA has been demonstrated to be similar in lymphocytes from old and young people. These data suggest that the membrane-cytoplasmic transduction of the proliferation signal is impaired during aging.

The depressed cytotoxic T-cell response and the decreased NK activity found in peripheral lymphocytes of the elderly were also evident when we analyzed homogeneous populations deriving from one clone. CD8+ and CD16+ clones of the old subjects showed less activity than did the young ones, and the NK cytotoxic activity of CD16+ clones was similar to that previously shown (Facchini et al., 1987) in peripheral Le11+-sorted lymphocytes.

As a whole, these results are consistent with the hypothesis that the decline in functional cytotoxic activity (T or NK dependent) found in the peripheral blood of aged subjects persists after in vitro selection when these cells are analyzed at a clonal level.

ACKNOWLEDGMENTS. This work was supported by grants from the National Research Council (CNR) P. F. "Medicina preventiva e riabilitativa" SP2 Meccanismi di invecchiamento and was made within the framework of Eurage.

REFERENCES

Adler, S. J., Morley, A. A., and Seshadri, R. S., 1982, Reduced lymphocyte colony formation with age, Clin. Exp. Immunol. 49:129–133.

Chrysostomou, A., Seshadri, R., and Morley, A. A., 1984, Decreased cloning of lymphocytes from elderly individuals, Scand. J. Immunol. 19:293–296.

Facchini, A., Mariani, E., Mariani, A. R., Papa, S., Vitale, M., and Manzoli, F. A., 1986a, NK cells during human ageing, in: Immunoregulation in Ageing, Vol. 9 (A. Facchini, J. J. Haaijman, and G. Labò, eds.), Topics in Ageing Research in Europe, Eurage Series, The Hague, pp. 227–237.

Facchini, A., Mariani, E., and Pazzaglia, M., 1986b, Immunological changes during ageing, IRCS Med. Sci. 14:859–862.

Facchini, A., Mariani, E., Mariani, A. R., Papa, S., Vitale, M., and Manzoli, F. A., 1987, Increased number of circulating Leu11c+ (CD16) large granular lymphocytes and decreased NK activity during human ageing, Clin. Exp. Immunol. 68:340–347.

Herberman, R. B., Nunn, M. E., and Larvin, D. H., 1975, Natural cytotoxic reactivity of mouse lymphoid cells against syngeneic and allogeneic tumors. 1. Distribution of reactivity and specificity, Int. J. Cancer, 16:216–229.

Inkeles, B., Innes, J. B., Kuntz, M. M., Kadish, A. S., and Weksler, 1977, Immunological studies of ageing. 3. Cytokinetic basis for the impaired response of lymphocytes from aged humans to planct lectins, J. Exp. Med. 145:1176–1187.

Kay, M. M. B., and Makinodan, T., 1981, Relationship between aging and the immune system, Prog. Allergy 29:139–181.

Kiessling, R., Klein, E., Pross, H., and Winzell, H., 1975, Natural killer cells in the mouse. 2. Cytotoxic cells with specificity for mouse Moloney leukemia cells. Characteristics of the killer cells, Eur. J. Immunol. 6:117–121.

Lefkovits, I., and Waldmann, H., 1979, Limiting dilution analysis of the cells of the immune system. 1. The clonal basis of the immune response, Immunol. Today 5:265–268.

Lightart, G., Corberand, J. X., Fournier, C., Galanoud, P., Hijmans, W., Kennes, B., Muller-Hermelink, H. K., and Steinmann, G. G., 1984, Admission criteria for immunogerontological studies in man: The SENIEUR protocol, Mech. Aging Dev. 28:47–55.

Mariani, E., Facchini, A., Miglio, F., Mazzetti, M., Leupers, T., Gasbarrini, G., Labò, G., and Astaldi, A., 1984, Analysis with OKT monoclonal antibodies of T lymphocytes subsets present in blood and liver of patients with chronic active hepatitis, Liver 4:22–28.

Mariani, E., Mariani, A. R., Mingari, M. C., Sinoppi, M., and Facchini, A., 1986a, Lymphokine production in normal old subjects, in: *Immunoregulation in Ageing,* Vol. 9 (A. Facchini, J. J. Haaijman, and G. Labò, eds.), Topics in Ageing Research in Europe, Eurage Series, The Hague, pp. 101–108.

Mariani, E., Mariani, A. R., Vitale, M., Papa, S., Manzoli, F. A. and Facchini, A., 1986b, Effect of interferon gamma (IFN-gamma) on NK activity in the elderly, *Mod. Trends Aging Res.* **147:**243–248.

Mariani, E., Mariani, A. R., Roda, P., Sinoppi, M., and Facchini, A., 1987, IFN-gamma production in elderly subjects, *Fed. Proc.* **46:**1090.

Miller, A. R., and Harrison, D. E., 1987, Clonal analysis of age associated changes in T cell reactivity, in: *Aging and the Immune Response: Cellular and Humoral Aspects* (E. A. Goidl, ed.), Dekker, New York, pp. 1–26.

Ortaldo, J. R., Bonnard, G. D., and Herberman, R. B., 1977, Cytotoxic reactivity of human lymphocytes cultured in vitro, *J. Immunol.* **119:**1351–1355.

Schwab, R., and Weksler, M., 1987, Cell biology of the impaired proliferation of T cells from elderly humans, in: *Aging and the Immune Response: Cellular and Humoral Aspects* (E. A. Goidl, ed.), Dekker, New York, pp. 67–80.

Taswell, C., 1981, Limiting dilution assay for the determination of immunocompetent cell frequencies. 1. Data analysis, *J. Immunol.* **126:**1614–1619.

Van de Griend, R. J., Van Krimpen, B. A., Bol, S. J. L., Thompson, A., and Bolhuis, R. H. L., 1984, Rapid expansion of human cytotoxic T cell clones: Growth promotion by a heat-labile serum component and by various types of feeder cells, *J. Immunol. Meth.* **66:**285–298.

29

Caloric Restriction and Longevity

RICHARD WEINDRUCH

1. INTRODUCTION

Studies in experimental animals (usually mice or rats) show that dietary restriction (DR) of caloric intake, but without essential nutrient malnutrition, generates many desirable biological outcomes (see Holehan and Merry, 1986; Masoro, 1988; Walford et al., 1987; Weindruch and Walford, 1988). In rodents, caloric restrictions of 30–70% reduce the incidence and delay the onset of many late-life diseases. The rates of change for almost all the age-sensitive biological parameters tested to date are slowed by DR. These effects of DR on rodents are unmatched by competitor methods. As a result, rodents subjected to DR are widely viewed as the best model available to study the biology of decelerated aging in homeothermic vertebrates.

Caloric restriction extends average and maximum life span in diverse species. Figure 1 shows survival curves from DR studies in four species: *Tokophyra* (a protozoan), *Daphnia* (the water flea), *Rattus* (the rat), and *Lebistes* (the guppy). The maximum life spans (10th decile survivals) were increased by DR by 40–85% in the first three species and by 5% in *Lebistes* (the guppies were on DR only for the first third of life). The present comments briefly highlight parts of an extensive collaborative analysis of DR retardation of aging and disease (Weindruch and Walford, 1988).

2. STUDIES IN INVERTEBRATES

Most of the work on DR in invertebrates was carried out during 1915–1965. These studies show that life-span extension by DR is phylogenetically widespread; therefore, DR is not merely a better diet for overfed underactive rodents in cages. In addition to *Tokyphyra* and *Daphnia* (Fig. 1), underfeeding is associated with increased longevity in rotifers, nematodes, *Drosophila*, mollusks, and spiders.

RICHARD WEINDRUCH • Biomedical Research and Clinical Medicine Program, National Institute on Aging, National Institutes of Health, Bethesda, Maryland 20892.

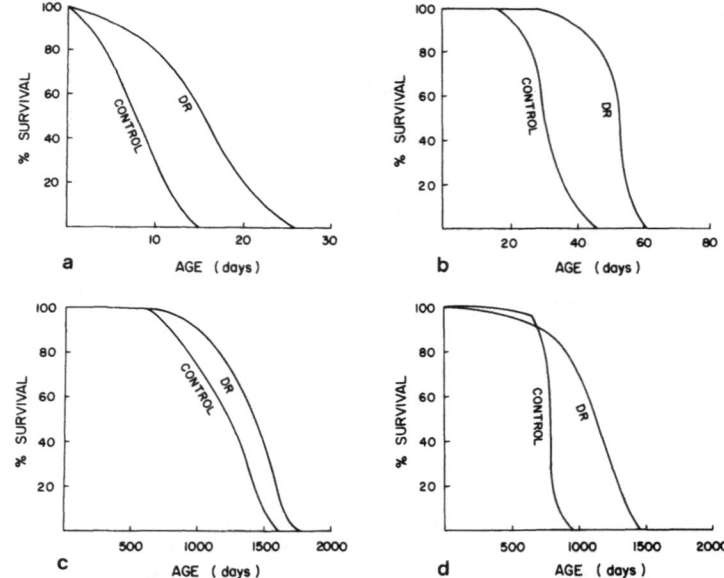

FIGURE 1. Survival curves for dietary restriction (DR) and control animals from four species. (a) Curves approximated from data of Rudzinska (1952) for *Tokophyra* (a protozoan). (b) Survival of *Daphnia* (a water flea) using the data of Ingle *et al.* (1937). (c) Survival of *Lebistes* (guppy) as studied by Comfort (1963). (d) Data for *Rattus* (the rat) reported by Yu *et al.* (1982). (From Weindruch and Walford, 1988.)

3. STUDIES IN VERTEBRATES

Mice and rats have been studied in the vast majority of DR longevity experiments. Most of these investigations tested early-onset DR, which retarded growth rates and delayed puberty onsets. Although less studied, adult-onset DR is far more relevant from the perspective of potential human use. The effect of DR on the longevity of primates is untested.

3.1. Early-Onset Dietary Restriction

In rodents, DR begun early in life (usually 3–6 weeks of age) slows the actuarial aging rate and/or decreases the population's initial vulnerability to mortality. The very longest life spans (50–55 months) have been observed in mice fed diets enriched in essential nutrients but in severely restricted amounts, with caloric intakes and peak body weights of DR animals being only 30–50% of those of controls. Figure 2 shows that for female mice of the long-lived C3B10RF$_1$ hybrid strain, the more severe the DR, the longer the life span. Likewise, longevity is increased by early-onset DR in short-lived disease-prone strains of mice and rats.

3.2. Adult-Onset Dietary Restriction

Caloric restriction first started in midadulthood can also increase longevity (Fig. 3) and often the results approach those of early-onset DR (Table I). It appears that much of the life-

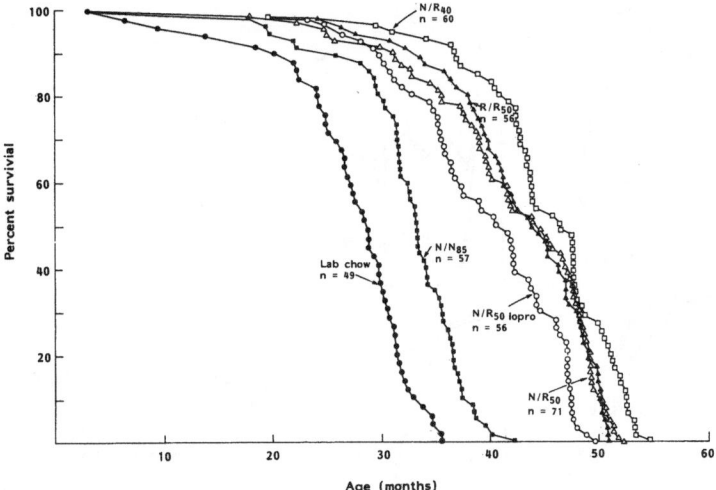

FIGURE 2. Influences of early-onset dietary restriction (DR) on the survival of C3B10RF$_1$ female mice. Each symbol represents an individual mouse. Diet groups: Lab Chow, Purina Lab Chow *ad libitum;* N/N$_{85}$, fed normally before and after weaning, postweaning diet fed at 85 kcal/week (25% less than *ad libitum*); N/R$_{50}$, fed normally before weaning, restricted postweaning to 50 kcal/week; R/R$_{50}$, restricted in feeding level both before and after weaning; N/R$_{50lopro}$, restricted after weaning to 50 kcal/week with a decrease with age in the protein content of the diet; N/R$_{40}$, restricted after weaning to 40 kcal/week. (From Weindruch *et al.*, 1986.)

span extension via DR does not depend on interrupting maturation. Studies in short-lived, disease-prone rodent strains show that adult-onset DR can retard the course of pre-existing disease (Good and Gajjar, 1986). Knowledge about age-sensitive biological measures in animals started on DR at or beyond mid-adulthood is largely limited to indexes of immune system aging and most of these stay "younger longer" with underfeeding.

TABLE I. Three Longevity Studies Testing Both Early- and Adult-Onset Dietary Restriction[a]

			Average life span[c]				Maximum life span[d]			
Investigators	Animal	Onset[b]	C	EDR[b]	ADR[b]	A:E	C	EDR[b]	ADR[b]	A:E
Cheney *et al.* (1983)	B10C3F$_1$ mice	1, 14	36	43	39	0.91	41	50	45	0.90
Yu *et al.* (1985)	F344 rats	1.5, 6	23	35	31	0.89	27	41	39	0.95
Beauchene *et al.* (1986)	Wistar rats	1, 12	31	38	35	0.92	39	46	41	0.89

[a]Adapted from Weindruch and Walford (1988).
[b]Onset (in months) for early-onset DR (EDR) and adult-onset DR (ADR) groups.
[c]Values are in months. C gives values for controls. A:E gives the ratio for the life spans of the ADR:EDR groups.
[d]The value given is the average life span (in months) for each group's longest-lived 10%.

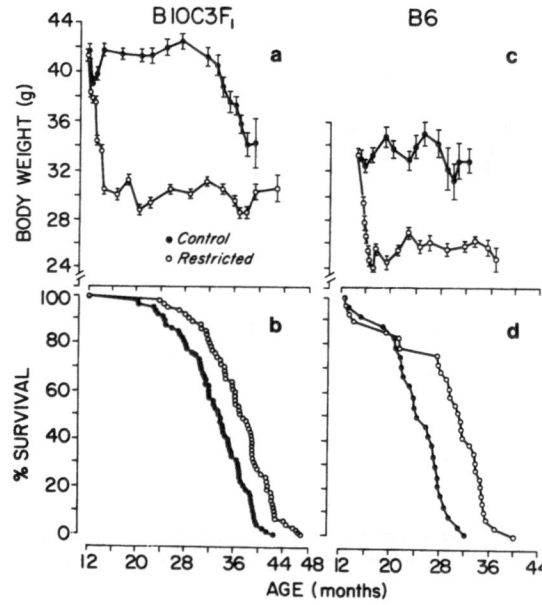

FIGURE 3. Body weights and survival curves of B10C3F$_1$ mice (a,b) and B6 mice (c,d) fed control or adult-onset dietary restriction (DR) diets. DR started at 12 months of age. Each point in the survival curves represents one male mouse. (From Weindruch and Walford, 1982.)

4. CONCLUDING QUESTIONS

Two major questions now face investigators of DR:

1. What is the mechanism whereby DR exerts its multisystem and multiprocess effects? Does DR work by affecting a single root process that causes aging, or are multiple factors involved? The fact that only dietary *energy restriction* retards aging in mammals suggests that effects on energy metabolism may underlie some of the actions of DR. Future work on mechanisms behind the effect of DR must do more than show by ever more advanced procedures that DR animals are functionally younger.
2. What is the effect of DR on the aging rate of primate species? This question has never been carefully asked but is the central issue of one recently started project and of others being planned.

Quite likely, question #2 will be much easier to answer. By the conclusion of the twentieth century there will likely be substantial information on the rate of aging in food-restricted monkeys and significant findings in humans (e.g., epidemiologic data on relationship of caloric intake, disease incidence, and longevity in various populations). Question #1 provides a far more complex challenge largely because the basic aging processes that DR must be affecting are as yet unidentified.

REFERENCES

Beauchene, R. E., Bales, C. W., Bragg, C. S., Hawkins, S. T., and Mason, R. L., 1986, Effect of age of initiation of feed restriction on growth, body composition, and longevity of rats, *J. Gerontol.* **41**:13–19.

Cheney, K. E., Liu, R. K., Smith, G. S., Meredith, P. J., Mickey, M. R., and Walford, R. L., 1983, The effect of dietary restriction of varying duration on survival, tumor patterns, immune function, and body temperature in B10C3F$_1$ mice, *J. Gerontol.* **38**:420–430.

Comfort, A., 1963, Effect of delayed and resumed growth on the longevity of a fish (*Lebistes reticulatus*, Peters) in captivity, *Gerontologia* **8**:150–155.

Good, R. A., and Gajjar, A. J., 1986, Diet, immunity and longevity, in: *Nutrition and Aging* (M. L. Hutchinson and H. N. Munro, eds.), Academic, Orlando, Florida, pp. 235–249.

Holehan, A. M., and Merry, B. J., 1986, The experimental manipulation of ageing by diet, *Biol. Rev.* **61**:329–368.

Ingle, L., Wood, T. R., and Banta, A. M., 1937, A study of longevity, growth, reproduction and heart rate in *Daphnia longispina* as influenced by limitations in quantity of food, *J. Exp. Zool.* **76**:325–352.

Masoro, E. J., 1988, Food restriction in rodents: An evaluation of its role in the study of aging, *J. Gerontol.* **43**:B59–64.

Walford, R. L., Harris, S., and Weindruch, R., 1987, Dietary restriction and aging: Historical phases, mechanisms, current directions, *J. Nutr.* **117**:1650–1654.

Weindruch, R., and Walford, R. L., 1982, Dietary restriction in mice beginning at one year of age: Effects on lifespan and spontaneous cancer incidence, *Science* **215**:1415–1418.

Weindruch, R., and Walford, R. L., 1988, *The Retardation of Aging and Disease by Dietary Restriction,* Charles C. Thomas, Springfield, Illinois.

Weindruch, R., Walford, R. L., Fligiel, S., and Guthrie, D., 1986, The retardation of aging by dietary restriction: Longevity, cancer, immunity and lifetime energy intake, *J. Nutr.* **116**:641–654.

Yu, B. P., Masoro, E. J., Murata, I., Bertrand, H. A., and Lynd, F. T., 1982, Life span study of SPF Fischer 344 male rats fed ad libitum or restricted diets: Longevity, growth, lean body mass, and disease, *J. Gerontol.* **37**:130–141.

30

Effect of Dietary Linolenate on the Pathogenesis of Fever

E. KENEDI and D. MENDELSOHN

1. INTRODUCTION

The effects of a reduction in the level of arachidonic acid $20:4(\omega6)$ by increases in linoleic acid $18:2(\omega6)$ and/or linolenic acid $18:3(\omega3)$ in a febrile condition, induced by gram-negative bacterial pyrogens, are unknown. Yet it is recognized that endotoxin fever in humans and rabbits is arachidonate dependent (Spawinski *et al.*, 1978). It is also recognized that increasing amounts of linolenate, $18:3(\omega3)$, reduce the metabolites of linoleic acid, $18:2(\omega6)$ (Machlin, 1962; Mohrhauer and Holman, 1963; Rahm and Holman, 1964; Anding and Hwang, 1986) by acting as a competitor for the same cyclo-oxygenase (Pace-Asciak and Wolfe, 1968), thereby not only influencing the formation of arachidonic acid but suppressing its metabolites as well. The metabolites of arachidonic acid have been implicated in the biochemical sequences leading to fever induced by bacterial endotoxin (Feldberg and Saxena, 1975; Milton, 1976; Skarnes *et al.*, 1981). Therefore, deficiency in arachidonic acid diminishes the fever response (Kenedi *et al.*, 1984), which, in the course of constant stimulation by endotoxin, leads to tolerance of the fever (Atkins, 1960; Kanoh *et al*, 1977). The physiological consequences of tolerance in the body, induced by increased intake in linolenate, together with chronic induction of fever, have not been associated with a diseased condition, as the biochemical mechanism leading to tolerance had been unknown until the present study. According to Bernheim *et al.* (1979), a "true" fever is a disorder of thermoregulation in which the body actively seeks to raise its temperature by increasing heat production (Bernheim *et al.*, 1979). Heat is the result of oxidative catabolism in the body, and there is a relationship between the amount of O_2 absorbed and the amount of CO_2 eliminated (Benedict, 1907; Fritz, 1961).

Excessive unsaturation of plasma by $18:2(\omega6)$ and $18:3(\omega3)$ induced by increased dietary linolenate results in decreased oxygenation (Stadie, 1945), which, coupled with increased phosphorylization (Stadie, 1945; Marco *et al.*, 1961), stimulates CO_2 production

E. KENEDI and D. MENDELSOHN • Department of Chemical Pathology, School of Pathology, Medical School, University of the Witwatersrand; and The South African Institute for Medical Research, Johannesburg 2000, Republic of South Africa.

via the long-chain fatty acids (Fritz, 1961). Heat is thus gained mainly by a change in the respiratory quotient (R.Q.), which in turn increases the body temperature (Harper, 1967). This illustrates both the biochemical importance and the physiological role of the essential fatty acids (Burr and Burr, 1930; Friedman, 1979). Excess or lack of the latter could impair R.Q. in such a way as to influence the body's mechanism for gaining or losing heat. Thus, body temperature depends on the equilibrium between unsaturated and polyunsaturated fatty acids. Fluctuation in the concentration of $18:2(\omega6)$ can thus alter the equilibrium between thermolysis and thermogenesis. Body temperature, which is the index of the resultant two factors, can be affected by either (Benedict, 1915). An increase in body temperature can therefore be equated with increased R.Q. induced by excessive formation of $18:2(\omega6)$ and the development of fever with rapid oxidation of polyunsaturates (eicosanoids) (Fritz, 1961), provided R.Q. remains constant.

Therefore, a deficiency in $20:4(\omega6)$ and its metabolites (Hwang and Carrol, 1980) in spite of an abundance in essential fatty acids, combined with chronic induction of fever, could contribute to a physiopathological condition that is diet-induced and not recognized. As lecithin constitutes 70% of human phospholipids (Frederickson and Gordon, 1958) and is rich in both unsaturated and polyunsaturated fatty acids, changes in essential fatty acids causes greater alterations in this class of lipids than in either free fatty acids or triglycerides (Ogburn et al., 1982).

The present work has been undertaken to clarify the effects of an increased intake in dietary linolenate on the specific distribution of fatty acids and consequently on the production of fever induced by gram-negative bacterial endotoxin and the pathological consequences of this alteration in thermoregulation.

2. MATERIALS AND METHODS

2.1. Experimental Model

Ten white New Zealand (NZ) rabbits weighing 2.20–2.80 kg were divided into two groups. Group A (N = 5), designated the control, received the standard commercial diet of rabbit pellets (Table I). Its fatty acid content included 50% linoleic acid. Group B (N = 5) received the standard diet supplemented with hay and contained fatty acids comprising 65% linoleic acid and 48% linolenic acid (Table II). Water was available to all rabbits ad lib. Both groups were injected once daily intravenously (IV) with 2.0 µg/kg body mass of the endotoxin Salmonella thyphosa for 7 days.

The animals were housed individually in stainless steel cages and kept on a 12-hr–12-hr photophase–scotophase regimen. To minimize the effect of sudden stress during the experimental period, the animals were acclimatized to their restraining boxes and to thermocouples for 1 week before the start of the experiment. Each animal was weighed daily before being given its injection and again 180 min thereafter.

2.2. Endotoxin

Purified lipopolysaccharide of S. thyphosa 0901 (Difco 3124-25-6) was suspended in pyrogen-free saline at 1.0 mg/ml and stored at −15°C. This stock solution was further diluted daily to a concentration of 15 µg/ml. Of this, 0.35 ml containing 5 µg endotoxin was injected daily into the marginal ear vein of each rabbit, giving the required quantity of 2.0 µg/kg endotoxin.

TABLE I. Composition of Standard
Commercial Diet

Composition	Normal maintenance diet
Fat	5% corn oil
Protein	20% milk powder (vitamin free)
Fiber	4% cellulose
Carbohydrate	64% sucrose
Salt	4% salt mix[a]
Vitamin mix	2%[b] (ICN Pharmaceuticals)

[a]As recommended by Jones and Foster (1942).
[b]ICN Pharmaceuticals, Inc. (Cleveland, Ohio) g/kg, vitamin A 90.2000 IU, vitamin D 100.000 IU, α-tocopherol 1.5 g, ascorbic acid 45.0 g, inositol 1.0 g, choline chloride 75.0 g, p-aminobenzoic acid 5.0 g, niacin 4.5 g, pyrodoxin hydrochloride 1.0 g, thiamine hydrochloride 1.0 g, calcium pentotenate 3.0 g, vitamin B_{12} 1.4 g, biotin 20.0 mg, folic acid 90.0 mg.

2.3. Temperature Measurements

The rectal temperature was measured using copper constant thermocouples covered with polyethylene tubing and inserted into the rectum to a depth of $\simeq 100$ mm. All thermocouples were calibrated by immersion in water against a certified mercury thermometer. Temperature measurement was accurate to within 0.2°C. The output from each thermocouple was recorded at 10-min intervals for 1 hr before and 3 hr after every injection, using a Solomat thermometer, model 335K (Ballainvillers, France). The temperature was compared with that

TABLE II. Fatty Acid Composition
of Rabbit Standard Diet and Hay Diet

Fatty acid	Standard diet[a]	Hay diet[a]
Unidentified	0.04	3.40
14:0	0.27	2.38
14:1	0.10	1.29
16:0	16.50	15.78
16:1	0.67	1.22
18:0	1.98	2.55
18:1	27.94	2.30
18:2 (ω6)	50.87	14.70
18:3 (ω3)	—	48.30
22:0	0.63	1.97
20:4 (ω6)	—	0.04
24:0	0.60	3.40
22:5 (ω6)	0.40	2.30

[a]Values are the mean of two lipid extractions expressed as a percentage of the respective fatty acids.

prevailing before the injections. All experiments were carried out at an ambient room temperature of $21° ± 1°C$.

2.4. Blood Sampling

Blood samples of 1.0–2.0 ml were drawn from the ear artery of each rabbit with a butterfly needle (21-gauge) into heparinized (vacutainer) tubes before the start of the experiment (baseline) and again at 60 min and 180 min after the first and seventh injections, respectively. Shortly after collection, the blood samples were centrifuged for 10 min at 1800 rpm. The resultant serum supernatant was centrifuged for a second time to remove any remaining blood cells. The serum was flushed with N_2 and stored at $-20°C$ for fatty acid analysis. Three control rabbits (group A) were injected with saline alone. Their temperatures were measured and serum lecithin fatty acids analyzed to eliminate any interference from the carrier solvent (Fig. 1, Table III). Two rabbits died during the course of the experiment; measurements for these two rabbits are not included in the results.

2.5. Extraction of Fatty Acids from Solid Food

Pulverized rabbit pellets of 2.50 g or hay were macerated in 32.0 ml 15% KOH in ethanol; the mixture was allowed to saponify overnight at 60°C. After cooling, 12.0 ml distilled water was added, mixed, and divided into four 11.0-ml aliquots. To each aliquot, 9.50 ml petroleum ether (40–60°C) was added, mixed on a vortex mixer for 60 sec, and the

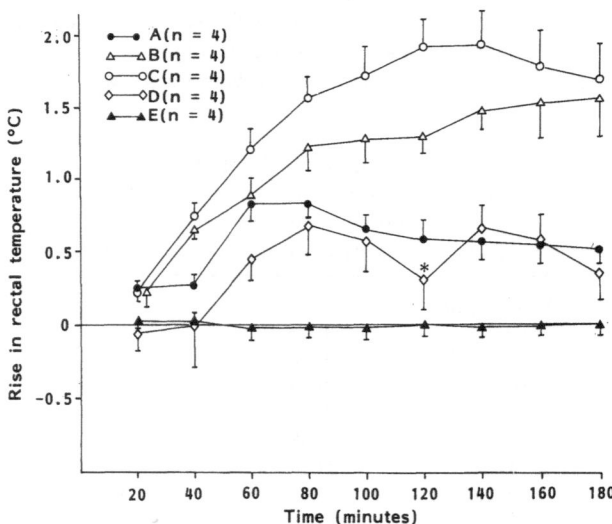

FIGURE 1. Rise in the rectal temperature in conscious rabbits following a single or seven consecutive intravenous (IV) injections of 2.0 µg/kg *S. thyphosa* (endotoxin). Each point represents a mean of four rabbits; error bars indicate SE ±SEM. (●) Single injection in rabbits on standard diet ($N = 4$). (△) Single injection in rabbits on hay-supplemented diet ($N = 4$). (○) Seven consecutive IV injections in standard diet group ($N = 4$). (◇) Seven consecutive IV injections in hay-supplemented group ($N = 4$). (▲) Pyrogen-free saline 0.35 ml alone ($N = 4$).

TABLE III. Effect of a Single Dose of Intravenous
Saline Injection at 180 min[a]

| Fatty acid | Group A[a] | |
	Control	Saline
16:0	24.07 ± 0.15	26.36 ± 1.00
18:0	15.38 ± 0.58	15.36 ± 0.40
18:1 (ω9)	15.99 ± 0.62	16.61 ± 0.63
18:2 (ω6)	30.96 ± 0.77	28.35 ± 0.63
18:3 (ω3)	0.76 ± 0.04	0.70 ± 0.70
18:3 (ω6)	0.40 ± 0.03	0.36 ± 0.05
20:3 (ω6)	0.40 ± 0.03	0.32 ± 0.04
20:4 (ω6)	3.97 ± 0.19	3.42 ± 0.04
20:5 (ω6)	0.64 ± 0.03	0.46 ± 0.17
22:4 (ω6)	1.20 ± 0.11	1.70 ± 0.29
22:5 (ω6)	3.94 ± 0.27	3.85 ± 0.13
Unidentified polyunsaturate	2.34 ± 0.28	2.21 ± 0.23

[a]Values represent the relative percentage of fatty acids measured on gas–
liquid chromatography (GLC) and the average of three determinations. Test
SE ± SEM of three rabbits.
[b]Group A control on standard diet.

resulting supernatant centrifuged (model TG 6 refrigerated centrifuge, Beckman Instruments, Palo Alto, California) at 3000 rpm for 5 min. The supernatant layer containing the non-saponifiable portion was then decanted. This extraction procedure was repeated twice.

The residue remaining from the rabbit pellets or hay was acidified to a pH of 2.0 with 3.75 ml concentrated HCl. The fatty acids were recovered by the addition of 9.50 ml petroleum ether (40–60°C) mixed on a vortex for 30 sec, and centrifuged as above for 5 min. The extracts were combined into one fraction. This recovery procedure was repeated twice. The pooled extract was dried over Na_2SO_4, and the solvent evaporated to dryness under N_2. The extracted total lipids were saponified and methylated the same way as serum fatty acids, the resultant fatty acid methyl esters were dissolved in 100 μl hexane and analyzed on a gas chromatograph (Packard 427) (see Table II).

2.6. Extraction of Serum Lipids

Serum of 0.20 ml was extracted with 1.0-ml AR grade MeOH–CHCl$_3$ (1:1, v/v) for 10 min by gentle stirring. After standing for 5 min at room temperature, the mixture was centrifuged for 10 min at 3000 rpm and the supernatant decanted into a clean test tube. The residue was further extracted with MeOH–CHCl$_3$ (1:1) following the same procedure. After separation of the two phases with 0.1 M NaCl, the CHCl$_3$ phase subnatant was filtered through solvent-washed filter paper (Whatman No. 1), dried under N_2 at 50°C, and immediately dissolved in 100 μl CHCl$_3$.

2.7. Thin-Layer Chromatographic Separation of Phospholipids

The 100 μl extracted lipid was separated on precoated silica gel G-plastic baked plates 20 × 20 cm, 0.25-mm layer (Machery-Nagel) prewashed in MeOH–CHCl$_3$ (1:1) and activated for 1 hr at 100°C. The solvent system CHCl$_3$–MeOH–CH$_3$COOH (glacial)–H$_2$O (50 : 25 : 7 : 1), (v/v) was used for the separation of phospholipid classes. After drying and exposure to iodine vapor, the lecithin fraction was outlined and the thin-layer chromatography (TLC) plate redried at 100°C for 15 min to remove the iodine.

2.8. Saponification and Methylation of Lecithin

The lecithin fraction was scraped off into a clean test tube, saponified, and methylated by the addition of 1.0 ml MeOH in 2.0 ml 0.2 M sodium methylate (CH$_3$NaO) in MeOH for 20 min in a 50°C water bath with frequent shaking. After cooling with 4.0 ml H$_2$O, the methyl esters were extracted twice with 1.0 ml hexane. The separated hexane layer was transferred to a clean test tube and evaporated under N$_2$ at 60°C. The plasma lecithin fatty acid methyl esters were dissolved in 100 μl hexane, capped in glass vials, and stored at −20°C until analyzed.

2.9. Gas Chromatography

A Packard 427 gas chromatograph fitted with a flame ionization detector and a glass column measuring 1.8 m × 4 mm (internal diameter) packed with 10% SP 2330 on 100/100 chromasorb WAW was used for the separation of the fatty acid methyl esters. The samples were run at 200°C with a carrier gas (N$_2$) flow rate of 25 ml/min. Both the detector heater and injector were set at 220°C. The fatty acid methyl esters were identified using retention volumes of known GLC standard Pufa-2, NHIF, RM3, 68A (animal source, Supelco, Inc., Bellefonte, Pennsylvania). Peak areas were measured using an SP 4100 (Spectrophysics) integrator.

3. RESULTS

3.1. Influence of Hay on Plasma Lecithin Fatty Acid Composition

The results shown in Table IV indicate that within 1 week, increased dietary linolenate affected the interrelationship between the unsaturated and polyunsaturated fatty acids. Prior to the fever experiment, an increase in levels of 18 : 2(ω6), 18 : 3(ω3), and 20 : 5(ω3) followed by a decrease in 20 : 4(ω6) was observed, together with an absence of 22 : 4(ω6) and 22 : 5(ω6).

3.2. Effect of Endotoxin on Fever Response and on the Composition of Serum Lecithin Fatty Acids

3.2.1. Single Dose of Endotoxin

A difference between the two groups in their response of fever to a single dose of endotoxin (2.0 μg/kg body mass) became apparent. In group A, the endotoxin produced a short monophasic fever with a delay of 20 min before its onset. Fever peaked after 60 min and had a duration of 80 min. In group B, the endotoxin evoked a magnified biphasic fever with the same delay to its onset as group A, but with its first peak at 80 min and a second at 140

TABLE IV. Effect of a Single Intravenous Injection of 2.0 μg/kg Endotoxin S. *thyphosa* on the Composition of Serum Lecithin Fatty Acid in Rabbits Fed Standard or Hay-Supplemented Diet[a]

Fatty acid	Group A[b]			Group B[c]		
		Postinjection			Postinjection	
	Preinjection	60 min	180 min	Preinjection	60 min	180 min
16:0	24.07 ± 1.15α	26.11 ± 2.37α	27.01 ± 1.92α	22.27 ± 1.44α	21.05 ± 1.61α	19.06 ± 1.74α
18:0	15.38 ± 0.58α	12.76 ± 1.36α	13.40 ± 0.74α	20.91 ± 0.35β	21.70 ± 0.50β	21.85 ± 0.67β
18:1 (ω9)	15.99 ± 0.62α	18.97 ± 1.38α	14.36 ± 1.15α	14.90 ± 1.68α	13.82 ± 1.62α	13.85 ± 1.02α
18:2 (ω6)	30.96 ± 0.77α	26.83 ± 0.48β	32.17 ± 0.43α	32.39 ± 0.91α	34.72 ± 0.17β	36.40 ± 0.93β
18:3 (ω3)	0.76 ± 0.04α	0.75 ± 0.04α	0.90 ± 0.03α	1.52 ± 0.44β	0.85 ± 0.12α	0.94 ± 0.08α
18:3 (ω6)	0.40 ± 0.03α	0.27 ± 0.05α	0.35 ± 0.05α	0.73 ± 0.13α	0.63 ± 0.11α	0.70 ± 0.22α
20:3 (ω6)	0.40 ± 0.03α	0.27 ± 0.04α	0.38 ± 0.01α	0.70 ± 0.17α	0.45 ± 0.06β	0.55 ± 0.08α
20:4 (ω6)	3.97 ± 0.19α	2.63 ± 0.35α	3.94 ± 0.71α	1.82 ± 0.40β	2.65 ± 0.38α	3.34 ± 0.21α
20:5 (ω3)	0.64 ± 0.03α	0.46 ± 0.09α	0.69 ± 0.18α	3.80 ± 0.98β	3.22 ± 0.38β	2.80 ± 0.30β
22:4 (ω6)	1.20 ± 0.11	1.96 ± 0.28	1.64 ± 0.20	—	—	—
22:5 (ω6)	3.94 ± 0.27	3.75 ± 0.31	2.90 ± 0.13	—	—	—
Rest. Poly.	2.34 ± 0.28α	2.71 ± 0.31α	1.42 ± 0.36α	0.62 ± 0.21β	0.76 ± 0.11β	0.88 ± 0.12β

[a]Values represent the relative percentage of fatty acids measured by gas–liquid chromatography (GLC) and the average of four or five determinations. β indicates significantly different from control (<0.05) ($p > 0.05$) by Duncan multiple range. Test SE ±SEM.
[b]Standard diet, $N = 4$.
[c]Hay-supplemented diet, $N = 5$.

min, and a duration of several hours (see Fig. 1). Changes in the serum lecithin fatty acid composition appear to coincide with alteration in the fever pattern.

In group A, decrease in the level of all the unsaturates and of the polyunsaturates $20:3(\omega6)$, $20:4(\omega6)$, $22:5(\omega6)$ occurred within minutes, together with an increase in $22:4(\omega6)$. No change in $20:5(\omega3)$ in the plasma levels occurred (Table IV). The return to normal in most of the fatty acids at 180 min coincided with the termination of the fever (Table IV).

In group B, an increase in levels of $18:2(\omega6)$ and $20:4(\omega6)$ occurred within minutes, followed by a decrease of the linolenate $18:3(\omega3)$ $18:3(\omega6)$, together with reduced levels of $20:3(\omega6)$ and $20:5(\omega3)$ while both docosatetraeonic acid $22:4(\omega6)$ and docosapentaeonic acid $22:5(\omega6)$ remained inhibited. These changes suggest heightened degree of lipolysis and decreased unesterification of fatty acids within the plasma (Table IV).

3.2.2. Multiple Doses of Endotoxin

The fever response by the seventh day to daily IV injections of endotoxin further emphasized the difference between the two groups. In group A, a monophasic fever was again evoked with increased magnitude and extended duration beyond 180 min (Fig. 1). This is reflected in the serum lecithin fatty acid composition (Table V). An increase in levels of $18:2(\omega6)$ and $20:4(\omega6)$, and a decrease in $22:4(\omega6)$ at 180 min indicates increasing combustion of fatty acids to meet increasing energy demands under the action of endotoxin (Table V). This did not affect the body temperature, which returned to normal at the end of each experiment (Fig. 2).

Conversely, in group B, the change in the pattern of fever by the seventh injection (see Fig. 1) resulted in a decrease in the size of the second fever peak. The characteristic retention of the first peak was not reversed even by the administration of a second injection at 120 min. This suggests that the animals had been made immune to the action of bacterial pyrogen not only by its continual administration (Fig. 1), but more so by the deficiency in the production of $20:4(\omega6)$ induced by increased intake in dietary $18:3(\omega3)$ (Tables IV and V). Tolerance to endotoxin in these animals did not prevent the rise in body temperature (Fig. 2), which

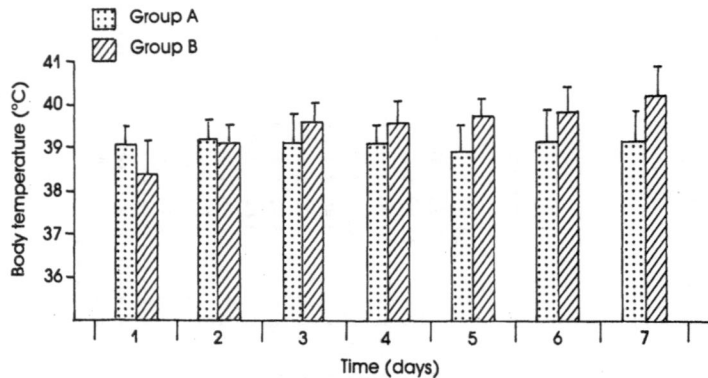

FIGURE 2. Body temperature of rabbits before injection of endotoxin *S. thyphosa*. Group A fed on standard diet ($N = 4$). Group B fed on hay-supplemented diet ($N = 4$). Error bars indicate SE ±SEM.

TABLE V. Effect of Seven Consecutive Intravenous Injections of 2.0 μg/kg Endotoxin S. thyphosa on the Composition of Serum Lecithin Fatty Acid in Rabbits Fed Standard or Hay-Supplemented Diet[a]

Fatty acid	Group A[b]			Group B[c]		
		Postinjection			Postinjection	
	Preinjection	60 min	180 min	Preinjection	60 min	180 min
16:0	22.98 ± 2.64α	25.90 ± 0.72α	23.17 ± 1.35α	20.37 ± 1.35α	20.60 ± 1.79α	19.91 ± 3.16α
18:0	15.73 ± 1.63α	13.12 ± 0.72α	14.14 ± 1.51	22.02 ± 1.94α	21.19 ± 2.98α	20.88 ± 1.90α
18:1 (ω9)	15.05 ± 0.95α	18.91 ± 1.64α	16.42 ± 1.92α	14.82 ± 1.71α	14.82 ± 1.71α	12.90 ± 1.99α
18:2 (ω6)	31.72 ± 0.77α	30.06 ± 0.33α	34.57 ± 0.92α	34.74 ± 1.65α	34.07 ± 0.72β	37.27 ± 0.26β
18:3 (ω3)	0.94 ± 0.03α	0.63 ± 0.02α	0.80 ± 0.09α	1.50 ± 0.52β	1.01 ± 0.18β	0.92 ± 0.26α
18:3 (ω6)	0.28 ± 0.06α	0.33 ± 0.06α	0.36 ± 0.06α	0.65 ± 0.16α	0.66 ± 0.25α	0.49 ± 0.31α
20:3 (ω6)	0.24 ± 0.05α	0.37 ± 0.07α	0.31 ± 0.07α	0.56 ± 0.18α	0.58 ± 0.20α	0.42 ± 0.15α
20:4 (ω6)	3.15 ± 0.53α	2.64 ± 0.69α	3.71 ± 0.38α	1.79 ± 0.08β	1.99 ± 0.59α	2.49 ± 0.48α
20:5 (ω3)	0.76 ± 0.17α	0.42 ± 0.04α	0.51 ± 0.10α	2.31 ± 0.55β	1.96 ± 0.64β	3.93 ± 0.40β
22:4 (ω6)	2.38 ± 0.45	1.19 ± 0.01	1.62 ± 0.34	—	—	—
22:5 (ω6)	4.47 ± 0.45	2.69 ± 0.01	3.26 ± 0.60	—	—	—
Rest. Poly.	2.03 ± 0.57	2.60 ± 0.45	1.53 ± 0.14	—	—	—

[a] Values represent the relative percentage of fatty acids measured by gas–liquid chromatography (GLC) and the average of four determinations in each group. Test SE ±SEM of four rabbits. β indicates significantly different from control (<0.05) (p > 0.05) by Duncan multiple range.
[b] Standard diet, N = 4.
[c] Hay-supplemented diet, N = 5.

increased daily from $39.2 \pm 0.05°C$ to $40.25 \pm 0.09°C$, and occurred simultaneously with an increase in levels of $18:2(\omega 6)$. This finding further supports the contention that essential fatty acids are involved in thermoregulation and polyunsaturates in endotoxin-induced fever.

4. DISCUSSION

Under normal physiological conditions, biochemical changes introduced by the diet and their effect on serum lipid composition can go unobserved. Under changed physiological conditions that are sensitive to differences in the amounts of arachidonic acid, absence of, excessive, or imbalanced arachidonic synthesis in the tissue can lead to irreversible pathological changes. As these changes are not recognized, they cannot be diagnosed clinically. In the present study, the existence of a sensitive balance between $18:2(\omega 6)$ and $18:3(\omega 3)$ is clearly defined by an abnormal response of fever to a single dose of endotoxin on the one hand, and the rabbit's tolerance to endotoxin within 7 days on the other, together with a gradual rise in the body temperature. This in turn governs the equilibrium between $18:(\omega 6)$ and $20:4(\omega 6)$. A change in this balance appears to influence not only the prognosis of fever but also the body temperature. A fall in levels of $18:2(\omega 6)$ and $20:4(\omega 6)$ under the stimulus of endotoxin indicates that fever is produced by the metabolites of arachidonic acid. Heat is thus mainly gained by peripheral polyunsaturates provided that R.Q. remains constant. However, if body heat is increased by either $18:2(\omega 6)$ or $18:3(\omega 3)$, or both, it is followed by a decrease in the formation of not only serum $20:4(\omega 6)$ but of cerebral arachidonite as well (Kenedi and Mendelsohn, unpublished results), thereby significantly increasing CO_2 production and in turn altering R.Q. (Splawinski *et al.*, 1978).

Since metabolism (R.Q.) and heat production go hand in hand (Benedict, 1907) in increasing oxidative catabolism by way of either $18:2(\omega 6)$ or $18:3(\omega 3)$, or both, increased peroxidation (Stadie, 1945; Marco *et al.*, 1961) and an alteration in the cerebral mitochondrial function occurs in the course of increasing intake in dietary linolenate (Marco *et al.*, 1961).

Thus, fluctuation in levels of $18:2(\omega 6)$ due to endotoxin influences the pattern of fever, which in turn indicates whether fever is centrally or peripherally initiated. It also defines the existence of tolerance to endotoxin in animals rendered resistant to the pyrogenic action of a bacterial pyrogen within a short time by the combination of increased amounts of $18:3(\omega 3)$ and regular induction of small doses of endotoxin. Two different mechanisms can be differentiated: (1) initiation by peripheral arachidonic acid and its metabolites, which induce fever; and (2) hyperthermia induced by peripheral $18:2(\omega 6)$ and $18:3(\omega 3)$. These results can therefore be regarded as further evidence that polyunsaturates are actively involved in the induction of fever.

Linoleic and linolenic acids appear to be involved in thermoregulation. A change in the thermoregulatory process reflects the rise or fall in the body temperature and can therefore be considered a change in the life process accompanied by increased or decreased heat production (Benedict, 1915). In the present study, an increase in body temperature can therefore be equated with increased heat production induced by an increased concentration of $18:2(\omega 6)$, in turn induced by an increase of $18:3(\omega 3)$ in the diet. Under the stimulus of *S. thyphosa,* the fever had less effect on the body temperature.

REFERENCES

Anding, R. H., and Hwang, D., 1986, Effect of dietary linolenate on the fatty acid composition of brain lipids in rats, *Lipids* **41:**697–701.

Atkins, E., 1960, Pathogenesis of fever, *J. Physiol. Rev.* **40**:580–646.

Benedict, F. G., 1907, Influence of inanitition on the metabolism, *Carnegie Inst. Wash.* **77**:96–101.

Benedict, F. G., 1915, A study on prolonged fasting. Carnegie Inst. Publ. No. 23.

Bernheim, H. A., Block, L. H., and Atkins, E., 1979, Fever: Pathogenesis, pathophysiology and purpose. *Ann. Intern. Med.* **91**:261–270.

Burr, G., and Burr, M., 1930, The nature and the role of fatty acids essential in nutrition, *J. Biol. Chem.* **86**:587–621.

Feldberg, W., and Saxena, P., 1975, Prostaglandins, endotoxin, and lipid A on body temperature, *J. Physiol.* **249**:601–615.

Frederickson, D. S., and Gordon, R. S., 1958, Transport of fatty acids, *Physiol. Rev.* **38**:585–630.

Friedman, Z., 1979, Polyunsaturated fatty acids in low-birth-weight infants, *Semin. Perinatol.* **3**:341–361.

Fritz, I. B., 1961, Factors influencing the rate of long chain fatty acid oxidation and synthesis of mammalian system, *Physiol. Rev.* **41**:52–129.

Harper, H. A., 1967, *Review of Physiological Chemistry*, Lange Medical, Los Altos, California, pp. 464–468.

Hwang, D. H., and Carrol, A. E., 1980, Decreased formation of prostaglandins derived from arachidonic acid by dietary linolenate in rats, *J. Clin. Nutr.* **63**:67–74.

Jones, J. H., and Foster, C. J., 1942, Salt mixture for use with basal diet either low or high in phosphorus, *Nutrition* **24**:245–256.

Kanoh, S., Nishio, A., and Kawasaki, H., 1977, Studies on the pyrogenic tolerance to bacterial lipopolysaccharide in rabbits, *Biken J.* **20**:69–75.

Kenedi, E., Norton, G., Abrahams, O., Mitchell, D., and Laburn, H., 1984, The role of arachidonic acid in fever, in: *Prostaglandins and Leukotrienes, Washington, D.C.* (abst.).

Machlin, L. J., 1962, Effect of dietary linolenate on the proportion of linoleate and arachinodate, *Nature (Lond.)* **194**:868–869.

Marco, G. J., Machlin, L. J., Emery, E., and Gordon, R. S., 1961, Dietary effects of fats upon fatty acid composition of mitochondria, *Arch. Biochem. Biophys.* **94**:115–120.

Milton, A. S., 1976, Modern views on the pathogenesis of fever and the mode of action of antipyretic drugs, *J. Pharm. Pharmacol.* **28**:393–399.

Mohrhauer, H., and Holman, R. T., 1963, Effect of linolenic acid upon the metabolism of linoleic acid, *J. Nutr.* **63**:67–74.

Ogburn, P. L., Sharp, H., Lloy-Still, J. D., Johnson, S. B., and Holman, R. T., 1982, Abnormal polyunsaturated fatty acid pattern of serum lipids in Reye's syndrome, *Proc. Natl. Acad. Sci. USA* **79**:908–911.

Pace-Asciak, C., and Wolfe, L. S., 1968, Inhibition of prostaglandin synthesis by oleic, linoleic and linolenic acids, *Biochem. Biophys. Acta.* **152**:784–787.

Rahm, J. J., and Holman, R. T., 1964, Effect of linoleic acid upon the metabolism of linolenic acid, *J. Nutr.* **84**:15–19.

Skarnes, R. C., Brown, S. K., Hull, S. S., and McCraken, J. A., 1981, Role of prostaglandin E in the biphasic fever response to endotoxin, *J. Exp. Med.* **154**:1212–1224.

Spawinski, J. A., Gorka, Z., Zacny, E., and Wojtaszek, B., 1978, Hyperthermic effects of arachidonic acid, prostaglandins E_2 and F_2 in rats, *Pflugers* **374**:15–21.

Stadie, W. C., 1945, The intermediary metabolism of fatty acids, *Physiol. Rev.* **25**:395–441.

31

Poor Early Growth and Adult Mental and Somatic Health

GEORGE A. CLARK, NICHOLAS R. HALL,
CAROLYN M. ALDWIN, ALLAN L. GOLDSTEIN,
and R. CLAYTON STEINER

1. INTRODUCTION

Early growth and adult psychoneuroimmunology are usually seen as two separate ends of the life course, but in some ways they may be inextricably linked. This chapter presents a rationale and preliminary evidence suggesting that poor early growth may be a factor in adult psychoneuroimmunology.

Research is emerging that suggests that early stress might permanently rearrange neuroendocrine and immune mechanisms (Pierpaoli, 1981). Bidirectional influences have now been documented involving neuroendocrine and immune function (Hall *et al.*, 1985). These studies have begun to detail the specific mechanisms whereby emotions might affect health and life span (Riley, 1981; Plaut and Friedman, 1981). Still, almost all the research in psychoneuroimmunology focuses on adults.

Fetal growth is extraordinarily sensitive to a wide variety of common environmental stressors, such as maternal malnutrition (Allen, 1986) and a wide variety of behavioral and socioeconomic factors (Gruenwald, 1968). The thymus gland is arguably the most sensitive organ to growth disruption, especially because of such common factors as protein malnutrition (Usher and McLean, 1974; Cooper *et al.*, 1974; Platt and Stewart, 1967). Unlike other factors affecting thymic function in the adult, if growth disruption outlasts the normal period of thymic development, its growth and performance appear to be chronically reduced (Chandra, 1981).

In humans, the thymus gland appears to cease growth and begins to involute by age 1 (Steinman, 1986). Development and maturation of many thymic-immune functions become

GEORGE A. CLARK and CAROLYN M. ALDWIN • Normative Aging Study, Veterans Administration Outpatient Clinic, Boston, Massachusetts 02108.   NICHOLAS R. HALL • Department of Psychiatry and Behavioral Medicine, and Center of Psychoimmunology, University of South Florida, Tampa, Florida 33613.   ALLAN L. GOLDSTEIN and R. CLAYTON STEINER • George Washington University Medical Center, Washington, D.C. 20037.

effective by early postnatal development (Cooper, 1983; Hayward, 1981). Between young and mid-adulthood, several aspects of thymic-immune function, such as serum thymic hormones, appear to accelerate their decline. This decline, in later life, may be associated with the diseases of aging (Fig. 1).

The pattern of thymic-immune development varies across species. Generally, maturation in lower animals, such as murine species, occurs later in development than in humans. The relationship between early stress and later thymic function may have been overlooked, because most animal studies examining stress effects in later functioning have not specifically targetted crucial developmental periods for the thymus. If stress does not persist throughout thymic-immune development, the effects may be reversible via catchup growth (Gerbase-DeLima et al., 1975). The few studies that have examined nutritional stress, through the period of thymic-immune development, have found that function is permanently depressed with decreased health and life span (McLeod and Liew, 1975).

In both humans (Brandt, 1978; Brooke et al., 1984) and animals (Winick, 1969; Dubos et al., 1967), brain development may also be permanently stunted in development and function if growth disruption outlasts its normal period of development. However, it does not appear to be as easily stunted as the thymus (Usher and McLean, 1974; Platt and Stewart, 1967). Nonetheless, poor early growth may affect both the brain and thymus later in life.

The thymus also appears to affect brain growth and function indirectly. It has long been established that normal development of the thymus is critical in programming the hypothalamus–pituitary (Pierpaoli et al., 1976). Thus, the potential pathways for poor early growth by which adult psychoneuroimmunology can be permanently changed are both direct and indirect.

The purpose of this chapter is to review relevant research on thymic-immune and neural development and function. We then present pilot studies linking poor early growth and adult psychoneuroimmunology in humans. Gaps in our understanding of this process are emphasized.

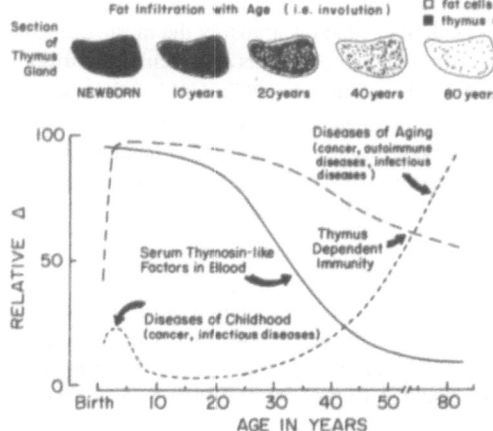

FIGURE 1. Changes in thymic involution and function with age. Note that thymic involution depicted here is in healthy adults, characterized by an increase in fat infiltration rather than a decrease in size or weight seen in malnourished or diseased individuals. (Based on Steinman 1986; Moore et al., 1983; Watts, 1969.)

2. THYMIC-IMMUNE DEVELOPMENT

The normal, much less abnormal, development of the thymic-immune system and its implication for overall immune system development are complex and still poorly understood. While some investigators suggest that stem cells coming from the bone marrow and liver cells already contain all the genetic information for potential immunologic functions (Silverstein, 1970), many others believe that certain stem cells coming from the bone marrow and liver must pass obligatorily through the thymic microenvironment for maturation and balanced immune function. This may be true even for stem cells undergoing additional "post" or "extra" thymic maturation (Haynes, 1984; Koninkx et al., 1984). Normal thymic development may also be critical to normal immunogenesis via germ-line theories of antibody formation (Hood and Talmage, 1971). Although some cells stay in the thymus, thymocytes, other immune cells migrate out of thymus and "seed" the lymphatic system including the spleen, intestine, appendix, liver, and mesenteric lymph nodes.

These peripheral sites also appear involved in the genesis and regulation of immune function (Stutman and Good, 1971; Guyton, 1982; Hess et al., 1967; Michalke et al., 1969). Some of these lymphoid cells appear to stay within these peripheral organs, such as the spleen. Others, such as T lymphocytes, circulate within the bloodstream and are pumped back periodically through these organs, where they may undergo further differentiation, functional "fine tuning," and repairing, i.e., morphostasis (Pierpaoli and Sorkin, 1972; Burch, 1976).

Exactly how this is done is unknown and is the subject of intense research. Gowans et al. (1961) and Porter and Cooper (1982) were among the first to suggest that a large number of T lymphocytes are short-lived nonstimulated cells that die in the thymus. Jerne (1971) suggested that the thymus is a breeding organ, while Zinkernagel (1978) hypothesized that the thymus is an obligatory selector of restriction specificity of effector T cells independent of the T cells original H-2 genotype.

Stem cells that undergo direct thymic maturation within the microenvironment apparently do so by direct cell–cell contact with the stroma. The thymus also produces soluble thymic hormones, which appear to promote T- and B-cell morphogenesis, lymphogenesis, and maturation, perhaps in the periphery as well (Steinman, 1986).

The epithelial cells of the thymus secrete several peptide hormone-like factors that may be secreted by different regions of the thymus gland (Hirokawa et al., 1980; Goldstein et al., 1981). In spite of their close origin, these factors may be biochemically distinct. Each type may act on specific aspects of immune development and function or on the programming of the bidirectional neuroendocrine circuitry. Thymic peptides, such as thymosin, fraction-5 (TF5), and its component thymosin α_1 (TSN-a_1), can induce differentiation of specific subsets of T lymphocytes. These include killer, helper, and suppressor cells, as indicated by induction of certain T-cell-associated markers, such as TdT, Thy-1, and Lyt-2. This suggests that specific hormone-like thymic peptides may exert a sequential, selective, and conditioning effect that causes proliferation of only specific thymic and peripheral T lymphocytes. Afterward, presumably clonal expansion occurs (Goldstein et al., 1983; Savino and Dardenne, 1972).

As Pierpaoli (1981) points out, normal thymic development must be crucial at some stage of fetal development, either inducing proliferation of certain lymphocytes or secreting hormones that promote cellular differentiation in other lymphoid tissues. This is unequivocal, because after neonatal thymectomy, or in congenital absence of the thymus, immunodeficiencies, and other pathological alterations occur.

In neonatal thymectomy, there is a virtual disappearance of T cells from the periarteriolar region of the spleen and the perifollicular paracortical areas of the lymph nodes and about a 50% reduction of T lymphocytes from the peripheral blood and peripheral thoracic duct. Cell-mediated immunity does not develop. There is also a decrease in hormone-like thymic peptides (Pierpaoli, 1981).

Studies that have examined the effects of poor early growth due to malnutrition on subsequent thymic development and function have called this nutritional thymectomy (Jose *et al.*, 1973; Keusch *et al.*, 1987), because the effects are similar to those seen when the thymus is surgically removed early in development. After normal thymic development, thymic involution or surgical thymectomy do not appear to have long-lasting effects (Steinman, 1986).

So-called "auto"-thymectomy may be diagnosed when the precise cause of thymic growth failure is not known (Watts, 1969). For example, Chandra (1981) found fetally growth retarded infants whose mothers had hypertension had chronically lowered thymic hormones and thymic-immune function, presumably due to poor thymic development.

Bone marrow and the liver are also easily stunted in development (Usher and McLean, 1974; Platt and Stewart, 1967; Gross and Newberne, 1980; Morley *et al.*, 1974; Mitchell *et al.*, 1969). This could result in defective immune cell development in stem cells, even before the effects of "nutritional thymectomy."

In poor thymic growth, there are several parallels to that seen in aging. There appears to be decreased perivascular space for stem cells within the epithelium to make contact in the stroma. The impact seems to be greatest in the more rapidly growing cortex, compared to the more slowly growing medulla (Boyd, 1936). A decrease in cortical mass of the thymus is associated with a dramatic decrease in thymocytes (Watts, 1969). There is decreased output of thymic hormones and in both the number and degree of differentiation of T cells. Thus, the stunted involuted thymus may alter its ability to generate normal immunocompetence (Chandra, 1975; Wilson *et al.*, 1985). These changes parallel many changes seen in aging (Steinman, 1986; Weksler *et al.*, 1978; Hirokawa and Makinodan, 1975; Andreasen *et al.*, 1949; Blau, 1972). However, unlike aspects of normal aging, or thymic damage after normal thymic development, if growth disruption outlasts the normal period of thymic development, immune imbalances might be permanent (Fig. 2).

3. STRESS AND NEUROENDOCRINE DEVELOPMENT

Winick (1969) showed in rats that surprisingly mild nutritional stress can permanently stunt brain growth. He was one of the first to demonstrate convincingly that, since various regions of the brain grow at different times, each has a "critical period" of development. Some of these are intense and brief, such as the hypothalamus. Consequently, growth disruption coinciding with their particular development can stunt brain development in specific ways (see also Zamenhof *et al.*, 1968; Winick and Rosso, 1969). Most of these studies focus on gross coordination and cognitive functions (McCormick, 1985; Brooke *et al.*, 1984; Brandt, 1978).

These specific deficits caused by poor early growth may, or may, not be functionally measurable, because of the integrated nature of thymic-immune and brain growth and function (Pierpaoli and Sorkin, 1972). From the perspective of public health, improving prenatal

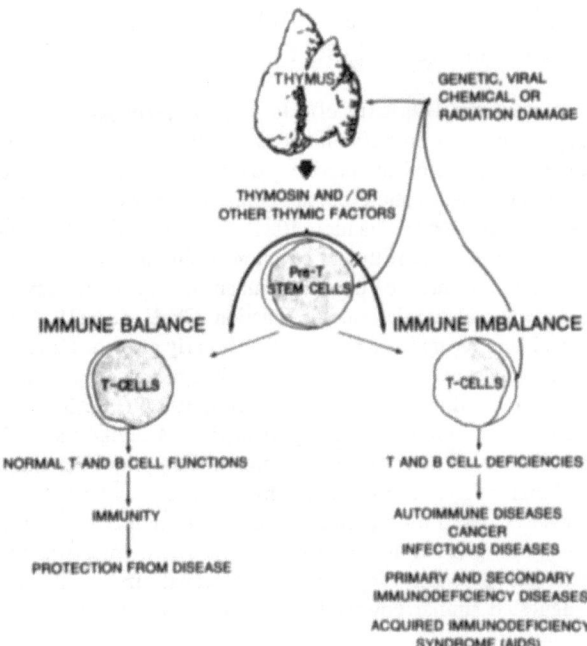

FIGURE 2. Factors that may cause involution (damage) of the thymus and result in decrease in output of thymosin-like factors causing immune imbalances.

protein nutrition may be effective in that it can generally improve postnatal health. However, from the perspective of biochemical intervention strategies, understanding the particular thymic-immune and neuroendocrine circuits is probably more critical, because changing one parameter may be deleterious to others, such as interleukin-2 (IL-2) (Smedley *et al.*, 1983).

The thymus programs a variety of neuroendocrine functions (Pierpaoli and Besedovsky, 1975), including the hypothalamus (Pierpaoli *et al.*, 1977), and pineal gland (Pierpaoli and Maestroni, 1981). Poor pineal development itself results in chronically lower serotonin levels, and the pineal gland is normally rich in serotonin. Serotonin is thought, at least by some, to be responsible for the negative feedback from ACTH and cortisol, and there is hypersecretion of cortisol and longer periods of secretion (Klein, 1978). Pinealectomy has been shown to result in chronic psychological and immune depression (Lapin, 1974).

There is also some evidence that early stress may accelerate the maturation of the neuroendocrine system. Rats handled in early infancy opened their eyes earlier, achieved locomotion and puberty earlier, and showed marked differences in neuroendocrine response to stress in adulthood. Infant-handled rats showed much greater increases in ACTH in response to stress but then returned to baseline levels much more rapidly than controls (cf. Denenberg, 1964.) Thus, while poorly understood, there is some evidence that early stress may affect neuroendocrine functioning in later life.

4. POOR EARLY GROWTH AND ADULT PSYCHONEUROIMMUNOLOGY

In humans, assessing the long-term effects of poor early growth on either thymic-immune or neural function has been difficult because of the long life span in humans. Most studies assessing the significance of intrauterine growth retardation (IUGR) tend to examine either neural or thymic-immune function (but not both), and they only follow up infants for a few years (e.g., McCormick, 1985; Chandra, 1981). We are aware of no studies assessing relationships between poor early growth and psychoneuroimmunology at any age.

To help overcome the obstacle of the long human life span, in studying relationships between poor early growth and thymic-immune function, Clark *et al.* (1986) suggested using the size of the vertebral neural canal as a marker of poor early growth. Canals grow primarily *in utero* and cease growth generally about age 4, although some portions may mature at earlier periods (Roaf, 1960; Hinck *et al.*, 1966; Barson, 1974) (Fig. 3).

Canals generally track brain and thymic growth (Fig. 4). Like the brain and thymic-immune system, canals are extremely sensitive to growth disruption. For example, studies in protein malnourished piglets have shown that the thymus, brain, and canals are among, if not the most, stunted features. Even mild protein malnutrition, induced at birth, was found to decrease canals size by 17% (Platt and Stewart, 1962). The thymus was the other greatly affected tissue (Platt and Stewart, 1967). Studies of canal size in human malnourished populations have suggested similar powerful effects (Clark *et al.*, 1985; Clark, 1987; and Pavitt, 1987).

Canals, the brain, and the thymus not only complete most of their growth *in utero* and cease growth in early childhood, but all respond to similar anabolic and catabolic hormones, such as growth hormones and cortisol (e.g., Vetter *et al.*, 1985; Fabris, 1977). Unlike the brain and thymic-immune system, after the canals cease growth, they are remarkably stable in size and shape (Porter *et al.*, 1980). Thus, in the adult, the canal may be an indelible marker of poor early neural and thymic-immune growth. In the adult, small (stunted) canals should be correlated with abnormal neuroendocrine and thymic-immune function, and con-

VERTEBRAL
NEURAL CANAL

VERTEBRAL
BODY

YOUNG CHILD (age 4)

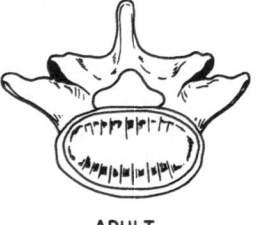

ADULT

FIGURE 3. Comparison of a vertebrae (cranial view) from a young child (age 4) and an adult. Note that the size of the vertebral neural canal is already fully grown by age 4.

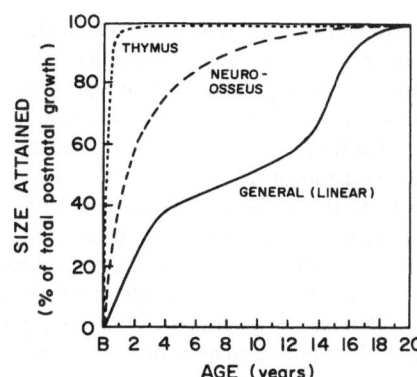

FIGURE 4. Thymus gland, neuro-osseous, and general (linear) growth from birth to adulthood. (Based on Scammon, 1930; Steinman, 1986.)

comitant morbidity and mortality. Initial research focused on a very gross test of this model—the relationship between canal size and age at death in a skeletal population.

More than 1000 vertebrae were measured from 90 adults between 15 and 55 years of age in an American Indian who lived in Illinois, 950–1300 AD. Age at death and sex were determined by accurate forensic techniques. Results showed that canals were independent of adult body size (general linear growth), suggesting that after canal growth ceased, catchup growth occurred in those features with remaining growth potential, such as height (Clark *et al.*, 1986). All vertebrae were involved. Coefficient α was above 80% for all canals up and down the vertebral column, suggesting systemic stunting effects. Regardless of time frame and environmental context, adults with small canals had significantly reduced life span.

Preliminary unpublished research was then conducted in another skeleton population of known age and sex, the Terry Collection. Results showed that adults with small canals also had a significant effect on age at death.

On the basis of these preliminary skeletal data, Porter and Pavitt (1987) examined relationships between canals, health, and academic status in living English populations. Canal size in adults was measured *in vivo* using ultrasound. Health records from birth were analyzed. Adults with smaller canal size had a significantly greater incidence of infection, while those with larger canals had significantly higher rates of autoimmune diseases.

In a related study, Porter *et al.* (1987b) measured canal size in high school freshman in two independent schools. In their senior year, they took standardized graduation examinations, the General Certificate of Education. In both school systems, students with small canals had significantly lower academic scores.

Academic performance is determined by a larger array of factors than brain development and function, such as personal motivation, missed school days possibly due to infection, family life, teaching quality, and a host of socioeconomic factors. Porter *et al.* (1987b) acknowledged these confounding factors. Indeed, there were a few excellent students with small canals, but generally students with small canals had lower scores.

In a preliminary test of these direct relationships between canal size and neuroendocrine and thymic-immune function, we collected data from a small group of men ($N = 13$–35) from the Normative Aging Study (NAS). The NAS was begun in 1963 to assess biological and social determinants of aging (Bell *et al.*, 1972).

Age, weight, height, and sitting height were measured. After an overnight fast, blood was drawn at 8:00 AM and measured for TSN-a_1, cortisol, and blood sugar. After the fasting serum was drawn, a 100-g glucose challenge test (GCT) was administered; 2 hr later, blood was drawn again and examined for the same serum variables. Men were measured each Monday morning, from May through August 1985. Canal size was measured with computed tomography (CT) in 16 of the men (Fig. 5).

Cortisol is a glucocorticoid that might be influenced by changes in blood sugar. Cortisol has been shown to decrease with blood sugar, at least in younger-level adults (Jialal and Joubert, 1982). Serum TSN-a_1 (and TF5) levels have been shown to covary with adrenal corticosteroids, at least in rats (Hall *et al.*, 1983) and monkeys (Healey *et al.*, 1983). The ability to handle blood sugar decreases significantly with age and weight in the NAS (Sparrow *et al.*, 1986). Thus, besides canal size, these factors might influence TSN-a_1.

Preliminary results on TSN-a_1 were published by Clark *et al.* (1988). The findings with cortisol are presented here for the first time. Table I demonstrated that all values were within the normal range and normally distributed (Naylor *et al.*, 1986; Liddle, 1965; Clark, 1985). After the GCT, there was a highly significant decrease in cortisol, but there was almost no effect on TSN-a_1.

Under both the fasting and glucose challenge test conditions, there was a significant

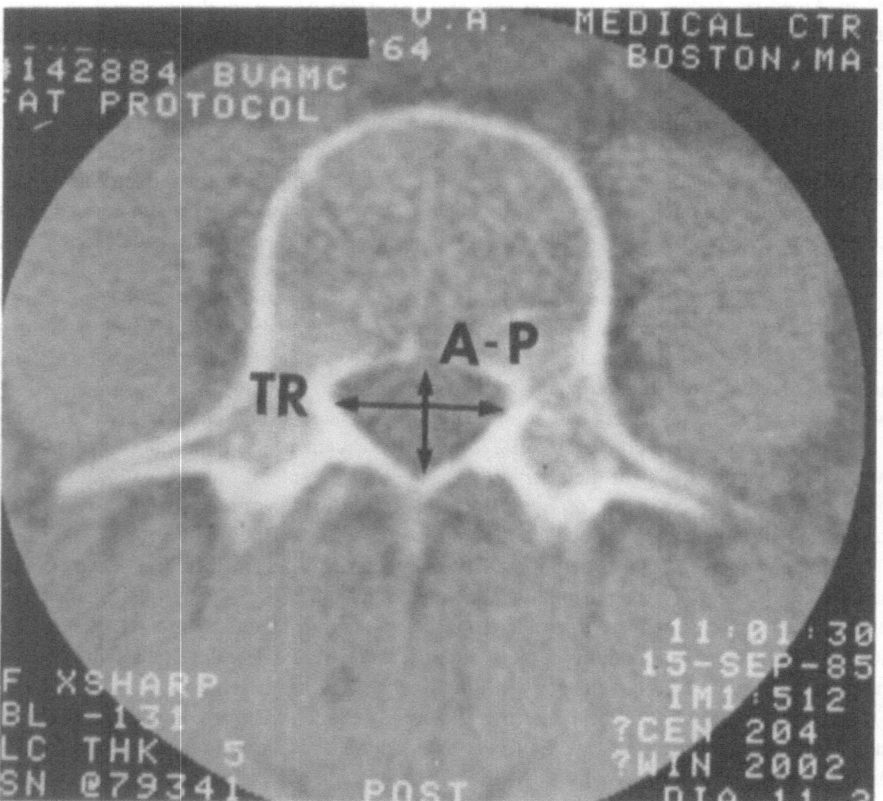

FIGURE 5. Computed tomography scan of the third lumbar (L3) vertebral neural canal. Both the anteroposterior (AP) and transverse (TR) diameters were measured.

TABLE I. Descriptive Statistics ($N = 16$)

Variable	Mean	SD	Skewness	Kurtosis
Spinal neural canals (mm)				
T7 anteroposterior	14.4	1.3	1.0	0.7
T7 transverse	16.3	2.4	0.4	−1.1
L3 anteroposterior	15.5	2.7	0.8	−0.2
L3 transverse	25.8	4.4	1.8	5.0
Anthropometry				
Age (years)	66.8	9.2	−0.8	−0.2
Weight (lb)	169.8	17.2	−0.2	0.8
Height (cm)	174.0	4.2	−0.4	0.8
Sitting height (cm)	89.7	2.6	−1.7	4.3
Thymosin-α_1 (ng/ml)				
Fasting	191.82	76.12	0.0	0.2
2-hr post-GCT[a]	202.24	66.48	−1.0	1.8
Cortisol (ng/ml)				
Fasting	185.4	31.4	−0.0	1.4
2-hr post-GCT[a]	139.8[b]	29.7	0.9	0.9
Glucose (ml/di)				
Fasting	97.2	10.6	0.7	0.4
2-hr post-GCT[a]	113.7	41.9	1.0	0.6

[a]GCT, glucose challenge test.
[b]$p < 0.001$.

correlation between canal size and TSN-α_1 ($r = 0.47$; $p < 0.05$). Canal size tended to be correlated ($r = 0.37$) with cortisol in the fasting, but not in the challenged, condition ($r = 0.06$). These outcomes for the fasting and glucose challenge test conditions among canal size, TSN-α_1, and cortisol makes sense, given that glucose depressed only cortisol and not TSN-α_1.

In the fasting state, TSN-α_1 and cortisol tended to be correlated ($r = 0.37$). After challenge, this tendency decreased ($r = 0.26$). However, fasting cortisol was significantly correlated with glucose challenged TSN-α_1 levels ($r = 0.44$; $p < 0.05$), suggesting that individuals with higher fasting cortisol levels had higher glucose challenged levels of TSN-α_1.

As many factors may influence TSN-α_1, stepwise multivariate analyses were performed to determine the best predictor of TSN-α_1. The predictor variables were age, cortisol, blood sugar, weight, height, and sitting height. Results showed the only two predictors to be sitting height and canal size, explaining 53% ($p < 0.05$) of the variance of fasting TSN-α_1 (Table II). After the GCT, canal size was the only predictor, explaining 22% ($p = 0.055$) of the variation in serum TSN-α_1.

We repeated the analyses to determine the best predictor of fasting cortisol. Among blood sugar, age, canal size, height, sitting height, weight, and TSN-α_1, the best predictor was canal size, explaining 28% ($p > 0.06$) of the variation in fasting cortisol. The only other predictor of cortisol that tended to predict cortisol reliably was weight ($R^2 = 0.14$; $p < 0.14$). It should be emphasized that this study was conducted in a small group of men ($N = 16$), and must be considered preliminary.

As provocative as these data were, the key question remained unanswered: Did small

TABLE II. Multiple Regression Equation Predicting Thymosin-α_1 Levels
(*N* = 16)

Equations	R^2	Delta R^2	β	*r*	*F*
Equation (1)					
Fasting condition					
Sitting height	0.37	0.37	−0.56	−0.61	8.46[b]
T7 AP diameter	0.53	0.16	0.40	0.47	4.39[c]
Equation (2)					
2-hr post-GCT[a]					
T7 AP diameter	0.22	0.22	0.47	0.47	4.32[c]

[a]GCT, glucose tolerance test.
[b]$p = 0.01$.
[c]$p = 0.056$.

canal size (i.e., poor early growth) permanently lower TSN-α_1 and cortisol levels? We re-examined available participants (*N* = 13) 2½ years later, reassessing the serum parameters to assess the stability of the relationship between canal size TSN-α_1 and cortisol.

Again, the men had blood drawn after overnight fast at 8:00 AM. Unfortunately, due to funding limitations, the GCT could not be conducted, but we were able to measure a wider number of thymic-immune functions.

Results showed (Fig. 6) that fasting TSN-α_1 still correlated ($r = 0.52$; $p < 0.05$). At time 1, 1 mm of canal size accounted for 249 ng/ml of TSN-α_1, and at time 2, 317 ng/ml. Canal size and cortisol also tended to be correlated ($r = 0.37$), but a larger sample size would be necessary to reject the null hypothesis with $p < 0.05$ and a power of 0.80 (Cohen and Cohen, 1975). These results suggested that canal size is associated with TSN-α_1 and cortisol

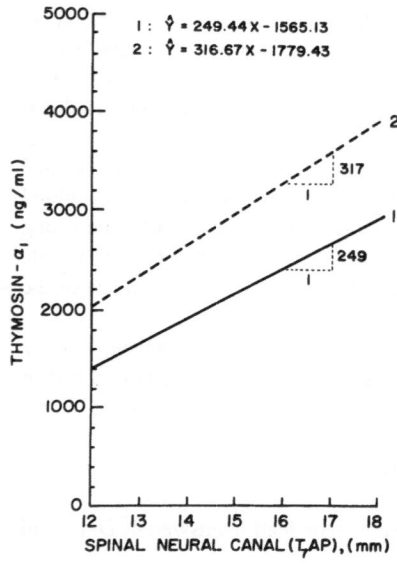

FIGURE 6. Linear relationships between time 1 and 2 TSN-α_1 and spinal (i.e., vertebral) neural canal (VNC) size. The difference in the intercepts, between time 1 and 2, is due to a new more sensitive antibody at time 2. However, the slopes are similar and both show that adults with smaller VNC have lower levels of TSN-α_1 at both time points. This suggests that early growth disruption (GD), implied by smaller VNC, leads to chronically lower TSN-α_1.

serum levels. Perhaps poor early growth can permanently alter these neuroendocrine and thymic-immune functions.

The same stepwise multiple regressions were conducted to assess the best predictor of fasting TSN-α_1. Age, height, sitting height, weight, and canal size were the predictors. Once again, only sitting height and canal size entered the equation. Together they explained 57% ($p < 0.01$) of the variation in TSN-α_1 serum levels. These results mirror those from time 1 (see Clark et al., 1989).

Other thymic-immune measures were also correlated with canal size, including Concanavalin A (Con A) ($r = 0.61; p < 0.01$), natural killer (NK) cell activity ($r = 0.67; p < 0.006$) and total white blood cells (WBC) ($r = -0.70; p < 0.003$). Interleukin-2 (IL-2) tended to be correlated with canal size ($r = 0.39$), as did total peripheral T lymphocytes ($r = 0.30$). To be tested with confidence of 0.80 and <0.05, a sample size of 46 is necessary (Cohen and Cohen, 1975).

Blood chemistry has been collected from the NAS men for more than 20 years. Data collected from the first data-collection cycle include some immune measures; these were correlated with the recent measurement of canal size. Canal size was still inversely correlated with WBC ($r = -0.25$) and positively with T lymphocytes ($r = 0.30$), collected more than 20 years earlier. Canal size was also correlated with other measures collected long ago, including monocytes ($r = 0.47$), hemoglobin ($r = 0.41$), hematocrit ($r = 0.46$), and total protein ($r = 0.52$). Larger sample sizes (<0.80) are necessary to test whether these were statistically significant with a power of 0.80 and $p < 0.05$ (Cohen and Cohen, 1975). Given that small canals presumably indicate "auto"-thymectomy, "growth-arrested T lymphocytes" should also be found (Watts, 1969).

We also measured TSN-β_4; it was not correlated with TSN-α_1 ($r = -0.10$). Furthermore, TSN-β_4 and cortisol tended to be strongly inverse ($r = -0.51; p < 0.07$). This was the opposite of TSN-α_1.

Goldstein et al. (1983) and Pazmino et al. (1978a,b) suggest that TSN-α_1 and thymosin β_4 (TSN-β_4) are produced by different regions of the thymus gland. TSN-β_4 may act on an earlier stage of T-cell differentiation than TSN-α_1, and TSN-β_4 may not covary with cortisol (corticosterone).

Hall et al. (1985) suggest that cortisol (corticosterone) and TSN-α_1 (and TF5) covary because functionally mature T cells are resistant to these steroids, and higher levels of thymic peptides cause their proliferation. Conversely, functionally immature steroid-sensitive T cells are suppressed. Thus, there is a more parsimonious and functional immune response.

These preliminary results support the observations and theories of Goldstein et al. (1983) and Hall et al. (1985). TSN-β_4 may be independent of TSN-α_1. Indeed, the given model suggests that there ought be inverse relationships between TSN-α_1 and TSN-β_4, and this was borne out. When cortisol stimulates TSN-α_1, if it also stimulated TSN-β_4 there could be proliferation of undifferentiated T cells. Given their model, one would also expect TSN-β_4 to decrease, to avoid immune imbalance. In this very limited study, this appears to be the case.

Even though TSN-α_1 and TSN-β_4 were themselves independent, canal size was also correlated with TSN-β_4 ($r = -0.64; p < 0.02$). The inverse correlation with canal size also suggests different pathways in early growth for TSN-β_4.

Mental health questionnaires (SCL-90-R) had been mailed and filled out at home over the same time period. The SCL-90-R measures various parameters of mental health (Derogatis, 1983). The primary mental health variable of interest was depression. Canal size tended to be significantly correlated with depression ($r = 0.32; p < 0.06$). It was more reliably correlated with somatization ($r = 0.39$; $p < 0.02$) and with interpersonal sensitivity ($r = 0.33$; $p < 0.05$). Fasting TSN-α_1 levels were not significantly correlated with any mental health measures. However, under the GCT conditions, TSN-α_1 levels were significantly correlated with depression ($r = 0.60$; $p < 0.009$), sensitivity ($r = 0.62$; $p < 0.006$), and psychoticism ($r = 0.54$; $p < 0.02$) (Aldwin et al., 1988). Cortisol was correlated with paranoia ($r = -0.50$; $p < 0.03$). As provocative as these relationships are, the sample size precludes multivariate analyses, much less firm conclusions. Moreover, it remains to be seen whether adults with small canals and altered neuroendocrine and thymicoimmune functions are more susceptible to increased morbidity and mortality.

It is worth mentioning, however, that since the start of the NAS in 1962, 235 men have died. Among 47 anthropometrics routinely collected (canal size is not), the single best predictor of mortality was sitting height and breadth (Borkan et al., 1985). When a variety of biological and behavioral factors are considered, the best predictor of mortality is the WBC (deLabry et al., 1988). Unfortunately, thymosins and other immune functions are not routinely measured.

5. SUMMARY

Psychoneuroimmunology has come a long way since it began as a hybrid discipline. It is challenging to integrate psychology, neurology, and immunology and assess their effects on health and life span. Determining the role of poor early growth in adult psychoneuroimmunology is still in its infancy. Yet the rewards to clinical and public health may be profound. Toward this end, it may be time to consider more closely the long-term effects of early stress for aging processes in late life.

ACKNOWLEDGMENT. We gratefully appreciate the secretarial help of Claire Leonardi and Marie Gill, and the statistical assistance of Dr. Avron Spiro III.

REFERENCES

Aldwin, C. M., Clark, G. A., Hall, N., Levenson, M. R., and Bosse', R., 1988, Immune regulation and psychological symptoms, Gerontologist. 28:155A (abstract).

Allen, L. H., 1986, Maternal nutrition and fetal outcome, in: Human Growth: A Multidisciplinary Review (A. Demirjian, ed.), Tayler and Francis, London, pp. 265–272.

Andreasen, E., and Christensen, S., 1949, Rate of mitotic activity in lymphoid organs of rat, Anat. Rec. 103:401–412.

Bach, J. F., LeBrigand, H., and Barois, M., 1972, Evidence for a serum thymic factor produced by the human thymus, Lancet 2:1056–1058.

Barson, A. J., 1974, Developmental pathology of the spine, in: Scientific Foundations of Pediatrics (J. A. Davis and J. Dobbing, eds.), W. B. Saunders, Philadelphia, pp. 759–785.

Bell, B., Rose, C. L., and Damon, A., 1972, The Normative Aging Study: An interdisciplinary study of aging, Aging Hum. Dev. 3:5–17.

Blau, J. N., 1972, DNA synthesis in the adult and aging guinea pig thymus, Clin. Exp. Immunol. 11:461–468.

Borkan, G. A., and Vokonas, P. S., 1986, Interaction between physique and mortality risk, Gerontologist 26:8 (abstract).

Boyd, E., 1936, Weight of the thymus and its component parts and number of Hassal corpuscles in health and disease, *Am. J. Dis. Child.* **51**:313.

Brandt, E., 1978, Growth dynamics of low-birth-weight infants with emphasis on the perinatal period, in: *Human Growth and Postnatal Growth* (F. Falkner and J. M. Tanner, eds.), Plenum, New York, pp. 557–617.

Brooke, O. G., Wood, C., and Butters, F., 1984, The body proportions for small-for-date infants, *Early Hum. Dev.* **10**:85–94.

Brown, R. E., 1965, Decreased brain weight in malnutrition and its implications, *E. Afr. Med. J.* **11**:584.

Burch, P. R. J., 1976, *The Biology of Cancer, A New Approach.* MTP Press, Lancaster, England.

Chandra, R. K., 1981, Serum thymic hormone activity and cell-mediated immunity in healthy neonates, preterm infants and small-for-gestational age infants, *Pediatrics* **67**:407–411.

Chandra, R. K., 1975, Fetal malnutrition and postnatal immunocompetence, *Am. J. Dis. Child.* **129**:450.

Clark, G. A., 1985, Heterochrony, Allometry, and Canalization in the Human Vertebral Column: Examples from Prehistoric Amerindian Populations, Doctoral dissertation, Department of Anthropology, University of Massachusetts, Amherst, Massachusetts, International Microfilms, #8509532, Ann Arbor, Michigan.

Clark, G. A., 1987, A new method for analyzing poor early growth and sexual dimorphism, *Am. J. Phys. Anthropol.* **77**:105–116.

Clark, G. A., Panjabi, M. M., and Wetzel, F. T., 1985, Can infant malnutrition cause adult vertebral stenosis?, *Spine* **10**:165–170.

Clark, G. A., Hall, N. R., Armelagos, G. J., Borkan, G. A., Panjabi, M. M., and Wetzel, F. T., 1986, Poor growth prior to early childhood: Decreased health and life-span in the adult, *Am. J. Phys. Anthropol.* **70**:145–150.

Clark, G. A., Hall, N. R., Aldwin, C. M., Harris, J. M., Borkan, G. A., and Srinivasan, M., 1988a, Measures of poor early growth are correlated with lower adult levels of thymosin alpha-1: Results from the Normative Aging Study, *Hum. Biol.* **60**:435–451.

Clark, G. A., Hall, N. R., Aldwin, C. M., Goldstein, A., and Armelagos, G. J., 1989, Measures of poor early growth are correlated with adult levels of thymosin alpha-1: A follow-up study in the Normative Aging Study, *Am. J. Hum. Biol.* **1**:331–337.

Cohen, J., and Cohen, P., 1975, *Applied Multiple Regression/Correlational Analysis For the Behavioral Sciences,* Lawrence Erlbaum Associates, Hillsdale, New Jersey.

Cooper, M. D., 1983, B-Cell differentiation, *Birth Defects* **19**:25–29.

Cooper, W. C., Good, R. A., and Mariani, T., 1974, Effects of protein insufficiency on immune responsiveness, *Am. J. Nutr.* **27**:647–664.

Cueto, S. M. C., Carmona-Buendia, P., and Cruz-Bolanos, J. C., 1985, Activity of serum thymic factor in undernourished new born infants, *Arch. Invest. Med.* **16**:199–207.

de Labry, L. L., Champion, E. W., Glynn, R. J., and Vokonas, P. S., 1988, Relation of white blood cell count and lymphocytes to mortality over 13 years, *Gerontologist,* **28**:110A (abstract).

Denenberg, V. H., 1964, Critical periods, stimulus input, and emotional reactivity: A theory of infantile stimulation, *Psychol. Rev.* **71**:335–357.

Derogatis, L., 1983, *SCL-90-R Revised Manual,* Johns Hopkins University School of Medicine, Baltimore.

Dubos, R., Lee, C., and Costello, R., 1969, Lasting biological effects of early environmental influences, *J. Exp. Med.* **130**:963–977.

Fabris, N., 1977, Hormones and aging, in: *Comprehensive Immunology.* Vol. I: *Immunology and Aging* (T. Makinodan and E. Yunis, eds.), Plenum, New York, pp. 73–89.

Fabris, N., Mocchegiani, E., Mariotti, S., Caramia, G., Braccili, T., Pacini, F., and Pinchera, A., 1987, Thymulin deficiency and low 3,5,3'-triiodothyronine syndrome in infants with low birth weight syndromes, *J. Clin. Endocrinol. Metab.* **65**:247–252.

Fauman, M. A., 1982, The central nervous system and the immune system, *Biol. Psychiatry* **17:**1459–1482.

Gerbase-Delima, M., Liu, R. K., Cheney, K. E., *et al.*, 1975, Immune function and survival in a long-lived mouse strain subjected to undernutrition. *Gerontologia* **21:**184.

Goldstein, A. L., Low, T. L. K., Zatz, M. M., Hall, N. R., and Naylor, P. H., 1983, Thymosins: Chemical and biological studies of thymosins, *Clin. Immunol. Allergy* **3:**119–132.

Gowans, J. L., Gesner, B. M., and McGregor, D. D., 1961, The immunological activity of lymphocytes, *Ciba Found. Study Group* **10:**32–40.

Gray, J. A., 1971, *The Psychology of Fear and Stress,* Weidenfeld and Nicolson, London.

Gross, R. I., and Newberne, P. M., 1980, Role of nutrition in immunologic function, *Physiol. Rev.* **60:**188–302.

Gruenwald, P., 1968, Fetal growth as an indicator of socioeconomic change, *Publ. Health Rep.* **83:**867–872.

Gunn, T., Reece, E., Metrakos, K., and Colle, E., 1981, Depressed T cells following neonatal steroid treatment, *Pediatrics* **67:**61–67.

Guyton, A. C., 1982, *Basic Human Physiology: Normal Function and Mechanisms of Disease,* W. B. Saunders, London.

Hall, N. R., and Goldstein, A. L., 1983, The thymus–brain connection: Interactions between thymosin and the neuroendocrine system, *Lymphokine Res.* **2:**1–5.

Hall, N. R., J. P., McGillis, B. L., Spangelo, D. L., Healy, and Goldstein, A. L., 1985, Immunomodulatory peptides and the central nervous system, *Springer Semin. Immunopathol.* **8:**153–164.

Hatotani, N., Nomura, K. Inoue, and Kitayama, I., 1979, Psychoendocrine model of depression, *Psychoneuroendocrinology* **4:**155–172.

Haynes, B. F., 1984, Phenotypic characterization and ontogeny of components of the human thymic microenvironment, *Clin. Res.* **32:**500–507.

Hayward, A. R., 1981, Development of lymphocyte responses and interactions in the human fetus and newborn, *Immunol. Rev.* **57:**39–60.

Healy, D. L., Hodgen, G. D., Schulte, H. M., Chrousos, G. P., Loriaux, D. L., Hall, N. R., and Goldstein, A. L., 1983, The thymus–adrenal connection: thymosin has corticotropin-releasing activity in primates, *Science* **222:**1353.

Hess, M. W., Stoner, R. D., and Cottier, H., 1967. Growth characteristics of mouse thymus in the neonatal period, *Nature (Lond.)* **215:**426–428.

Hinck, V. C., Clark, W. M., Hopkins, C. E., 1966, Normal interpediculate distance (minimum and maximum) in children and adults, *Radiology* **97:**141–153.

Hirokawa, L., and Makinodan, T., 1975, Thymic involution. Effect on T-cell differentiation, *J. Immunol.* **114:**1659–1664.

Hood, L., and Talmage, D. W., 1971, On the mechanism of antibody diversity: Evidence for the germ-line basis of antibody variability, in: *Developmental Aspects of Antibody Formation and Structure,* Vol. II (J. Sterzl and I. Riha, eds.), Academic, New York, pp. 935–962.

Jerne, N. K., 1971, The somatic generation of immune recognition, *Eur. J. Immunol.* **1:**1–9.

Jialal, I., and Joubert, S. M., 1982, Cortisol, glucagon and growth hormone responses to oral glucose in non-insulin dependent diabetes in the young, *S. Afr. Med. J.* **62:**549–552.

Jose, D. G., Stutman, O., and Good, R. A., 1973, Long term effects on immune function of early nutritional deprivation, *Nature (Lond.)* **241:**57–58.

Keusch, G. T., Cruz, J. R., Torun, B., Urrutia, J. J., Smith, H., Jr., and Goldstein, A. L., 1987, Immature circulating lymphocytes in severely malnourished Guatemalan children, *J. Pediatr. Gastro. Nutr.* **6:**265–270.

Klein, D. C., 1978, The pineal gland: A model of neuroendocrine regulation, in: *The Hypothalamus* (S. Reichlin, R. J., Baldessanni, and J. B. Martin, eds.), Raven, New York, pp. 303–327.

Koninkx, J. F. J. G., Schreurs, A. D. J. M., Penninks, A. H., and Seinen, W., 1984, Induction of postthymic T-cell maturation by thymic humoral factor(s) derived from a tumor cells of epithelial origin, *Thymus* **6**:395–409.

Lapin, F., 1974, Influence of simultaneous pinealectomy and thymectomy on the growth and formation of matastases of the Yoshida sarcoma in rats, *Exp. Pathol.* **9**:108–112.

Lewis, V. M., Twomey, J. J., Bealmear, P., Goldstein, G., and Good, R. A., 1978, Age, thymic involution, and circulating thymic hormone activity, *J. Clin. Endocrinol. Metab.* **47**:145–150.

Liddle, G. W., 1965, Assessment of pituitary and adrenal function, *Physicians* **3**:1–5.

McCormick, M. C., 1985, The contribution of low birth weight to infant mortality and childhood morbidity, *Engl. J. Med.* **312**:82–89.

McLeod, K. I., and Liew, F. Y., 1975, Maternal protein deficiency and the immune response of the progeny in the rat, *Proc. Nutr. Soc.* **34**:41A.

Michalke, W. D., Hess, M. W., Riedwyl, H., Stoner, R. D., and Cottier, H., 1969, Thymic lymphopoiesis and cell loss in newborn mice, *Blood* **33**:541–554.

Mitchell, G. F., and Miller, J. F. A. P., 1968, Cell-to-cell interaction in the immune response. II. The source of hemolysin-forming cells in irradiated mice given bone marrow and thymus or thoracic duct lymphocytes, *J. Exp. Med.* **128**:821–837.

Morley, A., Holmes, K., and Forbes, I., 1974, Depletion of B lymphocytes in chronic hypoplastic marrow failure (aplastic anaemia), *Aust. NZ. J. Med.* **4**:538–541.

Naylor, P. H. Friedman-Kien, A., Hersh, E., Erdos, M., and Goldstein, A., 1986, Thymosin alpha 1 and thymosin beta 4 in serum colon: Comparison of normal, cord, and homosexual and AIDS serum comparison, *Int. J. Immunol. Pharmacol.* **8**:667–676.

Owen, J. J. T., and Jenkinson, E. J., 1981, Embryology of the lymphoid system, *Prog. Allergy* **29**:1–34.

Pazmino, N. H., Ihle, J. N., and Goldstein, A. I., 1978a, Induction *in vivo* and *in vitro* of terminal deoxynucleotidyl transferase by thymosin in bone marrow cells from athymic mice, *J. Exp. Med.* **147**:708.

Pazmino, N. H., Ihle, J. N., McEwan, R. N., and Goldstein, A. L., 1978b, Control of differentiation of thymocyte precursors in the bone marrow by thymic hormones, *Cancer Treatm. Rep.* **62**:1749–1755.

Pierpaoli, W., 1975, Inability of thymus cells from newborn donors to restore transplantation immunity in athymic mice, *Immunology* **29**:802–803.

Pierpaoli, W., 1981, Integrated phylogenetic ontogenetic evolution of the neuroendocrine system and identity-defense, immune functions, in: *Psychoimmunology* (R. Arden ed.), Academic, Orlando, Florida, pp. 575–606.

Pierpaoli, W., and Besedovsky, H., 1975, Role of the thymus in programming of neuroendocrine functions, *Clin. Exp. Immunol.* **20**:323–338.

Pierpaoli, W., and Maestroni, M., 1981, *Proceedings XXVIII Inter. Cong. of Physiol. Sciences*, Budapest.

Pierpaoli, W., and Sorkin, E., 1972, Hormones, thymus and lymphocyte functions, *Experientia* **28**:1385–1389.

Pierpaoli, W., Kopp, H. G., and Bianchi, E., 1976, Interdependence of thymic and neuroendocrine functions in ontogeny, *Clin. Exp. Immunol.* **24**:501–506.

Pierpaoli, W., Haemmerli, M., Sorkin, E., and Hurni, H., 1977, Role of thymus and hypothalamus in ageing, in: *European Symposium on Basic Research in Gerontology*, Vergag Straube, Erlangen, pp. 141–150.

Platt, B. S., and Stewart, R. J. C., 1962, Transverse trabeculae and osteoporosis in bones in experimental protein-calorie deficiency, *Br. J. Nutr.* **16**:483–495.

Platt, B. S., and Stewart, R. J. C., 1967, Experimental protein-calorie deficiency: Histopathological changes in the endocrine glands of pigs. *J. Endocrinol.* **38**:121–143.

Plaut, S. M., Friedman, S. B., 1981, Psychosocial factors in infectious disease, in: *Psychoneuroimmunology* (R. Ader, ed.), Academic, Orlando, Florida.

Porter, K. A., and Cooper, E. H., 1962, Transformation of adult allogeneic small lymphocytes after transfusion into new born rats, *J. Exp. Med.* **115:**997–1007.

Porter, R. W., Hibbert, C., and Wellman, C., 1980, Backache and the lumbar spinal canal, *Spine* **5:**99–105.

Porter, R. W., and Pavitt, D., 1987, The vertebral canal. 1. Nutrition and development: An archaeological study, *Spine* **12:**901–906.

Porter, R. W., Drinkall, J. N., Porter, D. E., and Thorp, L., 1987b, The vertebral canal. II. Health and academic status, A clinical study, *Spine* **12:**907–911.

Riley, V., 1981, Psychoneuroendocrine influences on immunocompetence and neoplasia, *Science* **212:**110–1109.

Roaf, P., 1960, Vertebral growth and its mechanical control, *J. Bone Joint Surg.* **42B:**40–59.

Rose, N. R., Milgroom, F., and Von Oso, C., 1973, *Principles of Immunology*, Macmillan, New York.

Silverstein, A. M., 1970, Lymphogenesis, immunogenesis, and the generation of immunologic diversity, in: *Developmental Aspects of Antibody Formation and Structure*, Vol. I (J. Sterzl and I. Riha, eds.), Academic, New York, pp. 69–77.

Smedley, H., Katrak, M., Sikora, K., and Wheeler, T., 1983, Neurological effects of recombinant human interferon, *Br. Med. J.* **286:**262.

Sparrow, D., Borkan, G. A., Gerzof, S. G., Wisnniewski, C., and Silbert, J., *Diabetes* **35:**411.

Steinman, G. G., 1986, Changes in the thymus during aging, *Curr. Top. Pathol.* **75:**43–88.

Stutman, O., 1978, Intrathymic and extrathymic T cell maturation, *Immunol. Rev.* **42:**139–184.

Stutman, O., and Good, R. A., 1971, Immunocompetence of embryonic hemopoietic cells after traffic to thymus, *Transplant Proc.* **3:**923–925.

Usher, R. H., and McLean, F. H., 1974, Normal fetal growth and the significance of fetal growth retardation, in: *Scientific Foundations of Pediatrics* (J. A. Davis and J. Dobbing, eds.) W. B. Saunders, Philadelphia, pp. 69–80.

Vetter, V., Helbing, G., Heit, W., Pirsig, W., Sterzig, K., and Heinze, E., 1985, Clonal proliferation and cell density of chondrocytes isolated from human fetal epiphyseal, human adult articular and nasal cartilage, influence of hormones and growth factors, *Growth* **49:**229–245.

Watts, T., 1969, Thymus weights in malnourished children, *J. Trop. Pediatr.* **15:**155–158.

Weksler, M. E., Innes, J. B., and Goldstein, G., 1978, Immunological studies of aging. IV. The contribution of thymic involution to the immune deficiencies of aging mice and reversal with thymopoietin, *J. Exp. Med.* **148:**996–1006.

Wilson, M., Rosen, F. S., Schlossman, S. F., and Reinhoez, E. L., 1985, Ontogeny of human T-cells and B-lymphocytes during stressed and normal gestation: Phenotypic analysis of umbilical cord lymphocytes from term and preterm infants, *Clin. Immunol. Immunopathol.* **37:**1–12.

Winick, M., 1969, Malnutrition and brain development, *J. Pediatr.* **74:**657–679.

Winick, M., and Rosso, P., 1969, Head circumference and cellular growth of the brain in normal and marasmic children, *J. Pediatr.* **74:**774–778.

Xanthou, M., 1985, Immunologic deficiencies in small-for-date neonates, *Acta Paediatr. Scand. Suppl.* **319:**143–149.

Zamenhof, S., Van Marthens, E., and Margolis, F. L., 1968, DNA (cell number) and protein in neonatal brain: Alteration by maternal dietary protein restriction, *Science* **160:**322–323.

Zinkernagel, R. M., 1978, Thymus and lymphohemopoietic cells: Their role in T cell maturation, in selection of T cells' H-2-restriction-specificity and in H-2 linked Ir gene control, *Immunol. Rev.* **42:**224–270.

Immunological Components and Immunoregulation in Aging

Alterations in B Cells and Antibodies of Aged Mice

NORMAN R. KLINMAN, SYLVIA C. RILEY,
DORITH ZHARHARY, BARBARA G. FROSCHER,
GORDON D. POWERS,
and PHYLLIS-JEAN LINTON

1. INTRODUCTION

Among the immunologic defects associated with aging is a decrease in humoral immune responses. Much of this decrease in antibody production, particularly in response to T-dependent antigens, is the result of diminished T-cell helper function (Price and Makinodan, 1972; Nordin and Makinodan, 1974, Makinodan, 1972; Krosgrud and Perkins, 1977; Segre and Segre, 1976). However, multiple alterations in B-cell function have also been identified in aged individuals (Callard *et al.*, 1977; Goidl *et al.*, 1976; Kishimoto and Yamamura, 1971; Kishimoto *et al.*, 1976; Zharhary and Klinman, 1983; Zharhary and Klinman, 1986a; Zharhary and Klinman, 1986b). The alterations in B cells of aged mice are generally evidenced in two ways: (1) the decreased amount of antibody production after antigenic stimulation to many but not all antigens (Kishimoto and Yamamura, 1971; Kishimoto *et al.*, 1976; Zharhary and Klinman, 1983, 1986a); and (2) subtle but reproducible alterations in the antibody specificities expressed by immunized aged versus young animals (Goidl *et al.*, 1976, 1980; Zharhary and Klinman, 1983; Szewczuk and Campbell, 1980; Doria *et al.*, 1978). Such changes in B-cell function could be the result of intrinsic differences in the B cells generated in aged versus young individuals or alternatively may reflect the consequences of environmental modulation of expressed B cells that could differ in aged versus young individuals. An example of the latter effect is the well-demonstrated increase in anti-idiotypic reactivity that appears to accumulate as mice age (Klinman, 1981; Goidl *et al.*, 1980). This increase in anti-idiotypic reactivity dampens the responsiveness of all B cells—even those derived from young mice—when they are placed in the environment of an aged mouse (Klinman, 1981).

NORMAN R. KLINMAN, SYLVIA C. RILEY, DORITH ZHARHARY, BARBARA G. FROSCHER, GORDON D. POWERS, and PHYLLIS-JEAN LINTON • Department of Immunology, Scripps Clinic and Research Foundation, La Jolla, California 92037.

2. THE FREQUENCY OF HAPTEN-SPECIFIC SPLENIC B CELLS IN AGED MICE

To determine the cellular and environmental contributions to the B-cell alterations associated with aging, experimental methods that permit the stimulation and evaluation of clonal responses of isolated B cells at various developmental stages have been used (Zharhary and Klinman, 1983, 1986a,b). Table I summarizes the data obtained from an extensive analysis of the frequency of B cells obtained from aged versus young mice that respond to stimulation with the haptenic determinants 2,4-dinitrophenol (DNP), (4-hydroxy-3-nitro-phenyl) acetyl (NP), and (4-hydroxy-3,5-dinitrophenyl) acetyl (NNP). It can be seen that, on a per-B-cell basis, the frequency of mature splenic B cells responsive to these antigens is lower in aged mice than in young mice. It should be noted that there are no substantive differences in the amount, isotype, or affinity of antibodies produced by the clonal progeny of B cells derived from aged versus young individuals (Zharhary and Klinman, 1983). Thus, for most antigens, while the frequency of responsive B cells in aged mice is lower than in young mice, those B cells that do respond appear to be normal.

3. THE GENERATION OF BONE MARROW B CELL PRECURSORS IN AGED MICE

Also shown in Table I is the frequency of antigen-responsive surface immunoglobulin-negative (sIg^-) precursor cells obtained from the bone marrow of aged and young mice. It can be seen that the frequency of DNP-, NP-, and NNP-responsive cells in the newly generated B-cell pool of aged mice is very similar to that in young mice. Thus, the low frequency of B cells responsive to a variety of antigens in the mature splenic B-cell popula-

TABLE I. Antigen-Specific Precursor Cell Frequencies
Determined in Fragment Cultures[a]

Frequency	Antigen	Mouse strain	Spleen		sIg^- bone marrow	
			Old[b]	Young[c]	Old	Young
Reduced	DNP	BALB/c	1.1[d]	2.3	0.4	0.57
	NP	BALB/c	0.28	0.54	0.13	0.15
		B10.D2	0.39	0.75	—	—
	NNP	B10.D2	0.7	1.78	—	—
Normal	PR8	BALB/c	0.57	0.56	—	—
	PR8-HA	BALB/c	0.23	0.22	—	—
Elevated	PC	BALB/c	0.97	0.57	0.25 (58%)[e]	0.04 (38%)[e]

[a]Data abstracted from Zharhary and Klinman (1983, 1984, 1986a,b).
[b]Old mice were 23–25 months old.
[c]Young mice were 2–4 months old.
[d]Responses/10^6 injected cells.
[e]Percentage of monoclonal antibodies that were $T15^-$.

tion of aged mice does not reflect a reduced capacity of the stem cell population to generate normal number of antigen responsive B cells. Instead, the data are best interpreted as indicating a shortened functional half-life of newly generated B cells in aged individuals. Such a reduction in the functional half-life of B cells could be the result of either an intrinsic defect in the newly generated B cells or an environmental downregulation of B cells that results in an accelerated loss of their functionality.

4. THE RESPONSE TO PHOSPHORYLCHOLINE IN AGED BALB/c MICE

Although the frequency of splenic B cells responsive to most antigenic determinants is significantly lower in aged versus young mice, for certain antigens, e.g., influenza virus PR8 hemagglutinin (PR8-HA) (Zharhary and Klinman, 1984), the frequency is approximately equivalent (Table I). In addition, the frequency of phosphorylcholine (PC)-responsive splenic B cells is actually increased in aged individuals (Table I) (Zharhary and Klinman, 1986b). The increased frequency of PC-responsive B cells in aged mice is not indicative of a longer functional half-life as compared with cells responsive to DNP, NP, or NNP, since a dramatic increase in the frequency of PC-responsive B cells is also observed in the sIg$^-$ bone marrow precursor cell pool.

The murine response to PC is unique in that almost all antibodies obtained from all tested strains of young mice use the same heavy-chain variable-region segment, V_h-S107 (Lieberman et al., 1974; Kohler, 1975; Gearhart et al., 1975; Perlmutter et al., 1984). In BALB/c mice, the vast majority of B cells that respond to PC use not only V_h-S107 but also one light chain (Vκ T15) and thus share idiotype (Perlmutter et al., 1984). Using anti-idiotypic antibodies specific for the prototype TEPC-15 (T15) myeloma protein, the responses of splenic B cells and sIg$^-$ bone marrow precursor cells of aged and young mice were analyzed with respect to their level of expression of the predominant clonotype. As anticipated, most of the responses from both the spleen and bone marrow populations of young mice were T15$^+$. However, the majority of responses of sIg$^-$ cells of aged mice were T15$^-$ (Table I).

5. ALTERATIONS IN ANTIBODY VARIABLE REGION GENE UTILIZATION IN AGED MICE

One of the unique aspects of the murine response to PC is that even those PC-specific antibodies that are T15$^-$ tend to use V_h-S107. Thus, the potential molecular basis for the 6- to 10-fold increase in T15$^-$ PC-responsive precursor cells in the bone marrow of aged mice was investigated. In order to do this, two approaches have been employed. First, a series of hybridomas was constructed by the transfer-fusion protocol (Liu et al., 1984) using bone marrow B cells from either aged or young mice. These hybridomas were then analyzed for their V_h gene utilization. Eight hybridomas were obtained from the bone marrow of young mice, all of which use a V_h gene segment that hybridizes specifically to V_h-S107. By contrast, among 14 PC-specific hybridomas obtained from bone marrow cells of aged mice, only five use members of the V_h-S107 family. Seven of the nine remaining hybridomas use variable regions identified as members of other V_h-gene segment families, including V_h-7183, V_h-X24, and V_h-J558.

In order to analyze these responses more extensively, riboprobes specific for various V_h-gene segments were constructed. Using these riboprobes, V_h gene-segment utilization by the clonal progeny of B cells stimulated in fragment cultures was delineated. Preliminary results from these analyses indicate that more than 90% of splenic and sIg^- bone marrow precursor cells obtained from young mice use a heavy-chain variable-region segment that hybridizes with a riboprobe specific for V_h-S107. By the same analysis, a large proportion of monoclonal responses obtained from PC-responsive sIg^- precursors of aged mice were negative for the use of V_h-S107.

6. CONCLUSION

The analysis of the PC response of BALB/c mice has provided a graphic demonstration that one component of the immunologic alteration associated with aging is the expression of novel variable-region gene combinations in newly generated B cells of aged mice. Indeed, at least for the response to PC, repertoire diversity appears to be increased rather than decreased in aged BALB/c mice. Whether such changes in repertoire expression contribute to the increased autoimmunity and/or anti-idiotypic reactivity seen in aged mice has yet to be determined.

Importantly, this alteration in repertoire expression associated with aging apparently reflects an intrinsic change in the molecular mechanism responsible for the generation of B cells in aged versus young individuals. The cellular origin of this alteration is not yet known. For example, since newly generated B cells emanate from stem cells within the bone marrow, it has yet to be determined at which level of stem-cell development the novel V-region gene expression associated with aging occurs. Nonetheless, the demonstration of a reproducible alteration in B-cell repertoire generation that occurs in aged BALB/c mice provides a novel approach to the analysis of the control of variable-region gene expression in the immune system per se and may provide a valuable marker for the aging process.

ACKNOWLEDGMENTS. This work was supported by grant AG 01743 from the National Institutes of Health. SCR, BGF, GDP, and PJL were supported by NIH Training Grant AG-00080. SCR was also supported by a Frank L. Crocker Postdoctoral Fellowship from the Cancer Research Institute.

REFERENCES

Callard, R. E., Basten, A., and Waters, L. K., 1977, Immune function in aged mice. II. B cell function, Cell. Immunol. 31:26–36.

Doria, G., D'Agostaro, G., and Porette, A., 1978, Age dependent variations of antibody avidity, Immunology. 35:601–611.

Gearhart, P. J., Sigal, N., and Klinman, N. R., 1975, Heterogeneity of the BALB/c anti-phosphorylcholine antibody response at the precursor cell level, J. Exp. Med. 141:56–71.

Goidl, E. A., Innes, H. B., and Weksler, M. E., 1976, Immunological studies of aging. II. Loss of IgG and high avidity plaque-forming cells and increased suppressor cell activity in aging mice, J. Exp. Med. 144:1037–1048.

Goidl, E. A., Thorbecke, G. J., Weksler, M. E., and Siskind, G. W., 1980, Production of auto-anti-idiotypic antibody during the normal immune response: Changes in the auto-anti-idiotypic antibody response and the idiotype repertoire associated with aging, *Proc. Natl. Acad. Sci. USA* **77**:6788–6792.

Kishimoto, S., and Yamamura, Y., 1971, Immune responses in aged mice: Changes of antibody-forming cell precursors and antigen-reactive cells with aging, *Clin. Exp. Immunol.* **8**:957–962.

Kishimoto, S., Takahana, T., and Mizumachi, H., 1976, In vitro immune responses to the 2,4,6-trinitrophenyl determinant in aged C57BL/6J mice: Changes in the humoral immune response to, avidity for the TNP determinant and responsiveness to LPS effect with aging, *J. Immunol.* **116**:294–300.

Klinman, N. R., 1981, Antibody-specific immunoregulation and the immunodeficiency of aging, *J. Exp. Med.* **154**:547–551.

Kohler, H., 1975, The response to phosphorylcholine: Dissecting an immune response, *Transplant. Rev.* **27**:24–55.

Krosgrud, T. L., and Perkins, E. H., 1977, Age-related changes in T-cell function, *J. Immunol.* **118**:1607–1611.

Lieberman, R., Potter, M., Mushinski, W., Humphrey, W., Jr., and Rudikoff, S., 1974, Genetics of a new IgV$_H$ (T15 idiotype) marker in the mouse regulating natural antibody to phosphorylcholine, *J. Exp. Med.* **139**:983–1001.

Liu, F. T., Bohn, J. W., Ferry, E. L., Yamamoto, H., Molinaro, C. A., Sherman, L. A., Klinman, N. R., and Katz, D. H., 1980, Monoclonal dinitrophenyl-specific murine IgE antibody: Preparation, isolation, and characterization, *J. Immunol.* **124**:2728–2737.

Makinodan, T., 1972, Age-related changes in antibody forming capacity, in: *Tolerance, Autoimmunity and Aging* (M. Sigel and R. Good, eds.), Charles C. Thomas, Springfield, Illinois, pp. 3–17.

Nordin, A. A., and Makinodan, T., 1974, Humoral immunity in aging, *Fed. Proc.* **33**:2033–2035.

Perlmutter, R. M., Crews, S. T., Douglas, R., Sorensen, G., Johnson, N., Nivera, N., Gearhart, P. J., and Hood, L., 1984, The generation of diversity in phosphorylcholine-binding antibodies, *Adv. Immunol.* **35**:1–37.

Price, G. B., and Makinodan, T., 1972, Immunologic deficiencies in senescence. I. Characterization of intrinsic deficiencies, *J. Immunol.* **108**:403–412.

Segre, D., and Segre, M., 1976, Humoral immunity in aged mice. II. Increased suppressor T cell activity in immunologically deficient old mice, *J. Immunol.* **116**:735–738.

Szewczuk, M. R., and Campbell, R. J., 1980, Loss of immune competence with age may be due to auto-anti-idiotypic antibody regulation, *Nature (Lond.)* **286**:164–166.

Zharhary, D., and Klinman, N. R., 1983, Antigen responsiveness of the mature and generative B cell population of aged mice, *J. Exp. Med.* **157**:1300–1308.

Zharhary, D., and Klinman, N. R., 1984, B cell repertoire diversity to PR8-influenza virus does not decrease with age, *J. Immunol.* **133**:2285–2287.

Zharhary, D., and Klinman, N. R., 1986a, The frequency and fine specificity of B cells responsive to 4-hydroxy-3-nitrophenyl acetyl (NP) in aged mice, *Cell. Immunol.* **100**:452–461.

Zharhary, D., and Klinman, N. R., 1986b, A selective increase in the generation of phosphorylcholine specific B cells associated with aging, *J. Immunol.* **136**:368–370.

33

Molecular Genetic Analysis of Human Monoclonal Gammopathies

G. N. ABRAHAM, A. PERL, P. D. GOREVIC, J. M. WILLIAMS, G. JONES, AND R. A. KYLE

1. THE BENIGN MONOCLONAL GAMMOPATHIES

Numerous age-related alterations in immune function and regulation were defined and recently summarized by Makinodan and Hirokawa (1985), Hausman and Weksler (1985), and Siskind (1987). Among the most common are those abnormalities of immune function that are mediated by B lymphocytes. In their simplest form, this may be reflected as a gradual increase in the percentage of sera obtained from presumably healthy individuals from the fifth through and past the ninth decade, which contain monoclonal immunoglobulins. Analysis of sera from 27,000 consecutive blood donors showed that while monoclonal immunoglobulins occur with a frequency of 0.17% in the general population, their incidence increases progressively with age, rising from 0.025% to 0.5% between the ages of 18–29 and 50–60 years, respectively (Fine et al., 1979). Kyle (1984) and others (Radl et al., 1975) extended these observations and demonstrated the presence of serum paraproteins in 19% of individuals 90 years and older. These paraproteins (1) do not involve a particular subset of immunoglobulin; (2) are not confined to a particular immunoglobulin class, their distribution being similar to that noted for a random population of patients with multiple myeloma and for the frequency of occurrence of immunoglobulins of various classes and subclasses in a pool of healthy individuals; (3) do not generally have any demonstrable antigenic specificity; and (4) may be at serum concentrations similar to those found in multiple myeloma (Melistedy et al., 1984). It is presumed that these paraproteins are synthesized at an accelerated rate by an amplified clone of B cells, which may reflect an abnormal immune response.

While this condition was initially termed benign monoclonal gammopathy when the

G. N. ABRAHAM, A. PERL, J. M. WILLIAMS, and G. JONES • Departments of Medicine, and Microbiology and Immunology, and Clinical Immunology Unit, University of Rochester School of Medicine and Dentistry, Rochester, New York 14642. P. D. GOREVIC • Clinical Allergy and Rheumatology Unit, Department of Medicine, State University of New York at Stony Brook, Stony Brook, New York 11794. R. A. KYLE • Department of Medicine, Clinical Immunology Unit, Mayo School of Medicine, Mayo Clinic, Rochester, Minnesota 55905.

clinical course of 250 patients were followed from 4–14 years (Kyle, 1984), 47/250 (19%) developed either a lymphoid or plasma cell malignancy. Despite numerous studies (Mac-Kenzie, 1979; Bast *et al.*, 1982); Carmagnola *et al.*, 1983; Greipp and Kyle, 1983), there are no consistent morphological or biologic criteria to predict which "benign" gammopathy will undergo malignant degeneration. For the above reasons, Kyle (1984) has suggested that because of the inability to predict the clinical outcome, these asymptomatic immu-noglobulinopathies should be termed monoclonal gammopathies of undetermined signifi-cance (MGUS).

2. THE CRYOGLOBULINEMIAS

2.1. General Properties of the Cryoglobulinemias

Other syndromes with clinical manifestations also occur almost exclusively in middle to older individuals and are associated with the presence of a monoclonal serum immu-noglobulin. Among these are hypergammaglobulinemia purpura (Clark *et al.*, 1974), diffuse demyelinating polyneuropathy (Stefansson *et al.*, 1974; Steck *et al.*, 1983), and the idi-opathic cryo- and pyroglobulinemias (Meltzer and Franklin, 1966; Brouet, *et al.*, 1974; Abraham *et al.*, 1979a; Gorevic *et al.*, 1980; Mathison *et al.*, 1971; Grossman *et al.*, 1972). Cryoglobulins are proteins that precipitate from serum *in vitro* at temperatures below 37°C and that resolubilize after rewarming. While the cryoglobulinemias have been classified into three groups, (Meltzer and Franklin, 1966; Brouet *et al.*, 1974), based on the immu-noglobulin composition of the cryoprecipitate, the type 1 monoclonal IgG without defined antigenic specificity and type 2 monoclonal IgM with anti-IgG activity have been the focus of our investigations. The clinical signs in patients with cryoglobulinemia are attributable to the temperature- and concentration-dependent formation of circulating IgG : IgG (type 1) or IgM anti-IgG : IgG (type 2) immune complexes, which produce severe peripheral vascular insuffi-ciency and vasculitis. In type 2 cryoglobulinemia, the immune complexes can also cause severe renal disease and/or peripheral or central neuropathy and may be associated with multiple organ involvement. The clinical features of type 2 or mixed cryoglobulinemia have been recently summarized by Gorevic (1986). Both types may be complicated by the devel-opment of hematologic malignancies. As is characteristic of MGUS, an excessive amount of monoclonal cryoglobulin is present in serum, presumably synthesized at an accelerated rate by an expanded clone of B cells.

However, the two types are discriminated by the properties of the cryoimmunoglobulin produced. The monoclonal IgG are individually diverse in their primary structure; may contain unprecedented and inconsistent mutations of primary amino acid sequence through-out the V regions of both their light and heavy chains; comprise all γ-chain subclasses, light-chain types, and V-region subgroups; and have no defined antigenic specificity (Jones *et al.*; Abraham *et al.*, 1979b). By contrast, virtually all the IgM cryoglobulins contain κ-light chains, 90% of which belong to the VK-iii variable region subgroup, and from patient to patient, are almost all identical in primary structure. These κ-chains have recently been shown to be the product of a germline gene (Jirik *et al.*, 1986; Radoux *et al.*, 1986). The near-exclusive selectivity of the Vk-iii light chain in the IgM anti-IgG found in type 2 cryoglobulinemia contrasts with the spectrum of light-chain V regions found for the anti-IgG (rheumatoid factors) in the sera of patients with rheumatoid arthritis and related diseases (Williams *et al.*, 1987). Because of these differences, we propose that the B-cell clones producing type 1 and type 2 cryoglobulins may be activated at different developmental stages and represent different B-cell synthetic disorders.

Our studies have been directed toward clarifying the molecular genetic and biologic properties of the B cells involved in these diseases and in determining the basis for their excessive cryoimmunoglobulin synthesis and ensuing malignant degeneration. This information is of great relevance to understanding of other disorders of abnormal B-lymphocyte function in the elderly and of the development of B-cell malignancies in general.

2.2. Frequency and Immunoglobulin Synthetic Rate of Cryoglobulin-Producing B Cells

Previous investigations have demonstrated that B cells bearing the immunoglobulin idiotype comprise 0.05–4% of the peripheral blood B-lymphocyte pool of, and are amplified in, patients with MGUS (Bast *et al.*, 1979, 1982). However, the detection of an expanded population of idiotype-positive cells in the peripheral blood or bone marrow of patients with cryoglobulinemia has been difficult (Ono *et al.*, 1986) and findings have not been reported for the cryoglobulinemias. As an approach to this question, peripheral blood mononuclear cells from 12 patients with type 2 cryoglobulinemia were isolated by centrifugation through Ficoll-Hypaque and assayed by flow cytometry using antisera specific for B- and T-cell markers, the immunoglobulin classes, and light-chain types. Expansion of IgM-k-positive B cells was found in four patients. Two patients had κ/λ ratios of 3.5 and 14, which are significantly increased as compared with normal controls. No abnormalities have been noted in the frequency of cells bearing the CD3, CD8, or CD4 T-cell markers.

In addition, supernatants of cultures of peripheral blood lymphocytes from four type 1 and six type 2 cryoglobulinemia patients infected with Epstein–Barr virus (EBV) or stimulated with pokeweed mitogen (PWM) were analyzed by microtiter or spot enzyme-linked immunosorbent assay (ELISA) for the presence and frequency of cryoglobulin producing B-cells and for the quantity of specific cryoglobulin. Preliminary data suggest a frequency for cryoglobulin-producing B cells, in a range similar to that detected for the MGUS. It is apparent from this and other studies (Ono *et al.*, 1986) that B cells that synthesize the cryoparaproteins are capable of being stimulated and amplified *in vitro*. While the absolute synthetic rate of cryoglobulin per B cell has not as yet been determined, previous *in vivo* metabolic studies reported from these laboratories (Abraham *et al.*, 1979) demonstrated that nearly eight times as much IgG-k cryoglobulin as normal IgG was synthesized per day in a patient whose cryoglobulin-producing B cells were estimated as comprising 6–8% of the total peripheral B-lymphocyte pool.

2.3. Molecular Genetic Analysis

Genomic DNA was isolated from purified peripheral lymphocytes, B cells, or T cells, digested with appropriate restriction enzymes, and analyzed by Southern blotting (Southern, 1975) for the presence of immunoglobulin gene rearrangements. The normal peripheral blood B-cell pool contains a multitude of diverse immunoglobulin gene rearrangements, which are not individually detectable by Southern blotting (Korsmeyer *et al.*, 1982). When detected, specific immunoglobulin gene rearrangements are thought to indicate the presence of a malignant clone (or clones) of B cells (Hieter *et al.*, 1981). Our results are summarized in Table I. Four patients with type 1 and 12 patients with type 2 cryoglobulinemia were studied

TABLE I. Frequency of Gene
Rearrangements in Cryoglobulinemia

	Type 1	Type 2
No. patients	4	12
Ig gene	3/4	4/12
c-myc	2/3	1/4
Karyotype abnormality	1/4	0/3

and immunoglobulin gene rearrangements detected in the frequencies indicated. While DNA from all patients was assayed, rearrangement of the *c-myc* proto-oncogene was noted for two of the three type 1 and one of the four type 2 patients who demonstrated immunoglobulin gene rearrangements. In all experiments, DNA isolated from placenta and/or the patient's granulocytes was used as a germline control. Representative examples of the Southern blotting patterns obtained are shown in Fig. 1a,b for type 1 and type 2 cryoglobulins, respectively. Despite the presence of only one monoclonal protein in the sera of both patients, the multiple bands detected with the immunoglobulin gene probes [J_H, $C\mu$, and C-γ-4], indicate the presence of two or more distinct B-cells clones. While presumed to be non-secretory, these B cells may have the potential for production of paraprotein. These findings were previously detailed by Perl *et al.* (1987).

Because of the previously described association of chromosomal abnormalities in lymphocytes isolated from patients with cold agglutinin disease (Silberstein *et al.*, 1986) and other B-cell neoplasias (Croce and Nowell, 1986), karyotypic analysis was performed on the lymphocytes of four patients with type 1 and in three patients with type 2 cryoglobulinemia. Only lymphocytes from patient Br (Southern blot shown in Fig. 1a) demonstrated chromosomal aberrations. Three cells were detected that showed a deletion of the long arm of chromosome 8. One of these also contained 47 chromosomes with trisomy 17 (Perl *et al.*, 1987).

2.4. Correlation of Clinical Disease with Molecular Genetic Changes

In order to determine whether changes in the patterns of immunoglobulin gene rearrangements correlated with disease activity, blood samples were collected repeatedly from eight patients with type 2 cryoglobulinemia for up to 3 years. In five patients, no clonal patterns were ever detected. In two patients, whose clinical disease had either become quiescent or was markedly diminished in severity, and whose sera showed loss or diminished content of IgM cryoglobulin, the prominent immunoglobulin gene rearrangements that were previously found were no longer noted. Thus, clonally expanded B-cell populations were no longer present in peripheral blood. In a third patient, whose clinical course has been gradually

→

FIGURE 1. DNA was isolated from lymphocytes (L) of patients with (a) type 1 (BR) and (b) type 2 (CA) cryoglobulinemia, digested with the indicated restriction enzymes, hybridized to the indicated immunoglobulin gene probes, and analyzed by Southern blotting. Arrows, rearranged fragments; =, co-migrating bands as determined by sequential hybridization of the same blot to the probes shown.

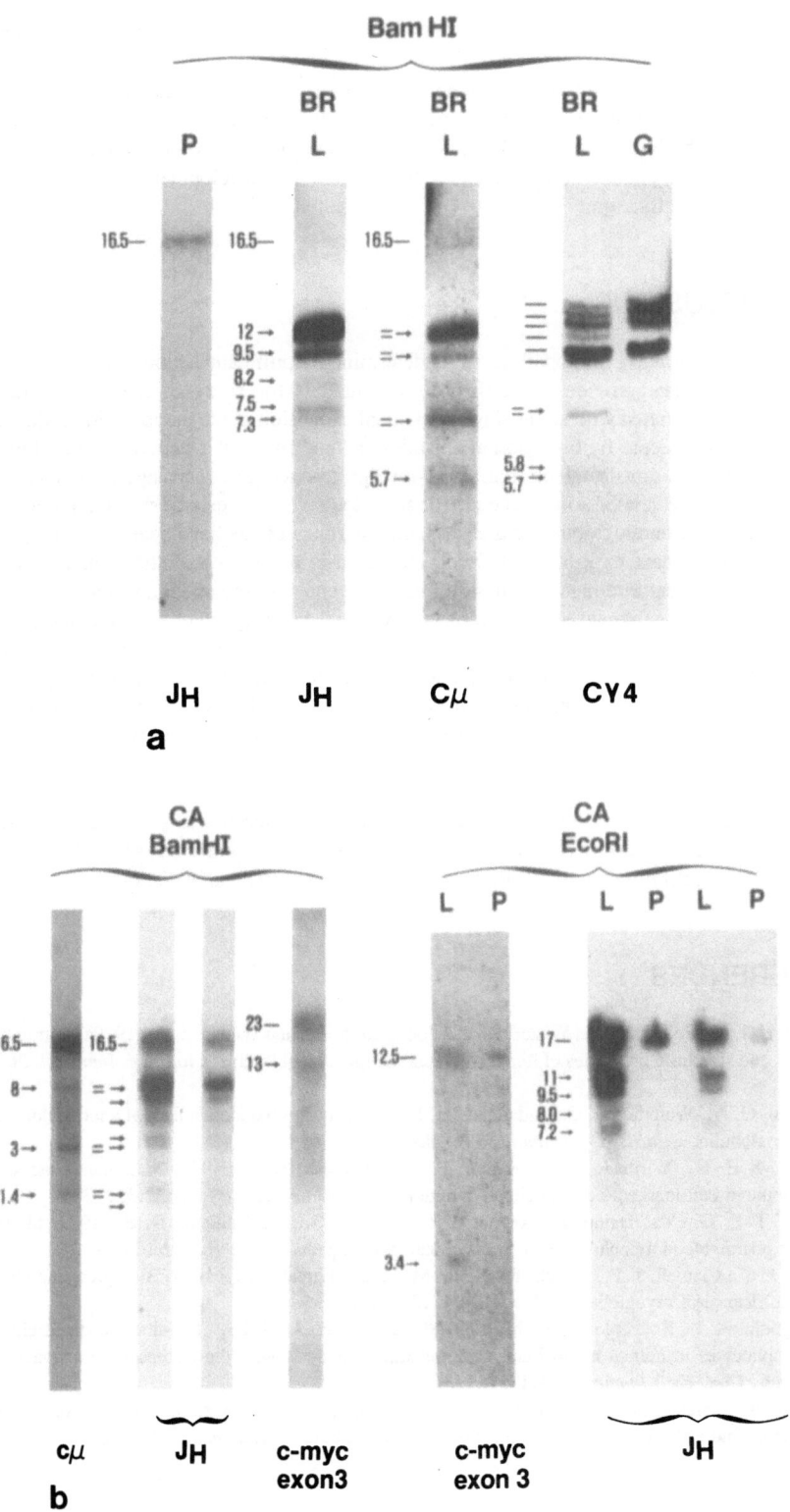

progressive, DNA isolated from lymphocytes 2 years previously showed only germline configurations, while current samples demonstrate both J_H and $C\mu$ rearrangements. Perhaps, the immunoglobulin gene rearrangements are indicative of an insidious increase in disease severity, and this patient may potentially be targeted for development of malignancy or marked disease activation.

3. CONCLUSIONS

The monoclonal gammopathies of undetermined significance, and the cryoglobulin-emias in particular, provide interesting disease models for study of the B-cell immune dysfunctions associated with advancing age. Clonal expansion of the paraprotein producing B cells has been detected by both immunohistological and molecular genetic means. Further-more, while not a consistent finding, the *c-myc* proto-oncogene rearrangements have been noted and may be related to or account for the excessive synthesis of immunoglobulin. In addition, while immunoglobulin and *c-myc* gene rearrangements have been previously asso-ciated with malignant expansion of B-cell clones, it is obvious that other conditions exist which may represent intermediate phases of cellular gene rearrangement and activation, from the benign to the malignant state. Clearly, *c-myc* gene rearrangement and activation, while potentially necessary, is not sufficient in and of itself for the development of a malignant B-cell neoplasm in these patients. Finally, the use of the molecular genetic techniques may provide a means of evaluating and following the clinical state of the patient. However, additional clinical correlative studies are required to prove the ultimate efficacy and predic-tive value of these techniques.

ACKNOWLEDGMENTS. The research described in this manuscript was supported by USPHS grants RO-1 AG-06350, AG-08177, AI-19658, AM-26588, and PO1-AI-21288, and the James P. Wilmot Foundation. A. Perl is a Wilmot Cancer Research Fellow.

REFERENCES

Abraham, G. N., Podell, D. N., Wistar, R., Jr., Johnston, S. L., and Welch, E. H., 1979a, Immunolog-ical and structural properties of human monoclonal IgG cryoglobulins, *Clin. Exp. Immunol.* 36:63–70.

Abraham, G. N., Waterhouse, C., and Condemi, J. J., 1979b, In vivo metabolism of a monoclonal IgG cryoglobulin, *Clin. Exp. Immunol.* 35:89–95.

Bast, B. J. E. G., Wiringa, G., VanCamp, B., and Ballieux, R. E., 1979, Malignancy associated lymphoid cell-markers in monoclonal gammopathy, *Protides Biol. Fluids* 27:351–355.

Bast, B. J. E. G., Van Damp, B., Reynaert, P., Wiringa, G., and Ballieux, R. E., 1982, Idiotypic peripheral blood lymphocytes in monoclonal gammopathy, *Clin. Exp. Immunol.* 47:677–682.

Brouet, J. C., Clauvel, J. P., Danon, F., Klein, M., and Seligmann, M., 1974, Biological and clinical significance of cryoglobulins, *Am. Med.* 57:775–788.

Carmagnola, A. I., Boccadoro, M., Massaia, M., and Pileri, A., 1983, The idiotypic specificities of lymphocytes in human monoclonal gammopathies: Analysis with the fluorescence activated cell sorter, *Clin. Exp. Immunol.* 51:173–177.

Clark, R. A., Abraham, G. N., Kyle, R. A., and Vaughan, J. H., 1974, Gamma globulin complexes in rheumatoid arthritis and hypergammaglobulinemia purpura, *J. Rheumatol.* 1:54–65.

Croce, C. M., and Nowell, P. C., 1986, Molecular genetics of human B-cell neoplasia, *Adv. Immunol.* **38**:245–274.

Fine, J. M., Lambin, P., and Derycke, C., 1979, Systematic survey of monoclonal gammopathies in a normal adult population, *Protides Biol. Fluids* **27**:351–355.

Gorevic, P. D., 1986, Mixed cryoglobulinemia: An update of recent clinical experience, in: *Antiglobulins, Cryoglobulins and Glomerulonephritis* (C. Ponticelli, L. Minetti, and G. D'Amico, eds.), Martinus Nijhoff, Dordrecht/Boston/Lancaster, pp. 179–192.

Gorevic, P. D., Kassar, H. J., Levo, Y., Kohn, R., Meltzer, M., Prose, P., and Franklin, E. C., 1980, Mixed cryoglobulinemia: Clinical aspects and long-term follow-up of 40 patients, *Am. J. Med.* **69**:287–308.

Greipp, P. R., and Kyle, R. A., 1983, Clinical, morphological and cell–kinetic differences among multiple myeloma, monoclonal gammopathy of undetermined significance, and smoldering multiple myeloma, *Blood* **62**:166–171.

Grossman, J., Abraham, G. N., Leddy, J. P., and Condemi, J. J., 1972, Crystalglobulinemia, *Ann. Intern. Med.* **77**:395–401.

Hausman, P. B., and Weksler, M. E., 1985, Changes in the immune response with age, in: *Handbook of the Biology of Aging* (C. E. Finch and E. L. Schneider, eds.), 1987, Van Nostrand–Reinhold, New York, pp. 414–432.

Hieter, P. A., Korsmeyer, S. J., Waldman, T. A., and Leder, P., 1981, Human immunoglobulin k light-chain genes are deleted or rearranged in lambda producing B-cells, *Nature (Lond.)* **290**:368–372.

Jirik, F. R., Sorge, J., Fong, S., Heitzmann, J. G., Curd, J. G., Chen, P. P., Goldfien, R., and Carson, D. A., 1986, Cloning and sequence determination of a human rheumatoid factor light-chain gene, *Proc. Natl. Acad. Sci. USA* **83**:2195–2199.

Jones, G., Abraham, G. N, and Podell, D. N., Structural properties of monoclonal IgG cryoglobulins, manuscript in preparation.

Korsmeyer, S. J., Hieter, P. A., Sharrow, S. O., Goldman, C. K., Keder, P. and Waldman, T. A., 1982, Normal human B-cells display ordered light-chain rearrangements and deletions, *J. Exp. Med.* **156**:975–985.

Kyle, R. A., 1984, "Benign" monoclonal gammopathy. A misnomer?, *JAMA* **251**:1849–1854.

MacKenzie, M., 1979, In vitro cytotoxic response to human myeloma plasma cells by peripheral blood leukocytes from patients with multiple myeloma and benign monoclonal gammopathy, *Blood* **54**:226–237.

Makinodan, T., and Hirokawa, K., 1985, Normal aging of the immune system, in: *Relations Between Normal Aging and Disease* (H. A. Johnson, ed.), Raven, New York, pp. 117–132.

Mathison, D. A., Condemi, J. J., Leddy, J. P., Callerame, M. L., Panner, B. J., and Vaughan, J. H., 1971, Purpura, arthralgia, and IgM–IgG cryoglobulinemia with rheumatoid factor activity. Response to cyclophosphamide and splenectomy, *Ann. Intern. Med.* **74**:383–390.

Melistedy, H., Holm, G., and Bjorkholm, M. 1984, Multiple myeloma, Waldenstrom's macroglobulinemia and benign monoclonal gammopathy: Characteristics of the B-cell clone, immunoregulatory cell populations and clinical implications, *Adv. Cancer Res.* **41**:257–289.

Meltzer, M., and Franklin, E. C., 1966, Cryoglobulinemia—A study of twenty patients, *Am. J. Med.* **40**:828–836.

Ono, M., Winearls, C. G., Grennan, D., Peters, D. K., and Sissons, J. G. P., 1986, Monoclonal antibodies to idiotypic determinants on monoclonal rheumatoid factors—Application to patients with type II cryoglobulinaemia, in: *Antiglobulins, Cryoglobulins, and Glomerulonephritis* (C. Ponticelli, L. Minetti, and G. D'Amico, eds.), Martinus Nijhoff, Dordrecht/Boston/Lancaster, pp. 161–176.

Perl, A., Wang, N., Williams, J. M., Hunt, M. J., Rosenfeld, S. I., Condemi, J. J., Packman, C. H., and Abraham, G. N., 1987, Aberrant immunoglobulin and c-myc gene rearrangements in patients with nonmalignant monoclonal cryoglobulinemia, *J. Immunol.* **139**:3512–3517.

Radl, R., Skvaril, J. M., Morell, A., and Hijams, W., 1975, Immunoglobulin patterns in humans over 95 years of age, *Clin. Exp. Immunol.* **22**:84–90.

Radoux, V., Chen, P. P., Sorge, J. A., and Carson, D. A., 1986, A conserved human germline Vk gene directly encodes rheumatoid factor light chain, *J. Exp. Med.* **164**:2119–2124.

Silberstein, L. E., Robertson, G. A., Hannam-Harris, A. C., Moreau, L., Besa, E., and Nowell, P. C., 1986, Etiologic aspects of cold agglutinin disease: Evidence for cytogenetically defined clones of lymphoid cells and demonstration that an anti-Pr cold autoantibody is derived from a chromosomally-aberrant B-cell clone, *Blood* **67**:1705–1709.

Siskind, G. W., 1987, Aging and the immune system, in: *Modern Biological Theories of Aging* (H. R. Warner, ed.), Raven, New York, pp. 235–242.

Southern, E. J., 1975, Detection of specific sequences among DNA fragments separated by gel electrophoresis, *J. Mol. Biol.* **98**:503–517.

Stefansson, K., Marton, L., Antel, J-P., Wollman, R. L., Roos, R. P., Chefec, G., and Arnason, B. G. W., 1983, Neuropathy accompanying IgM-lambda monoclonal gammopathy, *Acta. Neuropathol. (Berl).* **59**:255–261.

Steck, A. J., Murray, N., Meier, C., Page, N., and Perruisseau, G., 1983, Demyelinating neuropathy and monoclonal IgM antibody to myelin-associated glycoprotein, *Neurology (NY)* **33**:19–23.

Williams, J. M., Gorevic, P. D., Looney, R. J., and Abraham, G. N., 1987, Isoelectric focusing characterization of IgM-Vkiiib immunoglobulin light chains and their association with anti-IgG autoantibodies in essential mixed cryoglobulinemia, Sjogren's syndrome and rheumatoid arthritis, *Immunology* **62**:529–535.

34

Developmental Aspects of T Lymphocytes in Aging

A. GLOBERSON, R. EREN, L. ABEL, and D. BEN-MENAHEM

1. INTRODUCTION

Decline of immunity has been considered a major cause of increased incidence of disease in old age. In order to establish approaches to treatment that would lead to augmentation of immunological vigor, attempts were made to determine the mechanisms underlying the age-related changes in the immune system. Since reduced immune responses are most pronounced in the T-cell compartment (reviewed by Makinodan et al., 1987), it has been causally related to thymic involution. Consequently, studies on treatment with thymic hormones were carried out, showing that certain immunological responses of peripheral lymphoid cells can be enhanced (Friedman et al., 1974; Weksler et al., 1978; Grinblat et al., 1983; Frasca et al., 1985). In addition, decreased function of thymic microenvironment in inducing T-cell development was reported (Hirokawa and Sado, 1978; Hirokawa et al., 1982). It was thus postulated that developmental failures may be, at least in part, the basis of immunosenescence. Indications that immature T cells become abundant in aging were subsequently reported (Jensen et al., 1986), lending further support to this idea. In this respect, the increase in levels of PNA+ cells noted in aging mouse spleen (Globerson et al., 1981) seemed to conform to this notion. However, the precise nature of developmental failures has hardly been established. The main difficulty has been the fact that T-cell development is a complex stepwise process. It involves migration of stem cells from lymphohematopoietic tissues into the thymus, in which differentiation into various T-cell subsets occurs (Scollay et al., 1984), and T-cell receptor genes are rearranged (Snodgrass et al., 1985). Furthermore, although generation of T cells starts in early ontogeny and continues throughout the life span, the tissue origin of cells that seed the thymus changes with aging, in addition to the aging processes in the thymus itself. Thus, sequential changes have been described regarding the source of cells that can settle in the thymus in ontogeny and the adult, starting in the

A. GLOBERSON, R. EREN, L. ABEL, and D. BEN-MENAHEM • Department of Cell Biology, Weizmann Institute of Science, Rehovot, Israel 76100.

embryonic yolk sac, continuing in the fetal liver, with the bone marrow eventually becoming the major site of lymphohematopoietic stem cells throughout the life span. The question that then arose was whether any age-related changes in the bone marrow compartment may be manifested in the nature of T cells generated in old age. The problem with critically approaching this question is that it is hard to follow the cells *in vivo* from their initial origin via the circulation to the thymus and to evaluate their differentiation in the thymus, which is itself changing with age. In addition, the continuous influx of cells as well as emigration to the peripheral tissues represent further obstacles in identifying the origin and fate of the T cells appearing in the thymus and in evaluating the effects of this dynamic situation on the differentiating cells. Moreover, the stem cells in their different tissue origins, as well as cells in the thymus, may be subject to hormonal effects, which have not yet been elucidated. Consequently, the question of whether developmental changes continue within the bone marrow stem cell compartment throughout the life span and whether these changes may account, at least in part, for T-cell senescence, has been controversial (Farrar *et al.*, 1974; Tyan, 1977; Harrison *et al.*, 1978; Ross *et al.*, 1982; Astle and Harrison, 1984).

Ideally, for a proper analysis of age-related developmental failures in the T-cell compartment, each step needs to be examined separately, under critical conditions. This chapter presents a brief review of our studies in this area, focusing mainly on age-related changes in the potential of lymphohematopoietic cells to differentiate into T lymphocytes in the thymus.

2. EXPERIMENTAL STRATEGY

We have been studying possible developmental failures in T cells in aging, by combining *in vivo* and *in vitro* experimental systems. Using a mouse model, we investigated the potential of lymphohematopoietic stem cells to develop into T cells from early ontogeny to old age, by transferring them to irradiated recipients as well as by seeding them *in vitro* into fetal thymic stroma.

The *in vitro* experimental model was based on our early observations that fetal thymus, depleted of its lymphocytes by treatment with urethane, could be reconstituted *in vitro* by young adult bone marrow cells (Globerson and Auerbach, 1965). To achieve maximal depletion of thymocytes from the fetal thymus, we used 2-deoxyguanosine (Jenkinson *et al.*, 1982). The lymphocyte-depleted fetal thymus lobes were then reconstituted with cells from various lymphohematopoietic tissues, as described (Eren *et al.*, 1987b). To ascertain that the developing T cells were indeed of donor origin, and not thymus-generated cells, we used the Thy 1 congenic strains Thy 1.1 and Thy 1.2, for fetal thymus and donors of lymphohematopoietic stem cells. Accordingly, the conclusion that the T cells developed from the reconstituting cells was based on the observation that they expressed the donor Thy 1 allotype, and not the recipient thymus allotype. The advantage of this *in vitro* approach is that it enables focusing on the potential of the cells to develop in the thymus, uncoupled from the capacity to circulate and home to the thymus. This system was used to compare the potential of lymphohematopoietic cells from various tissue origins (including the spleen, which is hematopoietic in the mouse) to give rise to T lymphocytes. By this experimental strategy, we were able to evaluate the potential of the various tissue sources of T lymphocytes from early ontogeny to senescence, under the same conditions, and to distinguish between processes that occur within the thymus and events that may be associated with cell circulation and homing, or environmental effects *in vivo*.

3. DEVELOPMENT OF T LYMPHOCYTES IN ONTOGENY

3.1. Development of T Lymphocytes in Fetal Liver Radiation Chimeras

Studies designed to examine the potential of lymphohematopoietic stem cells to give rise to T lymphocytes were based chiefly on the reconstitution of irradiated mice with hematopoietic cells from donors of different age groups, and the T cells were assessed in the resulting chimeras. Using this approach, we demonstrated that 14-day fetal liver cells can differentiate into T lymphocytes, detectable in the peripheral lymphoid tissues of the chimeras (Rabinowich et al., 1983). Furthermore, we showed that when fetal liver and bone marrow chimeras were established in parallel, under the same experimental conditions, appearance of T cells in the spleen and lymph nodes of the fetal liver chimeras lagged behind that in the bone marrow chimeras. Development of the T lymphocytes in the chimeras depended on the presence of the thymus (Rabinowich et al., 1983). We subsequently examined the pattern of development in the thymus, of T lymphocytes from fetal liver as compared with donor-type bone marrow-derived cells. As shown in Table I, T lymphocytes from both fetal liver and bone marrow donors developed in the thymus of the irradiated recipients. The appearance of donor-type T cells was delayed in the fetal liver as compared with bone marrow chimeras, similar to our previous observations on the peripheral lymphoid tissues. In addition, it was noted in both cases, that the first wave of cells emerging in the thymus in both cases was of recipient type, as revealed from the Thy 1 allotype of the T cells (Table I). Under these in vivo experimental conditions, it was difficult to determine whether the results pointed to a lower potential of the fetal liver cells to give rise to T lymphocytes or to a different capacity of the cells to circulate and home to the thymus. To clarify this, further studies, based on an in vitro approach, were carried out.

TABLE I. Phenotypes of Cells in the Thymus of Fetal Liver and Bone Marrow Radiation Chimeras

Donor cells[a]	Age of the chimeras (weeks)	Cells per lobe ($\times 10^6$)	% positive cells (mean $\pm$SD)[b]				Lyt2+/ L3T4+
			Recipient type (Thy 1.1+)		Donor type (Thy 1.2+)		
			Lyt 2+	L3T4+	Lyt 2+	L3T4+	
Fetal liver	2	42 ± 10	55.7 ± 6.8	65.3 ± 5.8	10.0 ± 3.5	11.0 ± 4.1	ND[c]
	3	54 ± 11	2.3 ± 0.7	1.9 ± 0.5	62.4 ± 14	73.3 ± 4	43.8 ± 15
	4	79 ± 17	2.3 ± 0.4	3.7 ± 0.4	73.0 ± 3	94.1 ± 1	57.3 ± 8.5
Bone marrow	2	52 ± 15	23.3 ± 1.2	25.0 ± 4.3	40.5 ± 0.9	46.0 ± 1.4	ND[c]
	3	54 ± 22	2.2 ± 0.1	1.9 ± 0.2	73.0 ± 4.2	77.2 ± 0.4	50.7 ± 13
	4	70 ± 9	1.9 ± 0.1	2.9 ± 0.1	73.5 ± 1.3	95.0 ± 1.9	73.1 ± 7.5

[a]Donor cells were fetal liver from 14-day-old embryos and bone marrow from 2- to 3-month-old mice. Recipients were irradiated (950 R) 2- to 3-month-old mice.
[b]Mean values of five individuals in each group.
[c]ND, not determined.

3.2. *In Vitro* Studies on the Generation of T Lymphocytes from Fetal Tissues

Using the *in vitro* model, differentiation of T lymphocytes could be obtained from embryonic yolk sac as well as from fetal liver cells (Eren *et al.*, 1987a,b). To determine whether there is any difference in the T-cell developmental potential of the yolk sac as compared to the fetal liver, we examined the levels of T-cell subsets. The results showed a gradual age-related change in the levels of Lyt 2+ and L3T4+ subsets. However, it was noted that the levels of Lyt 2+ and L3T4+ cells in fetal thymuses reconstituted *in vitro* with the hematopoietic cells were different from those in intact fetal thymuses developing *in vitro* (Eren *et al.*, 1987b). We therefore performed additional experiments to analyze the different subsets more extensively. Double-color analysis of cells expressing the Lyt 2 and L3T4 membrane markers demonstrated that the difference between reconstituted and intact fetal thymus explants was actually in the levels of double-positive (Lyt 2+/L3T4+) and double-negative (Lyt 2−/L3T4−) cells (Table II). Regardless of the mechanisms underlying this difference, the results seem to indicate at least two possible pathways of T-cell subset development in the thymus. This is in line with the proposed scheme of T-cell development in the thymus suggested by Scollay and Shortman (1985).

It should be noted that, *in vivo*, the developmental potential of the fetal liver cells was inferior to that of the bone marrow. This may be related to the fact that the *in vitro* system preferentially supports T-lymphocyte differentiation, whereas *in vivo* erythroid and myeloid cells develop as well. Consequently, the *in vitro* system is a more critical indicator of the potential for T-cell development.

TABLE II. Developmental Patterns of Thymocytes in Fetal Thymus Explants Reconstituted with Stem Cells from Donors of Various Age Groups

Cell membrane marker	Adult[a] thymus	Cultured fetal thymus	% positive cells (mean ±SE)					
			Fetal thymus[b] reconstituted with:					
			YS	FL	YBM	OBM	YSP	OSP
Thy 1	90 ± 1	90 ± 4	90 ± 8	90 ± 6	92 ± 5	91 ± 7	48 ± 4	52 ± 3
Ly1	80 ± 2	75 ± 1	60 ± 1	70 ± 10	66 ± 2	55 ± 10	ND[c]	ND[c]
Lyt2+/L3T4+	60 ± 4	44 ± 12	23 ± 3	21 ± 6	14 ± 7	12 ± 7	8 ± 6	5 ± 4
Lyt2−/L3T4−	11 ± 1	17 ± 10	37 ± 3	49 ± 6	56 ± 17	55 ± 24	49 ± 21	58 ± 20
Lyt2+/L3T4−	14 ± 5	17 ± 7	22 ± 1	19 ± 5	14 ± 4	11 ± 1	19 ± 2	23 ± 4
Lyt2−/L3T4+	15 ± 2	22 ± 6	18 ± 1	11 ± 5	16 ± 6	23 ± 17	25 ± 16	14 ± 12

[a]Adult thymus cells were obtained from 2- to 3-month-old mice.
[b]Thymus lobes from 14-day mouse (C57BL/Ka) embryos were cultured without any treatment (cultured fetal thymus) or treated with deoxyguanosine and reconstituted with cells of 12-day embryonic yolk sac (YS), 12-day fetal liver (FL), 2- to 3-month-old mouse bone marrow (YBM) or spleen (YSP), and 24-month-old mouse bone marrow (OBM) or spleen (OSP) from C57BL/6 donors. Bone marrow and spleen cells were depleted of Thy1+ cells before reconstitution of the fetal thymuses. Cultures were assayed after 12 days of incubation. Values represent mean of results obtained from at least three repeated experiments.
[c]ND, not determined.

4. AGE-RELATED CHANGES IN THE BONE MARROW PROTHYMOCYTE COMPARTMENT

4.1. Studies on Bone Marrow Radiation Chimeras

Early studies designed to determine whether the bone marrow cells of aging mice have the same, or a different, capacity to give rise to T cells were based on transferring bone marrow cells from donors of various age groups to lethally irradiated recipients and measuring T-cell functions in the resulting bone marrow chimeras. No difference was noted in the levels of T-cell responses of the young and old bone marrow chimeras, when examined within the first 2 months after exposure (Friedman and Globerson, 1978a,b). However, 6–8 months following irradiation and reconstitution with the bone marrow, T-cell parameters measured in the spleen and lymph nodes of the old bone marrow chimeras were lower than those of the young (Gozes et al., 1982; Globerson, 1984). Obviously, under such conditions, it is difficult to dissociate changes in the capacity to migrate and home to the thymus and peripheral tissues, from the mere potential of the cells to differentiate within the thymus. Subsequent evaluation of age-related changes in the potential of the bone marrow to generate T lymphocyte was based on the in vitro model.

4.2. Bone Marrow-Derived T-Cell Development in Thymic Explants

The first studies focused on the in vitro development of T lymphocytes from young and old mouse bone marrow cells (Eren et al., 1988). We found both young and old mouse bone marrow to give rise to Thy 1^+ cells, at levels similar to those observed in intact fetal thymuses developing in vitro under similar conditions. Comparative analysis of phenotypes of the cells (See Table II) showed a similar pattern of T cells developing from young and old mouse bone marrow. Levels of Lyt2$^+$/L3T4$^+$ cells were similar to those observed in explants reconstituted with fetal cells, yet lower than those either found in intact fetal thymuses cultured without any treatment or uncultured adult thymus. Thus, the pattern of T-cell subsets developing in vitro in a lymphocyte-depleted fetal thymic stroma remains similar in principle throughout development, with respect to the origin of the cells. By contrast, generation of Lyt2$^+$/L3T4$^+$ cells seems to have essential requirements that are met in the intact thymus, in vitro or in vivo, and limited in the cultured fetal thymic stroma. Alternatively, there may be different pathways of differentiation of these cells in the thymus (Wilson et al., 1988), and the present experimental system represents distinct selective conditions.

5. CONTRIBUTION OF THE SPLEEN TO GENERATION OF T LYMPHOCYTES

5.1. Splenic Effects on Thymus Regeneration in the Adult

The contribution of the spleen to T-cell development has been documented in the past for various experimental systems. Early observations on splenic effects on developmental processes in the thymus were based on in vitro studies on spleen and thymus inductive tissue interactions in early ontogeny (Auerbach, 1965) and radiation recovery in the adult (Glober-

TABLE III. Radiation Recovery of the Thymus in Splenectomized or Sham-Operated Mice, Reconstituted with Bone Marrow or Spleen Cells after Exposure

Exp. No.	Reconstituting cells	Thymus weight (g)[a]				p value
		Splenectomized		Sham-operated		
1	None	14 ± 1.5	(9)	26.1 ± 2.1	(9)	0.0002
	Bone marrow	24.3 ± 2.7	(10)	22.8 ± 1.9	(10)	NS[b]
	Spleen	19.9 ± 2.2	(7)	20.8 ± 0.9	(9)	NS[b]
2	None	28.4 ± 4.6	(6)	51.1 ± 3.2	(7)	0.0017
	Bone marrow	40.5 ± 2.2	(3)	42.6 ± 5.8	(6)	NS[b]
	Spleen	45.6 ± 2	(6)	43.8 ± 4.5	(6)	NS[b]

[a]Values represent mean ±SE. Mice were exposed to a total-body dose of 850 R, and examined after 7 (Exp. 1) or 8 (Exp. 2) days. Numbers in parentheses represent number of mice.
[b]NS, not significant.

son, 1966). Thymic lymphoid development *in vitro* was shown to be enhanced in the presence of splenic explants. Subsequent *in vivo* studies revealed that spleen deprivation in neonatal mice had pronounced effects on the bone marrow and thymus (Battisto *et al.*, 1971; Russell and Golub, 1977). We have further studied age-related changes in this respect in the adult. To find out whether the spleen plays any role in thymic developmental processes in the adult, we examined radiation recovery of the thymus in (BALB/c × C57BL/6)F1 mice that have been splenectomized at the age of 8–10 weeks and exposed to total body irradiation (850 R) 4–10 days later. The results demonstrated that thymus recovery, as measured by weight, was delayed. The values at 7 and 8 days postexposure were significantly lower than those of sham-operated or intact irradiated controls (Table III). After the 10th day, there was no obvious difference between the various experimental groups (results not shown). In view of these results, the observations that the first wave of T cells emerging in the thymus of irradiated mice is of recipient origin (see Table I) could be related to their being radioresistant cells from the spleen or to the fact that the spleen indirectly induces radioresistant bone marrow cells to colonize the thymus, or intrathymic radioresistant T-cell precursors (Kadish and Basch, 1975) to replicate.

An indirect effect of the spleen on the thymus had been suggested from early organ culture studies (Auerbach, 1965). To examine whether the spleen contains any thymus reconstituting cells that can differentiate into T lymphocytes, we performed *in vitro* experiments as described below.

5.2. *In Vitro* Development of T Cells from Splenocytes

In view of observations on the *in vivo* effects of the spleen on thymus regeneration, we examined the capacity of spleen cells to differentiate into T cells, after seeding in the thymic stroma. The splenocytes were depleted of mature T cells, before reconstitution by treatment with anti Thy 1 antibodies and complement to distinguish between T-cell development and maintenance of already established T cells.

The results showed that under these conditions, T cells from the young and old donor splenocytes developed at similar levels, yet levels were lower as compared with those of bone marrow or fetal hematopoietic cells (see Table II).

6. AGE-RELATED DECLINE IN POTENTIAL FOR T-CELL GENERATION FROM DIFFERENT LYMPHOHEMATOPOIETIC TISSUES

Studies on *in vitro* reconstitution of fetal thymic stroma with lymphohematopoietic cells showed no significant difference in the levels of developing Thy 1$^+$ cells, whereas low values were observed in splenic derived T cells. For a critical evaluation of the relative reconstitution potential of cells from different tissue origins, we performed competitive reconstitution. In these experiments, fetal thymus stroma tissues were reconstituted with mixtures at equal doses of bone marrow cells from old and young donors of the different Thy 1 genotypes. Bone marrow cells of the old (Thy 1.2) were found inferior to those of the young (Thy 1.1), whereas there was no difference in levels of T cells when a mixture of young bone marrow cells from the two Thy 1 congenic mouse donor groups were used (Eren *et al.*, 1988). Thus, although both young and old mouse bone marrow can give rise to T cells, when induced on its own by the thymic microenvironment, age-related inferiority of the old mouse bone marrow is expressed under the competition conditions. Accordingly, competition experiments served as a tool to determine developmental changes in the different lymphohematopoietic tissues. Consequently, we examined T-cell development from the fetal liver, bone marrow, and spleens of young and old mice, using this approach. The results (Table IV) demonstrated that the fetal liver had a higher capacity for T-cell development than did the young mouse bone marrow, the spleen was inferior to the young bone marrow, and the old mouse spleen was inferior to the young. Thus, a gradual decline in the potential of cells from lymphohematopoietic tissues seems to be manifested from ontogeny on, throughout an animal's life span.

TABLE IV. Developmental Scale Expressed under Competitive Reconstitution of Fetal Thymus Explants

C57BL/Ka (Thy 1.1)	C57BL/6 (Thy 1.2)	Thy 1.1	Thy 1.2
Fetal liver	Bone marrow	66 ± 14	30 ± 2
Bone marrow	Young spleen	53	33
Young spleen	Old spleen	26	17
Bone marrow	Old spleen	65	6
Fetal liver	—	82 ± 2.5	0.3 ± 0.5
Bone marrow	—	86 ± 1	1 ± 0.3
—	Bone marrow	1 ± 1	87 ± 7
Young spleen	—	44 ± 6	ND[b]
—	Old spleen	ND[b]	43 ± 11

Column headers: Reconstituting cells[a] — C57BL/Ka (Thy 1.1), C57BL/6 (Thy 1.2); % positive cells[b] (mean ±SD) — Thy 1.1, Thy 1.2.

[a]Fetal liver cells were from 14-day-old mouse embryos; bone marrow and young spleen cells were from 2- to 3-month-old donors, and old spleen cells were from 24-month-old donors. Values represent results of 2 repeated experiments.
[b]ND, not determined.

7. DEVELOPMENTAL POTENTIAL OF SPLENIC CELLS SEPARATED BY PNA

The proportions of PNA⁺ cells in the old mouse spleen were shown to be increased (Globerson *et al.*, 1981). Furthermore, the PNA⁺ splenocytes were found to express low responses to the T-cell mitogens Concanavalin A (Con A) and phytohemagglutinin (PHA). The notion that the lectin PNA may be used as a marker for immature T lymphocytes, as shown for thymocytes (Reisner *et al.*, 1976), led us to examine whether PNA⁺ cells in the old mouse spleen have the capacity to differentiate into T cells, as well as their developmental status in relationship to that fraction of cells in the young. Reconstitution of fetal thymus with Thy 1⁺-depleted PNA⁺ and PNA⁻ spleen cells was then performed as in the previous experiments, using Thy 1.1 and Thy 1.2 congenic mice as donors for the competition. Equal numbers of cells from either the PNA⁻ or the PNA⁺ fractions of splenocytes from young and old mice were seeded. In both cases, competition of old and young PNA⁺ or PNA⁻ cell fractions resulted in low levels of T cells of the old donor origin, as compared with the young (Table V). Thus, while cells derived from young mouse spleens maintained the same capacity to develop in the thymus under competition conditions as without, PNA⁻ and PNA⁺ cell fractions originating from the old spleen lost this property.

Thus, our experiments on reconstitution of the fetal thymuses show that neither PNA⁻ nor PNA⁺ splenocytes originating in old mice are enriched with cells that are able to differentiate further, within the thymic microenvironment, as compared with their counterparts in the young. By contrast, cells of old mice are inferior, in this respect, to those of the young.

8. CONCLUDING REMARKS

The present study on developmental aspects of T lymphocytes in aging has elucidated some points with respect to the source of cells that may seed the thymus throughout the life

TABLE V. *In Vitro* Development of T Cells in Fetal Thymus Reconstituted with PNA-Separated Cells from Young and Old Mouse Spleens

Cells	C57BL/Ka (Thy 1.1)	C57BL/6 (Thy 1.2)	% positive cells[b] (mean ±SE)	
			Thy 1.1	Thy 1.2
PNA⁻	Young	—	46.5 ± 8.5	ND[b]
	—	Old	ND[b]	26.5 ± 14.5
	Young	Old	35.0 ± 8.0	0.5 ± 0.5
PNA⁺	Young	—	30.05 ± 5.0	ND[b]
	—	Old	ND[b]	16.5 ± 1.5
	Young	Old	43 ± 0	3.5 ± 3.5

[a]Spleen cells from young (2- to 3-month) and old (24-month) mice were separated by PNA. Values represent results of two repeated experiments.
[b]ND, not determined.

span. Our observations indicate that the capacity to give rise to T lymphocytes decreases with age, from the fetal liver, to young and eventually old bone marrow. We have not elaborated here on the basis for this age-related reduced potential. However, regardless of the mechanism involved, our studies show that the changes are actual manifestations of continuous developmental processes from ontogeny to ultimate senescence. In addition, the findings that splenic cells can give rise to T cells, and that this property is changed with age, provide a further insight into this developmental system. Whether T lymphocytes originating in the spleen represent a distinct category of cells is as yet an open question. The possible consequences of interactions of spleen and bone marrow cells that can develop in the thymus need to be critically evaluated.

Finally, based on our observations, one may speculate that T-cell development in the thymus actually depends on interactions between cells from different sources that seed the thymus simultaneously, from fetal liver and bone marrow or from bone marrow and the spleen. The contribution of these sources to the ultimate repertoire of the T cells needs to be properly evaluated. Our experimental strategy provides the tools for further elucidation of these points.

9. SUMMARY

Age-related changes in the development of T lymphocytes were investigated, using an *in vivo* and *in vitro* approach, to permit a comprehensive analysis of changes at various steps of the T-cell developmental processes. Particular attention was paid to the potential of lympho-hematopoietic stem cells from mice of different age groups to differentiate into T lymphocytes and to the effect of the spleen on developmental processes in the thymus. *In vivo* experiments focused on thymus recovery and on generation of T lymphocytes in total body irradiated mice. *In vitro* studies were based mainly on seeding the cells into fetal thymic stroma under conditions enabling T-cell differentiation. Bone marrow of aging mice gave rise to T cells in this system, yet these cells were inferior to those of the young, as shown when cells from both age groups were mixed and administered simultaneously to the thymus. A similar pattern was observed when Thy 1 +-depleted splenocytes from old and young mice were seeded into fetal thymuses. Furthermore, when PNA-separated splenocytes from the various age groups were examined, PNA+ as well as PNA− cells of the old were found inferior to those of the young in their capacity to develop into T lymphocytes under competitive conditions. Thus, in addition to age-related changes in the thymus itself, developmental failures are manifested in a decreased potential of bone marrow and spleen cells of the old to differentiate into T lymphocytes within the thymic microenvironment.

ACKNOWLEDGMENTS. This work was supported in part by a grant from the United States–Israel Binational Science Foundation, Jerusalem. A. G. is an incumbent of the Harriet and Harold Brady Chair for Cancer Research. We appreciate the technical assistance of S. Leib in the original research reported in this paper. We thank Mrs. M. Baer for editorial assistance.

REFERENCES

Astle, C. M., and Harrison, D. E., 1984, Effects of marrow donor and recipient age on immune responses, *J. Immunol.* **132:**673–677.

Auerbach, R., 1965, Experimental analysis of lymphoid differentiation in the mammalian thymus and spleen, in: *Organogenesis* (R. L. DeHaan and H. Ursprung, eds.), Holt, Rinehart, New York, pp. 539–557.

Auerbach, R., Globerson, A., and Umiel, T., 1982, The ontogeny of cellular immune reactivity in the mouse, in: *The Reticuloendothelial System*, Vol. 3, *Ontogeny and Phylogeny* (N. Cohen and M. Sigel, eds.), Plenum, New York, pp. 687–712.

Battisto, J. R., Borek, F., and Bucsi, R. A., 1971, Splenic determination of immunocompetence: Influence on other lymphoid organs, *Cell. Immunol.* 2:627–633.

Eren, R., Globerson, A., Auerbach, R., 1987a, T Cell ontogeny: Extrathymic and intrathymic development of embryonic lymphohemopoietic stem cells, *Immunol. Res.* 6:279–287.

Eren, R., Zharhary, D., Abel, L., and Globerson, A., 1987b, Ontogeny of T cells: Development of pre-T cells from fetal liver and yolk sac in the thymus, *Cell. Immunol.* 108:76–84.

Eren, R., Zharhary, D., Abel, L., and Globerson, A., 1988, In vitro development of T cells from old and young mouse bone marrow, *Cell. Immunol.* 112:449–455.

Farrar, J. J., Loughman, B. E., and Nordin, A. A., 1974, Lymphohemopoietic potential of bone marrow cells from aged mice: Comparison of the cellular constituents of bone marrow from young and aged mice, *J. Immunol.* 112:1244–1249.

Frasca, D., Adorini, L., and Doria, G., 1985, Enhancement of helper and suppressor T cell activities by thymosin α_1 injection in old mice, *Immunopharmacology* 10:41–49.

Friedman, D., and Globerson, A., 1978a, Immune reactivity during aging. I. T helper-dependent antibody responses to different antigens in vivo and in vitro, *Mech. Aging Dev.* 7:289–298.

Friedman, D., and Globerson, A., 1978b, Immune reactivity during aging. II. Analysis of the cellular mechanisms involved in the deficient antibody response in old mice, *Mech. Aging Dev.* 7:299–307.

Friedman, D., Keiser, V., and Globerson, A., 1974, Reactivation of immunocompetence in spleen cells of aged mice, *Nature (Lond.)* 251:545–546.

Globerson, A., 1966, In vitro studies on radiation lymphoid recovery of mouse spleen, *J. Exp. Med.* 123:25–32.

Globerson, A., 1984, Developmental aspects of altered immunoregulatory mechanisms in aging, in: *Lymphoid Cell Functions in Aging*, Vol. 3 (A. L. de Weck, ed.), Topics in Aging Research in Europe, EURAGE, Rijswijk, The Netherlands, pp. 17–27.

Globerson, A., Abel, L., and Umiel, T., 1981, Immune reactivity during aging. III. Removal of peanut-agglutinin binding cells from aging mouse spleen cells leads to increased reactivity to mitogens, *Mech. Aging Dev.* 16:275–281.

Globerson, A., and Auerbach, R., 1965, In vitro studies on thymus and lung differentiation following urethane treatment, *Wistar Inst. Monogr.* 4:3–15.

Gozes, Y., Umiel, T., and Trainin, N., 1982, Selective decline in differentiating capacity of immunohemopoietic stem cells with aging, *Mech. Aging Dev.* 18:251–259.

Grinblat, J, Schauenstein, K., Saltz, E., Trainin, N., and Globerson, A., 1983, Regulatory effects of THF on TCGF in aging mice, *Mech. Aging Dev.* 22:209–218.

Harrison, D. E., Astle, C. M., and Delaitre, J. A., 1978, Loss of proliferative capacity in immunohemopoietic stem cells caused by serial transplantation rather than aging, *J. Exp. Med.* 147:1526–1531.

Hirokawa, K., and Sado, T., 1978, Early decline of thymic effect on T cell differentiation, *Mech. Aging Dev.* 7:89–95.

Hirokawa, K., and Sato, K., and Makinodan, T., 1982, Influence of age of thymic graft on the differentiation of T cells in nude mice, *Clin. Immunol. Immunopathol.* 24:251–262.

Jenkinson, E. J., Franchi, L., Kingston, R., and Owen, J. J. T., 1982, Effect of deoxyguanosine on lymphopoiesis in the developing thymus rudiment in vitro: Application in the production of chimeric thymus rudiments, *Eur. J. Immunol.* 12:583–587.

Jensen, T. L., Hallgren, H. M., Yasmineh, W. G., and O'Leary, J. J., 1986, Do immature T cells accumulate in advance age?, *Mech. Aging Dev.* 33:237–245.

Kadish, J. L., and Basch, R. S., 1975, Thymic regeneration after lethal irradiation: Evidence for an intrathymic radioresistant T cell precursor, *J. Immunol.* **114**:452–458.

Makinodan, T., Chang, M. P., Norman, D. C., and Li, S. C., 1987, Vulnerability of the T cell lineages to aging, in: *Aging and the Immune Response: Cellular and Humoral Aspects* (E. A. Goidle, ed.), Dekker, New York, pp. 27–43.

Rabinowich, H., Umiel, T., and Globerson, A., 1983, T cell progenitors in the mouse fetal liver, *Transplantation* **35**:40–48.

Reisner, Y., Linker-Israeli, M., and Sharon, N., 1976, Separation of mouse thymocytes into two subpopulations by the use of peanut agglutinin, *Cell. Immunol.* **25**:129–134.

Ross, E. A. M., Anderson, N., and Micklem, H. S., 1982, Serial depletion and regeneration of the murine hematopoietic system, *J. Exp. Med.* **155**:432–444.

Russell, J. L., and Golub, E. S., 1977, Functional development of the interacting cells in the immune response. III. Role of the neonatal spleen, *Eur. J. Immunol.* **7**:305–309.

Scollay, R., and Shortman, K., 1985, Identification of early stages of T lymphocyte development in the thymus cortex and medula, *J. Immunol.* **134**:3632–3642.

Scollay, R., Bartlett, P., and Shortman, K., 1984, T cell development in the adult murine thymus: Changes in the expression of the surface antigens Ly2, L3T4, and B2A2 during development from early precursor cells to emigrants, *Immunol. Rev.* **82**:79–103.

Snodgrass, H. R., Demic, Z., Steinmetz, M., and von Boehmer, H., 1985, Expression of T-cell antigen receptor genes during fetal development in the thymus, *Nature (Lond.)* **315**:232–233.

Tyan, M. L., 1977, Age related decrease in mouse T cell progenitors, *J. Immunol.* **118**:846–851.

Weksler, M. E., Innes, J. B., and Goldstein, G., 1978, Immunological studies of aging. IV. The contribution of thymic involution to the immune deficiencies of aging mice and reversal with thymopoietin 32–36, *J. Exp. Med.* **148**:996–1006.

Wilson, A., D'Amico, A., Ewing, T., Scollay, R., and Shortman, K., 1988, Subpopulations of early thymocytes. A cross-correlation flow cytometric analysis of adult mouse Ly2⁻L3T4⁻ (CD8⁻CD4⁻) thymocytes using eight different surface markers, *J. Immunol* **140**:1405–1461.

35

Role of the Thymus in Aging of the Immune System

KATSUIKU HIROKAWA, MASANORI UTSUYAMA, and
MICHIYUKI KASAI

1. INTRODUCTION

The age-related decline of immune functions has been well documented in humans and rodents, although the onset, magnitude, and rate of the decline are different depending on species, strains, and immunological indices. There has been accumulating evidence that the age-related decline of immune functions is due mainly to T-cell insufficiencies caused primarily by an early decline in thymic function (Makinodan *et al.*, 1987; Hirokawa, 1985). This chapter attempts to describe the mechanism of the age-related thymic involution and its influence on the aging immune system.

The weight of mouse thymus increase rapidly after the birth, peaks at pubertal age (4 weeks), and progressively decreases thereafter showing about a 10-fold decrease at 26 months of age. The total number of thymocytes is about 400 million per lobe at the peak size, exponentially decreasing in number thereafter to a level of 8 million (about a 50-fold decrease) at 26 months of age. Along with the age-related change in the total number of thymocytes, the number of T-cell subsets also changes greatly. For example, the number of double-positive cells (L3T4$^+$Lyt-2$^+$) peaks at 1 month of age and decreases with age, while the number of double-negative (L3T4$^-$Lyt-2$^-$) cells shows an opposite pattern with a minimum level occurring at 1 month of age and an increase with age thereafter. These findings indicate that the age-related thymic involution mainly reflects a profound decrease in the number of thymocytes, but only a slight change in the number of stromal portion (Table I).

These changes in thymocytes could be dependent on the process of proliferation and differentiation of thymic T cells, starting with pro-T cells in the bone marrow. This process in turn could be dependent on some qualitative changes in the thymic microenvironment. Thus, we examine the following three points to determine the role of the thymus in the aging immune system: (1) age change of growth and differentiation of T cells, from pro-T cells to

KATSUIKU HIROKAWA, MASANORI UTSUYAMA, and MICHIYUKI KASAI • Department of Pathology, Tokyo Metropolitan Institute of Gerontology, 35-2, Sakaecho, Itabashi-ku, Tokyo 173, Japan.

TABLE I. Age Change in Thymus of C57BL/6 Male Mice[a]

	Age			
	2 days	1 month	3 months	26 months
Thymus weight (mg)	2.23 ± 0.03	81.86 ± 4.45	42.70 ± 0.52	8.83 ± 3.69
Total cell count × 10^6	6.01	414	226	7.53
L3T4−Lyt-2− (%)	10.43 ± 0.42	3.52 ± 0.04	4.74 ± 0.05	9.48 ± 2.44
L3T4+Lyt-2− (%)	10.67 ± 0.34	7.86 ± 0.29	8.95 ± 0.10	14.66 ± 2.79
L3T4−Lyt-2+ (%)	2.32 ± 0.18	3.37 ± 0.12	3.08 ± 0.05	4.77 ± 1.17
L3T4+Lyt-2+ (%)	75.80 ± 0.68	84.94 ± 0.38	82.83 ± 0.25	70.42 ± 6.52
Thy-1.2+PNA− (%)	7.65 ± 0.12	9.43 ± 0.80	7.77 ± 0.14	17.03 ± 4.81

[a]Thymus cells were analyzed by two-color flow cytometry, and the percentage of each subset was assessed.

thymocytes and mature T cells (for this purpose, we must understand how pro-T cells enter the thymus, proliferate within the thymus, and give rise to peripheral T cells); (2) age change of the thymic microenvironment in terms of the induction of T cells and their subset, and their immunological function; and (3) what can be expected if the thymic functions are artificially supplemented throughout life.

2. AGE CHANGE IN THE GROWTH AND DIFFERENTIATION OF T-CELL LINEAGE

2.1. Pro-T Cells in Bone Marrow

Precursor cells of thymocytes (pro-T cells) originate mainly in the bone marrow; their frequency in the bone marrow can be assessed by transplanting them in lethally irradiated mice or directly injecting them into the thymus. Katsura *et al.* (1986) employed the latter method of intrathymic injection of bone marrow cells; they reported that the frequency of pro-T cells was $1/10^3$ in young mice and did not change with age.

We produced radiation bone marrow chimera between young B10.Thy-1.1 as recipients, and young and old C57BL/6(Thy-1.2) mice as bone marrow donors, and compared the capacity of pro-T cells to give rise to thymocytes and splenic T cells between young and old mice (Hirokawa *et al.*, 1986). The results showed that the capacity of pro-T cells in old bone marrow was slightly depressed, about 1/1.5 (60–70%), as compared with that of young bone marrow (Table II, experiment A), and the difference between young and old appeared to be almost negligible as compared with 50-fold difference in the total thymocyte count between young and old mice.

We then assessed the age change of the thymic microenvironment in terms of the capacity to produce thymocytes and splenic T cells, using radiation bone marrow chimera between young and old C57BL/6 mice (Thy-1.2) as recipients and young B10.Thy-1.1 mice as bone marrow donors. The results showed that the production of thymocytes and splenic T cells decreased to 1/5 (20%) and 1/2.5 (40%), respectively, in old thymus, as compared with those in young one (Table II, experiment B). These results would indicate that the changes

TABLE II. Number of Donor-Type T Cells in the Thymus and Spleen of Bone Marrow Chimeras Produced between C57BL/6 (Thy-1.2) and B10.Thy-1.1 of Different Age[a]

	Experiment A[b]			Experiment B[c]		
	Young → young	Old → young	Ratio (%)	Young → young	Young → old	Ratio (%)
Thymus	19.8	14.3	72	17.2	3.42	20
Spleen	2.82	1.71	61	1.32	0.53	40

[a]Numbers indicated on the order of $\times 10^7$.
[b]Young B10.Thy-1.1 mice were sublethally irradiated and transplanted with either young bone marrow cells (young → young) or old bone marrow cells (old → young).
[c]Young B10.Thy-1.1 bone marrow cells were transplated into sublethally irradiated mice that were either young C57BL/6 (Thy-1.2) (young → young) or old (young → old).

occurring in the thymic environment are more responsible for the thymic involution than numerical and qualitative changes of pro-T cells in the bone marrow.

2.2. Entry of Pro-T Cells into the Thymic Microenvironment

In the radiation bone marrow chimeras, pro-T cells can smoothly enter and repopulate the thymic microenvironment, as most pre-existing thymocytes are destroyed by lethal irradiation. In the normal situation, however, the entry of pro-T cells into the thymic microenvironment appeared to be interfered with by pre-existing thymocytes. When bone marrow cells (2×10^7) of B10.Thy-1.1 mice were injected intravenously (IV) into 1-day-old newborn C57BL/6 (Thy-1.2) mice, a certain number of pro-T cells could enter the thymus. However, the number of donor-type T cells peaked at 4 weeks of age was only 2.5% (41.5×10^5) of total thymocytes. When the same number of bone marrow cells was injected into adult mice ranging in age from 1 to 24 months of age, the entry of pro-T cells appeared to be lower in number; i.e., the number of donor-type T cells in the thymus decreased to 1/7 in 1 month and to 1/15 in 24 months old mice as compared with that in newborn mice (Table III). However, it is interesting to note that even old atrophic thymus could accept entry of a small

TABLE III. Emigration of Pro-T cells into the Thymus of Various Ages[a,b]

	1 day	1 month	3 months	12 months	18 months	24 months
a	2.50 ± 0.17	0.40 ± 0.11	0.51 ± 0.25	2.14 ± 1.85	0.61 ± 0.44	1.16 ± 0.36
b	41.5×10^5	6.05×10^5	5.06×10^5	3.75×10^5	1.19×10^5	2.91×10^5
	(42.6–40.5)	(9.20–3.97)	(9.15–2.80)	(13.0–1.08)	(2.19–0.06)	(3.73–2.27)
c	100%	14.5%	12.9%	9.0%	2.9%	7.0%

[a]2×10^7 Thy-1.1 BM cells were injected intravenously into C57BL/6 mice of various ages; the number of donor-type thymocytes was assessed 4 weeks later.
[b]Line a indicates the percentage of donor-type thymocytes in the total number of thymocytes. Line b indicates the absolute number of donor-type thymocytes. The line c indicates the percentage of donor-type thymocytes in each age group as compared with that of 1-day-old thymus.

number of pro-T cells and allowed them to proliferate. The number of donor-type T cells did not increase in the thymus of 1-month-old C57BL/6, even when the number of transplanting bone marrow cells was increased fivefold. These results suggested that only a limited number of pro-T cells were allowed to enter the thymus of mice after the birth; most of thymocytes rapidly proliferating in the thymus appeared to be derived from pro-T cells that had entered the thymus before the birth.

2.3. Presence of Intrathymic Thymocyte Precursors

In contrast with the IV injection of bone marrow cells into newborn mice, a remarkable proliferation of donor-type T cells occurred in the thymus, when bone marrow cells (5×10^5) of B10.Thy-1.1 mice were injected directly into the thymus, by intrathymic injection (IT), of C57BL/6(Thy-1.2) newborn mice (Hirokawa *et al.*, 1988). The number of donor-type thymocytes peaked 6 weeks later, occupying 20% of the total thymocytes, and declined thereafter. However, a significant number of donor-type thymocytes remained to exist at the level of $5.8 \pm 3.1\%$, even 10 months after IT. As precursors of donor-type T cells were not found in the bone marrow of these experimental mice, these donor-type T cells continuing to proliferate in the thymus for a long time should be derived from pro-T cells injected directly into the thymus just after birth. Immunohistochemical examination demonstrated that in the case of IT, the proliferation of donor-type thymocytes started from the subcapsular layer, and this pattern is quite similar to the pattern of thymocytes proliferation observed in radiation bone marrow chimeras (Hirokawa *et al.*, 1985). In the case of IV injection of bone marrow cells, however, donor-type thymocytes were observed in a scattered manner in the inner cortex and were very sparse in number. These results have suggested that pro-T cells entering the thymus at perinatal stage give rise to a certain number of intrathymic thymocyte precursors in the subcapsular layer and that these precursors can replicate and differentiate into a large number of thymocytes. By contrast, pro-T cells entering the thymus of adult stage cannot give rise to long-lasting intrathymic thymocyte precursors and are short-lived in the thymus. The presence of intrathymic thymocytes precursors was reported as radioresistant thymocyte precursors, which initially repopulate the depleted thymus after radiation and bone marrow transplantation (Kadish and Basch, 1975; Hirokawa *et al.*, 1985). The above results suggest that intrathymic thymocyte precursors play an important role in maintaining the thymocyte pool in the normal physiological condition of the thymus, and most of these precursors appeared to have been derived from pro-T cells entering the thymus before birth.

2.4. Proliferation of Thymocytes within the Thymic Microenvironment

Experiment B using radiation bone marrow chimeras between young and old mice (Table II) showed that the capacity of the thymic microenvironment to support the proliferation of thymocytes declined with age. However, the results obtained in radiation bone marrow chimeras reflect the potential capacity of thymocyte precursors, but not necessarily their normal activity *in situ*.

The rate of incorporation of 5-bromodeoxyuridine (Budr) into *in situ* thymocytes would reflect more closely the physiological condition of proliferating thymocytes within the thymic microenvironment. The rate was most prominent in the newborn thymus (about 50%) (Table IV), declining thereafter with advancing age and reaching the level of 15% at 24 months of age. We believe that this decline in the proliferation of intrathymic thymocyte with age reflects the changes occurring in the thymic microenvironment.

TABLE IV. Percentage of Budr-Labeled Thymocytes in Aging C57BL/6 Mice[a,b]

Newborn	3 months	12 months	18 months	24 months
45.79 ± 5.71	26.63 ± 0.66	25.96 ± 1.72	28.83 ± 1.59	15.32 ± 2.99

[a]An injection of 0.2 mg/g body weight of Budr was given intraperitoneally to mice.
[b]Percentage of labeled cells was assessed 24 hr after injection by a flow cytometer.

Intrathymic injection of bone marrow cells (IT) is another method to see the capacity of thymic microenvironment to support the proliferation of thymocytes; i.e., bone marrow cells from B10.Thy-1.1 were injected directly into the thymus of untreated C57BL/6(Thy-1.2) mice of varying ages, and the number of donor-type thymocytes was assessed after various intervals (Hirokawa et al., 1988). The proliferation of donor-type thymocytes at 4 weeks after IT injection was most pronounced when the IT injection was performed in 7-day-old thymus, declining thereafter with the age of the thymus; i.e., about 1/4 in 4-week-old thymus and 1/30 in 18-month-old thymus (Table V). However, when the number was assessed at 8 weeks after IT injection, donor-type thymocytes were detected only in those thymuses treated by IT injection between 1 day and 2 weeks of age. The results suggest that the thymic environment until 2 weeks of age still has additional room for the development of longlasting intrathymic thymocyte precursors from pro-T cells, but the thymus after 4 weeks of age loses such space, and pro-T cells artificially injected into the thymus cannot differentiate into long-lasting intrathymic thymocyte precursors, hence disappear within a relatively shorter term.

2.5. Emigration of Thymic T Cells to the Peripheral Lymphoid Tissues

In the same experiment of IT injection mentioned above, the number of donor-type T cells was also assessed in the spleen to determine the magnitude of peripheral emigration (Hirokawa et al., 1988). The number of donor-type T cells was most pronounced when IT injection was performed in 1- to 7-day-old newborn mice (Table V). A detectable number of

TABLE V. Number of Donor-Type T Cells in the Thymus and Spleen after Direct Intrathymic Injection of Bone Marrow Cells[a,b]

Weeks after IT	Age of thymus at time of injection						
	1 day	3 days	7 days	2 weeks	4 weeks	6 months	18 months
				Thymus			
4	330	590	900	308	253	176	34
8	54	—	22	10	0	0	0
				Spleen			
4	10	21	19	4	6	7[c]	7[d]
8	37	—	30	13	0	0	0

[a]B10.Thy-1.1 bone marrow cells (5 × 10⁵) in 1 μl were directly injected into thymus of different age.
[b]Number of donor-type T cells in the thymus and spleen was assessed 4 and 8 weeks after the injection.
[c]Detected only 5 weeks after the injection.
[d]Detected only 6 weeks after the injection.

donor-type T cells were also observed in the spleen of IT-injected young adult and aged thymus. It is interesting to note that the donor-type T cells emigrated from 1 day to 2 weeks old thymuses were still present in the spleen 8 weeks after IT injection, but those from older thymuses were not detected at that time (Table V).

These results indicate that the peripheral emigration of thymic T cells was most pronounced in newborn mice, as previously reported by Scollay (1980), but a detectable number of the emigration, about one third to one fourth of the peak level, also occurred in the older thymus, and those T cells from newborn thymuses appeared to be long-lived and those T cells from older thymuses short-lived in the peripheral lymphoid tissues.

2.6. Role of Adult Thymus in Maintaining the Peripheral T-Cell Pool

An experiment was performed to see the extent to which adult thymus assisted in maintaining T-cell population in peripheral lymphoid tissues. When IT injection of bone marrow cells from B10.Thy-1.1 mice was performed in C57BL/6 (Thy-1.2) mice at 1 day of age, splenic cells contained 26.6% of host-type Thy-1.2 cells and 3.2% of donor-type Thy-1.1 cells 3 months later. When thymectomy was performed at 1 month of age, both host- and donor-type T cells were significantly reduced in the spleen at 3 months of age (Table VI). This would indicate that young adult thymus is necessary for the maintenance of the peripheral T-cell pool. By implanting newborn C57BL/6 thymus into those thymectomized C57BL/6 mice, almost complete recovery was observed in the number of host-type T cells, but not in the number of donor-type T cells. The fact that no increase in the number of donor-type splenic T cells was observed by the grafting C57BL/6 thymus would suggest that humoral factors secreted by the implanted C57BL/6 thymus did not influence the number of Thy-1.1[+] donor-type T cells in the spleen. Thus, the recovery in the number of host-type T cells could be mainly due to additional emigration of T cells from the implanted C57BL/6 thymus. These results suggest that (1) young adult thymus continues to export a significant number of T cells into the periphery for the maintenance of peripheral T-cell pool, and (2) thymic humoral factors do not directly influence the numerical increase of peripheral T cells.

TABLE VI. Effect of Thymus on the Peripheral
T-Cell Pool[a-c]

1 day IT	Splenic T cells (% in total nucleated cells)	
	Thy-1.2	Thy-1.1
Without TX	26.55 ± 0.27	3.20 ± 0.13
With TX	17.57 ± 0.67	0.91 ± 0.16
With TX + NTG	23.78 ± 0.11	0.87 ± 0.02

[a]Intrathymic injection of B10.Thy-1.1 bone marrow cells was performed in 1-day-old C57BL/6 mice (1 d-IT).
[b]Thymectomy (TX) was performed at 4 weeks of age.
[c]Newborn thymus from C57BL/6 mice was grafted within 24 hr after TX. Number of splenic T cells was assessed at 3 months of age.

2.7. Summary

Pro-T cells from bone marrow emigrate into the thymus primarily before birth, and then give rise to intrathymic thymocyte precursors. Only a limited number of pro-T cells can emigrate into the thymus after the birth. The proliferation of thymocytes from intrathymic thymocyte precursors declines with age, causing gradual atrophy of the thymus.

The emigration of the thymic T cells to the periphery is most pronounced at the neonatal stage, but continues to some extent throughout life for maintenance of the peripheral T-cell pool. T cells emigrated from the newborn thymus appear to be long-lived, while those from young adult and aged mice are short-lived.

3. AGING THYMUS INDUCE DIFFERENT SUBSETS OF T CELLS

Newborn thymus grafted into young nude mice can induce a sufficient amount of T cells necessary for most T-cell-dependent immunological functions. Thymus from young adult or aged mice grafted in young nude mice can also induce T cells, but only up to 60–80% as much as newborn thymus in terms of the number. More important is the observation that these T cells induced by the aged thymus were less active functionally. For example, in terms of number of T cells, thymus from 24-month-old BALB/C mice could generate as much as 70% of the T cells generated by the newborn thymus but, in terms of immunological activity, it could generate only 10% helper T cells and only 2% killer T cells, as compared with newborn thymus (Hirokawa et al., 1982).

The thymic lobe from 1-day, 1-week, 1-month, or 3-month-old C57BL/6 mice was grafted into young BALB/C nude mice, and the number of T cells and the ratio of T-cell subsets were assessed 12 weeks after the grafting. The number of splenic T cells induced by the grafted thymus decreased with age of thymus donor, showing about 75% of the peak level in nude mice with 3-month-old thymus graft (Table VII). A trend of an increased ratio of L3T4$^+$/Lyt-2$^+$ and decreased ratio of Lyt-1$^+$2$^-$/Lyt-1$^-$2$^+$ with advancing age of thymus donors was observed. As L3T4$^+$ cells and Lyt-2$^-$ cells contain a helper T-cell subset, and Lyt-2$^+$ cells contain a suppressor T-cell subset, the ratios of L3T4$^+$/Lyt-2$^+$ and

TABLE VII. Number of Splenic T Cells and the Ratio of T-Cell Subsets in Nude Mice with Thymus Graft of Various Ages[a-c]

Age of thymus graft	Number of splenic T cells ($\times 10^7$)	L3T4$^+$/Lyt-2$^+$	Lyt-1$^+$2$^-$/Lyt-1$^-$2$^+$
Control	0.5	4.3	4.1
1 day	4.0	3.1	10.5
1 week	3.2	3.4	9.2
1 month	2.3	3.6	8.6
4 months	2.6	4.1	7.4

[a]Young BALB/C nude mice were grafted with the thymus of C57BL/6 mice of various ages.
[b]Number of splenic T cells and the ratio of their subsets were assessed 12 weeks later.
[c]Control indicates values in nude mice without thymus graft.

TABLE VIII. Age-Related Change in the Ratio of T-Cell Subsets in the Spleen of C57BL/6 Mice

	3 days	7 days	2 weeks	1 month	3 months	12 months	24 months
Lyt-1$^+$2$^-$/Lyt-1$^-$2$^+$	1.97	1.80	3.48	3.58	5.85	1.59	1.99
L3T4$^+$Lyt-2$^+$	2.08	1.66	ND	1.46	1.30	ND	1.64

[a]Spleen cells were analyzed with two-color flow cytometry. FITC-labeled anti-Thy-1.2, and phycoerythrin labeled either anti-Lyt-1, anti-Lyt-2, anti-Lyt-1 + Lyt-2, or L3T4.
[b]Number and percentage of each T-cell subset were then calculated and the ratio between two subsets was assessed.
[c]Each value represents the mean of five to six samples.
[d]ND, not done.

Lyt-1$^+$2$^-$/Lyt-1$^-$2$^+$ are considered balances between helper and suppressor functions, reflecting different immune functions, respectively. When these ratios of T-cell subsets were assessed in the spleen of C57BL/6 mice ranging in age between newborn and 24 months of age, the spleen at 3 months of age showed the highest ratio of Lyt-1$^+$2$^-$/Lyt-1$^-$2$^+$ and the lowest ratio of L3T4$^+$/Lyt-2$^+$, while that at newborn and old age showed the reverse relationship (Table VIII). These results suggest that aging thymus is responsible for the altered ratio of T-cell subsets in the spleen (Utsuyama and Hirokawa, 1987) and that the altered ratio of T-cell subsets could be responsible for the immune deficiencies in aged mice.

4. SUPPRESSION OF T-CELL PROLIFERATION BY OLD THYMUS

Thymectomy (TX) performed in 4-week-old mice resulted in a decrease in the number of splenic T cells, but the reduced number could be increased by grafting newborn thymus (NTG) (Tables VI and IX). The reduced number of T cells could also be increased by grafting multiple old thymus (OTG × 5). The proliferative capacity of T cells assessed by phytohemagglutinin (PHA) response also decreased by TX but was recovered by NTG. How-

TABLE IX. Suppression of T-Cell Proliferation by Old Thymus Grafts[a–d]

	Control (sham TX + sham TG)	TX + sham TG	TX + NTG	TX + OTG × 5
Thy-1$^+$	5.76 × 10^7	2.81 × 10^7	5.93 × 10^7	5.18 × 10^7
cell count in spleen	(6.37–5.22)	(2.88–2.75)	(6.39–5.51)	(5.47–4.91)
PHA response	30.853	19,228	30,722	7,557
	(34,922)	(21,534)	(34,553)	(9,324)
	(27,258)	(17,169)	(27,316)	(6,124)

[a]Numbers in parentheses indicate range of standard error of the geometric means.
[b]C57BL/6 mice were thymectomized (TX) at 4 weeks of age and were grafted with either newborn thymus (NTG) or old thymus (OTG) within 24 hr after TX.
[c] In the case of grafting of newborn thymus, two lobes were grafted; in the case of grafting of old thymus, 10 lobes were grafted.
[d]Old thymuses were obtained from 24-month-old C57BL/6 mice.

ever, the depressed PHA response by TX was further depressed by OTG × 5, indicating that OTG was producing factor(s) suppressing the proliferation of T cells. It is interesting to note that old thymus not only loses the capacity to stimulate T-cell function, but also produces some detrimental substance suppressing T-cell proliferation.

5. ATTEMPTS TO RESTORE THE IMPAIRED IMMUNE FUNCTIONS OF AGING MICE

Enhancement of the immune functions and extension of the mean life expectancy were successfully performed in aging C57BL/6 and C3H mice by sequential multiple (syngeneic) newborn thymus grafting (MNTG), every 2 months, starting at 2 months of age (Hirokawa and Utsuyama, 1985). However, the enhanced level of immune functions was observed only at middle age and returned to the lower level in old age. This finding would also suggest that the involuting thymus had a suppressive effect on normal immunological function.

The same MNTG treatment was also performed in autoimmune-susceptible BW/F1 female mice; the effect on life span was compared with that for the group with grafting of newborn spleen and that treated with thymosin α_1 injection (Fig. 1). In autoimmune-suscepti-ble mice, MNTG accelerated the increase in the amount of urinary protein and shortened the life expectancy, as compared with control group grafted with newborn spleen instead of thymus. It was interesting to note, however, that thymosin α_1 treatment (10-μg/mouse, twice a week) decreased the rate of increase in the amount of urinary protein and extended the life

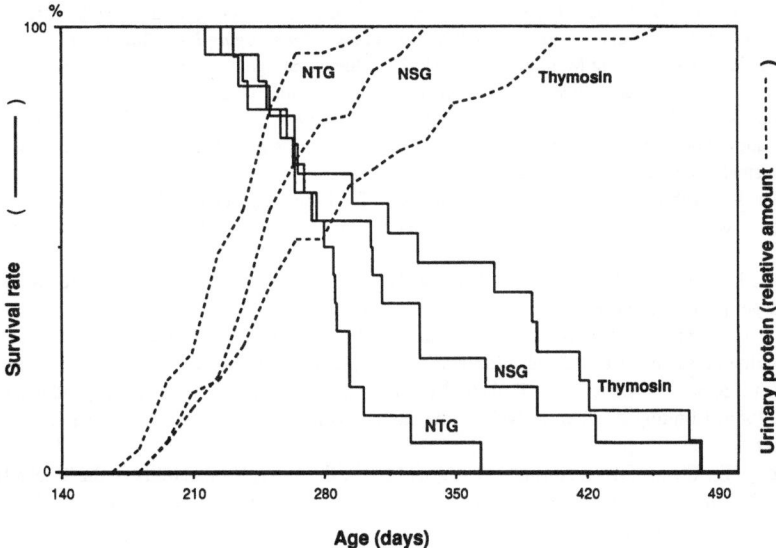

FIGURE 1. Survival rate of NZB/WF1 female mice, treated with sequential multiple graftings of newborn thymus from DBA/2 mice (NTG), newborn spleen from DBA/2 mice (NSG), or thymosin α_1 (Thymosin). Grafting of the organ was performed every month, starting at 2 months of age and ending at 330 days of age (10 times grafting in total). Thymosin α_1 (10 μg) was intra-peritoneally given 2 times per week. (-----) Relative amount of urinary protein of each group.

expectancy. Thymus grafting brings about a very complex effect on the host immune system, partly cellular and partly humoral. By contrast, chemically defined products such as thymosin α_1 make it relatively easy to see its effect on host pathophysiology, although the effect may be marginal in some cases. There have been accumulating data that various cellular components in the thymus (thymocytes, epithelial cells, macrophages, and dendritic cells) produced many kinds of products. Consequently, it would be obligatory to identify and purify each product to clarify their role in the aging thymus and immune system.

6. CONCLUDING REMARKS

Thymic involution is caused by intrinsic and extrinsic factors. One intrinsic factor is the alteration of the thymic microenvironment, which occurs early in life and results in a marked decrease in homing of pro-T cells to the thymus and a gradual decrease in proliferation of thymic T cells. Peripheralization of thymic T cells appears to be relatively well maintained in aging thymus, and qualitative changes occur in T-cell subsets produced by the aging thymus. Old atrophic thymus not only loses its capacity to produce T cells but also produces factor(s) that suppress immune function. Chemical and biological analysis of thymic products is clearly needed for further understanding of the mechanism of immunological aging.

REFERENCES

Hirokawa, K., 1985, Autoimmunity and aging, *Concepts Immunopathol.* **1**:251–262.

Hirokawa, K., and Utsuyama, M. 1984, The effect of sequential multiple grafting of syngeneic newborn thymus on the immune functions and life expectancy, *Mech. Aging Dev.* **28**:111–121.

Hirokawa, K., Sato, K., and Makinodan, T., 1982, Influence of age on thymic graft on the differentiation of T cells in nude mice, *Clin. Immunol. Immunopathol.* **24**:251–288.

Hirokawa, K., Sado, T., Kubo, S., and Kamisaku, H., 1985, Intrathymic T cell differentiation in radiation bone marrow chimeras and its role in T cell emigration to the spleen. An immunohistochemical study. *J. Immunol.* **134**:3615–3624.

Hirokawa, K., Kubo, K., Utsuyama, M., and Sado, T., 1986, Age-related change in the potential of bone marrow cells to repopulate the thymus and splenic T cells in mice, *Cell. Immunol.* **100**:443–451.

Hirokawa, K., Utsuyama, M., Katsura, Y., and Sado, T., 1988, Influence of age on the proliferation and peripheralization of thymic T cells, **112**:13–21.

Kadish, J. L., and Basch, R. S., 1975, Thymic regeneration after lethal irradiation: Evidence for an intrathymic radioresistant T cell precursor, *J. Immunol.* **114**:452–458.

Katsura, Y., Kina, T., Amagai, T., Tsubata, T., Hirayoshi, Y., Takaoki, T., Sado, T., and Nishikawa, S., 1986, Limiting dilution analysis of the stem cells for T cell lineage, *J. Immunol.* **137**:2434–2439.

Makinodan, T., Chang, M-P., Norman, D. C., and Li, S. C., 1987, Vulnerability of the T cells lineage to aging, in: *Aging and the Immune Response: Cellular and Humoral Aspects* (E. A. Goidl, ed.), Dekker, New York, pp. 27–43.

Scollay, R., Butcher, E., and Weissman, I., 1980, Thymus migration: Quantitative studies on the rate of migration of cells from the thymus to the periphery in mice, *Eur. J. Immunol.* **10**:210.

Utsuyama, M., and Hirokawa, K., 1987, Age changes of splenic T cells in mice. A flow cytometric analysis, *Mech. Aging Dev.* **40**:89–102.

36

Modulation of T-Cell Functions in Aging

GINO DORIA, CAMILLO MANCINI, and DANIELA FRASCA

1. INTRODUCTION

Aging is associated with marked changes in immunity characterized by a progressive decline of immune responsiveness to exogenous antigens and increasing incidence of autoimmune phenomena (Doria *et al.*, 1987a). These changes in immune reactivity may reflect multiple events affecting cell proliferation and differentiation in lymphoid tissues (Makinodan and Adler, 1975).

The onset, intensity, and duration of antibody responses are regulated by helper T cells (Th) and suppressor T cells (Ts). Expression of these antithetic T-cell functions involves activation of cell subsets and secretion of their soluble products, which amplify the interactions between the inducing signal and the expression of effector cells. Age-related alterations of immune responsiveness may result from changes in the activities of the Th- and Ts-cell populations, mainly as a consequence of thymus involution entailing a decreased secretion of thymic hormones that regulate the T-cell compartment.

2. MODULATION OF Th-CELL ACTIVITY

In our initial studies, the injection of immunodeficient old mice with synthetic thymosin α_1, a 28-amino acid peptide identified in a bovine thymus extract (fraction 5), was shown to restore Th-cell activity (Frasca *et al.*, 1982). This finding was confirmed and extended in our subsequent studies (Frasca *et al.*, 1985, 1986) as follows. Helper activity of spleen cells was induced *in vivo* by carrier priming and titrated *in vitro* 4 days later. Three days before carrier priming (C57Bl/$10 \times$DBA/2)F$_1$(BDF$_1$), mice were left uninjected or were injected with 10 μg thymosin α_1, 5 μg N$_{14}$ (N-terminal amino acid residues 1–14), or 5 μg C$_{14}$ (C-terminal amino acid residues 15–28) synthetic fragments of the α_1-molecule (all peptides were provided by A. L. Goldstein). Mice of different ages (3, 6, 12, 18, and 24 months) were assayed in separate experiments in each of which the Th-cell activities of all groups were referred, as percentages, to the helper activity of spleen cells from age-control 3-month-old carrier-

GINO DORIA, CAMILLO MANCINI, and DANIELA FRASCA • Laboratory of Pathology, C.R.E. ENEA, Casaccia, Rome, Italy.

primed mice. The results from five independent experiments reported in Fig. 1 illustrate that Th-cell activity is impaired by aging but is restored to a large extent by a single injection of 10 μg thymosin α_1. The injection of an equimolar amount of the N_{14} fragment is at least as effective as the entire α_1-molecule in restoring Th-cell activity in 6- to 24-month-old mice, whereas the injection of the C_{14} fragment has no effect. It is noteworthy that both thymosin α_1 and its N_{14} fragment are devoid of activity when injected in 3-month-old mice, suggesting that these molecules are effective only in T-cell-deficient mice.

The injection of thymosin α_1 appears to stimulate also a population of nylon wool-adherent, Lyt-2.2+, suppressor T cells that counteract Th-cell activity (Frasca *et al.*, 1985). Thus, thymosin α_1 injection in old mice enhances Th- and Ts-cell activities but, at the doses used, enhancement of helper activity is the prevailing effect.

The effect of thymosin peptide injection on interleukin-2 (IL-2) production by spleen cells from aging mice was also investigated, as described by Frasca *et al.* (1986): Spleen cells (1 × 10⁷) from aging BDF_1 mice, uninjected or injected with 10 μg thymosin α_1, 5 μg N_{14}, or 5 μg C_{14} fragment 3 days before sacrifice, were stimulated in 1 ml culture with 2 μg Concanavalin A (Con A) and 10 ng phorbol myristate acetate (PMA). After 48 hr, culture supernatants were collected and titrated for IL-2 activity as described by Sette *et al.* (1986). Data presented in Table I show that IL-2 production is reduced to 46% and 15% at 6 and 12 months of age, respectively, but is fully recovered by injection of thymosin α_1 or the N_{14} fragment. No recovery was induced by injection of the C_{14} fragment. The thymosin peptides were all ineffective when injected in 3-month-old mice (data not shown).

Thymosin α_1 and the N_{14} fragment, unlike the C_{14} fragment, enhance the expression of IL-2 receptors (IL-2R) in mitogen-activated spleen cells from old mice (Frasca *et al.*, 1986). These studies, performed by radioimmune assay (RIA) with anti-IL-2R monoclonal antibody (7D4), have been extended by use of a binding assay with radioiodinated IL-2. Radioiodina-

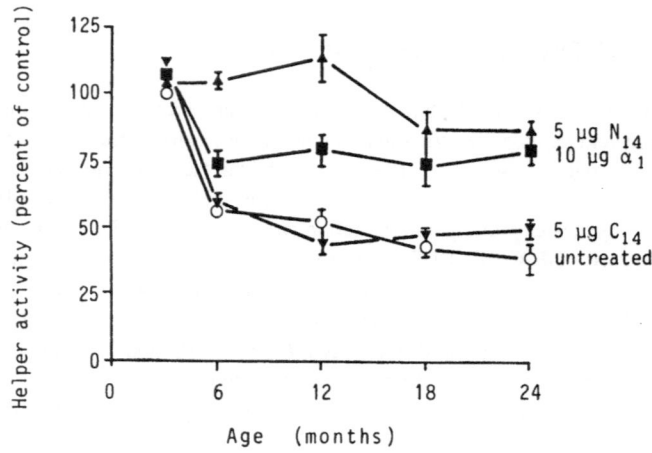

FIGURE 1. Effect of thymosin peptide injection on helper activity of spleen cells from carrier-primed mice of different ages. Vertical bars represent 1 SE.

TABLE I. Effect of Thymosin Peptide Injection on IL-2 Production
by Mitogen-Stimulated Spleen Cells

Exp. No.	Age (months)	Material injected	IL-2 production[a]	
			(U/ml)	%
1	3	None	11.53 (1.21)	100 (1.32)
	6	None	5.35 (1.22)	46 (1.32)
	6	α_1(10 μg)	9.98 (1.15)	86 (1.27)
	6	N_{14} (5 μg)	9.79 (1.19)	85 (1.29)
	6	C_{14} (5 μg)	2.56 (1.33)	22 (1.41)
2	3	None	6.59 (1.16)	100 (1.23)
	12	None	0.98 (1.23)	15 (1.29)
	12	α_1 (10 μg)	6.03 (1.06)	92 (1.17)
	12	N_{14} (5 μg)	6.50 (1.09)	99 (1.19)
	12	C_{14} (5 μg)	0.99 (1.22)	15 (1.28)

[a]Numbers in parentheses are error factors by which U/ml should be multiplied or divided to obtain the variations attributable to 1 SE.

tion of human recombinant IL-2 from Biogen was performed by the chloramine-T method as previously described (Robb et al., 1985). In the binding assay (Lowenthal et al., 1985), serial dilutions of radioiodinated IL-2 were incubated at 4°C for 1 hr with a constant number of mitogen-activated spleen cells from BDF_1 mice. Nonspecific binding was assessed by adding anti-IL-2R monoclonal antibody (PC61). High-affinity and total- (low- and high-) affinity IL-2R binding was determined using 0.002 pM or 2 pM ligand concentration, respectively. The data presented in Table II indicate that an injection of thymosin α_1 or N_{14} fragment in 12-month-old mice 3 days before sacrifice induces an increase in number of both low- and high-affinity IL-2R on mitogen-activated spleen cells. The C_{14} fragment appears devoid of a sizable effect.

Results from limiting dilution analysis of T-cell precursors in BDF_1 mice (Frasca et al., 1987) indicate that injection of thymosin α_1 or its N_{14} fragment increases the frequency of mitogen-responsive T lymphocytes in old, but not in young, mice, whereas injection of the C_{14} fragment is devoid of any effect in both young and old mice (Table III). Thus, active thymosin peptides amplify the pool of the T-cell precursors in immunodeficient old mice.

Our results altogether demonstrate that thymosin α_1 is a potent modulator of T-cell functions in aging mice, since it is able to recover Th-cell activity up to the level displayed by spleen cells from young mice. This effect of thymosin α_1 is restricted to the N-terminal half of the molecule and may depend not only on the increase in the precursor cell frequency of mitogen responsive T cells but also on the increased number of IL-2R-bearing T cells and on the enhanced production of IL-2 that, in turns, favors the expression of IL-2R on T cells.

3. MODULATION OF Ts-CELL ACTIVITY

B-cell clonal expansion and differentiation induced by antigen and amplified by Th-cell activity are controlled by Ts cells. Suppression of the antibody response is mediated by a

TABLE II. Effect of Thymosin Peptide Injection on the Expression
of IL-2-Binding Sites

Age (months)	Material injected	Bound [^{125}-I]-IL-2 molecules ($\times 10^3$) per cell	
		High affinity[a]	Low and high affinity[b]
3	None	21.2	47.0
12	None	8.7	17.3
12	α_1 (10 μg)	15.0	30.3
12	N_{14} (5 μg)	17.0	41.0
12	C_{14} (5 μg)	10.0	22.2

[a]Ligand concentration: 0.002 pM.
[b]Ligand concentration: 2 pM.

complex series of molecular and cellular interactions involving inducer (Tsi), transducer (Tst), and effector (Tse) cells, which are organized in cellular circuits.

Thymus involution and the increased frequency of autoimmune phenomena in aging suggest that the number of Ts cells decreases during senescence. Studies addressing this issue, however, have yielded controversial results, as immunosuppression appears to increase (Gerbase-De Lima et al., 1975; Goidl et al., 1976; Segre and Segre, 1976; Makinodan et al., 1976; Roder et al., 1978; De Kruyff et al., 1980; Callard et al., 1980; Liu et al., 1982; Amagai et al., 1982; Globerson et al., 1982; Doria et al., 1982; Gottesman et al., 1988), decrease (Amagai et al., 1982; Globerson et al., 1982; Barthoid et al., 1974; Krakauer et al.,

TABLE III. Effect of Thymosin Peptide Injection
on the Precursor Frequency of Proliferating T Cells

Exp. No.	Age (months)	Treatment	Precursors per 10^4 cells[a]
1	3	None	27 (1.35)
	3	α_1 (10 μg)	41 (1.28)
	19	None	9 (1.65)
	19	α_1 (10 μg)	23 (1.38)
2	3	None	79 (1.21)
	3	N_{14} (5 μg)	91 (1.20)
	19	None	24 (1.37)
	19	N_{14} (5 μg)	95 (1.19)
3	3	None	42 (1.28)
	3	C_{14} (5 μg)	51 (1.25)
	20	None	11 (1.57)
	20	C_{14} (5 μg)	13 (1.51)

[a]Numbers in parentheses are error factors by which precursor frequencies should be multiplied or divided to obtain the variations attributable to 1 SE.

1976; Halgren and Yunis, 1977; Thoman and Weigle, 1983; Gottesman *et al.*, 1984, 1988), or remain unchanged (Callard *et al.*, 1980) in aging mice and humans. This controversy reflects the large variety of experimental models and methods used that may deal with nonidentical parts of the same or different Ts-cell circuits and are therefore likely to provide dissimilar results. We found that the cell interactions involved in the 4-hydroxy-3-nitrophenyl acetyl (NP)-specific Ts-cell circuit are age-restricted as *in vitro* activation of Tst cells by Tsi cells is less effective if these cell populations are derived from mice of a different age (Doria *et al.*, 1987b). Moreover, age restriction was also found to operate in the interactions between Tst and Tse cells. Thus, aging appears to induce profound changes of the recognition repertoire expressed in the Ts-cell subsets of the NP-specific circuit. In our current studies, this analysis has been extended, by the use of Ts-cell products, to dissect out the molecular and cellular components of the circuit for a more precise identification of the network elements affected by senescence. As a major result from this approach, it has been found that if Ts cells and B cells are sampled from age-matched mice, *maximum* suppression of the antibody response is unaffected by aging. Thus, the age-related modulation of Ts-cell activity appears to stem from quantitative rather than qualitative changes, e.g., loss of Ts-cell subsets, leading to restrictions within the Ts-cell recognition repertoire. Yet, it is conceivable that during senescence a greater inducibility of Ts cells may compensate to some extent the decrease in Ts-cell subset frequency consequent to thymus involution.

4. CONCLUSION

The results from our studies on the modulation of Th- and Ts-cell activities may explain, at least in part, the decrease in immune responsiveness to exogenous antigens and the increased propensity to autoimmune phenomena as observed in aging. The use of thymosin peptides is promising but requires very accurate protocols to reach the antithetic objectives of stimulating helper or suppressor T cells. It is likely that the maintenance of a normal balance of immune functions may prolong the duration and improve the biological quality of life.

ACKNOWLEDGMENTS. This work was supported by a contract from ENEA-EURATOM and in part by Fondazione Pasteur-Cenci Bolognetti. This is publication No. 2546 of the Euratom Biology Division.

REFERENCES

Amagai, T., Nakano, K., and Cinader, B., 1982, Mechanisms involved in age dependent decline of immune responsiveness and apparent resistance against tolerance induction in C57BL/6 mice, *Scand. J. Immunol.* **16:**217–232.

Barthoid, D. R., Kysela, S., and Steinberg, A. D., 1974, Decline in suppressor T cell function with age in female NZB mice, *J. Immunol.* **112:**9–16.

Callard, R. E., de St. Groth, B. F., Basten, A., and McKenzie, I. F. C., 1980, The immune function in aged mice. V. Role of suppressor cells, *J. Immunol.* **124:**52–58.

De Kruyff, R. H., Kim, Y. T., Siskind, G. W., and Weksler, M. E., 1980, Age-related changes in the in vitro immune responses: Increased suppressor activity in immature and aged mice, *J. Immunol.* **125:**142–147.

Doria, G., Mancini, C., and Adorini, L., 1982, Immunoregulation in senescence: Increased inducibility of antigen specific suppressor T cells and loss of cell sensitivity to immunosuppression in aging mice, *Proc. Natl. Acad. Sci. USA* **79:**3803–3807.

Doria, G., Adorini, L., and Frasca, D., 1987a, Immunoregulation of antibody responses in aging mice, in: *Aging and the Immune Response: Cellular and Humoral Aspects* (E. Goidl, ed.), Dekker, New York, pp. 143–176.

Doria, G., Mancini, C., Frasca, D., and Adorini, L., 1987b, Age restriction in antigen specific immunosuppression, *J. Immunol.* **139:**1419–1425.

Frasca, D., Garavini, M., and Doria, G., 1982, Recovery of T cell functions in aged mice injected with synthetic thymosin α_1, *Cell. Immunol.* **72:**384–391.

Frasca, D., Adorini, L., and Doria, G., 1985, Enhancement of helper and suppressor T cell activities by thymosin α_1 injection in old mice, *Immunopharmacology* **10:**41–49.

Frasca, D., Adorini, L., Mancini, C., and Doria, G., 1986, Reconstitution of T cell functions in aging mice by thymosin α_1, *Immunopharmacology* **11:**155–163.

Frasca, D., Adorini, L., and Doria, G., 1987, Enhanced frequency of mitogen-responsive T cell precursors in old mice injected with thymosin α_1, *Eur. J. Immunol.* **17:**727–730.

Gerbase-De Lima, M., Meredith, P., and Walford, R. L., 1975, Age-related changes including synergy and suppression in the mixed lymphocyte reaction in long-lived mice, *Fed. Proc.* **34:**159–161.

Globerson, A., Abel, L., Barzilay, M., and Zan-Bar, I., 1982, Immunoregulatory cells in aging mice. I. Concanavalin A-induced and naturally occurring suppressor cells, *Mech. Ageing Dev.* **19:**293–306.

Goidl, E. A., Innes, J. B., and Weksler, M. E., 1976, Immunological studies of aging. II. Loss of IgG and high avidity plaque-forming cells and increased suppressor cell activity in aging mice, *J. Exp. Med.* **144:**1037–1048.

Gottesman, S. R. S., Walford, R. L., and Thorbecke, G. J., 1984, Proliferative and cytotoxic immune functions in aging mice. II. Decreased generation of specific suppressor cells in alloreactive cultures, *J. Immunol.* **133:**1782–1787.

Gottesman, S. R. S., Edington, J. M., and Thorbecke, G. J., 1988, Proliferative and cytotoxic immune functions in aging mice. IV. Effects of suppressor cell populations from aged and young mice, *J. Immunol.* **140:**1783–1790.

Halgren, H., and Yunis, E., 1977, Suppressor lymphocytes in young and aged humans, *J. Immunol.* **118:**2004–2008.

Krakauer, R. S., Waldmann, T. A., and Strober, W., 1976, Loss of suppressor T cells in adult NZB/NZW mice, *J. Exp. Med.* **144:**662–673.

Liu, J. J., Segre, M., and Segre, D., 1982, Changes in suppressor, helper, and B-cell functions in aging mice, *Cell. Immunol.* **66:**372–382.

Lowenthal, J. W., Corthesy, P., Tougne, C., Lees, R., Mac Donald, H. R., and Nabholz, M., 1985, High and low affinity Il-2 receptors: Analysis by IL-2 dissociation rate and reactivity with monoclonal antireceptor antibody PC 61, *J. Immunol.* **135:**3988–3994.

Makinodan, T., and Adler, W. H., 1975, Effects of aging on the differentiation and proliferation potentials of cells of the immune system, *Fed. Proc.* **34:**153–158.

Makinodan, T., Albright, J. W., Good, P. I., Peter, C. P., and Heidrick, M. L., 1976, Reduced humoral activity in long-lived old mice: An approach to elucidating its mechanisms, *Immunology* **31:**903–912.

Robb, R. J., Mayer, P. C., and Garlick, R., 1985, Retention of biological activity following radioiodination of human interleukin 2: Comparison with biosynthetically labelled factor in receptor binding assay, *J. Immunol. Methods* **81:**15–27.

Roder, J. C., Duwe, A. K., Bell, D. A., and Singhal, S. K., 1978, Immunological senescence. I. The role of suppressor cells, *Immunology* **35:**837–842.

Segre, D., and Segre, M., 1976, Humoral immunity in aged mice. Increased suppressor T cell activity in immunologically deficient old mice, *J. Immunol.* **116:**735–746.

Sette, A., Adorini, L., Marubini, E., and Doria, G., 1986, A microcomputer program for probit analysis of interleukin-2 (IL-2) titration data, *J. Immunol. Methods* **86:**265–277.

Thoman, M. L., and Weigle, W. O., 1983, Deficiency in suppressor T cell activity in aged animals. Reconstitution of this activity by interleukin 2, *J. Exp. Med.* **157:**2184–2189.

37

Age-Related Decline in Immunological Resistance to Infection

Murine Trypanosomiasis as a Model

JULIA W. ALBRIGHT and JOSEPH F. ALBRIGHT

1. INTRODUCTION

The health problems of the world's elderly population are now, and will continue to be, of global concern. According to World Health Organization (WHO) data, the population of elderly people will grow faster among the populations of the developing, rather than the developed, nations during the foreseeable future. Many of those developing nations may be referred to as "tropical"; in those nations, parasitic diseases have long been a major health problem. Is the prevalence of a parasitic diseases likely to be a significant factor affecting the health of emerging elderly populations in developing tropical countries? There is very little information with which to formulate an answer to that question. There has been almost no interest in the matter of parasitic infections in the aged; it was considered to be of moderate theoretical interest at best. Now, however, it appears that it could become a matter of considerably greater interest, both theoretical and pragmatic.

The studies discussed in this chapter appear to be the only reasonably comprehensive investigations of parasitic infections in the aged, so far. We have compared the ability of aged and young-adult mice to manage infections of *Trypanosoma musculi*, a highly specific murine parasite, and have found that aged mice are markedly defective in their ability to control such infections (Albright and Albright, 1982; Albright *et al.*, 1988). We present here a truncated account of our findings.

2. COURSE OF *TRYPANOSOMA MUSCULI* INFECTION IN YOUNG AND AGED MICE

Trypanosoma musculi are flagellated protozoa that live extracellulary in the bloodstream and peritoneal space of their murine hosts. A single trypansome is capable of establishing an infection in all strains of inbred mice, young or old. The course of typical infections in

JULIA W. ALBRIGHT and JOSEPH F. ALBRIGHT • Department of Microbiology, George Washington University School of Medicine, Washington, D.C. 20037.

young-adult and aged mice, as evaluated by parasitemia, is depicted in Fig. 1. Following
inoculation of the parasites, there is a phase of rapid growth that lasts about 1 week and ends
rather abruptly. The phase of growth gives way to a plateau, the duration of which varies with
the age of the host mice. In young-adult mice, the plateau lasts for about 1 week, but in aged
mice it continues for more than 2 weeks. The plateau ends with the onset of rapid elimination
of the parasites. It is obvious from Fig. 1 that the magnitude of parasitemia was more than
four times greater and the duration of infection twice as long in the aged C57BL/6 mice than
in the young-adult mice used in this study.

Parasitemia alone is not the most reliable index of trypansome infection because a
substantial number of parasites reside in the peritoneal space (PS) (Duffey *et al.*, 1985), and
that number varies with the strain and age of infected mice. Variation with age is demonstrated by the data in Table I. Data on parasitemia were converted to total numbers of
bloodstream parasites by adjusting for total blood volume (6.7% of body weight) (MacAskill
et al., 1980). The total number of bloodstream parasites was about four times greater in aged
than in young BC3F1 (C57BL/Cum female X C3H male) mice. There was about a 16-fold
difference in the number of PS *T. musculi* in old versus young mice when the comparison was
made at a time just preceding the phase of rapid elimination (day 12 in young mice, day 20 in
old mice). Thus, overall, the old mice experienced a parasite burden, at the time of maximum
infection, approximately 10 times greater than the burden in young mice. Table I also shows
that the degree of splenic enlargement (total splenocyte number) was significantly greater in
old than in young mice at the time of peak parasitemia.

Results similar to those presented in Table I have been obtained with young and aged
mice of several strains: A/He, C57BL/6, C3H, DBA, CBA, and BALB/c. Therefore,
heightened susceptibility to trypansomal infections appears to be characteristic of aged mice.
There is ample evidence that the greater susceptibility is a reflection of age-associated
deterioration of immunological competence as we show here and have described elsewhere
(Albright and Albright, 1982; Albright *et al.*, 1988).

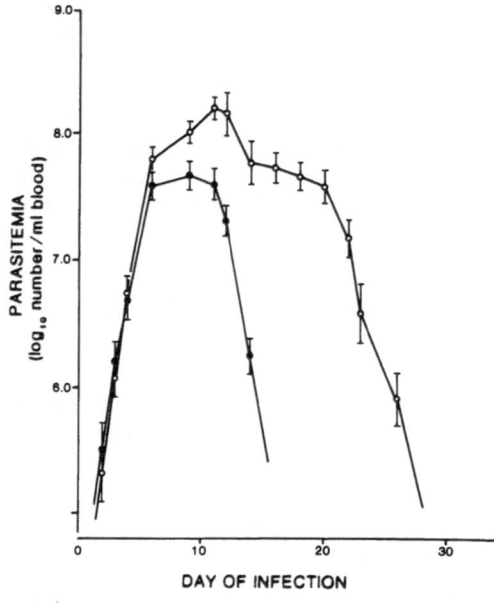

FIGURE 1. The course of *T. musculi* infection in young-adult (●) and aged (○)
BC3F1 mice as reflected by the profiles
of parasitemia.

DAY OF INFECTION

TABLE I. Distribution of *T. musculi* at Intervals during the Course of Infection
in Young-Adult and Aged BC3F1 Mice

Parameter	Age of mice (months)	Day of infection		
		12	16	20
Parasitemia (no./ml)	4	5.2×10^7	$<1 \times 10^4$	$<1 \times 10^4$
	30	1.6×10^8	1.2×10^8	1.9×10^8
Total blood trypanosomes	4	1.1×10^8	$<2 \times 10^8$	$<2 \times 10^4$
	30	3.9×10^8	2.9×10^8	4.7×10^8
Total PS trypanosomes	4	6.1×10^7	$<1 \times 10^4$	$<1 \times 10^4$
	30	2.3×10^8	6.9×10^8	1.0×10^9
Total trypanosomes/mouse	4	1.7×10^8	$<3 \times 10^4$	$<3 \times 10^4$
	30	6.3×10^8	9.8×10^8	1.5×10^9
Total splenic leukocytes	4	7.6×10^8	9.7×10^8	4.6×10^8
	30	9.0×10^8	1.2×10^9	2.3×10^9

3. MECHANISMS OF MURINE IMMUNITY TO *T. MUSCULI*

We will not attempt a review of this subject here, as a good recent review is available (Viens, 1985). A great deal of effort has been devoted to evaluating the relative importance of soluble antibodies, T cells, and phagocytes in the immunological cure of *T. musculi* infection and subsequent protective immunity to reinfection.

Studies by Viens *et al.* (1974), Targett and Viens (1975), Rank *et al.* (1977), and Brooks *et al.* (1982) have shown that, while thymus-derived T cells are required for immunity to *T. musculi,* a T-cell-mediated effector mechanism is not involved. The essential involvement of B cells and the antibodies they produce in the cure of *T. musculi* infections was demonstrated by Vargas *et al.* (1984) in mice treated from birth with antiserum against the μ chain of IgM. This has led to the current view, which is emphasized in this chapter, that the cure of *T. musculi* infections is primarily an antibody-dependent cell-mediated (ADCM) process (Albright and Albright, 1982; Wechsler and Kongshavn, 1984, 1986). Other mechanisms proposed as being involved in the cure of, and resistance to, reinfection by *T. musculi* include antibody-facilitated phagocytosis (Chang and Dusanic, 1976; Vincendeau *et al.,* 1986; Ferrante, 1986) and the action of natural killer (NK) cells on the trypanosomes (Albright and Albright, 1983). Our studies (unpublished observations) suggest that phagocytosis plays a minor role, if any, in the control of *T. musculi* infections. With regard to NK cells, we have shown that murine NK cells do not affect *T. musculi* (Albright *et al.,* 1984).

4. IMMUNITY TO *T. MUSCULI* IN YOUNG AND OLD MICE

4.1. Adoptive Immunity Assessed by Cell Transfer

The difference in the ability of young and old mice to control *T. musculi* infection was clearly displayed in early experiments involving the procedure of conferring immunity adoptively on irradiated mice by transfer of donor spleen cells (Albright and Albright, 1982). Young and old mice were inoculated with *T. musculi*. At intervals during the course of infection, they were used as donors of spleen cells. The latter, in graded numbers, were transferred to γ-irradiated syngeneic recipients, both young and old. A few hours later, the recipients were inoculated with *T. musculi,* and the course of infection was followed by estimates of parasitemia. The results are presented in Fig. 2. The transfer of 3×10^7 spleen cells from control uninfected donors (either young or old) failed to protect either young or old, irradiated (650-rad) recipients from fatal infection (Fig. 2). Spleen cells obtained from young donors on day 7 of infection were able only after prolonged residence in the recipients to provide eventual cure of infection, but only when transferred to young recipients. Spleen cells from infected old donors were ineffective. On day 14 of infection, the transfer of 3×10^7 spleen cells from young donors to young or old recipients suggested that active immunity against the parasites had developed in the infected donors. Thus, elimination of the parasites from the recipients began shortly after peak growth was achieved. Spleen cells from old infected donors were able to effect parasite elimination only after prolonged residence (and presumably growth and maturation) in young recipients. They were ineffective in aged recipients. Finally, 21 days after inoculation of parasites into donor mice, spleen cells from both young and old donors conferred protection on both young and old recipients. In fact, the course of infection in young or old recipients of young donor cells and in old recipients of young donor spleen cells was noticeably less severe and shortened in comparison with the

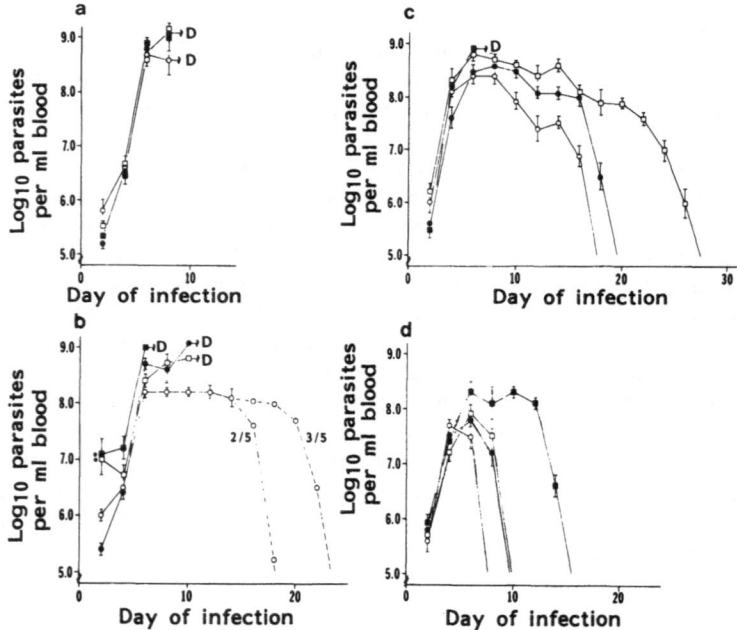

FIGURE 2. Course of parasitemia in irradiated recipients of 3×10^7 spleen cells. (a) Uninfected donors. (b) Donors on day 7 after trypanosomal inoculation (*indicates parasites at this time largely transferred as contaminants of donor spleen cell preparations). (c) Donors on day 14 after trypanosomal inoculation. (d) Donors on day 21 after trypanosome inoculation. Donor–recipient combinations: ○, young donors–young recipients; ●, young donors–aged recipients; □, aged donors–young recipients; ■, aged donors–aged recipients. Data from one of two replicate experiments, 5–6 samples per point. Bars = 1 SEM. (D, all were dead.)

course of primary infection in young or old normal mice. These results suggest that significant immunity to *T. musculi* did not develop until roughly 2 weeks after inoculation of *T. musculi* into young mice and after about three weeks in aged mice. Further evidence indicating a differential delay in the development of effective immunity in young and old mice is presented below.

4.2. Antibody Isotypes during the Course of Infection

It is well known that parasite infections (including trypanosomes) inhibit or interfere with immune responses to a variety of antigens; this is true of *T. musculi* infections (Albright and Albright, 1981). It was therefore important to determine by direct assay the course of appearance of antibodies against the trypanosomes themselves during the course of infections in young and old mice. In addition, given the evidence that trypanosome elimination is an antibody-dependent cell-mediated (ADCM) process, it was important to estimate the titers of antibodies of different isotypes directed against *T. musculi* epitopes. It has been demonstrated clearly by Wechsler and Kongshavn (1984, 1986) that the cure of *T. musculi* infections is effected by heat-labile antibodies of the IgG2a isotype. Other investigators (Olivier *et al.*, 1986) have shown that antibodies of the IgG2b, and possibly IgG1, isotypes protect nude mice against infection with *T. musculi*.

Titration of antibodies against *T. musculi* epitopes was performed by an immunofluorescence procedure, employing whole trypanosomes and specific goat antibodies against individual murine immunoglobulin isotypes (Albright *et al.*, 1988). The results are shown in Table II. There is an error of about one twofold dilution in these titrations. The development of antibodies appeared to be gradual, increasing over a period of 20 days after initial *T. musculi* inoculation into both young and old mice. However, the rise in IgM reached a peak after about 12 days. There were no obvious differences in the concentrations of antibodies of the different isotypes between young and aged mice, with one exception: the level of IgG2b appeared to decline between days 12 and 20 in old mice but to rise significantly in young mice over the same interval. The possible importance of this difference is unknown. The gradual, sluggish rise in antibodies against *T. musculi* epitopes in infected, young mice has been reported also by Wechsler and Kongshavn (1986). The absence of a detectable dif-

TABLE II. Immunofluorescent Estimation of Antibodies of Different Isotypes against *T. musculi* Antigens Present in Young-Adult and Aged Mice at Different Times after Trypanosome Inoculation

Age of mice	Day of infection	Titers[a] of antibodies of different isotypes					
		IgG	IgM	IgG1	IgG2a	IgG2b	IgG3
Young	8	5	3	4	5	5	3
Young	12	8	5	7	9	7	7
Young	20	10	6	9	10	9	7
Old	8	4	3	2	3	4	3
Old	12	8	7	6	8	8	7
Old	20	9	5	7	9	6	7

[a]Expressed as $\log_2$ reciprocal of the highest dilution giving detectable immunofluorescence in excess of background of normal serum controls.

ference between young and old mice in the isotypes of the bulk antibodies meant simply that our analysis was not sufficiently discriminating—or, in other words, we had to analyze for isotypic differences in the responses to certain, important antigens. Before embarking on that investigation, we needed to know more about the mechanism of immune elimination of *T. musculi*.

4.3. Antibody-Facilitated Hepatic Clearance of Trypanosomes

It has been demonstrated during the past few years that the most effective immune mechanism against African trypanosomes is antibody-enhanced hepatic clearance of the extracellular parasites from the bloodstream (MacAskill *et al.*, 1980; Dempsey and Mansfield, 1983), or, in other words, an ADCM process. We have conducted experiments to determine whether or not (1) the same process is involved in the elimination of *T. musculi* by young and old mice, (2) young and old mice differ in the efficiency of the process, and (3) antisera collected at intervals during *T. musculi* infection of young and old mice are equivalent with respect to enhancing parasite elimination.

Normal young or old mice were injected with excess volumes of blood serum collected at comparable times during the course of *T. musculi* infections of young or old donor mice. The same mice were injected 30 min after serum injections with 2×10^7 *T. musculi* that had been labeled with [^{75}Se]methionine (MacAskill *et al.*, 1980; Albright *et al.*, 1988). Elimination of these parasites from the bloodstream and uptake of radioactivity by various organs was assessed 2 hr later. Prospective enhancing antibodies were assessed in serum samples collected from young and old donor mice on days 7 and 12 of infection; day 7 is a time preceding rapid parasite elimination (Fig. 1) and preceding the appearance of effective antibody-producing cells in the spleens of infected mice as judged by the adoptive transfer procedure (Fig. 2.) Day 12 is a time just preceding rapid parasite elimination by young (but not old) mice (Fig. 1) and coincides (approximately) with the appearance of facilitating antibody-producing splenocytes in young (but not in old) mice (Fig. 2). The results of these experiments are summarized in Table III.

The extent of spontaneous elimination of bloodstream *T. musculi* in a 2-hr interval was the same in young and old mice. Similarly, spontaneous radioisotope uptake by liver and

TABLE III. Symbolic Representation of the Effects on *T. musculi* Elimination from Recipients of Serum Collected at Intervals during the Course of Infection in Young or Aged Donor Mice[a]

Serum donors		Effect of serum in recipient mice			
		Young		Aged	
Age (mo)	Day of infection	Liver	Spleen	Liver	Spleen
3–4	7	—	—	—	↓ ($p < 0.001$)
21–24	7	—	—	—	↓ ($p < 0.01$)
3–4	12	↑ ($p < 0.001$)	↑ ($p < 0.01$)	—	—
21–24	12	—	—	↓ ($p = 0.05$)	↓ ($p < 0.01$)

[a] —, no effect ($p < 0.05$) on *T. musculi* uptake in comparison with controls not treated with serum; ↑, enhanced uptake; ↓, depressed in comparison with untreated controls.

spleen was not different between young and old mice (uptake by kidney, heart, and gut was trivial in both normal and antibody-treated mice, so the data are not shown). The injection of even excessive volumes (one third of the total blood volume) of serum collected from mice on day 7 of infection did not enhance the spontaneous uptake of *T. musculi;* such serum from both young and old donors appeared to interfere with splenic clearance in old recipients. Serum from young donors on day 12 of infection clearly enhanced the uptake of trypanosomes by both liver and spleen of young, but not aged, recipients. By contrast, serum collected on day 12 of infection of old donor mice did not enhance uptake of parasites in young recipients and clearly inhibited uptake by the liver and spleen of aged recipients. These results reveal no apparent difference in the ability of organs of young and aged mice to sequester (and presumably destroy) the trypanosomes. However, young and old mice clearly differ in the ability to generate facilitating antibodies.

5. IMMUNOBLOT ANALYSES OF SPECIFIC ANTIBODIES DURING INFECTION OF YOUNG AND AGED MICE

At this point in the investigation, it seemed clear that our objective should be to identify one or a few key *T. musculi* antigens that elicited antibodies of the IgG2a isotype, the latter capable of facilitating efficient hepatic uptake of the trypanosomes. We have initiated a two-pronged approach to this objective. First, an immunoblotting (Western blotting) technique has been employed to identify *T. musculi* antigens against which antibodies of the IgG2a isotype appear around day 12 of infection, or later, in young-adult mice and later still in aged mice. The second approach has been to prepare monoclonal antibodies of the IgG2a isotype against key *T. musculi* antigens and to test the ability of such antibodies to effect efficient elimination of the trypanosomes from infected mice. The results of immunoblotting analyses are described here; the studies with monoclonal antibodies are not yet conclusive.

Extracts of *T. musculi* prepared by repeated freezing and thawing were resolved by electrophoresis in either 10% or 7.5% polyacrylamide gels including 0.1% sodium dodecyl sulfate (SDS). Resolved components were electroblotted on nitrocellulose sheets. After blocking with bovine serum albumin (BSA), the sheets were cut into strips and incubated in optimum dilutions of serum collected from young or old mice at different times during the course of *T. musculi* infections. Appropriate strips were exposed to isotype-specific peroxidase-conjugated antibodies, optimally diluted. Substrate–indicator reagent was added to permit visualization of colored bands.

We have analyzed serum samples collected from young and old mice on days 8, 12, 16, 20, and 30 following inoculation of *T. musculi* for antibodies against trypanosomal antigens. Although the immunoblot patterns were complex, as expected, several clear-cut results were obtained. First, the antigen-reactive patterns of IgM antibodies present on days 8, 12, and 20 after parasite inoculation were virtually identical in the case of young mice. The same was true of serum samples collected on days 8, 12, 20, and 30 of old mice. Thus, there was no change in the spectrum of antibodies from day 8 on, during the course of infection. Furthermore, the patterns of reactivity of antibodies from young and old mice were nearly identical. We concluded that the difference in resistance to infection by young and old mice was not related to antibodies of the IgM isotype. Second, among the IgG isotypes, there were interesting and reproducible differences in the spectrum of antibodies of the IgG2a and IgG2b isotypes between young and old mice. Figure 3 compares the immunoblots of serum collected

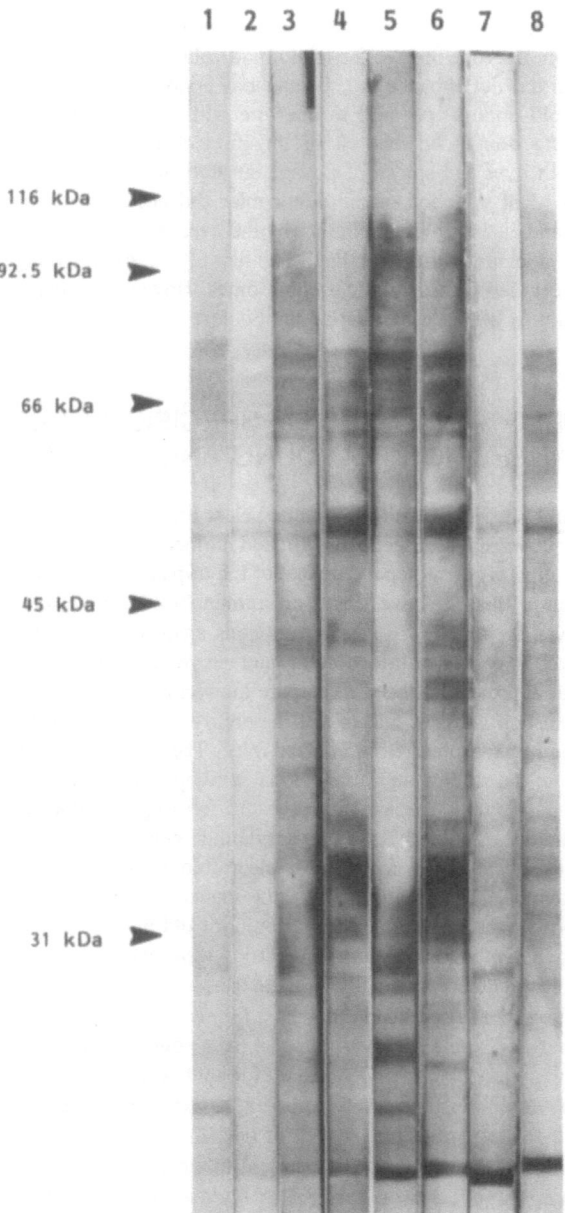

FIGURE 3. Immunoblots showing a comparison of antibodies produced by young-adult (lanes 1, 3, 5, and 7) and aged (lanes 2, 4, 6, and 8) mice on day 20 after *T. musculi* inoculation of isotypes IgG1 (lanes 1 and 2), IgG2a (lanes 3 and 4), IgG2b (lanes 5 and 6), and IgG3 (lanes 7 and 8).

from young and old mice on day 20 following *T. musculi* inoculation. The most striking differences are in the relatively high molecular weight region (>100 kDa) of the IgG2a patterns (lanes 3 and 4) and the IgG2b patterns (lanes 5 and 6) (see legend, Fig. 3). Although this region is not resolved in Fig. 3, it is clear that there were antibodies in the serum of young mice, but not old mice, on day 20 that reacted with *T. musculi* components of >100 kda.

Currently, we are performing electrophoresis of *T. musculi* extract in 7.5% SDS–polyacrylamide gels that provide reasonable resolution of components at 100–200 kDa. The unresolved, blurred bands shown in Fig. 3 has been resolved into three components having molecular weight values of approximately 130, 117, and 91 kDa. Antibodies of the IgG2a and IgG2b isotypes (but not IgG1 or IgG3) are present on days 16 and 20 of infection in young-adult mice, but not on day 12. Clearly, these three antigens are prime targets for further study.

6. CONCLUSIONS

The difference between young-adult and aged mice in their ability to control *T. musculi* infections appears to lie in the belatedness of old mice to generate antibodies of the IgG2a (and possibly IgG2b) isotypes against certain key antigens of the parasites. These key antigens appear to be relatively large (>100 kDa) and probably are situated on the external surface of the trypanosomes. The importance of the IgG2a (and IgG2b?) isotype of antibodies against these antigens lies in the efficiency with which this (these?) isotype(s) promote(s) phygocytosis of the trypanosomes, especially by the Kupffer cells of the liver. The spontaneous uptake of parasites by the liver is about the same in young and old mice. There could be a defect in the Fc receptors for IgG2b and IgG2b on the Kupffer cells of aged mice, a possibility suggested by the failure of young donor antiserum, that enhanced uptake by the livers of young mice, to facilitate uptake by the livers of aged mice.

We presume that the results of this investigation are of broad significance in, at least, two respects. First, the rodent trypanosome model should be archetypic for any type of infection in which the major immune defense is of the ADCM type, especially when the Kupffer cells are the effector cells. Therefore, the age-associated decline in ability to control *T. musculi* infections may reflect a similar decline in the ability to manage numerous infections. Second, the age-associated decline in immunological defense against *T. musculi* may be typical of the defense against many parasites. If it is, this model system may prove quite useful in evaluating the potential impact of the prevalence of parasites on the emerging elderly populations in developing tropical nations.

ACKNOWLEDGMENTS. This research was supported by grant DBC-8417637 from the National Science Foundation and by grant AG06278 from the National Institute on Aging.

REFERENCES

Albright, J. W., and Albright, J. F., 1981, Inhibition of murine humoral immune responses by substances derived from trypanosomes, *J. Immunol.* **126:**300–303.

Albright, J. W., and Albright, J. F., 1982, The decline of immunological resistance of aging mice to *Trypanosoma musculi*, *Mech. Ageing Dev.* **20:**315–350.

Albright, J. W., and Albright, J. F., 1983, Age-associated impairment of murine natural killer activity, *Proc. Natl. Acad. Sci. USA* **80:**6371–6375.

Albright, J. W., Hatcher, F. M., and Albright, J. F., 1984, Interaction between murine natural killer cells and Trypanosomes of different species, *Infect. Immun.* **44:**315–319.

Albright, J. W., Matusewicz, N. M., and Albright, J. F., 1988, comparison of the ability of young-adult and aged mice to manage infectious with *Trypanosoma musculi* and to produce antibodies of different isotypes against the spectrum of parasite antigens, *J. Immunol.* **141:**1318–1325.

Brooks, B. O., Wassom, D. L., and Cypess, R. H., 1982, Kinetics of immunoglobulin M and G responses of nude and normal mice to *Trypanosoma musculi, Infect. Immun.* **36:**667–671.

Chang, S., and Dusanic, D. G., 1976, *In vitro* phagocytosis of *Trypanosoma musculi* by mouse macrophages, *Chin J. Microbiol.* **9:**73–82.

Dempsey, W. L., and Mansfield, J. M., 1983, Lymphocyte function in experimental African Trypanosomiasis. V. Role of antibody and the mononuclear phagocyte system in variant-specific immunity, *J. Immunol.* **130:**405–411.

Duffey, L. M., Albright, J. W., and Albright, J. F., 1985, *Trypanosoma musculi:* population dynamics of erythrocytes and leukocytes during the course of murine infections, *Exp. Parasitol.* **59:**375–389.

Ferrante, A., 1986, The role of the macrophage in immunity to *Trypanosoma musculi, Parasite Immunol.* **8:**1178–1182.

MacAskill, J. A., Holmes, P. H., Whitelaw, D. D., McConnell, I., Jennings, F. W., and Urguhart, G. M., 1980. Immunological clearance of ^{75}Se-labelled *Trypanosoma brucei* in mice. II. Mechanisms in immune animals, *Immunology* **40:**629–635.

Olivier, M., Tijssen, P., and Viens, P., 1986, Participation of IgG2b antibodies in the initial control of *Trypanosoma musculi* infection, *Parasite Immunol.* **8:**27–29.

Rank, R. G., Robert, D. W., and Weidanz, W. P., 1977, Chronic infection with *Trypanosoma musculi* in congenitally athymic nude mice, *Infect. Immun.* **16:**715–716.

Targett, G. A. T., and Viens, P., 1975, The immunological response of CBA mice to *Trypanosoma musculi:* Elimination of the parasite from the blood, *Int. J. Parasitol.* **5:**231–234.

Vargas, F. del C., Veins, P., and Kongshavn, P. A. L., 1984, *Trypanosoma musculi* infection of B-cell-deficient mice, *Infect. Immun.* **44:**162–167.

Viens, P., 1985, Immunology of nonpathogenic trypanosomes of rodents, in: *Immunology and Pathogenesis of Trypanosomiasis* (I. Tizard, ed.), CRC Press, Boca Raton, Florida, pp. 201–217.

Viens, P., Targett, G. A. T., Leuchars, E., and Davies, A. J. S., 1974, The immunological response of CBA mice to *Trypanosoma musculi.* I. Initial control of the infection and the effect of T-cell deprivation, *Clin. Exp. Immunol.* **16:**279–294.

Vincendeau, P., Daeron, M., and Daulouede, S., 1986, Identification of antibody classes and F receptors responsible for phagocytosis of *Trypanosoma musculi* by mouse macrophages, *Infect. Immun.* **53:**600–604.

Wechsler, D. S., and Kongshavn, P. A. L., 1984, Cure of *Trypanosoma musculi* infection by heat-labile activity in immune plasma, *Infect. Immun.* **44:**756–759.

Wechsler, D. S., and Kongshavn, P. A. L., 1986, Heat-labile IgG2a antibodies effect cure of *Trypanosoma musculi* infection in C57BL/6 mice, *J. Immunol.* **137:**2968–2972.

38

The Clinical Significance of Immune Senescence

Advantages and Disadvantages

MARC E. WEKSLER, YOUNG TAI KIM,
GREGORY W. SISKIND, and RISE SCHWAB

1. INTRODUCTION

It is now 20 years since Walford proposed an immunologic theory of aging (Walford, 1969). According to this theory, changes in the anatomy and physiology of the immune system lead to the alterations in the organism with time that are known as aging. Thus, immune senescence was suggested to be the basic mechanism underlying the process of aging.

Today, a primary role of immune senescence in the aging process remains speculative. However, there is considerable evidence that immune senescence plays an important role in the pathogenesis of the diseases that accompany aging. Furthermore, considerable progress has been made in understanding the cellular and molecular mechanisms underlying immune senescence. The predominant change in the immune system with age is the involution of the thymus gland that begins at sexual maturity and results in alterations in the function of thymic-derived lymphocytes. With age, T lymphocytes lose their response to mitogens that stimulate their proliferation and secretion of lymphokines (Schwab *et al.*, 1989). These changes are associated with a progressive decrease in the response to "foreign" determinants on, for example, bacteria, viruses, or tumor cells and a progressive increase in the response to "self" determinants on autologous cells. The latter leads to autoreactive humoral and cell-mediated immunity.

What are the clinical consequences of immune senescence? It is likely that changes in the immune system with age lead to the higher incidence and greater severity of viral diseases, such as influenza and herpes zoster, and to bacterial diseases, such as urinary tract infections, pneumonia, and tuberculosis. It has also been suggested that immune senescence contributes to the increased incidence of cancer in the elderly. Finally, it is possible that autoimmune damage to the arterial wall may contribute to the increasing frequency of

MARC E. WEKSLER, YOUNG TAI KIM, GREGORY W. SISKIND, and RISE SCHWAB • Department of Medicine, Cornell University Medical College, New York, New York 10021.

cardiovascular disease with age. These are some of the clinical consequences of immune senescence.

The primary purpose of this presentation, however, is to raise the possibility that immune senescence may also convey benefits to the elderly organism. This point of view is particularly relevant at this time, when an increasing number of immunopharmacological approaches are being used to potentiate immune function. Several reports have been made that it is possible to augment the impaired antibody response of elderly subjects to vaccines (see Chapters 51 and 52, this volume).

Some time ago, we suggested the possibility that immune senescence might benefit the organism by limiting the level of auto-immune reactions in the elderly (Weksler, 1981). A direct test of this hypothesis, the effect of augmenting immune reactivity in older individuals on the frequency or severity of autoimmune reactions has not, to my knowledge, been carried out. However, recently we have begun to study the possible beneficial effect of immune senescence on the rate of tumor growth in old subjects.

Clinical observations have suggested that tumors grow more slowly in old as compared to young patients (Tsuda *et al.*, 1987). Furthermore, there was experimental support for "immunopotentiation" of tumor growth (Prehn, 1972). If the immune system could augment the rate of tumor growth, it was our conjecture that immune senescence might lead to slower growth of tumors in older as compared with younger subjects.

We have tested the hypothesis by studying the rate of growth of the B16 tumor in young and old mice. Ershler and colleagues previously showed that the B16 tumor, a tumor that arose spontaneously in a C57Bl/6 mouse, grew more slowly in old as compared with young mice (Ershler *et al.*, 1984). In collaboration with Ershler, we asked whether the slower tumor growth in old mice was related to the loss of thymic-dependent immune function associated with immune senescence. If so it was predicted that the rate of growth of the B16 tumor in young mice would be slowed if T-cell function were compromised in young mice prior to inoculation with the B16 tumor.

The results of our initial studies (Tsuda *et al.*, 1987) indicated that the rate of growth of the B16 tumor is slower in young adult thymectomized C57Bl/6 mice and even slower in young adult thymectomized mice given anti-theta antiserum as compared with young control mice. In addition, experiments showed that spleen cells were able to transfer the characteristic slow or rapid tumor growth rate of old or young donors, respectively, to young, irradiated, syngeneic recipients. These experiments did not identify either the specific cell in the spleen that regulated the rate of tumor growth and, perhaps more important, whether immune activity in old animals suppressed the rate of tumor growth or whether immune activity in young animals stimulated the rate of tumor growth.

Experiments now underway allow us to give tentative answers to these two important questions. Only T lymphocytes isolated from spleens of young or old mice appear capable of transferring the faster or slower rate of tumor growth characteristic of the young and old donor animals, respectively, to young, irradiated, syngeneic recipients. Furthermore, mixed-transfer experiments in which T lymphocytes from young or old are given, alone or in combination, to reconstitute young, irradiated, syngeneic young mice indicate that the tumor growth rate was as rapid in recipients of a mixture of T lymphocytes from young and old donors as in recipients of only T lymphocytes from young donors. These data suggest that T lymphocyte activity in young mice potentiate the rate of B16 tumor growth.

Thus, in this model system of tumor growth, immune senescence appears to benefit the host. It remains to be determined how general is the phenomenon of immunologically mediated enhancement of tumor growth. However, our findings suggest caution in augmenting immune function in older humans, especially in the presence of a tumor or even a history of neoplastic disease.

ACKNOWLEDGEMENTS. This work was supported in part by grants AG 00239 and AG 00541 from the U.S. Public Health Service.

REFERENCES

Ershler, W. B., Stewart, T. A., Hacker, M. D., Moore, A. L., and Tindle, B. H., 1984, Murine melanoma and aging: Slower growth and longer survival in old mice, *J. Natl. Cancer Int.* **72:**161–164.

Prehn, R. T., 1972, The immune reaction as a stimulator of tumor growth, *Science* **176:**170–171.

Schwab, R., Walters, C. A., and Weksler, M. E., 1989, Host defense mechanisms and aging, *Semin. Oncol.* **16:**20–27.

Tsuda, T., Kim, Y. T., Siskind, G. W., DeBlasio, A., Schwab, R., Ershler, W., and Weksler, M. E., 1987, The role of the thymus and T cells in slow growth of B16 melanoma in old mice, *Cancer Res.* **47:**3097–3100.

Walford, R., 1969, *The Immunologic Theory of Aging,* Copenhagen, Munksgaard.

Weksler, M. E., 1981, The senescence of the immune system, *Hosp. Pract.* **16:**53–64.

39

Immunosenescence and Human NK Cells

RAJABATHER KRISHNARAJ

1. INTRODUCTION

Of the three major cellular components of the lymphoid system, both T- and B-cell systems have been fairly well investigated with special reference to senescence-related changes in man and experimental animals (Makinodan and Kay, 1976; Weksler, 1982). It is widely believed that a general decline in immune competence (as seen in aging) is related to the high incidence of cancer. Despite the fact that the natural killer (NK) cells are known to play a role in immunosurveillance against malignancy and viral infection, and the regulation of hematopoiesis (Herberman and Holden, 1978, Trinchieri and Perussia, 1984), there are no strong data linking a vigorous NK cell system with healthy cancer-free survival to old age in humans. Peripheral blood NK activity is known to increase gradually from birth to adulthood (Herberman and Holden, 1978). However, the dynamics of the NK system from adulthood to old age (aging effect?) have not been studied systematically in healthy volunteers. Previously available literature showed equivocal results or had some methodological problems. In trying to investigate the quantitative and qualitative aspects of the immunosenescent changes in the NK cell system, we have asked three major questions:

1. Is it possible to demonstrate experimentally, an age-associated, but not necessarily an age-dependent change (see Chapter 11 *this volume*), in human peripheral blood NK activity by a multitechnique approach? The resulting pattern of NK cell dynamics should be qualitatively consistent with different traditional as well as unconventional techniques and experimental conditions used to quantitate the NK activity.
2. Would such a functional change in NK activity—whether positive or negative—have a cellular basis? If so, would those phenotypic alterations be unique to the aging process?

RAJABATHER KRISHNARAJ • Division of Geriatric Medicine, Department of Medicine, College of Medicine, University of Illinois at Chicago, Chicago, Illinois 60612, and Center on Aging/Northwestern University, McGaw Medical Center, Chicago, Illinois 60611.

3. Are there parallel immunosenescent changes in the non-null cell (T and B) systems? Do the NK cells have an immunoregulatory influence on the non-NK cell immune systems of an aging individual?

2. QUANTITATION OF AGE-ASSOCIATED ALTERATIONS IN NK CYTOLYSIS BY A MULTIPARAMETER ANALYSIS

We have examined the peripheral blood lymphocytes (Fiscoll-Paque purified, nonadherent cells freed of monocyte–macrophages with carbonyl iron treatment) from more than 200 healthy volunteers (20–94 years) for the NK activity in a standard ^{51}Cr-release assay using the K562 (erythroleukemic) target cell line (Krishnaraj and Blandford, 1987). Great care should be taken in selecting healthy volunteers. Our elderly donors were recruited from a retirement community, living independently in apartments.

2.1. Conventional Chromium-Release Assay

Our results clearly show (Table I) that the peripheral blood lymphocytes in elderly donors (>80 years of age) possess a statistically significant higher mean NK activity compared with healthy young adults (<40 years of age), the magnitude of increase varying with the parameter of expression of results. A similar trend has been reported by others based on a much smaller sample size (Batory et al., 1981; Onsurd, 1981; Tilden et al., 1986). Inconsistent results (over such an increase in NK activity with age) reported by others can sometimes be traced to either the differences in methodologies, e.g., the use of total mononuclear cell preparations (Nagel et al., 1981; Murasco et al., 1986), criteria used for donor selection, the range and upper age limit of the age group tested, and the gender mix. Also, a definition of "elderly" as >60 years of age would reduce the mean NK activity of the "elderly" group and, depending on the number, gender (males express slightly higher activity), or health status of those individuals, the statistically significant higher mean NK expression by the

TABLE I. Human Peripheral Blood NK Activity
as a Function of Age

Age group (years)	N	NK activity (mean ±SEM)		
		% cytotoxicity at 5 : 1 E : T	$LU_{30}/10^6$ lymphocytes	Area under titration curve (cm²)
<40	105	25.5 ± 1.3	19.8 ± 1.7	26.6 ± 1.1
40–59	64	31.6 ± 2.5	26.0 ± 2.7	30.0 ± 1.9
60–79	37	31.3 ± 2.6	26.2 ± 3.7	30.6 ± 2.1
>80	34	37.2 ± 2.6	32.0 ± 3.8	35.7 ± 2.0
Comparison of <40 years versus >80 years				
% increase		45.9	61.6	34.2
t value		4.0[a]	2.9[a]	4.0[a]

[a]Highly significant.

>80 year group ("oldest old") could be diluted and might become less significant when compared with young adults, <40 years of age.

2.2. Kinetic Determination of Maximal Cytotoxic Potential (V_{max})

Very few laboratories have explored the analysis of the NK cell-mediated cytotoxic phenomenon based on Michaelis–Menton kinetic behavior. A high degree of correlation exists between V_{max} values and other parameters of functional expression of NK cells (%[51]Cr release, % kill, area under titration curve, and lytic units) and the number of CD16+ (an NK cell marker) lymphocytes (Callewaert et al., 1983; Krishnaraj and Blandford, 1987, 1988). As expected, the existence of up to fourfold higher maximal oncolytic capacity (V_{max}) in the elderly became apparent by this approach (Fig. 1). While kinetic analysis can yield supportive data in NK studies by virtue of its ability to amplify subtle differences in NK activity, it cannot help reduce the coefficient of variation observed in conventional chromium release assay.

2.3. Dissection of Cytolytic Steps by the Agarose Immobilization Assay

Natural killer cytolysis is a multistep process (Hiserodt et al., 1982). First, an effector NK cell recognizes certain target structures and binds to it. This is a rapid, temperature-insensitive, and Mg^{2+}-dependent process. The second step includes a series of biochemical changes that result in the activation of NK cells and programming of NK-sensitive targets.

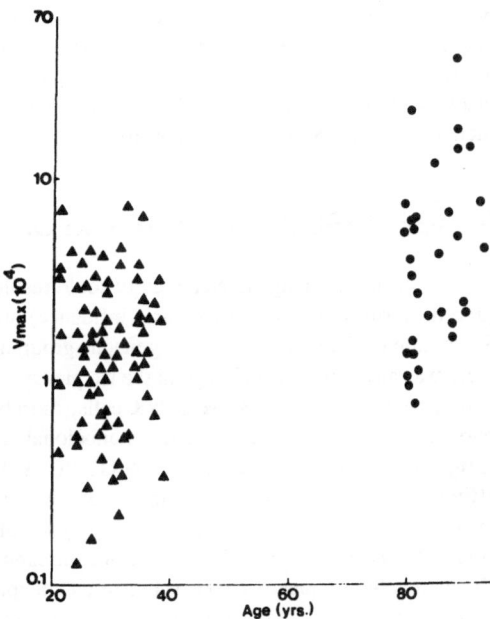

FIGURE 1. Maximal NK cytotoxic potential (V_{max}) of young and elderly donors. Each point represents maximal number of K562 targets that would be lysed at an infinite concentration of targets by NK cells present amongst the one tenth of a million effector lymphocytes from a donor. The mean V_{max} values for the young (28.4 ± 0.5 years) and old (84.8 ± 0.8 years) age groups are 1.9 ± 0.2 × 10⁴ and 7.2 ± 1.6 × 10⁴, respectively.

TABLE II. Correlation among Age and Target Recognition, Target
Killing, and NK Cell Frequency Determined at the Single-Cell Level

Parameter tested	Number of donors (N)	Correlation coefficient (r)	Significance (p)
Age vs. % TBC	84	0.2426	0.0262[a]
Age vs. % kill	83	0.3397	0.0017[b]
Age vs. % active killers (NK frequency)	83	0.3999	0.0002[b]
Age vs. absolute no. of killers per ml blood	78	0.2431	0.0320[a]

[a]Significant.
[b]Highly significant p value.

Once activated, NK cell lethally hits the target (secretes cytotoxic factors) and can detach from the target and recycle, while the target lysis can proceed to completion. Thus, the NK activity measured *in vitro* in a conventional chromium release assay is a cumulative result of a number of events. Using the single-cell assay (Bondavia *et al.*, 1983), we were able to dissect the influence of aging on discrete steps involved in NK-mediated cytolysis viz. target recognition state (% TBC, i.e., target-bound cells) and oncolysis by target bound lymphocytes (percentage kill i.e., dead conjugates) and thereby determine the NK cell frequency (% active killers, a product of the above two) in 84 individuals of all ages (Table II). Our cross-sectional study shows that there is a slight but significant increase in the number of circulating lymphocytes capable of recognizing the (target) tumor cell line (% TBC). What about the efficiency of killing? The results suggest that among the tumor target bound lymphocytes, perhaps more efficient NK subsets are present in the elderly group because the % kill is positively related with age of the lymphocyte donors ($r = 0.34$, $p = 0.0017$). Finally, there is a strong age-associated increase in the frequency of active killers, leading us to look for changes in the profile of NK subsets that might have been responsible for th age-associated increase in the NK functional capacity.

3. AGE-ASSOCIATED EXPANSION OF NK SUBSETS

Basically, a change in NK activity could result from (1) altered cytolytic activity per cell (due to intrinsic activity or extrinsic influence) and/or (2) a change in NK cell frequency. Since human NK cells are a heterogeneous group of cells, it was pertinent to inquire whether there was any significant change in the frequency of expression of NK cell surface markers in aging, healthy individuals. Most NK cells, morphologically defined as large granular lymphocytes, can be identified by many monoclonal antibodies that define the cell-surface CD16 antigen (Leu 11a, 11b, 11c), Leu-7, NKH-1 (Leu-19), and so forth. The CD16, i.e., the low-affinity receptor for the Fc domain of immune-complexed IgG, is a well-defined marker expressed on NK cells, and not on other types of lymphocyte subsets (Perussia and Trinchieri, 1984). By the use of the two-color immunofluorescence staining procedure, it can be shown that the frequency of NK subsets that coexpress the two gene products, viz. Leu-7 and Leu-11a (CD16) has a positive association with age (Krishnaraj and Blandford, 1985; 1986,

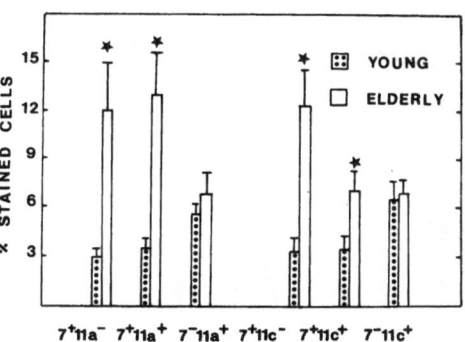

FIGURE 2. Selective expansion of NK subsets in the elderly. Values are mean ±SEM of young (N = 16–41) and elderly (N = 14–20) donors. In the case of Leu-11c, elderly ≥70 years of age. Asterisk (*) indicates statistical significance by Student's t test (t values = 2.37–4.37).

1988). Furthermore, the 7^+11a^- subset, unlike the 7^-11a^+ subset, appears to undergo parallel expansion with the 7^+11a^+ subset (Fig. 2). These changes are the same regardless of whether the results are expressed in relative percentage or in absolute number of lymphocytes per milliliter blood. It was also possible to confirm these trends in age-associated expansion of the null cell compartment by the use of Leu 11c (Fig. 2), another monoclonal antibody that recognizes a different epitope on the CD-16 antigen present on freshly isolated human peripheral blood NK cells (Perussia *et al.*, 1983).

4. HYPERACTIVE NK SYSTEM DESPITE A DOWNREGULATED T- AND B-CELL SYSTEM

A general decline in T- and B-cell reactivity is a common observation in aged humans and animals (Krishnaraj and Blandford, 1987; Weksler, 1982). An important question is whether the NK cell compartment behaves in concert with the T- and B-cell compartments. For examples, the proliferative (and other) responses of peripheral blood B lymphocytes, to pokeweed mitogen (PWM), decline with age (Fig. 3), despite a tendency to express a higher mean NK activity by the elderly. Furthermore, the inverse relationship between the frequency of 7^+11a^- subsets and the sensitivity to PWM (Krishnaraj and Blandford, 1988) strengthens a potential regulatory role for the NK system on B cells. This is consistent with the proposed negative immunomodulatory role for NK cells on blastogenesis and immunoglobulin synthesis by PWM-triggered B lymphocytes (Albruzzo and Rowley, 1983).

5. CONCLUSIONS

Healthy elderly, especially the "oldest old," tend to express a higher mean NK cell activity as a group. Although this is not a homogeneous group, which is not unusual, the use of a combination of different techniques shows a similar trend in age-associated NK dynamics. Our results are also supported by reports from other laboratories (Tilden *et al.*, 1986). Some possible reasons for the inconsistency (in NK dynamics) reported by other investigators (Nagel *et al.*, 1981) have already been discussed (see also Krishnaraj and Blandford, 1987, 1988).

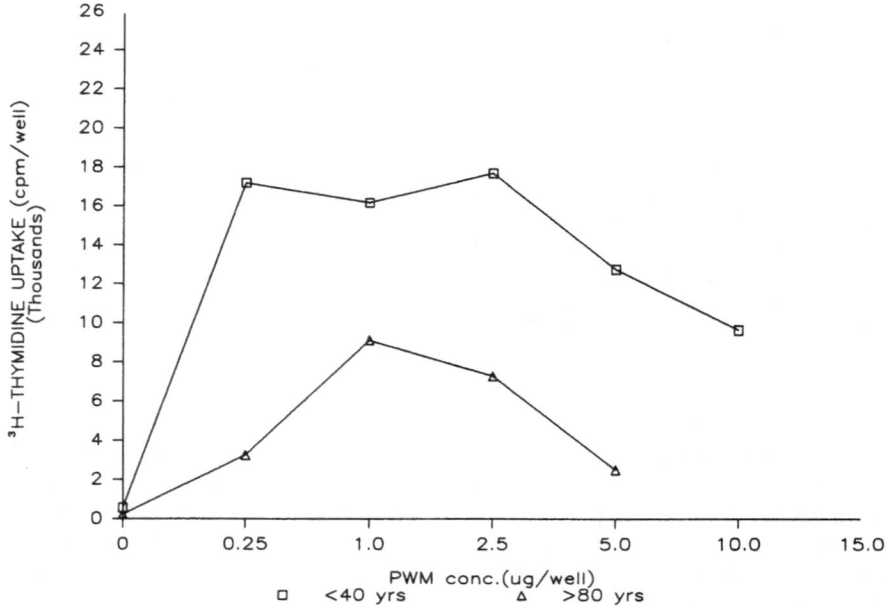

FIGURE 3. Decline in mitogen-induced proliferation of lymphocytes from the elderly. Three-day cultures of lymphocytes (±T-cell-dependent B-cell mitogen, PWM) from young adults ($N = 22$–40) or elderly ($N = 9$–13) were assessed to monitor B cell proliferative activity. The difference between young and the elderly is statistically significant ($t = 2.62$–4.16). Qualitatively similar results were obtained with the T-cell mitogen, Con A. (From Krishnaraj and Blandford, 1987.)

In nonhuman species, a consistent and combined decline in T-, B-, and NK cell activities has been demonstrated in aged murines (Roder and Kiessling, 1978; Herberman and Holden, 1978). It should be pointed out that spleen has been the source and focus of such studies, primarily because of practical reasons rather than immunological reasoning. This has resulted in a wrong notion that one should expect a defective NK system in aging humans as well. Hence, conclusions based on murine splenic NK cell activities have been widely and directly extrapolated to human senescence studies. However, early work by Lanza and Djeu (1982) has clearly shown that mouse peripheral blood NK activity is maintained throughout a major portion of adult life unlike that in the spleen. While murine peripheral blood NK activity is about twice that of the spleen, the strain distribution, surface phenotype, and most biological properties of murine NK cells suggest that the two effector populations stem from the same source (Kiessling *et al.*, 1975). Thus, the vigor of expression of human peripheral blood NK system (activity and $7-11a^+$ phenotype expression) is comparable to that observed for NK cells in murine peripheral blood; i. e., in both species we see strong evidence of preservation of the NK cell system during normal senescence.

What do these results tell us? First, the study of quantitative changes in Leu-7^+11a^-, 7^+11a^+, and 7^-11a^+ cells (and the corresponding combinations of 7 and 11c) within the framework of healthy biological aging, provides us an additional tool to investigate the differentiation pathways available for the cells of NK lineage under natural conditions over a period of several decades. The results might complement those obtained with experimentally induced short-term proliferation and differentiation of fresh, resting NK cells or their precursors with humoral factors such as interleukin-2 (IL-2) (Lainer *et al.*, 1985) or tumor cell lines of T and B lymphoid origin (Phillips and Lainer, 1985; Perussia *et al.*, 1987). Morphometric analysis (Arancia *et al.*, 1986) and biochemical evidence (Lainer *et al.*, 1986) on the rearrangement of genes encoding the T-cell antigen receptor strongly suggests that Leu-7$^+$11a$^-$ and Leu-11a$^+$ cells belong to different cell lineage. Second, the Leu-7$^-$11a$^+$ subset, believed to be the precursor for lymphokine-activated killer cells in the peripheral blood (Itoh *et al.*, 1985), is highly preserved through human senescence.

What causes the selective and progressive changes in these subsets? There can be several interpretations for our observations on the age-associated increase in NK activity and expansion of 7$^+$11a$^-$ and 7$^+$11a$^+$ subsets (for discussion, see Krishnaraj and Blandford, 1987, 1988). The hypothesis that these may be important predictive factors contributing to longevity (by virtue of enhanced nonspecific protection against cancer and viral infection) needs to be tested and confirmed by a longitudinal study on a larger scale with a wider population base. Perhaps a more fundamental question would be to ask whether there is an age-associated change at all. Are we measuring genetically predetermined levels of NK activity and subsets in this cross-sectional study rather than detecting chronobiological changes in NK cell number and function? Longitudinal studies combined with familial studies of inheritance of NK system (at functional and phenotypic levels) may be able to distinguish immunosenescent changes from a genetic dosage effect.

ACKNOWLEDGMENTS. This work was supported by grant R01 AG05717-03 from the National Institutes of Health, the Retirement Research Foundation, Inc., and the DEE and Moody Research Fund of the Evanston Hospital.

REFERENCES

Abruzzo, L. V., and Rowley, D. A., 1983, Homeostasis of the antibody response: Immunoregulation by NK cells, *Science* **222:**581–585.

Arancia, G., Fiorentini, C., Ferrari, C., De Panfilis, G., and Manara, G. C., 1986, Morphometric characterization of NK cell subset expressing the Leu-11 antigen in comparison to Leu-7 positive, 11 negative cells, *Cell Biol. Int. Rep.* **11:**845–853.

Batory, G., Benczur, M., Varga, M., Garam, T., Onody, C., and Petranyi, G. Gy., 1981, Increased killer cell activity in aged humans, *Immunobiology* **158:**393–402.

Callewaert, D. M., Mahle, J. G., Dayner, S., Koreniewski, C., and Schult, S., 1983, Simultaneous determination of the concentration and lytic activity of effector cells that mediate natural and antibody-dependent cytotoxicity, *Scand. J. Immunol.* **17:**479–487.

Herberman, R. B., and Holden, H. T., 1978, Natural cell-mediated immunity, *Adv. Cancer Res.* **27:**305–377.

Hiserodt, J. C., Britvan, L. J., and Targan, S. R., 1982, Characterization of the cytolytic reaction mechanism of the human natural killer (NK) lymphocyte: Resolution into binding, programming and killer cell-independent steps, *J. Immunol.* **129:**1782.

Itoh, K., Tilden, A. B., Kumagai, K., and Balch, C. M., 1985, Leu-11$^+$ lymphocytes with natural killer (NK) activity are precursors of recombinant interleukin-2 (rIL-2)-induced activated killer cells, *J. Immunol.* **134:**802–807.

Krishnaraj, R., and Blandford, G., 1985, Natural killer cell activity in human aging: A phenotypic, kinetic and functional assessment, *Fed Proc.* **43:**593.

Krishnaraj, R., and Blandford, G., 1986, An Analysis of Human NK cell features that change with age, in: *Immunoregulation in Aging* (A. Facchini, J. J. Haaijman, G. Labo, eds.), EURAGE, The Netherlands, pp. 239–245.

Krishnaraj, R., and Blandford, G., 1987, Age-associated alterations in human natural killer cells. 1. Increased Activity as per conventional and kinetic analysis, *Clin. Immunol. Immunopathol.* **45:**268–285.

Krishnaraj, R., and Blandford, G., 1988, Age-associated alterations in human natural killer cells. 2. Increased frequency of selective NK subsets, *Cell. Immunol.* **113:**001–0012.

Lanier, L. L., Benike, C. J., Phillips, J. H., and Engleman, G., 1985, Recombinant interleukin 2 enhanced natural killer cell-mediated cytotoxicity in human lymphocyte subpopulations expressing the Leu 7 and Leu 11 antigens, *J. Immunol.* **134:**794.

Lanier, L. L., Cwirla, S., Federspiel, N., and Phillips, J. H., 1986, Human natural killer cells isolated from peripheral blood do not rearrange T cell antigen receptor B chain genes, *J. Exp. Med.* **163:**209–214.

Lanza, E., and Djeu, J. T., 1982, Age-independent natural killer cells activity in murine peripheral blood, NK cells and other natural effector cells, in: *NK Cells and Other Natural Effector Cells* (R. B. Herberman, ed.), Academic, Orlando, Florida, pp. 335–340.

Makinodan, T., and Kay, M. M. B., 1980, Age influence on the immune system, *Adv. Immunol.* **29:**287–330.

Murasco, D. M., Nelson, B. J., Silver, R., Matour, D., and Kaye, D., 1986, Immunologic response in an elderly population with a mean age of 85, *Am. J. Med.* **81:**612–618.

Nagel, J. E., Collins, G. D., and Adler, W. H., 1981, Spontaneous or natural killer cytotoxicity of K562 erythroleukemic cells in normal patients, *Cancer Res.* **41:**2284–2288.

Onsrud, M., 1981, Age dependent changes in some human lymphocyte sub-populations, *Acta Pathol. Microbiol. Immunol. Scand. [C]* **89:**55–62.

Perussia, B., Ramoni, C., Anegon, I., Cuturi, M. C., Faust, J., and Trinchieri, G., 1987, Preferential proliferation of natural killer cells among peripheral blood mononuclear cells cocultured with B lymphoblastoid cell lines, *Nat. Immun. Cell Growth Regul.* **6:**171–188.

Perussia, B., Starr, S., Abraham, S., Fanning, V., and Trinchieri, G., 1983, Human natural killer cells analyzed by B73.1, a monoclonal antibody blocking Fc receptor function. I. Characterization of the lymphocyte subset reactive with B73.1, *J. Immunol.* **130:**2133–2141.

Phillips, J. H., and Lanier, L. L., 1985, A model for the differentiation of human natural killer cells: Studies on the in vitro activation of Leu-11+ granular lymphocytes with a natural killer-sensitive tumor cell, K562, *J. Exp. Med.* **161:**1464–1482.

Roder, J. C., and Kiessling, R., 1978, Target–effector interaction in the natural killer cell system. I. Covariance and genetic control of cytolytic and target-cell-binding subpopulations in the mouse, *Scand. J. Immunol.* **8:**135–144.

Tilden, A. B., Grossi, C. E., Itoh, K., Cloud, G. A., Dougherty, P. A., and Balch, C. M., 1986, Subpopulation analysis of human granular lymphocytes: Associations with age, gender and cytotoxic activity, *Nat. Immun. Cell Growth Regul.* **5:**90–99.

Trinchieri, G., and Perussia, B., Human natural killer cells: Biologic and pathologic aspects, *Lab. Invest.* **50:**489–513.

Weksler, M. E., 1982, Age-associated changes in the immune response, *J. Am. Geriatr. Soc.* **30:**718–723.

40

Regulation of the Expressed Idiotypic Repertoire in the Normal Immune Response of the Aged

EDMOND A. GOIDL, SUSAN J. MARTIN McEVOY, FRANCISCO A. BONILLA, AZAD KAUSHIK, and CONSTANTIN A. BONA

1. INTRODUCTION

Aging is accompanied by a gradual decline of certain physiological functions. Not the least of these are the effector functions of the immune system. Most aging animals demonstrate a progressive decline in their capacity to mount primary immune responses when compared in magnitude and heterogeneity of antibody affinity with that seen in the immune response of young adult animals.

We have demonstrated the progressive changes in the immune response of the aged (Goidl *et al.*, 1976a). This experimental model has facilitated our dissection of the mechanisms that contribute to the decreased responsiveness to both T-dependent (TD) and T-independent (TI) antigens. We and others (Goidl *et al.*, 1976; Zharhary *et al.*, 1977) have published data supporting the age-associated decrease in the heterogeneity of antibody affinity. This decrease is characterized by a profound diminution in medium- to high-affinity antibody. This is of considerable portent to the aging host's capacity to defend itself against microbial infectious agents. Since the experiments of Talmage and Maurer (1953), high-affinity antibody has been thought to provide increased resistance to infectious agents.

We also showed that the normal immune response of the aged animals is characterized by a relative increase in the production of auto-anti-idiotypic antibody (auto-anti-id) (Goidl *et al.*, 1980; Kim *et al.*, 1985). This finding was independently confirmed in the mouse model by Szcewczuk and Campbell (1980) and Klinman (1981). Further evidence was also obtained in the immune response of man by Geha (1982). An unexpected finding arose when the auto-

EDMOND A. GOIDL and SUSAN J. MARTIN McEVOY • Department of Microbiology and Immunology, School of Medicine, University of Maryland at Baltimore, Baltimore, Maryland 21201.   FRANCISCO A. BONILLA, AZAD KAUSHIK, and CONSTANTIN A. BONA • Department of Microbiology, Mount Sinai School of Medicine, New York, New York 10037.

anti-id obtained during the normal immune response to 2,4,6-trinitrophenyl-lysyl-Ficoll (TNP-F) by mice of different ages were used as probes for idiotype (id) expression. Mice of different ages express a different idiotypic antibody (Ab_1) repertoire in response to the same antigen (TNP-F) (Goidl et al., 1980). Therefore, there is an age-associated change in idiotypic antibody repertoire expression. We shall describe the kinetics and characteristics of the production of autoanti-id during the normal immune response of the aged.

The increase in auto-anti-id and our earlier finding of restricted heterogeneity of antibody affinity led us to re-evaluate the recruitment of B cells during the primary immune response of the aged mouse. We present evidence that B-cell recruitment during the primary immune response of the aged mouse appears to be as efficient as it is during the primary immune response of the young adult mouse. Expression of the idiotypic repertoire recruited during the normal immune response of the aged mouse seems to be downregulated by auto-anti-id. This is particularly noteworthy in the medium to high-affinity Ab subpopulations. In view of the level of degeneracy of the primary immune response of the aged mouse, we have analyzed the idiotype repertoire of the aged at the monoclonal antibody level (MAb). The implications of degeneracy of the immune response of the aged will be discussed in the context of anti-self-reactivity.

2. MATERIALS AND METHODS

All methods have been described extensively (Schrater et al., 1979; Goidl et al., 1979; Gibbons et al., 1985). Where changes have been made, descriptions are supplied in the footnotes of tables and figures.

3. RESULTS

3.1. Magnitude of the Immune Response to Thymus-Dependent Antigens in the Immune Response of the Aged Mouse

The magnitude and heterogeneity of the antibody response to dinitrophenylated bovine gamma-globulin (DNP-BGG) were compared between aged and young mice. All animals received 500 μg DNP-BGG emulsified in complete Freund's adjuvant (CFA, 2 mg/ml *Mycobacterium butyricum*) contained in final volume of 0.2 ml. Animals were immunized by intraperitoneal injection. The immune response was measured at the cellular level using an inhibition of plaque-forming cell assay (Goidl et al., 1976). The primary and secondary responses of 24-month-old mice were markedly diminished in magnitude and were of restricted heterogeneity of antibody affinity for the DNP hapten compared with the response of 2-month-old mice. IgG anti-DNP antibody response was more severely depressed than IgM anti-DNP antibody response in 2-year-old mice (Table I).

Following the demonstration by Gronowicz et al. (1974) that a sequential acquisition of mitogenic responsiveness to dextran sulfate, bacterial lipopolysaccharide (LPS), and purified protein derivate from *Mycobacterium tuberculosis* (PPD) occurs during ontogeny, we showed that these mitogens could accelerate maturational development and increase heterogeneity of antibody affinity early in ontogeny (Goidl et al., 1976b). We therefore administered LPS at the time of immunization to aged mice. This resulted in a further decrease in heterogeneity of antibody affinity as compared to that seen in untreated immune 12- and 24-

TABLE I. Comparison of the Immune Responses
of Young and Aged Mice[a]

Strain	Age (months)	Direct PFC	Indirect PFC	Heterogeneity[b] index
C57BL/6	2	2,500	8,000	2.8
	12	3,200	6,400	2.3
	25	900	1,200	1.6
BALB/c	2	9,600	11,000	2.8
	24	1,900	2,000	1.8

[a]Mice were immunized with DNP-BGG in complete Freund's adjuvant and sacrificed 2 weeks later.
[b]Heterogeneity index with respect to avidity is based on the Shannon function.

month-old mice (Goidl et al., 1976). It would seem that the effector mechanisms affected by LPS in early ontogeny are different or no longer exist in the immune response of the aged mouse. In conclusion, the effect of immunomodulators on the expressed immune response is dependent on the developmental stage of the host.

3.2. Relative Increase of Auto-Anti-Idiotypic Antibody in the Normal Immune Response of the Aged Mouse and the Age-Related Change in Idiotypic Antibody Repertoire Expression

A relative increase in the production of auto-anti-id occurs with respect to age, causing a further decrease in the magnitude of the expressed immune response of the aged mouse (Goidl et al., 1980; Szewczuk and Campbell, 1980). This can be assayed by enumerating hapten-augmentable PFC cells whose secretion of antibody is specifically inhibited by surface-bound auto-anti-idiotypic antibody (auto-anti-id) that can be displaced by free hapten. The percentage of hapten-augmentable plaque-forming cells (PFC) present in the normal immune response of mice increases with age (Table II).

The effect of age on the expression of immunoglobulin idiotype was also determined. Hapten-reversible inhibition of plaque formation was used as an assay for idiotype-bearing antibody-secreting cells. Sera from aged (21- to 22-month-old) C57BL/6$_{NNIA/CHR}$ mice immunized with 2,4,6-trinitrophenyl-lysyl-Ficoll (TNP-F) significantly inhibited plaque formation, in a hapten-reversible manner, by spleen cells of 81% of TNP-F immunized age-matched mice. However, these sera inhibited plaque formation by cells from only 50% of similarly immunized young adult (6- to 8-week-old) mice and 20% of immature (3- to 4-week-old) syngeneic mice. In the same manner, sera from TNP-F immune young adult or immature mice inhibited plaque formation by cells from immune donors of the same age as the mice from whom the immune serum was obtained but only rarely inhibited plaque formation by cells from mice of other age groups (Goidl et al., 1980). This suggests that the expression of the anti-TNP-specific idiotype repertoire in response to immunization with TNP-F changes with age. This has now been independently confirmed by Zharhary et al. (1988) and N. R. Klinman (personal communication). In conclusion, an age-related change in idiotype repertoire expression exists.

TABLE II. Effect of Age on Production of
Auto-Anti-Id Antibody[a]

Strain	Age (months)	Overall average of hapten-augmentable PFC (%) (x = SEM)
C57BL/6	2	39 ± 16
	3	12 ± 9
	20	532 ± 256
BALB/c	2	15 ± 6
	7	37 ± 20
	25	49 ± 25
AKR/J	2	17 ± 6
	6–7	110 ± 21
CBF$_1$	2–3	20 ± 6
	20	190 ± 94

[a]Mice were immunized with 10 μg TNP-F intravenously
and sacrificed 7 days later.

3.3. Normal Immune Response of the Aged Mouse is Characterized by Anti-Self Cross-Reactivity

We hypothesized that one possible function of the increased production of the immune response of the aged was to downregulate the expression of antibodies that cross-react with self-antigens. To test this, we measured anti-self reactivity against a panel of self-antigens, including bromelain-treated autologuous erythrocytes (Br-MRBC), mouse transferrin (M Transf), and mouse albumin (Table III).

Mice aged 6–8 weeks and 19 months were immunized with a single injection of 10 μg TNP-F administered intravenously (IV). Seven days later, single-cell suspensions obtained from their spleens were tested for plaque formation against TNP-sheep erythrocytes (SRBC)

TABLE III. Immune Reactivities of Young and Old Mice 7 Days after Immunization with TNP-Ficoll

Age (months)	N	TNP x̄ ±SE	Plaque formation against					
			Br-MRBC		M. transferrin		M. albumin	
			x̄ ±SE	%[a]	x̄ ±SE	%[a]	x̄ ±SE	%[a]
3–4	14	11,500 ± 450	5,035 ± 270	44	3,465 ± 27	30	900 ± 70	9
19	14	7,230 ± 290	4,620 ± 230	64	3,540 ± 200	49	1,100 ± 80	7

[a]Percentage of anti-self cross-reactivity obtained when compared with the magnitude of the antinominal antigen, antibody response. It should be noted that cross-reactivities are being measured at the single-cell level by plaque-forming cell assays.

(Goidl *et al.*, 1976), bromelain-treated autologous erythrocytes (Br-MRBC) (Zharhary *et al.*, 1988), and mouse transferrin chromium chloride (Cr_2Cl_3) conjugated to SRBC (Goding, 1976) and mouse albumin Cr_2Cl_3 conjugated to SRBC. (No reactivity was ever noted to mouse albumin•SRBC). Table III reports the degree of anti-self reactivity obtained following TNP-F immunization in mice aged 6–8 weeks and 19 months. Two dramatic findings can be seen: (1) the absolute magnitude of anti-self reactivity does not change between 2-month-old and 19-month-old mice, and (2) the percentage of the antinominal antigen cross-reactive to self-increases dramatically with the age of the animal. This may be caused by the age-related diminution of anti-TNP response following TNP-F immunization of young and aged mice.

However, it is not possible to tell whether this increase in anti-self cross-reactivity is the result of subpopulations of lymphocytes turned on through a "bystander" mechanism or is attributable to antinominal antigen antibody which directly cross-reacts with self-antigens.

It is remarkable that the absolute magnitude of anti-self cross-reactivity does not change with the age of the animal. This indicates that the age-associated rise in auto-antibodies must be under strict regulation whatever mechanism is responsible for its incept. In conclusion, anti-self cross-reactivity is an earmark of the immune response of young and aged mice. The percentage of the antinominal antigen antibody response devoted to anti-self cross-reactivites increases dramatically with age.

3.4. Normal Immune Response of the Aged Mouse is Highly Degenerate When Analyzed at the Monoclonal Antibody Level

In order to determine whether anti-self cross-reactivity observed in the normal immune response of the aged mouse was the result of "bystander" activation or increased degeneracy of antinominal antigen response, we established libraries of monoclonal antibody level (MAb) from immune young and aged donors. Table IV lists the reactivities observed in plaque-forming assays of MAb obtained from young and aged donors. More than 60% of MAb obtained from immune aged donors display multiple cross-reactivity toward self-antigens. The patterns of cross-reactivity range from reactivities to all three antigens tested (TNP+, BrMRBC+, and MTransf.SRBC+) to reactivity to TNP+, BrMRBC+, and MTransf.SRBC− to TNP+, BrMRBC−, and MTransf.SRBC+ and also TNP+, BrMRBC−, and MTransf.SRBC−. The surprising finding is that more than 50% of MAb obtained from aged donors bear the same idiotype. This idiotype is the AD8 major cross-reactive idiotype (CRI) of the anti-arsonate antibody response. This has been characterized by Hornbeck and Lewis (1983) as the nonspecific parallel set of the anti-TNP antibody system. In conclusion, anti-self cross-reactivity is a characteristic of the immune response of the aged. It is further characterized by a greater degeneracy of the antibody response and by an increase in cross-reactivity.

3.5. V_H and V_K Gene Usage of Anti-TNP MAb Obtained from Young and Aged Donors

Until now, the autoantibodies reactive to BrMRBC have been shown to be relatively monospecific and encoded exclusively by V_{H11} (which is a new V_H family (Reininger *et al.*, 1988) and by V_{K9} (Kaushik *et al.*, 1986; Kaushik *et al.*, 1988). Preliminary evidence indicates that some of the MAb obtained from aged donors, and that are extensively cross-

TABLE IV. Immune Reactivities of MAb Obtained from Aged and Young C57BL/6 Mice: Direct PFC Reactivity to Target Antigens[a]

MAb[b]	Anti-TNP	Anti-bromelain MRBC	Anti-mouse transferrin	AD8[c] id
		Aged		
20-1-A	+	+	+	+
20-3-A	+	+	+	+
19-9-A	+	+	+	+
19-8-A	+	+	+	+
19-7-A	+	+	+	−
19-6-A	+	+	+	−
19-5-A	+	+	+	±
19-4-A	+	+	+	−
19-2-A	+	−	−	+
19-1-A	+	+	−	+
20-4-A	+	−	+	+
		Young		
18-1-Y	+	−	−	−
18-4-Y	+	−	−	−
18-6-Y	+	−	−	−
18-7-Y	+	±	−	−

[a] The following target antigens were used in the plaquing assay: (1) TNP-SRBC by the method of Rittenberg and Pratt (1969); (2) bromelian-treated autologous erythrocytes (Br-MRBC) by the method of Naor et al. (1976); (3) mouse transferrin-SRBC (MTr-SRBC) by the chromium chloride method (Goding, 1976). For example, hybridoma #20-1-A demonstrated 43% cross-reactivity versus Br-MRBC and 41% cross-reactivity versus MTr-SRBC, when compared with anti-TNP reactivity. Similarly #19-2-A showed 22% cross-reactivity against Br-MRBC and 12% against MTr-SRBC. Cross-reactivities below 30% were considered nonsignificant.
[b] MAb obtained following fusion of immune spleen cells from aged mice are identified by the final letter A in the identification code of the cloned hybridoma; similarly, those from young animals by the letter Y.
[c] The monoclonal rat antimouse AD8 used in the plaquing assay was a reagent developed by Hornbeck and Lewis (1983).

reactive and possess anti-BrMRBC reactivity, are encoded by the V_{K8} gene. This is the first known example of a polyspecific reactive monoclonal antibody with antibromelain reactivity encoded by V_{K8}. Work is proceeding that should identify the usage of the V_H gene families of these MAb. In conclusion, a new class of anti-BrMRBC anti-self reactive MAb is reported. These multireactive anti-self MAbs use the V_{K8} gene. This is in contrast to all MAb anti BrMRBC, which have so far used the V_{K9} gene.

4. DISCUSSION

Jerne (1974) proposed a network of interacting elements as a model for the regulation of the immune system. The basic scheme of such a network is presented in Fig. 2. Antigenic determinants (idiotopes) on the combining site of the antibody molecules (idiotypes) that are produced in response to an antigen are regulated by other antigen combining sites (anti-idiotypic antibodies or Ab_2) arising in response to the newly produced idiotypic immu-noglobulins. The same reasoning can be applied to the newly produced Ab_2, which would then lead to anti-anti-idiotypic antibodies (anti-anti-id or Ab_3). In the original model, this is the "open network." Once the "antigenic perturbation" is over, the system reaches a new steady state. One aspect of this model is the prediction of nonspecific parallel sets. That is, some idiotopes may be shared between antibodies of different specificities.

Therefore, immunization with one antigen may alter the response to a totally unrelated antigen. This will result in primed Ab_2s, which will be restimulated with ever-increasing frequency with regard to the age of the animal. We propose that such events accumulate throughout the life of the individual and that following a multitude of "antibody-sins," the crossover at the nonspecific parallel sets will be stimulated repeatedly. Intuitively, this must lead to a restriction in the diversity of the idiotypic repertoire expressed in the immune response of the aged individual. The expressed idiotypic repertoire of the aged will be composed of the few Ab_1 that have not been recruited before, and the nonspecific parallel sets that will be activated will be downregulated by the primed Ab_2s.

The phenotype of the diversity of the antibody repertoire of the aged is remarkably similar to the one elicited during the early ontogeny of the immune response (Goidl et al., 1976). It is restricted in heterogeneity of antibody affinity and characterized by low- to medium-affinity antibodies and absence of high-affinity antibodies.

The data obtained by Vakil et al. (1986) following fusion of fetal liver cells lead to the conclusion that Ab_n is the progenitor set of the V_H region genes, which leads to the stimula-tion of Ab_{n-1}, and so on, until the acquisition of full diversity of the immune response, which occurs between 2 and 4 weeks of age in most inbred strains of mice (see Fig. 1). At this

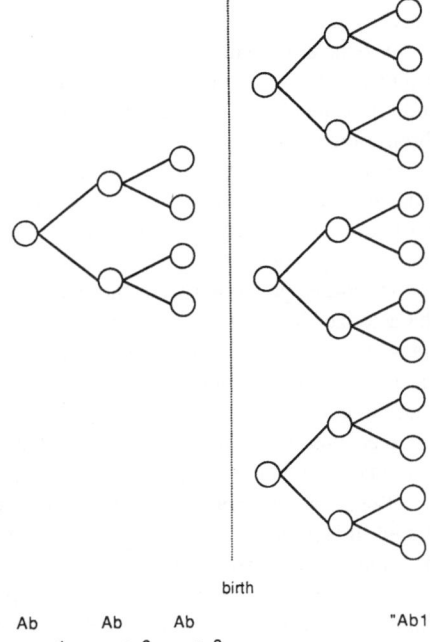

FIGURE 1. Ontogeny of the human network. Possible scheme fitting the data gathered by Vakil and Kearney (1986) and by Vakil et al. (1986). Presumably Ab_{n-1} is the "progenitor" element of the immune network. Ab_{n-1} leads to the activation of Ab_{n-2}, and so forth, until the actual full expression of the idiotype repertoire available and expressed in the young adult animal: the available idiotypic repertoire expressed in response to antigenic challenges (Ab_1).

birth

Ab   Ab   Ab   "Ab1"
n-1   n-2   n-3

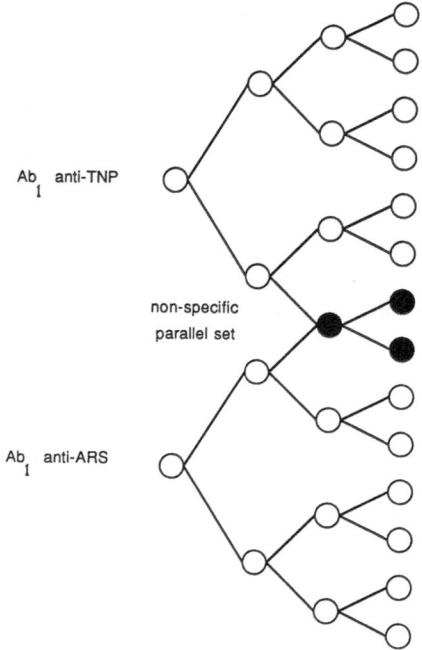

Ab$_1$ anti-TNP

non-specific
parallel set

Ab$_1$ anti-ARS

FIGURE 2. The one aspect of the immune network that precedes the expressed idiotypic repertoire of the immune response of the aged. The
two "families" of antibodies depicted here (○)
are the anti-TNP and the anti-ARS antibody systems, which following antigenic challenge, proliferate in a clonal fashion. (●) Nonspecific parallel set of antibodies, which share antigenic
determinants (idiotopes) on their combining
sites.

stage, antibodies produced in response to an antigen are arbitrarily referred to as Ab$_1$ (see
Fig. 2).

We have presented experimental evidence which supports our hypothesis that the aged
immune response expresses fewer and fewer idiotypes and that these idiotypes arise from
different gene usage. These probably will prove to be the more distal V_H genes present on the
chromosomal locus.

It is important to note that recruitment following antigenic stimulation is apparently as
efficient in the aged as it is in the young adult's response (McEvoy et al., 1988). What is
most severely affected in the immune response of the aged is the expression of the recruited
idiotypic repertoire.

A further prediction from the model is that the immune response of the aged will be
characterized by an increased degeneracy of specificity of the antibody response. This degeneracy has been characterized and documented in the immune response of the young by
Liacopoulos (Liacopoulos et al., 1971, 1976) and by Sperling et al. (1983). It has been a
transient event early in the immune response of the young adult. In the immune response of
the aged this degeneracy is long-lasting and is not limited to the early period following
antigenic stimulation.

We show that there are different modalities by which the phenotype of the aged can be
altered. It is possible through immunological manipulations to express a full heterogeneity of
the immune response in the aged. Therefore, a ruler exists that may be moved in both
directions—toward a more restricted idiotype expression or toward a more diverse idiotypic
expression. This ruler can be moved throughout the life of the individual, but its effects are

most noticeable at the developmental and aging stages, when restricted expression of the idiotypic repertoire is observed.

The model we propose affords an insight into the physiological processes leading to the immune response of the aged. It explains mechanistically the events that may account for the paucity of responsiveness seen in the expressed immune response of the aged. Furthermore, it permits a series of immunological manipulations that lead to alteration of the phenotype of the response of the aged.

This model is triggered by antigenic stimulations. It is a system that is antigen driven, a system whose internal self-stimulatory contribution pertains to only a fraction of the stochastic process encompassed in what we may call "the original antibody sins" representative of all the antigenic stimulations encountered throughout the lifetime of the individual (Fig. 3). Nevertheless, for whatever artifactual reasons, germfree and axenic animal models yield a low level of gammaglobulins. This level of production of immunoglobulins is perhaps in part endogenously driven. The inherent property of the model is that the "original antibody sins" are acquired in a stochastic manner. When an infinite number of events are generated randomly, this stochastic event, by definition, leads to the appearance of a pattern. The patterns of expression will be shared among individuals of the same ecological niche who will have been exposed to similar infections, environmental and food antigens, during their lifetimes. Different ecological niches will lead to patterns that will be idiosyncratic to these environments.

Our finding that more than 60% of the monoclonal anti-2,4,6-trinitrophenyl (TNP) antibodies (MAb) obtained following fusion of immune spleen cells from aged donors carry one single idiotype (the AD8 CR1) can be readily explained by our model. We cannot yet tell whether these clones represent idiotypes that cannot be expressed in the normal immune response of the aged mouse (i.e., they are blocked by Ab_2) or represent the remaining Ab_1, which have never been recruited before. It seems probable that these MAb may belong to the first set. This conclusion is supported by the extent of anti-self cross-reactivity displayed by these MAb (Table IV).

Evidence that a ruler exists has been provided by three lines of evidence. First, in studies on the ontogeny of B cell function we have used a syngeneic lethally irradiated cell transfer in which 14-day gestation fetal liver cells are transferred within the context of adult thymus cells. At this developmental stage, B cells express only IgM anti-DNP antibodies of restricted heterogeneity of antibody affinity. They are of low to medium affinity, and high-affinity antibody production is missing (Goidl et al., 1976). Administration of dextran sulfate at the time of cell transfer permits expression of a full heterogeneous IgM anti-DNP antibody response. Therefore, the ruler may be moved forward by stimulating lymphoid precursor cells obtained from a fetal liver donor or by stimulation with polyclonal B-cell mitogens that would not be encountered environmentally until after birth. Similarly, using day-18 fetal liver cells in the same cell-transfer system, LPS administration leads to a highly heterogeneous IgG anti-DNP antibody response. This is in contrast to the restricted heterogeneity of affinity of the IgG anti- DNP antibody repertoire obtained in the control group without LPS treatment (Goidl et al., 1976).

Second, after immunization with TNP-F, as we have shown above, mice produce both anti-TNP and auto-anti-Id antibody. Aged mice produce more auto-anti-Id than do young animals (Goidl et al., 1980; Kim et al., 1985; Szewczuk and Campbell, 1980). Mice exposed to a normally lethal dose of irradiation while their bone marrow (BM) was shielded survived and slowly regained their immune function (Kim et al., 1985). Recovery is presumably the

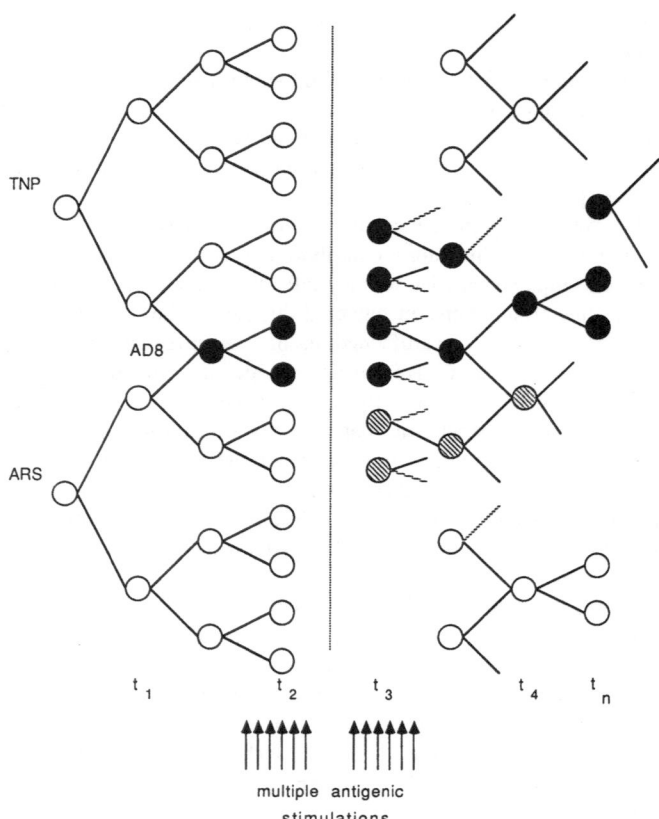

FIGURE 3. (Left) Young adult immune network at the level of Ab_1 (as seen in Fig. 2). (Right) Schematic representation of the immune network of the immune response of the aged. Most daughter cells have been omitted as well as any network at the Ab_2 level, for the sake of increased clarity. t_1, $t_2 \rightarrow t_4$ represent different ages from $t_2 \rightarrow t_3$. (Arrows) Stochastic events of multiple antigenic challenges leading to what we have described as the life-long accumulation of "original antibody sins." Some proliferative events are displayed by discontinuous lines; they are meant to depict hypothetical disappearances from the expressed repertoire of idiotypic antibodies. These antibodies for reasons as yet unclear may not be allowed to continue to proliferate or persist. This may occur as depicted in an unequal manner. By time t_4, the network is heavily represented by new Ab_1 (O) that have never been expressed before in the life of the individual; nonspecific parallel sets (●) recruited during the immune response and downregulated by memory Ab_2, some relatively newly arisen nonspecific parallel sets (◑) that may or may not be downregulated by Ab_2.

result of repopulation of the peripheral lymphatic system by cells originally in the BM. After recovery, old mice produce low auto-anti-id responses, similar to those of young animals.

Third, the transfer of splenic T cells into mice irradiated with their BM shielded also provides evidence that the magnitude of the auto-anti-id response is controlled by the peripheral T cells. Thus, mice that received splenic T cells from aged donors produced high levels of auto-anti-id, while those that received splenic T cells from young donors produced low levels of auto-anti-id. Therefore, the "ruler" may be moved backward by removing from the aged animal those cells that have been repeatedly stimulated by previous exposure to environmental antigens, throughout the lifetime of the individual.

5. CONCLUSION

We propose a model that explains the physiological mechanisms leading to the observed characteristics of the immune response of the aged. Furthermore, through immunological interventions, this model allows us to alter the restriction of the idiotypic repertoire expression and perhaps move profitably toward a greater diversity of the expression of the immunoglobulin repertoire.

An important aspect remains to be assessed. It is not certain that acquisition of the capacity to express an extensively diverse repertoire by the aged will be of immediate or long-lasting benefit to the individual. One must establish which of the immunological manipulations used to move the "ruler" proposed leads to a use of a repertoire characteristic of a "young-like" expressed repertoire. It seems reasonable to assume that full expression of the repertoire of the aged may lead to the production of highly degenerate anti-self cross-reactive antibodies. This may lead to nefarious consequences for the host.

ACKNOWLEDGMENTS. This work was supported in part by grants AG 04042 (to E.A.G.) and Al 18316 (to C.A.B.) from the U.S. Public Health Service. We acknowledge the expert technical assistance of Nancy Martinez and Andrea Harris. Special thanks go to Judith B. Innes, whose incomparable skills enabled us to carry out the original experiments described herein.

REFERENCES

Geha, R. S., 1982, Presence of auto-anti-idiotypic antibody during the normal human immune response to tetanus toxoid antigen, *J. Immunol.* **129:**139–144.

Gibbons, J. J., Goidl, E. A., Shepherd, G. M., Thorbecke, G. J., and Siskind, G. W., 1985, Production of auto-anti-idiotypic antibody during the normal immune response. XII. An enzyme-linked immunosorbant assay for auto-anti-idiotypic antibody, *J. Immunol. Methods* **79:**231–237.

Goding, J. W., 1976, The chromic chloride method of coupling antigens to erythrocytes: Definition of some important parameters, *J. Immunol. Methods* **10:**61–66.

Goidl, E. A. Innes, J. B., and Weksler, M. E., 1976a, Immunological studies of aging. II. Loss of IgG and high avidity plaque-forming cells and increased suppressor cell activity in aging mice, *J. Exp. Med.* **144:**1037–1048.

Goidl, E. A., Klass, J., and Siskind, G. W., 1976b, Ontogeny of B-lymphocyte function. II. Ability of endotoxin to increase the heterogeneity of affinity of the immune response of B lymphocytes from fetal mice, *J. Exp. Med.* **143:**1503–1520.

Goidl, E. A., Schrater, A. F., Siskind, G. W., and Thorbecke, G. J., 1979, Production of auto-anti-idiotypic antibody during the normal immune response to TNP-Ficoll. II. Hapten reversible inhibition of anti-TNP plaque-forming cells for auto-anti-idiotypic antibody, *J. Exp. Med.* **150:**154–165.

Goidl, E. A., Thorbecke, G. J., Weksler, M. E., and Siskind, G. W., 1980, Production of auto-anti-idiotypic antibody during the normal immune response: Changes in the auto-anti-idiotypic antibody response and the idiotype repertoire associated with aging, *Proc. Natl. Acad. Sci. USA* **77:**6788–6792.

Gronowicz, E., Coutinho, A., and Moller, G., 1974, Differentiation of B cells: Sequential appearance of responsiveness to polyclonal activators, *Scand. J. Immunol.* **3:**413–421.

Hornbeck, P. V., and Lewis, G. K., 1983, Idiotype connectance in the immune system. I. Expression of a cross reactive idiotype on induced anti-p-azophenyl-arsonate antibodies and on endogenous antibodies not specific for arsonate, *J. Exp. Med.* **157:**1116–1136.

Jerne, N. K., 1974, Towards a network theory of the immune system, *Ann. Immunol.(Paris)* **125C:**373–389.

Kaushik, A., Poncet, P., and Bussard, A., 1986, Autoantibodies against bromelainized mouse erythrocyte: Strain distribution of serum idiotype expression and relative peritoneal cell activity, *Cell. Immunol.* **102:**323–334.

Kaushik, A., Lim, A., Poncet, P., Ge, X.-R., and Dighiero, G., 1988, Comparative analysis of natural antibody specificities among hybridomas originating from spleen and peritoneal cavity of adult NZB and BALB/c mice, *Scand. J. Immunol.* **27:**461–471.

Kim, Y. T., Goidl, E. A., Samarut, C., Weksler, M. E., Thorbecke, G. J., and Siskind, G. W., 1985, Bone marrow function. I. Peripheral T cells are responsible for the increased auto-anti-idiotypic response of older mice, *J. Exp. Med.* **161:**1237–1242.

Klinman, N. R., 1981, Antibody-specific immunoregulation and the immunodeficiency of aging, *J. Exp. Med.* **154:**547–551.

Liacopoulos, P., Amstutz, H., and Gille, G., 1971, Early antibody forming cells of double specificity, *Immunology* **20:**57–66.

Liacopoulos, P., Couder, J., and Bleux, C., 1976, Evidence for multipotentiality of antibody synthesizing cells, *Ann. Immunol. (Paris)* **127C:**519–530.

McEvoy Martin, S. J., and Goidl, E. A., 1988, Studies on immunological maturation. II. The absence of high-affinity antibody producing cells early in the immune response of the aged is only apparent, *Aging Immunol. Infect. Dis.* **1:**47–54.

Naor, D., Bonavida, B., Robinson, R. A., Shibata, I. N., Percy, D. E., Chia, D., and Barnett, E. V., 1976, Immune response of New Zealand mice to trinitrophenylated syngeneic mouse red cells, *Eur. J. Immunol.* **6:**783–789.

Reininger, L., Kaushik, A., Izui, S., and Janton, J., 1988, A member of a new V_H gene family encodes anti-bromelinized mouse red blood cell autoantibodies, *Eur. J. Immunol.* **18:**1521–1526.

Rittenberg, M. B., and Pratt, K. L., 1969, Anti-trinitrophenyl (TNP) plaque assay. Primary response of Balb/c mice to soluble and particulate immunogen, *Proc. Soc. Exp. Biol. Med.* **132:**575–581.

Schrater, A. F., Goidl, E. A., Thorbecke, G. J., and Siskind, G. W., 1979, Production of auto-anti-ididiotypic antibody during the normal immune response to TNP-Ficoll. I. Occurrence in AKR/J and Balb/c mice of hapten-augmentable anti-TNP plaque-forming cells and their accelerated appearance in recipient of immune spleen cells, *J. Exp. Med.* **150:**138–153.

Sperling, R., Francus, T., and Siskind, G. W., 1983, Degeneracy of antibody specificity, *J. Immunol.* **131:**882–885.

Szewczuk, M. R., and Campbell, R. J., 1980, Loss of immunocompetence with age may be due to auto-anti-idiotypic antibody, *Nature (London)* **286:**164–166.

Talmage, D. W., and Maurer, P. H., 1953, I[131]-labelled antigen precipitation as a measure of quantity and quality of antibody, *J. Infect. Dis.* **92:**288–300.

Vakil, M., and Kearney, J., 1986, Functional characterization of monoclonal auto-anti-idiotypic antibodies isolated from the early B-cell repertoire of BALB/c mice, *Eur. J. Immunol.* **16:**1151–1158.

Vakil, M., Sauter, H., Paige, C., and Kearney, J., 1986, *In vivo* suppression of perinatal multispecific B-cells results in a distortion of the adult B-cell repertoire, *Eur. J. Immunol.* **16:**1159–1165.

Zharhary, D., Segev, Y., and Gershon, H., 1977, The affinity and spectrum of cross-reactivity of antibody production in senescent mice: The IgM response, *Mech. Aging. Dev.* **6:**385–392.

Zharhary, D., Wu, G., and Paige, C., 1988, Utilization of immunoglobulin V_H gene families in B cell colonies from aged mice, *J. Cell. Biochem.* **12B:**102.

41

Analysis of the Ability of Spleen Cells from Aged Mice to Produce Allospecific Cytotoxic Cells

SUSAN R. S. GOTTESMAN and J. M. EDINGTON

1. INTRODUCTION

The ability of aged rodents and humans to respond to foreign antigenic challenge decreases with age (Makinodan, 1977; Gottesman, 1987). This age-related deficiency is particularly severe in the T-cell system, as evidenced by the involution of the thymus, the decline in T-proliferative response to mitogens and specific antigens (Meredith and Walford, 1977; Miller and Stutman, 1981), the defeat in the ability to generate specific T-suppressor cells (Gottesman et al., 1984; Yin et al., 1988), and the inability of T cells to provide help for antibody production and cell-mediated immune responses (Miller and Stutman, 1981; Zharhary et al., 1984). Although many of these defects are contributed to by reduced lymphokine production by cells from aged donors (Miller and Stutman, 1981; Thoman and Weigle, 1982; Chang et al., 1982; Gilman et al., 1982), these activities are not all totally restored by addition of exogenous lymphokines (Gottesman et al., 1985). Cytotoxic T-lymphocyte (CTL) activity, a vital function for survival of the organism, shows an age-related decrease when assayed in bulk cultures (Gottesman et al., 1981). Limiting dilution analysis show a deficiency in a proportion of aged mice tested in CTL precursor frequency, under conditions in which helper cell function and interleukin-2 (IL-2) production are not limiting (Miller, 1984; Gorczynski and Chang, 1984; Zharhary et al., 1984).

Aged animals therefore have both a decrease in CTL precursor frequency and defects in their ability to generate functional cells due to reduced helper cell function and lymphokine production. The lytic activity of the sensitized cells, however, has not been directly measured. Here, data on bulk culture cytotoxic assays are reviewed and compared with the single-cell conjugation assay. This single-cell assay permits evaluation of the functioning of individual CTL after the sensitization period, dividing the lytic process into separate steps that are directly visualized (Zagury et al., 1975; Grimm and Bonavida, 1977).

SUSAN R. S. GOTTESMAN and J. M. EDINGTON • Department of Pathology, New York University Medical Center, New York, New York 10016.

2. BULK CULTURE CYTOTOXIC ASSAYS

Initially, C57Bl/6 (B6) mice of various ages were tested for the ability of their spleen cells to generate allospecific CTLs *in vitro* in bulk culture sensitization with irradiated DBA/2 (H-2^d) spleen cells. After 5 days, the cells were harvested, adjusted to the appropriate concentrations, and assayed in 4-hr chromium-release assays with chromium-labeled P815 (H-2^d) tumor target cells in microtiter plates. Sixty percent of the middle-aged (14–20 months old) and 79% of the aged (26–30 month old) mice tested generated significantly less cytotoxic activity than did the young control mice (3–8 months old) assayed simultaneously (Table I). The average effector-to-target cell ratio required for 33% lysis of targets increased with age (Table I); however, there was considerable overlap between the young and middle aged animals.

Most middle-aged and aged mice that gave normal responses in the CTL assay still had markedly reduced proliferative responses in mixed lymphocyte cultures (MLC) with DBA/2 stimulators (Gottesman *et al.*, 1981). The proliferative response in the MLC was measured by [^{3}H]thymidine uptake after a 4- to 5-day culture in 0.2-ml volumes in microtiter plates, in contrast to the bulk culture sensitization for CTL studied in 2-ml volumes. Therefore, to facilitate direct comparison of the two assays, cytotoxicity was also measured by adding chromated P815 target cells directly to the microtiter plates of B6 responders and irradiated DBA/2 stimulators at the end of the 5-day culture period. This method proved suboptimal for the generation of CTL by spleen cells from young control mice, as they gave a maximum response of 50% lysis. Differences in the generation of cytotoxicity between young and middle-aged mice that were not evident when measured under optimal conditions were revealed when these suboptimal sensitization conditions were applied. A representative experiment is shown in Table II in which three mice of different ages are compared for their activities in the three assays.

TABLE I. Effector–Target Cell Ratio for 33% Lysis in Bulk Culture
Chromium-Release Assays[a]

Age of mice	N	Average	Range of effectors–1 target cell	SD	% animals tested showing significant difference from young control[b]
Young (3–8 mo.)	16	0.8:1	0.2–2.2	0.58	—
Middle-aged (14–20 mo.)	14	1.0:1	0.2–2.1	0.6	60%
Aged (26–30 mo.)	19	3.2:1	0.2 → 10	3.1	79%

[a]Spleen cells were tested for their ability to lyse chromated P815 target cells in a 4-hr assay after a 5-day sensitization to H-2^d alloantigens. Spleen cells were tested at four ratios with target cells (10, 5, 1, 0.5:1) and the ratio required for lysis of 33% of the target cells extrapolated from the curves.
[b]Student's *t*-test analysis was used to compare the middle-aged or aged animal tested to its young control run simultaneously.

TABLE II. Activities of Three Mice of Different Ages in Three Different Assays

A. Mixed lymphocyte culture: ^{3}H-thymidine incorporation

Responding cells/ well ($\times 10^{-4}$)[b]	Age of spleen cell donor[a]		
	Young (cpm ± SE)	Middle-aged (cpm ± SE)	Aged (cpm ± SE)
2.5	3210 ± 1032	410 ± 111	272 ± 168
5.0	8700 ± 1192	1990 ± 607	1260 ± 478
7.5	15640 ± 2205	3100 ± 711	2160 ± 412
10.0	23920 ± 2402	7680 ± 653	5940 ± 1071
15.0	31100 ± 3295	11570 ± 1668	9230 ± 599

B. Cytotoxicity in bulk culture: chromium-release assay

Effector–target cell ratio[d]	Age of spleen cell donor[c]		
	Young (% lysis)	Middle-aged (% lysis)	Aged (% lysis)
0.5 : 1	12	10	3
1 : 1	24	17	4
5 : 1	72	76	35
10 : 1	77	87	44

C. Cytotoxicity in microtiter plates: chromium-release assay

Responding cells/ well ($\times 10^{-4}$)[f]	Age of spleen cell donor[e]		
	Young (% lysis)	Middle-aged (% lysis)	Aged (% lysis)
2.5	5	0	0
5.0	14	0	1
7.5	22	7	3
10.0	49	5	11

[a] Young: 5-month-old; middle-aged: 19-month-old; aged: 27-month-old.
[b] All cultures were stimulated with 2 × 10⁵ irradiated DBA/2 spleen cells in microtiter plates and incubated for 5 days. ^{3}H-thymidine was added for the last 8 hr of culture.
[c] Spleen cells stimulated for 5 days with irradiated DBA/2 spleen cells in 2-ml volumes.
[d] Cytotoxic cells were harvested after sensitization and incubated at the designated ratios with P815 target cells in a 4-hr chromium-release assay.
[e] Spleen cells were stimulated for 5 days with irradiated DBA/2 spleen cells in microtiter plates. Chromated P815 targets were added directly to the microtiter plates for the 4-hr assay.
[f] Number of B6 spleen cells in wells of microtiter plates at initiation of sensitization.

3. SINGLE-CELL CONJUGATION ASSAY

The single-cell conjugation assay was used to study the activity of individual sensitized cells in the different stages of lysis. Spleen cells from B6 mice were sensitized for 5 days in 24 well plates with an equal number of irradiated DBA/2 or (B6 × DBA/2)F1 spleen cells. Cells were harvested and first separated on lymphoprep to eliminate dead cells and debris. They were incubated with P815 cells at 30°C for 10 min, a temperature permissive for binding or conjugate formation but not for lysis. The conjugates were then spun and the tubes kept on ice while the samples were counted using a hemacytometer. The conjugates did not dissociate in this liquid phase, provided they were kept on ice. They were gently resuspended immediately prior to being counted. All samples were done with six replicates, and all tubes were blinded. Conjugates were quantitated as the number of lymphocytes with a bound target divided by 200 lymphocytes counted.

There is considerable day-to-day variability in the conjugation assay; however, when several individual young mice were assayed simultaneously, they gave essentially equivalent results. The values for three individual young mice assayed simultaneously were 32, 33, and 35% conjugate formation, for an average of 33.3% and a standard deviation of 1.5. The entire group of 20 young mice tested gave an average conjugate formation of 35.7% with a standard deviation (SD) of 3.7. Unsensitized spleen cells from young or aged mice formed fewer than 5% conjugates, and sensitized cells also formed fewer than 5% conjugates with EL-4 cells, as a nonspecific target.

Spleen cells from a series of individual young and aged mice were compared for their ability to be sensitized to form conjugates. The aged mice were always tested simultaneously with a paired young control as a control for the day-to-day variability in the assay. Sensitized cells from aged mice formed 20–36% conjugates, whereas cells from young mice formed 30–42% conjugates. The results for the first 15 aged mice tested are shown in Fig. 1 and are compared with the young controls assayed simultaneously. The difference between the young and the old was significant by Student's t-test analysis for 8 of the 15 pairs. None of the aged mice formed significantly more conjugates than did their young control-paired animals. The Wilcoxon signed rank analysis for paired values was used to analyze the entire series, and the difference between the young and aged populations was found to be significant ($p < 0.01$).

4. ADDITION OF EXOGENOUS IL-2 TO SENSITIZATION CULTURES

Recombinant murine IL-2 (10 U/ml, Cetus Corp., Emeryville, California was added to the sensitization cultures for the generation of CTL between responder cells from B6 mice of various ages and DBA/2 or (B6 × DBA/2)F1 stimulators. Sensitized cells were assayed for conjugate formation and for cytotoxicity by chromium-release assays. Exogenous IL-2 had previously been shown to increase, but not restore, the proliferative response of cells from aged mice to alloantigens (Gottesman et al., 1985). The lymphokine appeared to be effective in restoring functional responses. The exogenous IL-2 increased the number of conjugates formed by cells from aged mice without affecting the number formed by cells from young mice. The difference in conjugate formation between young and aged mice disappeared with the inclusion of IL-2 (Fig. 2). Similarly, in the bulk culture chromium-release assay, the

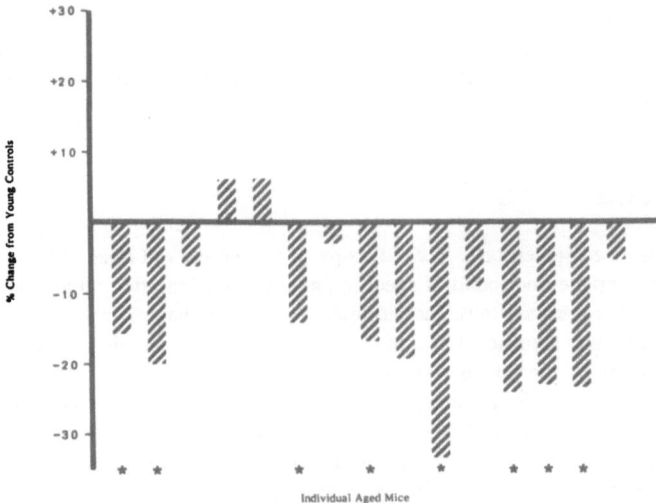

FIGURE 1. Conjugate formation by individual aged mice in comparison with their young controls run simultaneously. Spleen cells from young and aged B6 mice were sensitized to H-2^d alloantigens and then tested for their ability to form conjugates with P815 (H-2^d) tumor target cells. Conjugate formation for cells from the entire series of young mice ranged from 30 to 42% and for cells from the entire series of aged mice from 20 to 36%. Asterisks (*) denote significant difference ($p < 0.01$) between the aged mouse and its paired young control.

FIGURE 2. Ability of exogenous IL-2 in sensitization cultures to improve conjugate formation by cells from aged mice. Spleen cells from individual young and aged mice were sensitized to H-2^d alloantigens in the presence (+) or absence (−) of 10 U/ml exogenous rIL-2. Range of conjugate formation: young − IL-2, 31–42% young + IL-2, 30–41%; old − IL-2, 24–35%; old + IL-2, 31–43%. (*) Significant difference between old − IL-2 and young − IL-2. x, Significant difference between old + IL-2 and old − IL-2.

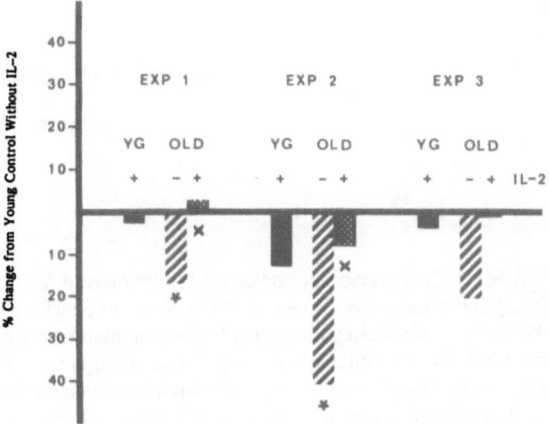

addition of IL-2 increased the percentage lysis by cells from aged mice without altering the activity of cells from young mice. Control experiments in which sensitized cells from old mice were incubated for 1 hr with IL-2, washed, and then tested for conjugate formation showed no effect of preincubation in IL-2.

5. SINGLE-CELL LYSIS

Single sensitized spleen cells from 10 pairs of young and old mice were compared for their ability to complete one round of specific target cell killing after conjugation. In all 10 pairs, the cells from the aged mice formed fewer conjugates than their young controls (Fig. 3). This difference was significant in 6 of the 10 pairs. For the complete series, the average conjugate formation by the young was 34.3% and by the aged was 26.2%.

The single-cell lysis within conjugates from these same 10 pairs of mice is shown in Fig. 3. Cells from an equal number of old mice showed slightly more or less lysis than did cells from their young partners, whether the differences in the conjugation assays were significant or not. The average percentage lysis by the young was 37.6% with a range of 35–42% and the average for the old was 36.2% with a range of 24–41%. Therefore, an equivalent percentage of cells that formed conjugates could go on to lyse their targets in young and aged mice.

6. CONCLUSIONS

Fewer CTL precursors exist in the spleens of aged mice (Miller, 1984; Zharhary *et al.*, 1984; Gorczynski and Chang, 1984), as shown by limiting dilution analysis in the presence of supplemental helper T cells and exogenous lymphokines. In bulk culture sensitization and

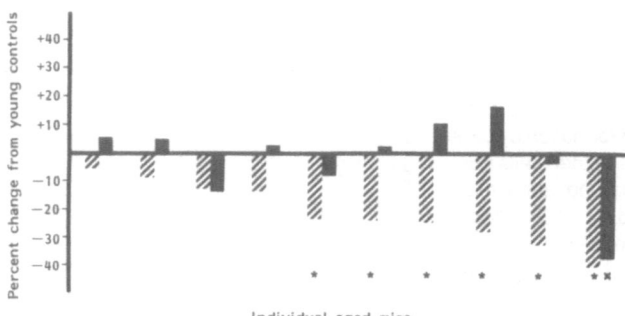

FIGURE 3. Comparison of conjugate formation and lytic ability of sensitized spleen cells from young and aged mice. Conjugate formation by sensitized cells from aged mice was compared with that by cells from young mice tested simultaneously and the difference found to be significant for 6 of the 10 pairs of mice (*). Those conjugates formed were allowed to lyse their bound target, and the aged were compared with their young control for lytic efficiency. For only one pair was the difference between young and aged significant (x). Range of lytic efficiency: young, 35–42%; old, 24–41%.

chromium-release assays, optimal sensitization conditions exist and effector cells are allowed to lyse and recycle to more than one target cell. Under these conditions, differences in the activity of cells from young and middle-aged or aged mice are sometimes difficult to demonstrate. Suboptimal conditions using low cell numbers and probably limiting lymphokine production facilitate demonstration of differences in cytotoxic activity between cells from young and aged mice.

Using the single-cell assay, we were able to investigate the functioning of sensitized effector cells and study the ability of the individual cell to bind and lyse targets. We found the number of conjugates generated from spleen cells of aged mice to be significantly lower than the number generated from cells of young animals. However, an equivalent proportion of sensitized effector cells from young and aged mice went on to lyse their bound targets in single-cell assays.

Addition of IL-2 to the sensitization cultures increased the percentage conjugates formed by cells from aged mice without affecting that for young mice. This exogenous IL-2 must act by supplementing the deficient helper cell function in the cultures and allowing the maximum proliferative burst of the CTL precursors that do exist in aged mice. It is possible that this expression of maximum proliferation in bulk cultures overcomes any deficiency in CTL precursor number. Proliferation by cells from young mice might already be at maximal levels and therefore unaffected by further addition of IL-2. In limiting dilution assays, negative wells would remain negative because of the absence of a precursor cell, and the standard supplementation with IL-2 would not alter the results. By contrast, it is possible that in limiting dilution assays, a second lymphokine that is not supplied becomes limiting in IL-2-supplemented cultures of cells from aged mice. Diminished supplies of this lymphokine may not be a factor under bulk culture sensitization conditions.

Although a smaller number of cells capable of forming conjugates with the specific targets are produced by spleen cells from aged mice, the same proportion of those that bind the target can go on to lyse them. Therefore, the progeny of CTL precursors that exist in aged mice have intact lytic machinery and function at control levels for at least the first round of lysis.

REFERENCES

Chang, M., Makinodan, T., Peterson, W. J., and Strehler, B. L., 1982, Role of T cells and adherent cells in age-related decline in murine interleukin 2 production, J. Immunol. 129:2426–2430.

Gilman, S. C., Rosenberg, J. S., and Feldman, J. D., 1982, T lymphocytes of young and aged rats. II. Functional defects and the role of interleukin-2, J. Immunol 128:644–650.

Gorczynski, R. M., and Chang, M.-P., 1984, Peripheral (somatic) expansion of the murine cytotoxic T lymphocyte repertoire. II. Comparison of diversity in recognition repertoire of alloreactive T cells in spleen and thymus of young or aged DBA/2J mice transplanted with bone marrow cells from young or aged donors, J. Immunol. 133:2381–2389.

Gottesman, S. R. S., 1987, T cell function in aging—An update, in: Review of Biological Research in Aging, Vol. 3 (W. H. Adler, ed.), Liss, New York, pp. 95–110.

Gottesman, S. R. S., Kristie, J. A., and Walford, R. L., 1981, Proliferative and cytotoxic immune functions in aging mice. I. Sequence of decline of reactivities measured under optimal and suboptimal sensitization conditions, Immunology 44:607–616.

Gottesman, S. R. S., Walford, R. L., and Thorbecke, G. J., 1984, Proliferative and cytotoxic immune functions in aging mice. II. Decreased generation of specific suppressor cells in alloreactive cultures, J. Immunol. 133:1782–1787.

Gottesman, S. R. S., Walford, R. L., and Thorbecke, G. J., 1985, Proliferative and cytotoxic immune functions in aging mice. III. Exogenous interleukin-2 rich supernatant only partially restores alloreactivity in vitro, *Mech. Aging Dev.* **31**:103–113.

Grimm, E. A., and Bonavida, B., 1977, Studies on the induction and expression of T cell mediated immunity. VI. Heterogeneity of lytic efficiency exhibited by isolated cytotoxic T lymphocytes prepared from highly enriched populations of effector–target conjugates, *J. Immunol.* **119**:1041–1047.

Makinodan, T., 1977, Immunity and Aging, in: *Handbook of the Biology of Aging* (C. E. Finch and L. Hayflick, eds.), Von Nostrand–Reinhold, New York, pp. 379–408.

Meredith, P., and Walford, R., 1977, Effect of age on response to T- and B-mitogens in mice congenic at the H-2 locus, *Immunogenetics* **5**:109–128.

Miller, R. A., 1984, Age-associated decline in precursor frequency for different T cell-mediated reactions, with preservation of helper or cytotoxic effect per precursor cell, *J. Immunol.* **132**:63–68.

Miller, R. A., and Stutman, O., 1981, Decline, in aging mice, of the anti-2,4,6-trinitrophenyl (TNP) cytotoxic T cell response attributable to loss of Lyt-2⁻, interleukin 2-producing helper cell function, *Eur. J. Immunol.* **11**:751–756.

Thoman, M. L., and Weigle, W. O., 1982, Cell mediated immunity in aged mice: An underlying lesion in IL-2 synthesis, *J. Immunol.* **128**:2358–2361.

Yin, J. -Z., Gottesman, S. R. S., Bell, M. K., and Thorbecke, G. J., 1988, Resistance to low dose tolerance and enhanced antibody repsonses of aged as compared to young mice immunized with pneumococca; polysaccharides, *Aging: Immunology and Infectious Disease* **1**:131.

Zagury, D., Bernard, J., Thierness, N., Feldman, M., and Berke, G., 1975, Isolation and characterization of individual functionally reactive cytotoxic T lymphocytes: Conjugation, killing, and recycling at the single cell level, *Eur. J. Immunol.* **5**:818–822.

Zharhary, D., Segev, Y., and Gershon, H. E., 1984, T-cell cytotoxicity and aging: Differing causes of reduced response in individual mice, *Mech. Aging Dev.* **25**:129–140.

The Brain, Neuroendocrine Circuits, Pathology, and Plasticity

Neuronal Populations in Normal and Abnormal Aging

ROBERT D. TERRY

1. INTRODUCTION

During the course of development, both structure and function in any organ or cellular system increase at a rate that varies according to the particular function, species, or even individual. A plateau is reached and maintained, again for a variable time. Following this second phase, there is a decrease in structure and function, which again follows a differing slope. Under normal circumstances, death would occur somewhere along the course of this downward slope before most functions reach that decreased level at which symptoms might be displayed. With disease, however, the functional decrease is exaggerated. A disease occurring at maturity can be more severe without pushing the function down to that symptomatic threshold than would be the same disease occurring in old age, where the distance between the negative slope and the threshold of symptoms is narrowed. This concept can be applied to many circumstances in the human, as, for example, glomerular filtration, cardiac output, muscle strength, and some aspects of cognition. This presentation will illustrate the declining slope of several structural aspects of the central nervous system in health and in Alzheimer's disease, and will illustrate the threshold concept by demonstrating the difference between Alzheimer's disease in the younger adult as compared with that in the older. Mild cerebral decrements occur in normal aging without major cognitive losses, as exemplified by Picasso, Casals, Rebecca West, George Burns, and countless other wise and witty elderly people.

2. RESULTS AND DISCUSSION

Both brain weight and cortical thickness decline as a function of normal aging (Fig. 1). Although neocortical neurons have been counted on many occasions, there is still considerable dispute as to the extent of loss in the normal elderly. The best known data are those of Brody (1955), who counted cells by hand and eye with the light microscope. The number of

ROBERT D. TERRY • Department of Neurosciences, School of Medicine, University of California–San Diego, La Jolla, California 92093.

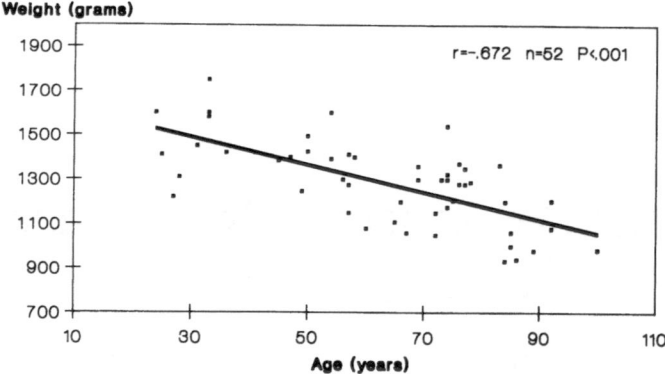

FIGURE 1. Age versus brain weight in normals. Brain weight falls in normal aging with a correlation coefficient of −0.67, accounting for 45% of the variance.

specimens he had available to him was small, and the tissue was apparently examined only with cresyl violet preparations, which cannot reveal either plaques or tangles indicative of Alzheimer disease. Neither were other disorders that might affect cortical populations sought by histologic study.

Our own normative data (Terry *et al.*, 1987) involve about 50 specimens, and reveal that there is a loss of large neurons; that is, cells greater than 90 μm^2 in cross-sectional area (in formalin-fixed paraffin-embedded cresyl violet-stained tissue) (Fig. 2). However, we also find by our techniques of image analysis that the number of smaller neurons (i.e., those between 40 and 90 μm^2) increases to an extent equal to the loss of large neurons (Fig. 3). We conclude that in normal aging neocortical large neurons shrink but are not lost in significant numbers. These data differ from those of Brody and from many other cell counters. To ensure that our data are reliable, we have examined these specimens with great care at both gross and

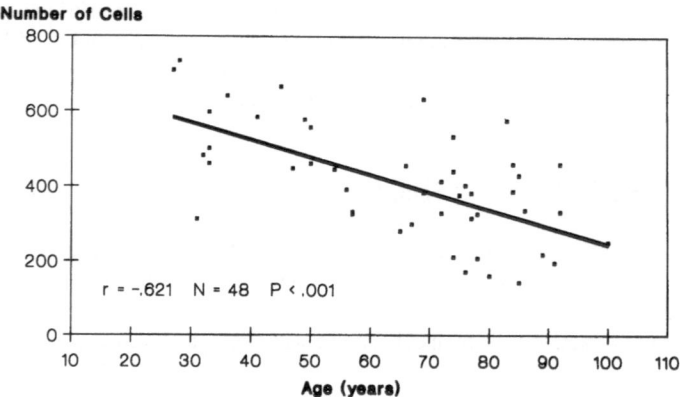

FIGURE 2. In normal aging, large neurons (>90 μm^2) decrease in the midfrontal cortex with a correlation coefficient of −0.62 accounting for 39% of the variance.

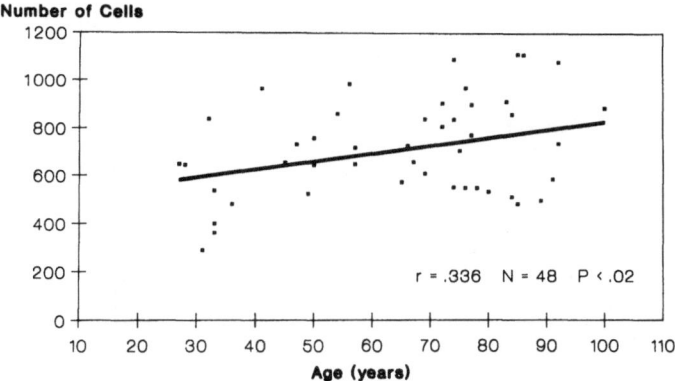

FIGURE 3. Small neurons in the frontal cortex increase slightly in the course of normal aging. The average increase in the elderly group equals the average decrease of large neurons in that group. (Cells 40–90 μm^2.)

microscopic levels, using several special stains, and looking especially to rule out cases of Alzheimer's disease, anoxia, Parkinson's disease, and so forth. Furthermore, our image analysis apparatus is used with extensive video editing, because without it there are significant errors. These can be created by contiguity of cells and understaining of part of the cell body, vessel walls, and vascular contents. Without editing, image analysis is not reliable in our experience (Terry and DeTeresa, 1982).

In Alzheimer's disease, the brain weight is inversely related to the duration of disease but is not correlated with age. In the well-diagnosed situation, i.e., with both clinical and histologic abnormalities, the concentrations of both plaques and tangles decline with age. This implies that the disease need not be as intense in the elderly patient as it is in the younger patient to produce symptoms, following the threshold concept as described above.

Neocortical neurons were counted by image analysis in the midfrontal, superior temporal, and inferior parietal regions. In each area, there was a highly significant diminution in the number of large neurons as compared with age-matched normals (Terry et al., 1981). This diminution is to be noted as a function of neuronal density or as to the number of neurons in the full thickness of the cortex. Patients dying between ages 50 and 69 displayed a greater loss than did those dying after age 70 (Hansen et al., 1988) (Fig. 4). In comparison with age-matched normals, a significant difference in the number of large neurons is to be found in Alzheimer patients at any age, even those who die after age 85. Small neurons do not appear to be significantly affected. By contrast, frontal lobe glia are increased in number or density in the younger patients (age 50–69), while they are decreased in those patients dying at age 70 or older (Fig. 5).

Major neuronal loss is not confined to the neocortex. It has been reported as highly significant in the CAl region of the hippocampus (Ball, 1977) and in the entorhinal area, especially layer 2 (Hyman et al., 1984). Loss of neurons from the entorhinal cortex effectively isolates the hippocampus in that the former serves as the major input and output relay station to and from the hippocampus. Neurons are also lost from the basal nucleus of Meynert (Whitehouse et al., 1984). These neurons synthesize choline acetyltransferase (ChAT), which is then transported to the axonal terminals, where it synthesizes acetylcholine (ACh).

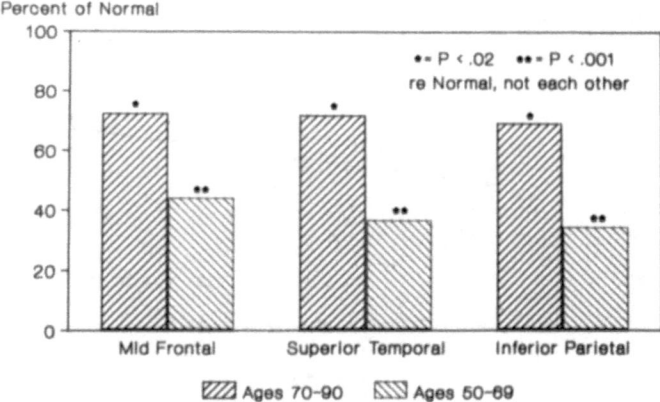

FIGURE 4. In Alzheimer's disease, the number of large neurons (>90 μm^2) is significantly decreased in all three neocortical areas. There is a greater decrease in the younger patients than in the older, but both groups are significantly different from normal.

The basal nucleus is therefore the major source of cholinergic activity in the neocortex and other parts of the forebrain. Many cases of Alzheimer's disease display a loss of the neuroadrenergic neurons of the locus ceruleus (Bondareff et al., 1981) and also of the serotonergic neurons of the dorsal raphe (Mann and Yates, 1983).

A loss of large neurons leads, obviously, to loss of brain weight—the number of large neurons in the superior temporal cortex correlates directly with brain weight—and more importantly, to a significant decrease in the interconnectivity by which the brain maintains its higher cognitive functions. There is a concomitant loss of specific neurotransmitters due to

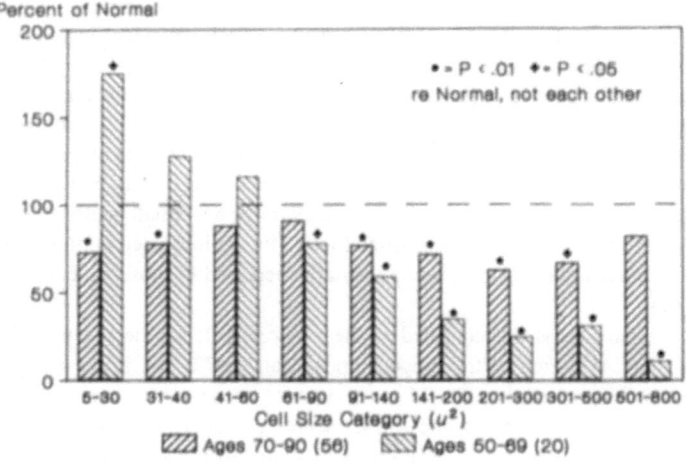

FIGURE 5. It can be seen that glia increase in the younger Alzheimer patients but not in the elderly, while large neurons are decreased in both groups.

TABLE I. The Anatomical Reserve

Cognition	Normal[a]	Normal with plaques[b]	Demented with plaques[c]
Blessed[d]	4	4	23
Age	84	87	86
Brain weight[e]	100	109[f]	97
Plaques[e]	100	1500	1900
Large neurons[e]	100	133[f]	79
ChAT[e]	100	65	44
Somatostatin[e]	100	74	100

[a]Group tested as cognitively normal; had no neocortical plaques.
[b]Cognitively normal group, but had neocortical plaques.
[c]Typical Alzheimer's dementia and neocortical plaques.
[d]Score on test of cognition, modified from Gary Blessed (1968); a higher
score = poorer cognition.
[e]Normalized to the first group (normal with neocortical plaques).
[f]Increased significantly, indicating anatomical reserve.

these neuronal decrements. These deficits give rise to the cognitive losses that characterize the disease.

We recently reported on a group of patients tested for cognitive ability in life and found to be normal, but whose brain tissue contained a concentration of plaques quite consistent with the diagnosis of Alzheimer's disease (Katzman *et al.*, 1988). In comparing a group of normal aged specimens from patients with normal cognition and no cortical plaques with this group of cognitively normal specimens with plaques, we find that the latter have heavier brains and a higher concentration of large neurons (Table I). We infer that this represents an anatomical reserve, so that incipient Alzheimer's disease is slower to reveal itself. These findings add to our confidence in the significance of neuronal populations.

ACKNOWLEDGMENTS. This work was supported by grants AGO5386 and AGO5131 from the National Institutes of Health and by the McKnight Foundation.

REFERENCES

Ball, M. J., 1977, Neuronal loss, neurofibrillary tangles and granulovacular degeneration in the hippocampus with aging and dementia. A quantitative study, *Acta Neuropathol. (Berl.)* **37**:111–118.

Blessed, G., Tomlinson, B. E., and Roth, M., 1968, The association between quantitative measures of dementia and of senile changes in the cerebral grey matter of elderly subjects, *Br. J. Psychiatry* **114**:797–811.

Bondareff, W., Mountjoy, C. Q., and Roth, M., 1981, Selective loss of neurones of origin of adrenergic projection to cerebral cortex (nucleus locus coeruleus) in senile dementia, *Lancet* **1**:783–784.

Brody, H., 1955, Organization of the cerebral cortex III. A study of aging in the human cerebral cortex, *J. Comp. Neurol.* **102**:511–556.

Hansen, L. A., DeTeresa, R., Davies, P., and Terry, R. D., 1988, Neocortical morphometry, lesion counts, and choline acetyltransferase levels in the age spectrum of Alzheimer's disease, *Neurology (NY)* **38**:48–54.

Hyman, B. T., Van Hoesen, G. W., Damasio, A. R., and Barnes, C. L., 1984, Alzheimer's disease: Cell-specific pathology isolates the hippocampal formation, *Science* **225:**1168–1170.

Katzman, R., Terry, R., DeTeresa, R., Brown, T., Davies, P., Fuld, P., Renbing, X., and Peck, A., 1988, Clinical, pathological, and neurochemical changes in dementia; a subgroup with preserved mental status and numerous neocortical plaques, *Ann. Neurol.* **23:**138–144.

Mann, D. M. A., and Yates, P. O., 1983, Serotonin nerve cells in Alzheimer's disease, *J. Neurol. Neurosurg. Psychiatry* **46:**96.

Terry, R. D., and DeTeresa, R., 1982, The importance of video editing in automated image analysis in studies of the cerebral cortex, *J. Neurol. Sci.* **53:**413–421.

Terry, R. D., Peck, A., DeTeresa, R., Schechter, R., and Horoupian, D. S., 1981, Some morphometric aspects of the brain in senile dementia of the Alzheimer type, *Ann. Neurol.* **10:**184–192.

Terry, R. D., DeTeresa, R. D., and Hansen, L. A., 1987, Neocortical cell counts in normal human adult aging, *Ann. Neurol.* **21:**530–539.

Whitehouse, P. J., Price, D. L., Clark, A. W., Coyle, J. T., and DeLong, M. R., 1981, Alzheimer's disease: Evidence of selective loss of cholinergic neurons in the nucleus basalis, *Ann. Neurol.* **10:**122–126.

43

An Optimistic View of the Aging Brain

MARIAN C. DIAMOND

1. INTRODUCTION

How much influence do brains have in controlling their own destiny during aging? On the one hand, brains can predict the negative sides of the fate of aging with more dementia, more illness, and more social problems over the years and decades ahead. Or, on the other hand, brains can develop a more positive point of view after learning the facts about their potential and applying these in creating a more optimistic path toward the process of attaining old age.

When one speaks of old age, one commonly refers to the chronological age of the total individual, not necessarily the biological age of various cellular constituents. Different cells and regions of the body age at different rates. The processes of development and aging are occurring simultaneously in various parts of the body during a total lifetime. In fact, although nerve cells are forming during embryogenesis, at the same time the greatest loss of nerve cells occur before the individual is born. Yet most people are primarily concerned about losing cells in the later years of life. Thus, it becomes clear that in order to understand the processes of old age, it is necessary to follow the steps that preceded it and, in doing so, to examine not only one structure but other structures that have a close relationship to it. What, then, are some of the findings during the past decades that offer representative samples of morphological changes that occur in a mammalian forebrain as it progresses toward an old chronological age?

The majority of developmental and aging studies in our laboratory have dealt with environmental influences on the anatomy of the forebrain of a lower mammal, the rat. Such studies must take into consideration numerous variables, including age, sex, brain region, right or left side, cell number, and size. This chapter examines patterns of development and aging in cerebral cortical thickness of male and female Long-Evans rats. Such patterns are then compared with the thickness of the male hippocampus and entorhinal cortex, offering examples of aging in neo-, paleo-, and archicortical samples. Neuron and glial counts in cortical area 18 between the ages of 26 and 904 days are discussed. With these basic values obtained from our standard laboratory conditions, results from cortical measures in rats exposed to differential environments, both enriched and impoverished, are offered. Much of

MARIAN C. DIAMOND • Department of Integrative Biology, University of California–Berkeley, Berkeley, California 94720.

this information has been presented previously (Diamond et al., 1964, 1985; Diamond, 1967, 1984, 1985a,b; Diamond, 1986); the data gained from old female rats are new.

2. FOREBRAIN DEVELOPMENT AND AGING

Our data on gender-based differences in the developing and aging cerebral cortex can be offered from two perspectives: cortical thickness measurements combining both hemispheres, and providing left-right differences separately. For the male values, the following age groups and numbers of Long-Evans animals in parentheses were examined: 6 (15), 10 (15), 14 (17), 20 (15), 41 (16), 55 (25), 77 (15), 90 (15), 108 (15), 185 (15), 300 (15), 400 (15), 650 (16), and 904 (7). For the females, the age and numbers of animals were as follows: 7 (14), 14 (15), 21 (18), 90 (15), 180 (11), 390 (17), and 800 (6).

2.1. Cerebral Cortical Thickness

From microslide projected images (22.5×) of 20-μm transverse sections stained with thionin, cortical thickness measurements were taken of samples from the frontal, somatosensory, and occipital cortices, using subcortical landmarks to ensure uniformity in sampling. In the male, all cortical regions grew very rapidly from an undeveloped stage at birth to the maximum thickness, somewhere between 26 and 41 days of age. The increases in cortical thickness were between 28% and 46% before the peaks were reached, after which the cortex began to decrease slowly throughout the ages studied. Between 650 and 904 days of age, the occipital cortical sample decreased at a greater rate than did the other two cortical areas (Diamond, 1985b). In the female, the developmental pattern was not identical to that of the male. All three cortical sections measured showed more advanced development at birth, with different patterns of growth. For example, the female frontal cortex was fairly well developed and grew postnatally by about 11% before reaching its maximum thickness. Area 39 in the lateralmost portion of the occipital cortical sample (so called because it contained several visual cortical areas) increased as much as 45%. Just as different cortical areas developed at different rates, they also aged at different rates. For example, between the ages of 26 and 390 days of age, cortical areas 4 and 18 decrease in thickness by 22% and 31%, respectively. At the same time, areas 10, 2, and 3 decrease only by one half as much by 11% and 15%. We learned that after 390 days of age, all cortical areas displayed a slight decrease until 800 days of age, the last group measured (Fig. 1).

In our 1975 study, we reported our findings on right–left cortical thickness differences in male rats, showing that the right cortex was thicker than the left in 92 of 98 areas measured on the brains from rats 6–650 days of age (Diamond et al., 1975). In 1983, we provided the levels of significance of these differences and more detailed information about the right–left findings (Diamond et al., 1983). By 1985, we could add the results from the 904-day-old rats (Diamond et al., 1985). From 6 to 904 days of age, the male right cerebral cortex is thicker than the left in 62 areas measured, except for one reversal found in area 2. In fact, area 2 does not develop a statistically significant right dominance until around 185 days of age. What this finding means is not clear, especially when area 3 adjacent to area 2 shows strong significant differences at all ages except 900 days. A consistent result throughout the cortex was also noted in the 904-day-old animals. In this group, even though the right cortex was thicker than the left, at no time were the differences significantly different. Evidently, in old males, cortical thickness dominant patterns become markedly reduced.

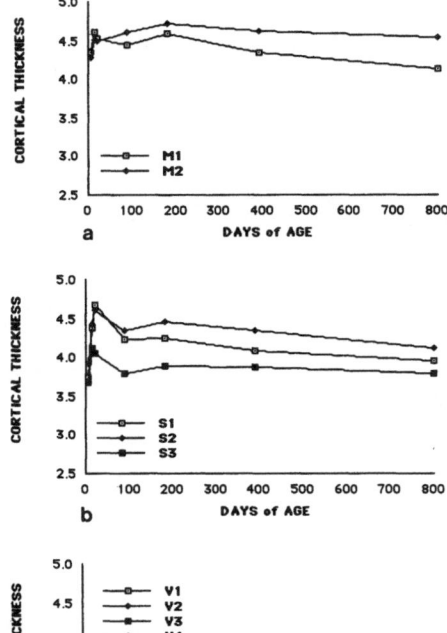

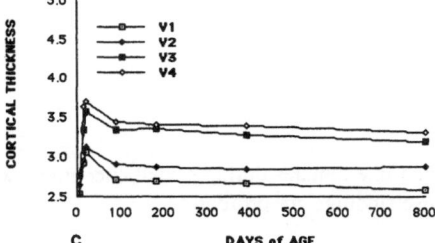

FIGURE 1. Changes in cerebral cortical thickness (in centimeters from microslide projected images) during development and aging (from 7 to 800 days) in Long-Evans female rats in (a) frontal cortex, (b) somatosensory cortex, and (c) visual context (occipital cortical sample). In (a) M1 and M2 represent medial and lateral area 10, in (b) S1, S2, and S3 represent areas 4, 3, and 2, in (c) V1, V2, V3, and V4 represent areas 18, 17, 18a, and 39.

In the female, cortical asymmetry is not as well defined as in the male. In 33 of 54 areas measured in rats between the ages of 7–390 days, the left cortex was thicker than the right, but the differences were significant in only two of these areas (Fig. 2). It is of interest to point out that the measurements from the occipital cortical sample showed the right hemisphere to be greater than the left at the end of the first postnatal week. Then, not until 180 and 390 days, did these right-greater-than-left differences appear again. In fact, in our most recent data on the 800-day-old female rats, the right occipital cortical samples showed a marked dominance over the left, becoming statistically significantly different in two areas. Is it possible that the old male cortex more closely resembles the earlier pattern of the female, while at the same time the old female asymmetry pattern becomes more similar to that of the young male? Asymmetrical patterns have been noted to change under other experimental conditions as well.

In one study, the left cerebral cortex of neonatal male rats had become larger than the dimensions of the right cortex (Fleming *et al.*, 1986). In other words, the usual right-thicker-than-left cortical asymmetry pattern was not evident. These males were born from mothers who were mildly stressed during the last days of pregnancy. Not only had the left male cortex increased in thickness, representing a pattern similar to that found in females, but these males

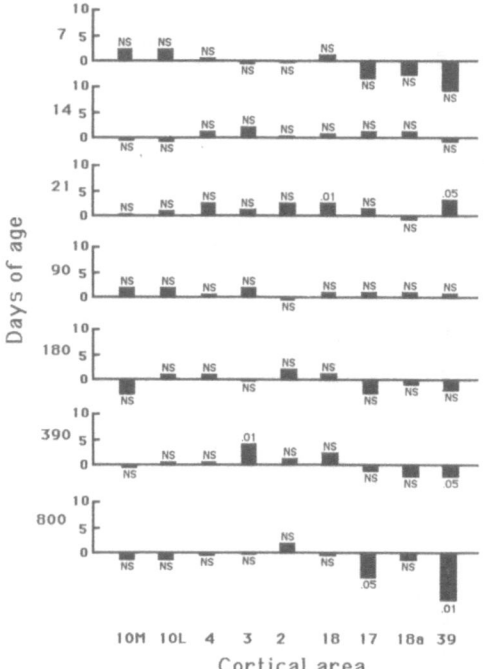

FIGURE 2. Percentage differences between left and right cerebral cortical thickness in young, adult, and old aged female Long-Evans rats. Above (0) signifies that left is greater than right.

acted like females during sexual encounters with right dominant males. The implications of these findings are profound.

2.2. Hippocampus, Entorhinal Cortex, and Amygdaloid Nucleus

The thickness of the hippocampus and entorhinal cortex between the ages of 26 and 904 days was measured for comparison with the occipital cortical sample (Diamond, 1986). The area of the amygdaloid nucleus was also measured between 26 and 400 days of age (Melone *et al.,* 1984). The measurements were taken on the same sections used for the cerebral cortical measures. For these studies, the rats lived 3 per colony cage (34 × 20 × 20 cm). The results indicted that the hippocampus continued to grow from 26 to 904 days of age. One wonders whether the same growth pattern will eventually be found in the human hippocampus. Since this structure has been proven to be related to recent memory and since recent memory processing frequently suffers during old age, an apparent paradox exists with our present data. In contrast to the hippocampus, both the entorhinal and occipital cortical samples showed a decrease in dimensions after a period between 26 and 41 days of age. Thus, comparing an archicortical sample, the hippocampus, with both a paleo- and neocortical sample, it is clear that different aging patterns exist in several of the forebrain structures.

The amygdaloid nucleus offered a more erratic aging pattern than did the cortical samples (Melone *et al.,* 1984). The developmental peak at 26 days was followed by a statistically significant decrease to 90 days, amounting to 13% ($p < 0.002$). An increase then occurred from 90 to 185 days by 16% ($p < 0.002$). In other words, the growth of the amygdala expressed as ($R + L/2$) did not show a continuous linear growth with time, but if one looks at its overall postnatal changes in dimension between 6 and 400 days, it increased by as much as 44% ($p < 0.001$). No amygdaloid measurements were taken after this date.

Since both the male and female right and left cortices changed the direction of thickness differences over time, we were interested in learning if the hippocampus followed suit. By about 400 days of age, the respective dominance patterns in both males and females were reduced and became nonsignificant. One can conclude that in the cerebral cortex as well as in the hippocampus, the asymmetrical patterns do change with aging.

2.3. Cerebral Cortical Cell Counts

Because of the lack of a large neuropil in the rat cerebral cortex before 26 days of age, differential cell counts cannot easily be made before this time. In our studies, such counts were made on 10 micra, luxol-fast blue-cresylecht violet-stained sections from male Long-Evans rats at 26, 41, 108, 650, and 904 days of age (Diamond et al., 1985). With the aid of standardized criteria, neurons and glia were counted on 46-cm montages of enlarged photographs (640×), including cortical cells from layer II through layer VI. We learned that there was no significant loss of neurons in the medial occipital cortex (area 18) between 108 and 904 days of age. It was amazing to discover the consistency of counts between 650 and 904 days because the counts were done 5 years apart. In support of our findings, a nonsignificant loss of neurons in the adjacent area 17 was reported in 1983 (Peters et al., 1983). In addition, in the somastosensory area, both Brizzee et al. (1968) and Curcio and Coleman (1982) found no significant loss of neurons in rats over 700 days of age.

With the cell counts being so consistent and the cortex decreasing in thickness with aging, one can assume that the shrinkage of the cortex with aging is primarily due to a decrease in the size of the cells, not the number. Altering the environmental input to the cortex can readily induce measurable changes in the dimensions of the neurons, from soma to dendrites to postsynaptic thickening (Diamond, 1988). Since the dendritic trees account for a large part of the cortical mass, it is likely that a decrease in number and length of these branches occurs with aging.

3. ENRICHMENT AND IMPOVERISHMENT

3.1. Prenatal

Having established periods of cortical increase and decrease during the lifetime of the Long-Evans laboratory rat, we can now ask how the environment alters these basic patterns. From the prenatal brain to the old aged brain, cortical measurements have been taken after rats have experienced enriched or impoverished conditions for varying periods (Diamond et al., 1964, 1985; Diamond, 1976, Malkasian and Diamond, 1971). These conditions are basically the same for the animals after weaning, but before this event the experimental design is constructed to meet specific requirements. Although we had no cortical thickness baseline on three generations of standard colony rats, we attempted to learn whether exposing parents to enriched conditions would affect the brains of their offspring. In these experiments, the male and female Long-Evans rats were separated by sex into enriched environments at 60–90 days of age. (Enrichment consists of 12 rats living in a large cage, 70 × 70 × 46 cm, containing many types of movable objects or "toys." The animals can climb, sniff, and explore the objects, thus receiving a good deal of sensory information.) The "enriched" animals were paired for mating into separate standard colony cages and the pregnant females returned to their enriched cage during gestation. For delivery, the mothers were again separated into standard cages, where they continued to live while nursing. At weaning at 21 days of age, all pups of like sex were placed three per standard cage to allow for growth until 60 days of age. At this time, one half of the pups were sacrificed to serve as the F1 generation, and 12 of the remaining F1 males and 12 F1 females were placed back into their separate enriched conditions to repeat the experimental cycle used for the F1 generation. Eventually they would provide for the 60-day-old F2 generation experimental groups. F3 generations were obtained as well, but these animals were different from the F1 and F2 groups because they experienced enrichment directly, not only that received indirectly through the parents. We found significantly greater thickness in the male F2 cortex than in the F1 in some areas in all three cortical sections sampled: frontal, somatosensory, and occipital. There was a nonsignificant trend showing F2 greater than F1 in all other male cortical areas sampled. The cortical differences between generations were greater in the males than in the females.

A recent experiment by Kiyono et al. (1985) demonstrated that enriching the environment of the pregnant rat can enhance the maze-learning ability of the offspring. Their results suggest that the thicker cortex found in the successive generations in our experiments may contribute to better maze learning. With our experimental design, we do not know whether the enrichment before pregnancy had any effect. We hypothesize that the high levels of sex steroid hormones during pregnancy might cross the placental barrier more readily if the mother is a physically active "enriched mother," thereby priming the cortex of the developing fetus. These experiments will have to be repeated in the future, when many of the variables can be individually examined.

3.2. Preweaned

In studying the brains of the postnatal but yet preweaned rats, we had to design appropriate enriched conditions (Malkasian and Diamond, 1971). The rat pups lived with their mothers (three mothers with three pups each) in the large enrichment cage with their "toys." At the same time, to serve as a control, one mother with three pups (each with a littermate in the enriched condition) lived in the standard colony cages. After only 8 days (from 6 to 14 days) in their respective conditions, the enriched pups had significantly thicker cortices in some areas (4, 3, 2, and 39) compared with the nonenriched. The visual cortical areas did not change. Normally the rat eyes do not open until 14 days of age. With the enriched condition, however, the eyes opened 1 day earlier, but evidently they were not open long enough to create a visual cortical difference. If, however, the animals lived until 19 or 28 days of age in the enriched condition, the visual cortex was also significantly thicker in the enriched than in the nonenriched animals.

3.2. Postweaned

Numerous experiments have been carried out over several decades with postweaned rats, either enriched or impoverished (one rat/standard cage) at many ages and for many different durations. We have learned that 1 day in the enriched environment is not sufficient to cause a measurable cortical thickness change, but in 4 days the enriched cortex in area 18 is significantly greater by 4% than in the nonenriched rat. After 30 days in the respective environmental conditions, at 60–90 days of age, most of the cortex, not just area 18, has changed dimensions. Enrichment increases cortical thickness compared with the standard colony condition; whereas, impoverishment decreases it (Diamond, 1967).

3.3. Neuron–Glial Counts

Neuron and glial counts were taken in a manner similar to that reported previously for the aging studies. We found, as expected, that no significant changes in neuronal number had taken place, but a significant increase in glial cells was noted, particularly the oligodendrocytes. In plotting the distribution of nerve cells through the cortical layers, it was evident in both an initial and replication experiment that the greatest changes were occurring in layers II, III, and IV (Diamond et al., 1964). The neurons were farther apart in these layers, signifying more neuropil between the cells. In later experiments it was learned that the enriched animals had more dendrites, more dendritic spines, and longer postsynaptic thickenings than did the nonenriched animals. Since the outer layers are the last to develop embryologically, the cells here may retain more "adaptability" to environmental input than the lower layers. At least this is suggested by our experimental results.

3.4. Age

Much of the early work dealing with enriched and impoverished environments was carried out with younger animals. We later learned that the environmental conditions could alter the cortices of young adults, as well as the brains of rats two thirds the way through their laboratory life span, at 630 days of age. Our ultimate challenge was to attempt to raise rats beyond this age and to see the effects of enrichment on the very old cortex.

We thought that by giving the rats a little more attention, by holding them several times each week, we might provide a more satisfying life-style. For whatever reason, the rats lived until 766 days in the standard colony environment before being separated into enriched and new standard colony cages (Diamond et al., 1985). After 138 days in their respective environments, when the rats reached the very old age of 904 days, the experiment was terminated. Upon examining the cortical thickness, once again we found that the enriched animals had a thicker cortex than the nonenriched, especially in area 18, where the difference reached 10% ($p < 0.05$). In fact, many of the differences were as great as those seen in the young rats, but it is essential to point out that in the experiments with old rats the duration of the experiment was 138 days and not 30 as with the young rats. The important message gained from this experiment was that even in the very old male, the cerebral cortex could still respond positively to an enriched living condition.

For these aging Long-Evans male rat experiments, the rats were raised from birth in the departmental colony, which had previously been in existence for decades. The animals were very healthy throughout their lifetime. (At the present we have to purchase our animals from local distributors.) While raising our female Long-Evans rats from these colonies, we ran into some difficulties during the aging study (Van Gough et al., 1988). After 1 year, many of the rats became ill with upper respiratory infections. Rather than taking a chance in losing all the precious rats, we put tetracycline into the drinking water of one half the group in hopes of saving at least one half the animals.

At 685 days of age, the rats were separated into enriched ($N = 9$) and standard colony (N

= 9) conditions. Five who had tetracycline in their drinking water and four who had access to nonmedicated water were placed in each experimental condition, where only tap water was available. These old female rats were also handled like the males as they aged. At about 800 days of age, the females had spent 115 days in their respective conditions, and the experiment was terminated. At autopsy, from the standard colony condition, three of the animals previously on tetracycline and three of the animals previously on water had survived. From the enriched condition, five of the animals previously on tetracycline and one of the animals previously on water had survived. It appeared that in the enriched living condition, those who had previously been on tetracycline survived well. But there were also disadvantages to such treatment. It has been shown that tetracycline has a catabolic effect, evidently dampening any influences of the enriched environment on cortical development. In young adult enriched females, cortical differences have been shown as compared with nonenriched females.

Whether we can gain access to female animals as healthy as our original males remains to be seen. If possible, we will try to repeat this experiment with healthy females free of any antibiotic influence. Our research project is a continual progress report of the morphological cortical responses to various kinds of inputs. Each step informs us of new variables to consider. From these recent female rat experiments, we have learned that prolonged use of tetracycline is not beneficial to enhanced brain development during exposure to enriched living conditions. This in itself is a useful finding.

4. CONCLUSIONS

Our experimental results have indicated that in the occipital region of the cerebral cortex there is no significant loss of nerve cells between 108 and 904 days of age. Since our cortical thickness measurements indicate that the cortex is decreasing during this period, it is likely that the decrease is due to a reduction in the size of the nerve cells, especially the dendritic branches. In male rats, we have been successful in demonstrating the effects of enriched experiential environments on cortical dimensions at any age, from prenatal to 904 days of age. The enriched animals have thicker cortices than those of nonenriched animals. Other investigators have demonstrated that the enriched rats have better maze-learning capacities than do the nonenriched. If we can extrapolate from this information about the potential of rat nerve cells to human nerve cells, and I think we can, then we have reason to be optimistic about living to an old age. We are genetically programmed at present to live about 100 years; so the active, healthy brain apparently does have the capacity to plan for a satisfying destiny throughout its lifetime.

REFERENCES

Brizzee, K. R., Sherwood, N., and Timiras, P., 1968, A comparison of various depth levels in cerebral cortex of young adults, and aged Long-Evans rats, *J. Gerontol.* **23**:289–297.

Curio, C. A., and Coleman, P. D., 1982, Stability of neuron number in cortical barrels of aging mice, *J. Comp. Neurol.* **212**:158–172.

Diamond, M. C., 1967, Anatomical brain changes induced by environment, in: *Knowing, Thinking, and Believing* (L. Petrinovich and J. L. McGaugh, eds.), Plenum, New York, pp. 215–241.

Diamond, M. C., 1984, Age, sex and environmental influences, in: *Cerebral Dominance-The Biological*

Foundations (N. Geschwind and A. M. Gallaburda, eds.), Harvard University Press, Cambridge, Massachusetts, pp. 134–146.

Diamond, M. C., 1985a, Rat forebrain morphology: Right–left; male–female; young–old; enriched–impoverished, in: *Cerebral Lateralization in Nonhuman Species* (S. Glick, ed.), Academic, Orlando, Florida, pp. 73–86.

Diamond, M. C., 1985b, Experience related morphological changes in the aging rat cerebral cortex, In: *Recent Advances in Psychogeriatrics,* (T. Arie, ed.) Churchill Livingston, London, pp. 5–16.

Diamond, M. C., 1986, Aging and environmental influences on the rat forebrain, in: Biological Substrates in Alzheimer's disease, Vol. 27 (A. B. Scheibel and A. Wexler, eds.), Academic, Orlando, Florida, pp. 55–63.

Diamond, M. C., 1988, *Enriching Heredity,* The Free Press, New York, pp. 60–79.

Diamond, M. C., Johnson, R. E., and Ingham, C. A., 1975, Morphological changes in the young, adult and aging rat cerebral cortex, hippocampus and diencephalon, *Behav. Biol.* **14**:163–174.

Diamond, M. C., Johnson, R. E., Young, D., and Singh, S. S., 1983, Age-related morphologic differences in the rat cerebral cortex and hippocampus: Male–female, right–left, *Exp. Neurol.* **81**:1–13.

Diamond, M. C., Johnson, R. E., Protti, A. M., Ott, C., and Kajisa, L., 1985, Plasticity in the 904-day-old-rat, *Exp. Neurol.* **87**:309–317.

Diamond, M. C., Krech, D., and Rosenzweig, M. R., 1964, The effects of an enriched environment on the histology of the rat cerebral cortex, *J. Comp. Neurol.* **123**:111–120.

Fleming, D. E., Anderson, R. H., Rhees, R. W., Kinghorn, E., and Bakaitis, J., 1986, Effects of prenatal stress on sexually dimorphic asymmetries in the cerebral cortex of the rat, *Brain Res. Rev.* **16**:395–398.

Kiyono, S., Seo, M. L., Shibagaki, M., and Inouye, M., 1985, Facilitative effects of maternal environmental enrichment on maze learning in rat offspring, *Physiol. Behav.* **34**:431–435.

Malkasian, D., and Diamond, M. C., 1971, The effect of environmental manipulation on the morphology of the neonatal rat brain, *Int. J. Neurosci.* **2**:161–170.

Melone, J. H., Teitelbaum, S. A., Johnson, R. E., and Diamond, M. C., 1984, The rat amygdaloid nucleus: A morphometric right-left study, *Exp. Neurol.* **86**:293–302.

Peters, A., Feldman, M. L., and Vaughn, D. W., 1983, The effect of aging on the neuronal population within area 17 of adult rat cerebral cortex, *Neurobiol. Aging* **4**:273–282.

Van Gough, J., Clouse, S., Greer, E. R., and Diamond, M. C., 1988, Asymmetry, tetracycline and the 800-day-old female rat cerebral cortex.

44

Complex Maze Learning in Rodents

Progress and Potential for Modeling Age-Related Memory Dysfunction

DONALD K. INGRAM

1. RESEARCH GOALS

An extensive body of research findings supports the view that normal aging in humans is associated with a defined dysfunction in memory processing. When sensorimotor performance requirements of tasks can be equated across age groups, the most salient age-related change appears in the ability to use *secondary memory* systems which represent the unlimited permanent store of newly acquired information (Poon, 1985). Age differences in *sensory memory*, which refers to the brief storage of sensory information; in *primary memory*, which refers to the temporary, limited capacity repository available for immediate recall; and in *tertiary memory*, which refers to memory for remote events, appear less robust (Poon, 1985). Much of the age-related impairment in retrieval of information from secondary memory can be attributed to deficient encoding processes, including organizational skills, visual imagination, depth of processing, and attention, as well as problems of equating motivational factors (Kausler, 1982; Poon, 1985). In terms of a storage-deficit hypothesis of age-related memory dysfunction, reviews of the literature have indicated that age differences in forgetting rates are minimal or nonexistent when effort is made to equate the original level of learning (Poon, 1985).

This perspective of the human literature can be contrasted to the emphasis in research on animal models of age-related memory dysfunction that has been focused on primary memory deficits and forgetting rates (Bartus *et al.*, 1983; Kubanis and Zornetzer, 1981). The focus of the present review will be on the age-related impairment observed in rodents during learning of a complex 14-unit T maze (Ingram, 1985, 1988). This paradigm can be classified as a task involving encoding of information into secondary memory.

Research with this paradigm has been directed toward three goals in our laboratory. The

DONALD K. INGRAM • Molecular Physiology and Genetics Section, Laboratory of Cellular and Molecular Biology, Gerontology Research Center, National Institute on Aging, National Institutes of Health, Francis Scott Key Medical Center, Baltimore, Maryland 21124.   The Gerontology Research Center is fully accredited by the American Association for the Accreditation of Laboratory Animal Care.

primary goal is to develop a reliable and valid test of learning that reflects aging at a psychobiological level of analysis in rodents. This objective is directed toward constructing a battery of behavioral tests that can measure biological aging in animal models (Ingram, 1985, 1984; Ingram and Reynolds, 1986) and, thus, can be used to test treatments (pharmacological, nutritional, surgical, environmental) that purport to affect aging rate. In this sense, the paradigm is used primarily to model functional aging in the rodent.

The secondary goal involves the investigation of possible psychological and neurobiological mechanisms regulating performance in this task. Elucidation of these mechanisms could suggest treatments to alter the observed age-related learning deficit. In this sense, the paradigm is used to model possible causal relationships between learning performance and specific neurobiological systems and to test these relationships with specific manipulations.

The tertiary goal is to determine the relevance of our observations in maze learning to human performance during aging. In this sense, this rodent paradigm is used to model the phenomenon of age-related impairment in secondary memory processing observed in humans. On the surface, the relevance of findings from these studies of maze performance in rodents appears far removed from the type of experimental results obtained in human studies. However, a possible convergence of findings is beginning to emerge. As is emphasized in this chapter, an initial agreement between human and nonhuman paradigms can be derived from the emphasis placed on age-related dysfunction in secondary memory processes with particular focus on defects in encoding.

2. BACKGROUND ON MAZE PARADIGM

Many paradigms have been used to assess age-related differences in learning and memory performance in rodents (Arenberg and Robertson-Tchabo, 1977; Kubanis and Zornetzer, 1981). The focus of this paper is on the use of a 14-unit T maze which can be recommended because of several distinct advantages that it offers. First, maze performance in general has great ecological validity for rodent models. Laboratory rodents easily adapt performance to such tasks. Second, this 14-unit T maze has an established history of use and has proven to be a robust paradigm for demonstrating age differences in learning performance in rodents.

Stone (1929) introduced the configuration of a 14-unit T maze (some modifications in design), shown in Fig. 1, hereinafter referred to as the *Stone maze*. Using a very small sample of aged rats, he found little evidence of an age-related decline in performance. Using the Stone maze, Verzar-McDougall (1957) reported an age-related decrease in maze-learning ability in female rats.

The strongest and most consistent evidence of an age-related decline in Stone maze performance appeared in a series of parametric studies of male and female rats by Goodrick (1968, 1972, 1973, 1975). Results from one study (Goodrick, 1973) are shown in Fig. 2. The age difference in maze learning is very apparent even under two conditions of training. Aged rats exhibited a slower rate of learning compared to young counterparts. The young rats perfected the maze, whereas the age group exhibited numerous errors at the end of training.

The procedure that Goodrick applied involved body weight reduction over several weeks and food rewards provided in the goal box during maze training. Using similar food-motivation procedures, Goodrick's observed age differences in Stone maze performance of rats have been replicated by others (Berman *et al.*, 1988; Michel and Klein, 1978). In food-motivated tasks, the issue of equivalent motivational levels across age groups is a critical one

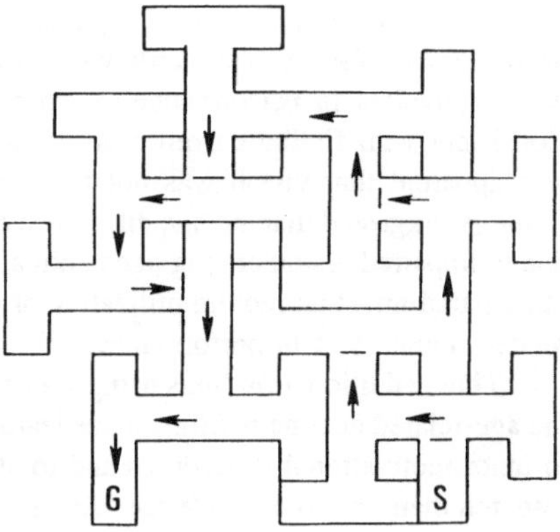

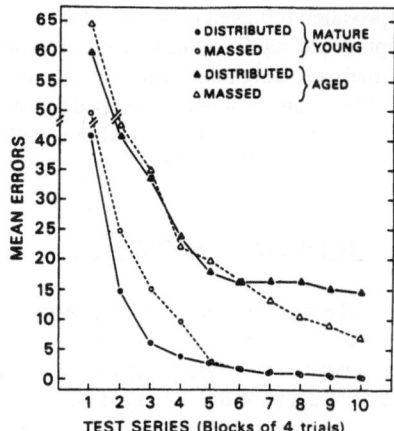

FIGURE 1. Configuration of Stone maze: S denotes start box; G denotes goal box; arrows denote correct path; straight lines in maze denote guillotine doors.

FIGURE 2. Comparison of mean errors of young (6-month-old) and aged (26-month-old) male Wistar rats during acquisition training in the Stone maze under distributed (one trial per day) and massed (four trials per day) practice conditions (n = 16).

to consider because baseline body weights and fat distribution can also vary with age. Attempting to equate motivational levels across age groups in such tasks, Goodrick (1980) would subject the older, heavier rats to a relatively greater degree of weight loss to increase motivation relative to younger, lighter counterparts, and still he would observe an age-related decline in maze learning.

Thus, it would appear from observations made in several laboratories that the Stone maze paradigm offers a robust demonstration of age differences in learning by laboratory rodents. However, Ingram (1985) argued that additional evidence was necessary to establish the specificity of the cognitive impairment and the generalization of the observations as a behavioral manifestation of biological aging. The specificity of the impairment was tested by experiments dealing with different motivational and sensory demands. Water deprivation and rewards were suggested as a better motivational manipulation to use in aging studies because it could be demonstrated that aged rodents manifested greater physiological demand for water (Ingram, 1985). Yet aged rats and mice still evidenced impaired Stone maze performance compared with young counterparts when fluid deprived and trained for water rewards (Ingram, 1985).

Sensory demands were manipulated by training rats and mice under darkened conditions. Trained for water rewards without access to visual cues in the maze, young animals were equivalent in performance to those trained under lighted conditions (Ingram, 1985). Consistent with findings from classic maze studies using enucleated rats (Munn, 1950), it was apparent that vision was not necessary for learning complex enclosed mazes. These findings suggested that the age difference observed in Stone maze performance was not likely due to impaired vision among aged animals. Attention to this issue is even more important to other paradigms that require utilization of visual cues external to the maze and report an age-related impairment in performance.

Thus, additional findings using water deprivation provided evidence of the robustness of the age-related decline in Stone maze learning by demonstrating the generality of the findings to other motivational procedures and to at least one other species, mice. The next phase of research then was to characterize further the nature of the behavioral deficit and to search for neurobiological mechanisms. To these ends, it was desirable to design a Stone maze paradigm that departed from that used by past studies. Previous protocols called for food or fluid deprivation followed by weeks of pretraining in a straight runway and in the Stone maze for appropriate reinforcement. Such extended protocols appeared to be stressful for the aged animal, and a high rate of mortality (e.g., 25–50%) was not uncommon. Therefore, a shock-avoidance protocol was developed for the Stone maze that required minimal pretraining and training sessions and that would expand the generalization of the observed age-related impairment (Ingram, 1985, 1988).

3. GENERAL METHODS

The sources and husbandry of rats and mice used for maze-learning experiments have been described previously (Ingram, 1985, 1988; Spangler et al., 1986). All animals were acclimated to the vivarium at least 2 weeks before testing. All training was conducted during the light cycle of the photoperiod.

The configuration of the 14-unit Stone maze was presented in Fig. 1. The only other apparatus is a straight runway, which is used for pretraining. Details of the construction and general laboratory environment for both have also been provided previously (Bresnahan et al., 1988; Spangler et al., 1986). The maze is constructed of translucent plastic walls with high wooden walls surrounding its perimeter. With only the ceiling and overhead lighting visible from the floor of the maze, the objective was to minimize intramaze and extramaze cues. The floor of the maze contains a diagonally placed stainless grid that is wired to deliver scrambled footshock. The maze is divided into five segments by guillotine doors as indicated in Fig. 1. What is not presented in the figure is the layout of the infrared photosensors that are interfaced to a microprocessor to record the movement of the animal through the maze. A computer program is used to score errors in the manner described by Goodrick (1968). White noise generators are used in both the straight runway and Stone maze to mask extraneous sounds from the maze environment.

The procedures for straight runway and maze training have been described previously (Bresnahan et al., 1988; Ingram, 1985; Spangler et al., 1986). The typical protocol involves three sessions of pretraining for one-way active avoidance in the straight runway with 10 trials per daily session and a 2-min intertrial interval. The animal is trained to run from the black startbox within 10 sec to an identical black goal box about 2 m away to avoid scrambled footshock (0.6–1.0 mA). All animals meeting a criterion of 8/10 avoidances on the last training day are then submitted to maze training the following day. The response contingency in the Stone maze is identical to that in pretraining. The animal must move through each segment of the maze within 10 sec, to avoid scrambled footshock (0.6–1.0 mA). The animal is not punished expressly for making errors, i.e., departing from the true path of the maze, but footshock is activated after 10 sec to be terminated when the animal moves through the next gate in the maze. The trial is terminated when the animal enters the black goal box at the end of the last segment, and another trial is initiated after a 2-min intertrial interval. Between trials, a pulley system is activated to hoist the maze from the grid floor, which is then mopped with an ethanol solution to mask possible odor cues. The typical maze-training protocol involves a 10-trial session on each of two consecutive days. However, other protocols have been used including having pretraining and maze training all in one day (Walovitch et al., 1987) or distributing 16 maze-training trials over 4 days (Ingram et al., 1987).

4. GENERALIZATION OF AGE EFFECT

The generalization of the age-related impairment in Stone maze learning involving the shock-motivated protocol described is demonstrated in Fig. 3. Increased error performance across age is evident in two strains of rats and three strains of mice involving both inbred and outbred lines. These data further emphasize the robustness of the age-related decline in learning demonstrated in this task. Age-related impairments have been observed with food, water, and shock motivation under a variety of conditions, apparatus, and training procedures. Although other data on age differences in the performance of male Fischer (F-344) rats will be shown subsequently, the data in Fig. 3 also demonstrate the sensitivity of the paradigm even with relatively young groups.

Further evidence that the paradigm might reflect aging rate at a behavioral level of analysis was provided in a study using C3B10RF$_1$ mice (Ingram et al., 1987). Aged (33-mo-old) mice from this strain subjected to a chronic regimen of caloric restriction had lower error rates compared with aged counterparts fed a more conventional diet (Ingram et al., 1987). This type of dietary manipulation is known to increase mean and maximum life span of these mice and other rodents (Weindruch, 1984).

5. NEUROBIOLOGY OF MAZE LEARNING

To pursue neurobiological analysis of the age-related impairment observed in the Stone maze, we have been guided by the logical and empirical strength of the cholinergic hypothesis of geriatric memory dysfunction (Bartus et al., 1982). However, much of the research aimed at testing this hypothesis has used paradigms emphasizing age-related differences in primary memory processing and forgetting rates.

5.1. Pharmacological Manipulations

Cholinergic involvement in Stone maze learning has been established in three separate studies from our laboratory that have used the muscarinic antagonist, scopolamine hydrochloride. Spangler et al. (1986) demonstrated a dose-related disruption of acquisition when scopolamine was given (i.p.) to young (3- to 4-month-old) male F-344 rats 30-min prior to maze training. The major disruption at a dose of 1.0 mg/kg was to error performance, as no

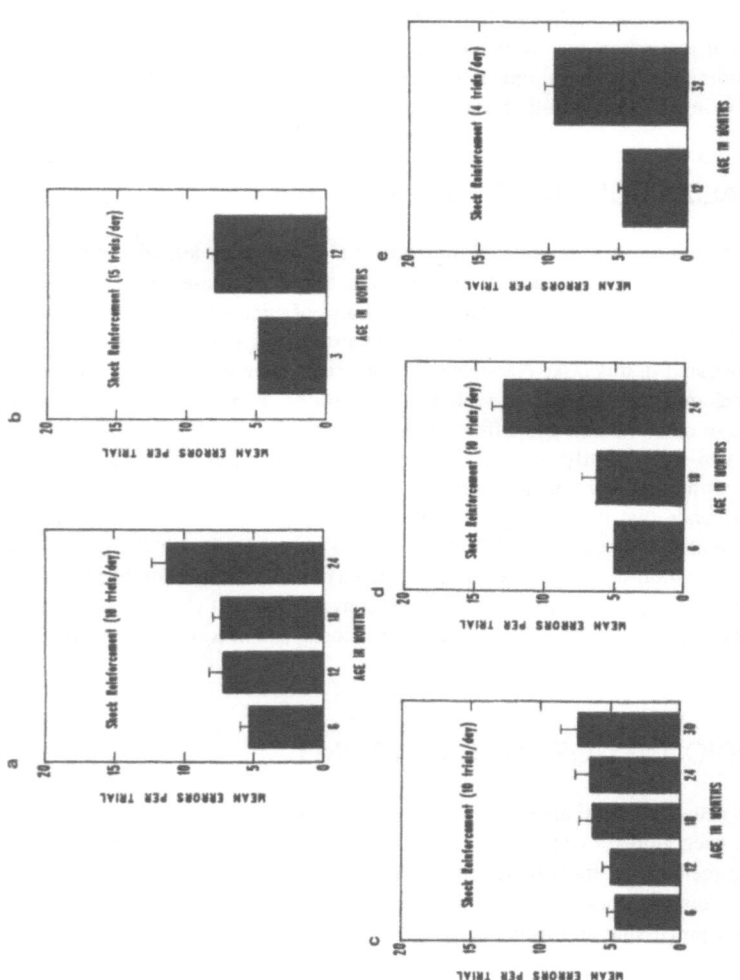

FIGURE 3. Age effects on mean (SEM) errors per trial made by (a) male Wistar rats, (b) male F-344 rats, (c) male C57BL/6J mice, (d) male A/J mice, and (e) female C3B10RF$_1$ mice during acquisition training in the Stone maze (ns = 6–10).

effects on shock avoidance were observed with this dose at the end of training (Fig. 4). Furthermore, the effect could be attributed to cholinergic antagonism in the central nervous system (CNS) because the primarily peripherally-acting antagonist, methylscopolamine, had no significant effects on maze performance.

In a follow-up study, Spangler *et al.* (1988) established that cholinergic antagonism with a dose of 1.0 mg/kg scopolamine hydrochloride (i.p.) impaired encoding processes primarily. Scopolamine had no effect on storage and retrieval processes, because retention performance was not significantly impaired in young (3- to 4-month-old) male F-344 rats when provided the drug immediately after brief acquisition training (five trials) or 30-min prior to retention training on the following day (Fig. 5). Even if they received scopolamine prior to acquisition, rats were not impaired during retention testing unless they had also received another treatment with the drug before this session. It is important to note that the observed impairment could not result from nonspecific effects of the drug on maze performance because no significance performance deficit was observed among the group receiving scopolamine only prior to retention training.

The results of these investigations supported many others noting the detrimental effects of scopolamine on learning and memory performance in animals and humans (Spencer and Lal, 1983) and suggest cholinergic involvement in geriatric memory dysfunction (Collerton, 1986). However, as emphasized by Spencer and Lal (1983) in their review of this extensive literature, the most salient effect of muscarinic antagonism appears to be on encoding processes.

With the established effects of scopolamine on maze learning in young rats, the next study (Spangler *et al.*, 1989) assessed age-related differences in response to cholinergic

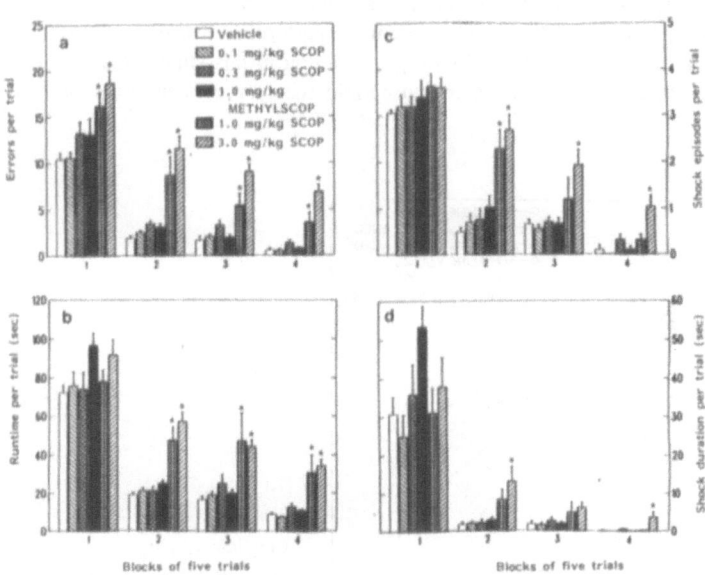

FIGURE 4. Effects of scopolamine (SCOP) or methylscopolamine (METHYLSCOP) on performance of young (3-month-old) male F-344 rats (NS = 6–7) during acquisition training in the Stone maze: (a) errors, (b) runtime, (c) shock episodes, (d) shock duration. Asterisk (*) significantly different from saline vehicle controls according to Dunnett's test, $p < 0.01$.

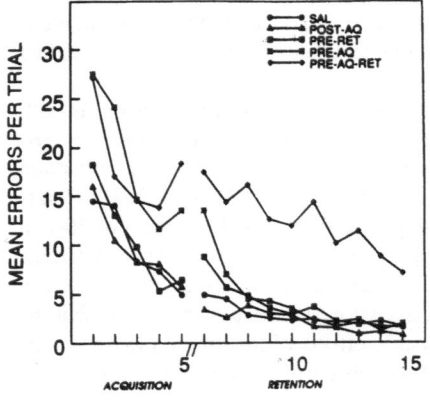

FIGURE 5. Mean error performance of young (3-month-old) male F-344 rats (n = 9–12) in the Stone maze according to scopolamine (1.0 mg/kg i.p.) treatment: saline controls (SAL); scopolamine immediately after acquisition (POST-AQ: after trial 5); scopolamine 30 min before retention (PRE-RET: before trial 6); scopolamine 30 min before acquisition (PRE-AQ: before trial 1); and scopolamine 30 min before acquisition and retention (PRE-AQ-RET: before trials 1 and 6).

blockade at doses lower than the 1.0-mg/kg dose used in the previous studies but higher than the 0.3-mg/kg dose that had not produced a significant impairment (Spangler *et al.*, 1986). To this end, young (6-month-old) and aged (22- to 24-month-old) male F-344 rats were administered either saline, 0.5, or 0.75 mg/kg scopolamine hydrochoride (i.p.) 30 min prior to training. The age-related and drug-related impairment in error performance is clearly evident (Fig. 6); however, the statistical analysis did not reveal a significant age by drug interaction. No other performance variable including runtime or shock avoidance measures was significantly affected by scopolamine treatment in either age group, an observation that indicated the specificity of the drug on cognitive performance at these doses.

The lack of a significant age by drug interaction in this study (Spangler *et al.*, 1989) would imply that age differences in muscarinic receptor concentration probably do not

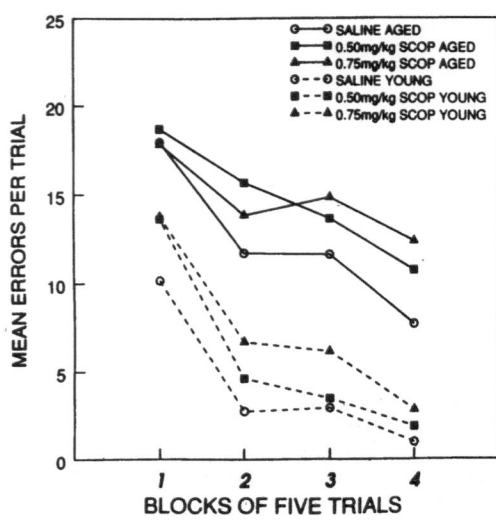

FIGURE 6. Effects of age and scopolamine (SCOP) on mean error performance of young (6-month-old) and aged (24-month-old) male F-344 rats during acquisition training in the Stone maze (n = 7–11).

account for the age-related impairment. Reviews of the literature have noted that evidence of age differences in muscarinic receptor concentrations in F-344 rats has been inconsistent (Bartus *et al.*, 1982; Decker, 1987). How, then, can the scopolamine-induced impairment in Stone maze learning among young rats represent a pharmacological model of the age-related impairment? Perhaps aging affects other aspects of the receptor, such as its sensitivity (Lippa *et al.*, 1985) or other aspects of neurotransmission at the cholinergic synapse (Decker, 1987).

Although cholinergic mediation of Stone maze acquisition was evident, additional research is necessary to establish the specificity or lack of specificity of the involvement of this neurotransmitter system. Several investigators have questioned the overemphasis on an exclusive role for the cholinergic system in geriatric memory dysfunction by pointing to the involvement of the ascending noradrenergic system in age-related memory deficits observed in several tasks (Collier *et al.*, 1985; Zornetzer, 1985). To examine this alternative hypothesis regarding Stone maze performance, we have initiated a series of experiments applying the neurotoxin, *N*-2-chloroethyl-*N*-ethyl-2-bromobenzylamine hydrochloride (DSP-4), which depletes forebrain norepinephrine (Sara, 1985). When young (3- to 4-month-old) male F-344 rats were treated with DSP-4 (50 mg/kg i.p.) 2 weeks prior to maze training, no significant effects on maze acquisition were observed as compared with untreated controls (Fig. 7). This dose resulted in a severe depletion of forebrain norepinephrine, as was manifested in greatly enhanced postdecapitation reflex times among the group treated with DSP-4 (Sara, 1985). Other studies with this compound are being conducted to determine its effects on retention performance; however, from this preliminary experiment, a tentative conclusion would be that an intact forebrain norepinephrine system is not vital to efficient learning in the Stone maze.

5.2. Lesion Manipulations

After demonstrating cholinergic involvement in Stone maze acquisition, the next step was to begin searching for the neuroanatomical loci of this involvement. Because of numerous studies documenting the detrimental effects of fimbria–fornix lesions on learning and

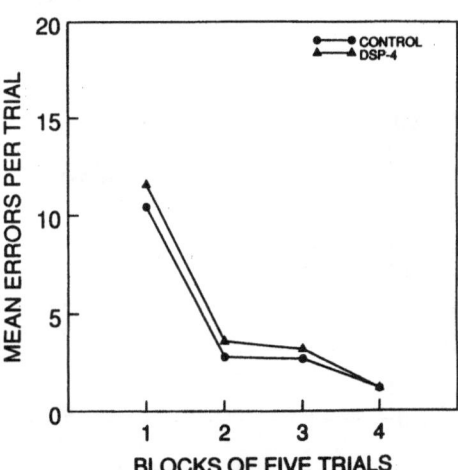

FIGURE 7. Effect of *N*-(2-chloroethyl)-*N*-ethyl-2-bromobenzylamine hydrochloride (DSP-4) on mean error performance of young (3- to 4-month-old) male F-344 rats during acquisition training in the Stone maze (*n* = 8 and 32 for controls and DSP-4 treated groups, respectively).

memory performance, an initial study has addressed the involvement of the septohippocampal system in Stone maze performance (Bresnahan *et al.*, 1989). Young (3- to 4-month-old) male F-344 rats were given bilateral electrolytic lesions to the fimbria–fornix 1 week prior to maze training. There was no difference between this experimental group and a control group composed of sham-operated and unoperated animals in straight runway pretraining to indicate that avoidance behavior was unaffected by this treatment. However, learning performance was impaired in lesioned animals compared with controls (Fig. 8). Whether this impairment was attributable to disruption of the septohippocampal cholinergic system exclusively will require additional experimentation. The fimbria–fornix carries both hippocampal afferents and efferents with other neurotransmitter fibers present. One study will focus on the medial septal nucleus which is the major source of cholinergic innervation to the hippocampus. Other studies in our laboratory are focusing on a different forebrain cholinergic system involving the nucleus basalis magnocellularis (NBM), which provides major cholinergic innervation to the frontal cortex. Damage to this neuronal population has been associated with impairment in a variety of learning and memory tasks in rats (Bartus *et al.*, 1984; Olton and Wenk, 1987), although behavioral recovery is possible with this lesion.

In addition, a preliminary experiment in our laboratory has focused on the effects of damage to specific hippocampal neuronal populations. Figure 9 compares Stone maze error performance between normal young (3- to 4-month-old) male F-344 rats and groups treated with trimethyltin, a toxic metal compound that produces cholinergic receptor loss and damage to hippocampal pyramidal neurons (Loullis *et al.*, 1985). The dose-related impairment is very evident and appears similar to that observed in animals treated with scopolamine or with fimbria–fornix lesions.

5.3. Therapeutic Manipulations

Most of the research described thus far has demonstrated that the performance of young rats can be made to simulate that of aged rats through various pharmacological and lesion manipulations. Although strong evidence of cholinergic involvement in Stone maze learning has been provided through this strategy, manipulation geared to improving the performance of aged rats in this task would strengthen the cholinergic hypothesis considerably. Thus far, we have experienced little success in several pilot studies using various direct and indirect

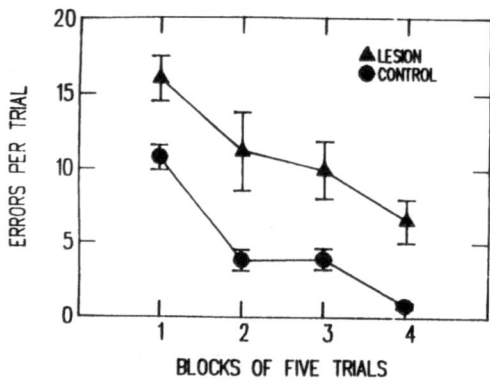

FIGURE 8. Mean (SEM) error performance of young (3-month-old) male F-344 rats during acquisition training in the Stone maze associated with bilateral fimbria–fornix lesions (*n* = 13 and 10 for the control and lesion groups, respectively).

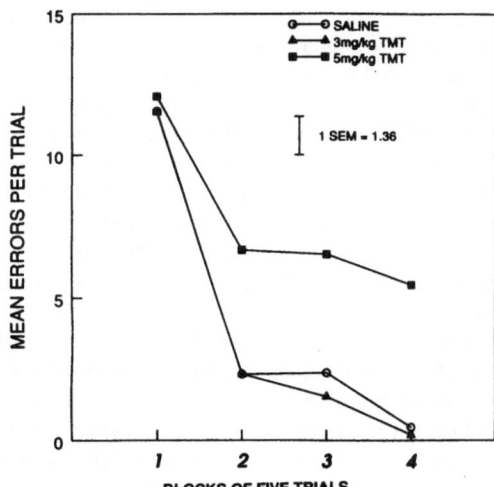

FIGURE 9. Effect of trimethyltin (TMT) on mean error performance of young (3- to 4-month-old) male F-344 rats during acquisition training in the Stone maze (n = 7-9).

cholinergic agonists in aged rats. Also, when the nootropic agent, co-dergocrine, was provided in an acute treatment, no beneficial effect on the Stone maze performance of middle-aged (12-month-old), male F-344 rats was observed, even though the drug stimulated glucose metabolism in hippocampus and subiculum (Walovitch *et al.*, 1987).

A new direction concerning therapeutic intervention taken in our laboratory involves application of the technology of fetal neural tissue grafts. Other researchers have reported success in improving the performance of aged rats in learning and memory tasks following the intracerebral grafting of fetal cells (Gage *et al.*, 1984).

6. NEUROPSYCHOLOGY OF MAZE LEARNING

According to the taxonomy of memory described at the outset of this chapter, secondary memory processes appear to be most affected by aging, and Stone maze learning clearly involves these processes. However, while the modal model of memory (Murdock, 1967), which conceptually divides memory into sensory, short-term, or primary (Waugh and Norman, 1965) memory, and long-term or secondary (Craik, 1977) memory, has proved useful for comprehending differences in the psychology of these phenomena, much additional theorization has fractionated each of these processes even more or has created new models altogether (Baddeley, 1988; Kesner, 1986). It is difficult to reconcile Stone maze learning within these other conceptualizations.

6.1. Working Memory/Reference Memory

Regarding the neuropsychology of hippocampal function, Olton *et al.* (1979, 1980) suggested a conceptual dichotomy between *reference memory* tasks that tax trial-independent memory events and *working memory* tasks that tax trial-dependent memory events. Damage to hippocampal circuitry affected the performance of rats in working memory tasks but not in reference memory tasks. Using this conceptualization, Knowlton *et al.* (1985) classified the Stone maze as a reference memory task. Combined lesions to the basal forebrain cholinergic system, including the medial septal nucleus and the NBM did not significantly affect the performance of young (3- to 4-month-old) rats in a Stone maze; however, this treatment did impair performance in a radial arm maze, which was classified as a working memory task. These results are difficult to reconcile with those from our laboratory, which indicated that fimbria–fornix lesions (Fig. 8) and trimethyltin damage to hippocampal cell populations impaired Stone maze performance in rats (Fig. 9).

Applying the Olton *et al.* (1979, 1980) conceptualization of hippocampal function, Ingram (1985) argued that both working and reference memory systems would be taxed during acquisition training in the Stone maze. Working memory would be necessary for retaining information about within-trial choices, while reference memory would be operational for organizing and retaining information across trials to result in the acquired knowledge about the maze configuration. Thus, the age-related impairment in maze acquisition could result in dysfunction to both reference and working memory systems. This hypothesis was supported in a previous study applying a two-component T-maze task in which both reference and working memory systems were operationally defined unambiguously (Lowy *et al.*, 1985). However, in this study it appeared to be the complexity of the task itself that was associated with impairment in reference memory performance. Moreover, results from other studies have questioned the conceptual dichotomy between working and reference memory systems with regard to hippocampal function. For example, Harrell *et al.* (1987) reported that damage to the medial septal nucleus, which provides cholinergic innervation to the hippocampus, was associated with impaired performance in both working and reference components of a radial arm maze task.

6.2. Spatial Memory

Barnes (1988) emphasized the importance of hippocampal circuitry in *spatial memory* tasks. Age-related impairment in many spatial tasks has also been observed and related to hippocampal electophysiological responses (Barnes, 1988). Ingram (1988) discussed the conceptual difficulty of classifying the Stone maze as a spatial memory task. The animal is required to learn a series of successive position discriminations. However, unlike operationally defined spatial memory tasks, which deliberately enrich the maze environment to provide abundant visual cues to use for spatial orientation, the Stone maze environment is designed with minimal visual cues available. Indeed, rats and mice can learn this maze under darkened conditions (Ingram, 1985). The behavior of a well-trained animal suggests that the response sequence becomes internalized. Toward the end of a training schedule of 20 trials, an animal can be observed to move quickly through the maze, rapidly negotiate each choice point, direct its vision ahead and almost never look upward while moving directly to the goal. An egocentric response algorithm appears to be internalized and driving the animal's behavior through kinesthetic and proprioceptive cues rather than reliance on externally available stimuli. Thus, a deficit in spatial memory processes associated with hippocampal aging would not appear to fit our observations either.

6.3. Representational Memory/Dispositional Memory

The conceptual model of Thomas (1984) appears to fit our observations more closely than others mentioned thusfar. Tasks that are controlled by external stimulus events at the time of choice, as in a visual discrimination task, are considered to involve *dispositional memory*, whereas tasks in which responses are required in the absence of external sensory cues at the time of choice, as in a delayed nonmatching-to-sample (DNMTS) task, are considered to involve *representational memory*. Therefore, regarding performance in the Stone maze as development of an internalized response algorithm that is not dependent on external cues at the time of choice would classify this paradigm to involve representational memory. In addition, our results indicating impaired Stone maze performance associated with FF or hippocampal damage would be consistent with observations from experiments testing this conceptual model. Rats with lesions to the posterior septal nucleus presumably affecting hippocampal innervation were reported to be deficited in a DNMTS task but unimpaired in a sensory discrimination task in the identical apparatus (Thomas and Gash, 1986). Moreover, regarding age differences in performance, it can be noted that when simple two-choice situations requiring visual or position discriminations are applied, age differences in performance are not typically observed (Goodrick, 1972; Lowy *et al.*, 1985). Thus the age difference in Stone maze performance could be classified as a representational memory task with hippocampal involvement.

6.4. Declarative Memory/Nondeclarative Memory

Research in the neuropsychology of human amnesia has also produced a fractionalization of long-term memory processes as related to hippocampal function. One such conceptual dichotomy has been described by Squire and Zola-Morgan (1988). When a task requires the storage of information in an explicit manner that is later available for conscious recollection, *declarative memory* is required. When information is accessible only during performance of a task, this implicit memory ability is referred to as *nondeclarative memory*. The former is impaired when hippocampal damage is present, while the latter is not. Because of the emphasis on "conscious" recollection of this model, it is difficult to apply to nonhumans; however, the descriptions of this model have also emphasized the stored representation of information (Morris *et al.*, 1988). Thus, if representation of the information is the operative description, then this model does not depart dramatically from that of Thomas described above. Stone maze acquisition would therefore be considered as involving declarative memory processes. However, it has also been recognized that with repetition a transformation of declarative memory to nondeclarative memory can occur (Morris *et al.*, 1988). So it is probably too simplistic to consider that only one component of secondary memory processing is involved in Stone maze learning.

6.5. Other Models

Many other neuropsychological models of memory processes related to hippocampal function exist, and several will have to be considered in light of the age-related impairment observed in Stone maze performance. For example, Kesner (1986) has emphasized the multistructural nature of memory processing. Winocur (1980) emphasized the role of interference in memory impairments associated with hippocampal damage and aging. We plan to assess these models using strategies described previously (Ingram, 1988).

6.6. Learning Strategies/Encoding Processes

If the age-related impairment in Stone maze learning can be considered to involve deficient encoding processes and this deficiency is assumed to be related to cholinergic mechanisms, some attention should also be paid to a very salient feature of performance in this task. Goodrick (1968, 1972, 1973, 1975, 1980) reported the high frequency of perseverative errors among aged rats in the Stone maze. Further analysis revealed that aged animals were making errors at the same locations in the maze probably because of the maintenance of an alternation strategy (Ingram, 1985). From the outset of training, all animals would have a response bias manifested as a left–right response pattern. Errors would occur at a high frequency at those choice points that required a response in same direction, e.g., right–right or left–left. Thus, an alternation strategy might be useful during initial learning but would have to be abandoned to perfect the maze. Relinquishing this strategy earlier in training is possibly how young rats manifest a faster learning rate in the Stone maze. Ingram (1988) presents data from several Stone maze studies that demonstrate a greater probability to maintain an alternation strategy in aged rats and in young rats with cholinergic antagonism or FF lesions. Investigators using other sequential maze paradigms have also noted alternation strategies among rats with hippocampal damage (Winocur and Breckenbridge, 1973). Thus, any neuropsychological model accommodating our observations of age-related impairment in Stone maze performance must deal with the issue of response biases and strategies. This issue might not be far removed with the perspective developed in the human literature that age-related impairment in encoding processes may result from decline in skills of elaboration, organization, and depth of processing during acquisition (Poon, 1985).

7. MODEL OF THE HUMAN CONDITION

The extent to which the age-related impairment in Stone maze performance observed in rodents is relevant to the age-related impairment in secondary memory processing observed in humans remains debatable. There is little apparent similarity between maze paradigms for rodents and learning paradigms used in human geropsychology. However, geropsychologists have recently suggested the relevance of using more real-world, three-dimensional spatial environments instead of small, two-dimensional stimulus arrays typically applied in laboratory environments (Kausler, 1982). Mazelike environments have been used to assess cognitive development in children (Aadland et al., 1985; Gauvain and Rogoff, 1986). In addition, several gerontological studies have reported an age-related decline in performance in real-world spatial environments (Evans et al., 1984; Sharps and Gollin, 1987; Waddell and Rogoff, 1981). Therefore, the possibility exists for greater convergence of human paradigms toward those used in rodent research.

8. CONCLUSIONS

Using one of the oldest behavioral paradigms in psychobiological research, we have made progress in developing a model of age-related memory impairment in rodents. Distinct advantages of the Stone maze paradigm for this effort can be identified as follows: (1) a robust age effect, (2) reduction of sensory and motivational confounds, (3) possibility for reliable automated tracking and scoring, (4) reduction of experimental time to less than 1 week for each subject, (5) establishment of muscarinic cholinergic involvement, and (6) establishment of hippocampal involvement. This progress must be weighed against the following current disadvantages of the paradigm: (1) requirement of a large space for the maze (about 3×3 m), (2) lack of specificit, of stimulus control of the behavior, (3) lack of opportunity for within-subject analysis, (4) incomplete neuropsychological characterization of performance in the task, (5) lack of comparison to other popular maze paradigms in psychobiological research, (6) lack of thorough characterization of neurotransmitter and neuroanatomical systems involved, and (7) unestablished relevance to human paradigms. Thus, the potential of this paradigm will emerge from further research conducted in our laboratory and elsewhere to address these deficiencies and, it is hoped, move forward in the effort to develop models of age-related memory dysfunction.

ACKNOWLEDGMENTS. This report was aided by the valuable contributions of Elaine Bresnahan, Mark Chachich, Hideki Kametani, Satoru Kobayashi, Pamela Rigby, Kenneth Smith, Edward Spangler, Philip Wise, and William Yee in specific maze studies and of Richard Hiner, Maurice Zimmerman, Gunther Baartz, Richard Zichos, and Raymond Bannar for construction of maze equipment.

REFERENCES

Aadland, J., Beatty, W. W., and Maki, R. H., 1985, Spatial memory of children and adults assessed in the radial maze, *Dev. Psychobiol.* **18:**163–172.

Arenberg, D., and Robertson-Tchabo, E. A., 1977, Learning and aging, in: *Handbook of the Psychology of Aging* (J. E. Birren and K. W. Schaie, eds.), Van Nostrand–Reinhold, New York, pp. 421–449.

Baddeley, A., 1988, Cognitive psychology and human memory, *Trends Neurosci* **11:**176–181.

Barnes, C. A., 1988, Selectivity of neurological and mnemonic deficits in aged rats, in: *Neural Plasticity: A Lifespan Approach* (T. Petit and G. O. Ivy, eds.), Liss, New York, pp. 235–264.

Bartus, R. T., Dean, R. L., Beer, B., and Lippa, A. S., 1982, The cholinergic hypothesis of geriatric memory dysfunction, *Science* **217:**408–412.

Bartus, R. T., Flicker, C., and Dean, R. L., 1984, Logical principles for the development of animal models of age-related memory impairments, in: *Assessment in Geriatric Psychopharmacology* (T. Crook, S. Ferris, and R. Bartus, eds.), Mark Powley Associates, New York, pp. 263–269.

Berman, R. F., Goldman, H., and Altman, H. J., 1988, Age-related changes in regional cerebral flow and behavior in Sprague–Dawley rats, *Neurobiol. Aging* **90:**691–696.

Bresnahan, E., Kametani, H. Spangler, E., Chachich, M., Wiser, P., and Ingram, D., 1988, Fimbria-fornix lesions impair acquisition performance in a 14-unit T-maze similar to prior observed performance deficits in aged rats, *Psychobiology* **16:**243–250.

Collerton, D., 1986, Cholinergic function and intellectual decline in Alzheimer's disease, *Neuroscience* **19:**1–28.

Collier, T., Gash, D. M., Bruemmer, V., and Sladek, J. R., 1985, Impaired regulation of arousal in old age and the consequences for learning and memory: Replacement of brain norepinephrine via neuron transplants improves memory performance in aged F-344 rats, in: *Homeostatic Function and Aging* (B. B. Davis and W. G. Wood, eds.), Raven, New York, pp. 99–110.

Craik, F. I. M., 1977, Age differences in human memory, in: *Handbook of the Psychology of Aging* (J. E. Birren and K. W. Schaie, eds.), Van Nostrand–Reinhold, New York, pp. 384–420.

Decker, M. W., 1987, The effects of aging on hippocampal and cortical projections of the forebrain cholinergic system, *Brain Res. Rev.* **12:**423–438.

Evans, G., Brennan, P., Skorpanich, M. A., and Held, D., 1984, Cognitive mapping in elderly adults: Verbal location memory for urban landmarks, *J. Gerontol.* **39:**452–457.

Gage, F. H., Bjorklund, A., Stenevi, U., Dunnett, S. B., and Kelley, P. A. T., 1984, Intrahippocampal septal grafts ameliorate learning impairments in aged rats, *Science* **255:**533–536.

Gauvain, M., and Rogoff, B., 1986, Influence of the goal on children's exploration and memory of large-scale space, *Dev. Psychol.* **22:**72–77.

Goodrick, C. L., 1968, Learning, retention, and extinction of a complex maze habit for mature-young and senescent Wistar albino rats, *J. Gerontol.* **23:**298–304.

Goodrick, C. L., 1972, Learning by mature-young and aged Wistar rats as a function of test complexity, *J. Gerontol.* **27:**353–357.

Goodrick, C. L., 1973, Maze learning of mature-young and aged rats as a function of distribution of practice, *J. Exp. Psychol.* **98:**344–349.

Goodrick, C. L., 1975, Behavioral rigidity as a mechanism for facilitation of problem solving for aged rats, *J. Gerontol.* **30:**181–184.

Goodrick, C. L., 1980, Problem solving and age: A critique of rodent research, in: *Age, Learning Ability, and Intelligence* (R. L. Sprott, ed.), Van Nostrand–Reinhold, New York, pp. 5–25.

Harrell, L. E., Barlow, T. S., and Parsons, D., 1987, Cholinergic neurons, learning, and recovery of function, *Behav. Neurosci.* **101:**644–652.

Ingram, D. K., 1983, Toward the behavioral assessment of biological aging in the laboratory mouse: Concepts, terminology, and objectives, *Exp. Aging Res.* **9:**225–238.

Ingram, D. K., 1984, Biological age: A strategy for assessment, in: *Gerontology and Geriatrics Yearbook (U.S.S.R.)* (D. F. Cherbotarev, A. V. Tokar, and V. P. Voitenko, eds.), Institute for Gerontology, Kiev, pp. 30–38.

Ingram, D. K., 1985, Analysis of age-related impairments in learning and memory in rodent models, *Ann. NY Acad. Sci.* **444:**312–331.

Ingram, D. K., 1988, Complex maze learning in rodents as a model of age-related memory impairment, *Neurobiol. Aging,* **9:**475–486.

Ingram, D. K., and Reynolds, M. A., 1986, Assessing the predictive validity of psychomotor tests as measures of biological age in mice, *Exp. Aging Res.* **12:**155–162.

Ingram, D. K., Weindruch, R., Spangler, E. L., Freeman, J. R., and Walford, R. L., 1987, Dietary restriction benefits learning and motor performance of aged mice, *J. Gerontol.* **42:**78–81.

Kausler, D., 1982, *Experimental Psychology and Human Aging,* Wiley, New York.

Kesner, R. P., 1986, Neurobiological views of memory, in: *Learning and Memory: A Biological View* (J. L. Martinez and R. P. Kesner, eds.), Academic, Orlando, Florida, pp. 389–438.

Knowlton, B. J., Wenk, G., Olton, D. S., and Coyle, J. T., 1985, Basal forebrain lesions produce a dissociation of trial-dependent and trial-independent memory performance, *Brain Res.* **345:**315–321.

Kubanis, P., and Zornetzer, S. F., 1981, Age-related behavioral and neurobiological changes: A review with an emphasis on memory, *Behav. Neural. Biol.* **31:**115–172.

Lippa, A. S., Loullis, C. C., Rotrosen, J., Cordasco, D. M., Critchett, D. J., and Joseph, J. A., 1985, Conformational changes in muscarinic receptors may produce diminished cholinergic neurotransmission and memory deficits in aged rats, *Neurobiol. Aging* **6:**317–323.

Loullis, C. C., Dean, R. L., Lippa, A. S., Clody, D. E., and Coupet, J., 1985, Hippocampal muscarinic receptor loss following trimethyl tin administration. *Pharmacol. Biochem. Behav.* **22:**147–151.

Lowy, A. M., Ingram, D. K., Olton, D. A., Waller, S. B., Reynolds, M. A., and London, E. D., 1985, Discrimination learning requiring different memory components in rats: Age and neurochemical comparisons, *Behav. Neurosci.* **99:**638–651.

Michel, M. E., and Klein, A. W., 1978, Performance differences in a complex maze between young and aged rats, *Age* **1:**13–16.

Morris, R. G. M., Kandel, E. R., and Squire, L. R., 1988, The neuroscience of learning and memory: Cells, neural circuits, and behavior, *Trends Neurosci.* **11:**125–127.

Munn, N. L., 1950, *Handbook of Psychological Research on the Rat,* Houghton-Mifflin, Boston.

Murdock, B. B., Jr., 1967, Recent developments in short-term memory, *Br. J. Psychol.* **58:**421–433.

Olton, D. S., Becker, J. T., and Handelmann, G. E., 1979, Hippocampus, space, and memory, *Behav. Brain Sci.* **2:**313–365.

Olton, D. S., Becker, J. T., and Handelmann, G. E., 1980, Hippocampal function: Working memory or cognitive mapping?, *Physiol. Psychol.* **8:**239–246.

Olton, D. S., and Wenk, G., 1987, Dementia: Animal models of the cognitive impairments produced by degeneration of the basal forebrain cholinergic system, in: *Psychopharmacology: The Third Generation of Progress* (H. Y. Meltzer, ed.), Raven, New York, pp. 941–953.

Poon, L. W., 1985, Differences in human memory with aging: Nature, causes, and clinical implications, in: *Handbook of the Psychology of Aging* (J. E. Birren and K. W. Schaie, eds.), Van Nostrand–Reinhold, New York, pp. 427–462.

Sara, S. J., 1985, The locus coeruleus and cognitive function: Attempts to relate norandrenergic enhancement of signal/noise in the brain to behavior, *Physiol. Psychol.* **13**:151–162.

Sharps, M. J., and Gollin, E. S., 1987, Memory for object locations in young and elderly adults, *J. Gerontol.* **42**:336–341.

Spangler, E. L., Rigby, P., and Ingram, D. K., 1986, Scopolamine impairs learning performance of rats in a 14-unit T-maze, *Pharmacol. Biochem. Behav.* **25**:673–679.

Spangler, E. L., Chachich, M. E., and Ingram, D. K., 1988, Scopolamine in rats impairs acquisition but not retention in a 14-unit T-maze, *Pharmacol. Biochem. Behav.* **30**:949–955.

Spangler, E. L., Chachich, M. E., Curtis, N. J., and Ingram, D. K., 1989, Age-related impairment in complex maze learning: Relationship to neophobia and cholinergic antagonism, *Neurobiol. Aging* **10**:133–141.

Spencer, D. G., Jr., and Lal, H., 1983, Effects of anticholinergic drugs on learning and memory, *Drug Dev. Res.* **3**:489–502.

Squire, L. R., and Zola-Morgan, S., 1988, Memory: Brain systems and behavior, *Trends Neurosci.* **11**:170–175.

Stone, C., 1929, The age factor in animal learning. I. Rats in the problem box and the maze, *Genet. Psychol. Monogr.* **5**:1–130.

Thomas, G., 1984, Memory: Time binding in organisms, in: *Neuropsychology of Memory* (L. Squire and N. Butters, eds.), Guilford, New York, pp. 374–384.

Thomas, G., and Gash, D. M., 1986, Differential effects of posterior septal lesions on dispositional and representational memory, *Behav. Neurosci.* **100**:712–719.

Verzar-McDougall, E., 1957, Studies in learning and memory in ageing rats, *Gerontologia* **1**:65–85.

Waddell, K. J., and Rogoff, B., 1981, Effect of contextual organization on spatial memory of middle-aged and older women, *Dev. Psychol.* **17**:878–885.

Walovitch, R. C., Ingram, D. K., Spangler, E. L., and London, E. D., 1987, Co-dergocrine, cerebral glucose utilization and maze performance in middle-aged rats, *Pharmacol. Biochem. Behav.* **26**:95–101.

Watts, J., Stevens, R., and Robinson, C., 1981, Effects of scopolamine on radial maze performance in rats, *Physiol. Psychol.* **26**:845–851.

Waugh, N. C., and Norman, D. A., 1965, Primary memory, *Psychol. Rev.* **72**:89–104.

Weindruch, R., 1984, Dietary restriction and the aging process, in: *Free Radicals in Molecular Biology, Aging, and Disease* (D. Armstrong, R. S. Sohal, R. G. Cutler, and T. F. Slater, eds.), Raven, New York, pp. 67–85.

Winocur, G., 1980, The hippocampus and cue-utilization, *Physiol. Psychol.* **3**:280–288.

Winocur, G., and Breckenridge, C. B., 1973, Cue-dependent behavior of hippocampally damaged rats in a complex maze, *J. Comp. Physiol. Psychol.* **82**:512–522.

Zornetzer, S. F., 1985, Catecholamine system involvement in age-related memory dysfunction, *Ann. NY Acad. Sci.* **444**:242–254.

45

Age-Related Changes in Brain Protein Kinase C and Serotonin Release

H-Y. WANG and E. FRIEDMAN

1. INTRODUCTION

Maintenance of controlled synaptic concentrations of neurotransmitters in the central and peripheral nervous systems is essential for the survival of the organism. Aging in mammals is associated with change in neurotransmission that may underlie some of the age-related deficits, such as those in psychomotor performance, cognitive function, and other physiological functions subserved by the peripheral autonomic systems. The mechanisms involved in neurotransmitter release and its regulation in response to a changing internal and external environment are not well understood (Cooper and Meyer, 1984). Recent work has demonstrated a role for the enzyme protein kinase C (PKC) in modulating the release of various neurotransmitter substances in the brain and in the periphery (Nishizuka, 1984; Wakade *et al.*, 1985; Zurgel and Zisapel, 1985; Nichols *et al.*, 1987; Wang and Friedman, 1987).

Protein kinase C has been found to be highly localized in presynaptic nerve endings of cortical and hippocampal brain cells (Worley *et al.*, 1986; Wood *et al.*, 1986). The enzyme is Ca^{2+}- and phospholipid-dependent and is activated by diacylglycerol (DAG), which is generated by the hydrolysis of phosphatidylinositol (Berridge, 1984). This action of DAG that can be simulated by the phorbol esters (Castagna *et al.*, 1982) lowers the Ka for Ca^{2+} at physiological concentrations of the ion and thus regulates the activity of PKC (Kishimoto *et al.*, 1980; Inoue *et al.*, 1977; Kikkawa *et al.*, 1986; Rasmussen *et al.*, 1985).

Protein kinase C is distributed in cells in both cytosolic and membranous fractions; upon activation, translocation of the enzyme occurs (from cytosol to membrane) (Wolf *et al.*, 1985; Kraft and Anderson, 1983). In the brain, the enzyme phosphorylates synaptosomal, presynaptic membranous, and various microtubular proteins that may be related to excitation–release coupling mechanisms.

In earlier studies from this laboratory, cortical S_1 and S_2 serotonin (5-HT) receptors were found to be reduced in 24- versus 6-month-old Fischer 344 rats (Friedman *et al.*, 1986). To understand the mechanisms contributing to this reduction in brain serotonin receptors, the

H-Y. WANG and E. FRIEDMAN • Division of Neurochemistry, Departments of Psychiatry and Pharmacology, Medical College of Pennsylvania, Philadelphia, Pennsylvania 19129.

effects of age on serotonin release was investigated. It was predicted that the release of brain serotonin may be elevated in senescent animals and that this may cause the postsynaptic receptor changes. This was reinforced by our earlier work in aged mice, which indicated age-related elevation in hippocampal 5-HIAA/5-HT ratios (Brennan et al., 1981). This chapter describes age-associated changes in the regulation of PKC-mediated serotonin release and in its relationship to the translocation of the enzyme.

2. METHODS

Release was studied in superfused cortical and hippocampal brain slices obtained from 6-, 12-, and 24-month-old Fischer 344 rats as described previously (Friedman and Wang, 1988). Brain slices were incubated with 10^{-7} M [^{3}H]-5-HT, washed, and perfused with physiological solution at a rate of 1 ml/min. Release was evoked by a 30-sec K^+ pulse (65 mM) and calculated as the percentage of tissue [^{3}H]-5-HT content at the time of stimulation.

To study the effect of age on PKC and its translocation, brain slices were incubated in Krebs–Ringer solution with or without phorbol 12-myristate 13-acetate (PMA) for 20 min. The supernatant was decanted, and the slices were homogenized in cold 0.32 M sucrose buffer containing 20 mM Tris HCl, pH 7.5, 2 mM EDTA, 0.5 mM EGTA, 50 ng/ml leupeptin, 0.2 mM phenylmethylsulfonyl fluoride, and 0.1% 2-mercaptoethanol and centrifuged at 800g for 10 min at 4°C. The supernatant was sonicated and centrifuged at 25,000g for 15 min. The supernatant (cytosol) was applied onto Whatman DE52 columns and washed with 5 ml buffer, followed by 0.5 ml of buffer with 0.1 M NaCl. The enzyme was eluted with 1.5 ml of the salt-containing buffer; PKC activity was determined by a modification of the method described previously by Kikkawa et al. (1982) and Zatz et al. (1983). The pellet obtained by centrifugation at 25,000g was employed in determining membrane-bound activity. It was solubilized for 1 hr in 200 μl of buffer containing 1% Nonidet P-40, diluted, and recentrifuged at 25,000g, the supernatant was treated as above for determination of PKC. Enzymatic activity was expressed as picomoles of ^{32}P incorporated in 1 min per microgram protein (Lowry et al., 1951).

3. RESULTS AND DISCUSSION

Potassium-stimulated [^{3}H]-5-HT release from cortical slices in 12-month-old (5.77 ± 0.11% release; $p < 0.005$) and 24-month-old (5.17 ± 0.11; f > 0.005) rats showed decreases as compared with 6-month-old rats (6.88 ± 0.10% release). In the hippocampus, age of the animals did not seem to affect K^+-induced [^{3}H]-5-HT release (7.48 ± 0.12%, 7.32 ± 0.15%, and 7.22 ± 0.16% released in slices of 6-, 12-, and 24-month-old animals, respectively).

In the same experiments, Ca^{2+}-independent spontaneous efflux of [^{3}H]-5-HT from cortical and hippocampal brain slices has also been compared. No age-related differences in efflux were observed in parietal cortex. However, a 30% elevation in the basal serotonin efflux was noted in hippocampal slices of 24-month-old rats as compared with 6- or 12-month-old animals. No differences in basal efflux were noted between 6- and 12-month-old animals. Thus, it appears that the postsynaptic receptor changes that occur during aging (Friedman et al., 1986) are not secondary to alteration in presynaptic neurotransmitter release.

The sensitivity of the presynaptic serotonin autoreceptors was assessed on the basis of the response of parietal cortical slices to the serotonin receptor agonist LSD. Slices were perfused with physiological solution containing various concentrations of lysergic acid diethylamide (LSD) 20 min before stimulation, and the inhibition of release was calculated. LSD exhibited dose-dependent inhibition of K^+-evoked [^{3}H]-5-HT release in 6-, 12-, and 24-month-old animals ($p < 0.01$, ANOVA). However, the inhibitory potency of LSD in cortical brain slices did not change with age, indicating that prejunctional serotonin receptor sites are not altered during senescence (Table I). Similar findings were also observed in hippocampal brain slices.

Previous investigations have shown that depolarization of neuronal preparations with high K^+ increases neurotransmitter release and phosphorylation of a 87-kDa protein, which is a known substrate for PKC (Wu et al., 1982; Nichols et al., 1987). We have shown that stimulation of PKC with phorbol esters can facilitate the release of serotonin in cortical brain slices (Wang and Friedman, 1987). Furthermore, we have observed age-related changes in PKC stimulation-induced neurotransmitter release (Friedman and Wang, 1989). The effect of age on phorbol ester-induced serotonin release in hippocampal slices are shown in Fig. 1. Hippocampal brain slices obtained from 6-, 12-, and 24-month-old Fischer 344 animals were preloaded with [^{3}H]-5-HT and stimulated with K^+ to obtain the control response and were subsequently preincubated for 20 min before the second K^+ stimulation with 81 or 162 nM of the active phorbol ester, PMA. The results demonstrate (1) dose-dependent effects of PMA on [^{3}H]-5-HT release in the three age groups examined, and (2) facilitation of release by the phorbol ester in 6- and 12-month-old animals (but the 12-month-old animals exhibited a

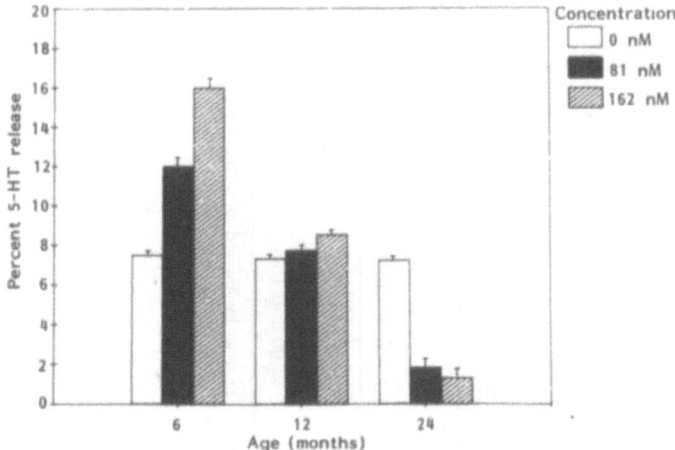

FIGURE 1. Hippocampal slices were preloaded with [^{3}H]-5-HT, washed, and superfused with physiological solution. Control release was evoked by a 30-sec K^+ pulse (65 mM). A second pulse was delivered following 20-min exposure to the indicated concentration of phorbol muristate acetate (PMA). Release was calculated as the percentage of tissue [^{3}H]-5-HT content. Significant dose-dependent effects were obtained at both PMA doses ($p < 0.001$). Each bar represents the mean ±SEM of 10–14 determinations.

TABLE I. Effect of Age on the Sensitivity of Presynaptic Serotonin Autoreceptors in Parietal Cortex[a]

LSD	6 months		12 months		24 months	
	% release	% inhibition	% release	% inhibition	% release	% inhibition
5×10^{-8} M	—	—	$3.97 \pm 0.23(4)$	31.3	$3.87 \pm 0.34(4)$	25.1
5×10^{-7} M	$3.60 \pm 0.14(4)$	47.6	$3.96 \pm 0.37(4)$	43.5	$3.08 \pm 0.40(4)$	40.4
5×10^{-6} M	$2.90 \pm 0.10(4)$	57.8	$2.23 \pm 0.34(4)$	61.5	$2.08 \pm 0.41(4)$	59.8

[a]Assessed after [³H]serotonin loading and after 20-min preincubation of slices with LSD at concentrations of 5×10^{-8} to 5×10^{-6} M. There were no significant differences among the three age groups.

reduced PMA facilitation of release as compared with the effect of PMA on 6-month-old animals), and (3) the response to PMA in 24-month-old animals involved inhibition of the K^+-evoked transmitter release.

In attempt to test whether the effects of PMA on [^{3}H]-5-HT release are mediated by stimulation of PKC, we examined the effect of the putative enzyme inhibitor, H-7 (Kawamoto and Hidaka, 1984), on PMA-elicited responses in 6- and 24-month-old animals. The results summarized in Table II show that the facilitory response exerted by the phorbol ester in 6-month-old animals was completely inhibited by preincubation with the inhibitor. In the 24-month-old animals, the characteristic inhibition of release seen with PMA was also prevented by the putative PKC inhibitor. The data therefore support the idea that both actions of the phorbol ester—stimulation (in 6- and 12-month-old animals) and inhibition (seen in 24-month-old animals)—are mediated by PKC phosphorylation. In addition, it can be seen that the putative PKC inhibitor reversed the age-related decrease in 5-HT release observed in the cortical slices of 24-month-old animals. These results further imply that PKC is involved in modulation of 5-HT release.

In an attempt to explore the potential mechanism underlying the changes in serotonin release observed during aging, we have examined the activity of PKC in senescent rats. The results shown in Table III indicate that enzymatic activity decreases with age in the cortex, but not in the hippocampus. Furthermore, PKC translocation induced in brain slices by PMA is decreased with age in cortical, but not in hippocampal, slices. These results appear to dissociate between age-related changes in serotonin release and PKC activity or its translocation. However, an alteration in phosphorylation mechanism in senescent animals cannot be discounted as involved in the mechanism responsible for the age-associated differential modulation of serotonin release. The phosphorylation mediated by PKC is dependent on a number of factors in the cellular environment of the enzyme, which may be affected by the

TABLE II. Effect of PKC Inhibitor-H7 on PMA-Induced Changes in Cortical and Hippocampal 5-HT Release[a]

	6 months	24 months
Exp. I: Cerebral cortex		
Control	6.74 ± 0.21	5.53 ± 0.17
PMA (162 nM)	11.77 ± 0.22[b]	3.87 ± 0.26[c]
H7 (10 μM)	6.62 ± 0.25	6.66 ± 0.51[d]
H7 (10 μM) + PMA (162 nM)	7.08 ± 0.25	6.43 ± 0.23[d]
Exp. II: Hippocampus		
Control	7.19 ± 0.16	6.96 ± 0.31
PMA (162 nM)	12.47 ± 0.41[b]	3.02 ± 0.13[b]
H7 (10 μM)	6.45 ± 0.31	7.72 ± 0.08[d]
H7 (10 μM) + PMA (162 nM)	6.92 ± 0.26	6.96 ± 0.20

[a]Cortical and hippocampal brain slices from 6- and 24-month-old rats were assessed after [^{3}H]serotonin loading and 20-min preincubation of slices with PMA, H7, or H7 + PMA. Release was initiated by exposure to 65 mM K^+ for 30 sec. Each value represents the mean ±SEM of four to eight individual experiments.
[b]$p < 0.001$ as compared with respective control group.
[c]$p < 0.01$ as compared with respective control group.
[d]$p < 0.05$ as compared with respective control group.

TABLE III. Protein Kinase C in Subcellular Cortical and Hippocampal Fractions of Aged Rats[a]

	6 months		12 months		24 months	
	Cytosol	Membrane	Cytosol	Membrane	Cytosol	Membrane
Exp. I: Cerebral cortex						
Control	3.63 ± 0.13	2.76 ± 0.16	3.96 ± 0.34	2.42 ± 0.21	2.00 ± 0.14[b]	1.56 ± 0.12[b]
	(56.8 ± 2.0%)	(43.2 ± 2.5%)	(62.1 ± 5.3%)	(37.9 ± 3.3%)	(56.2 ± 3.9%)	(43.8 ± 3.4%)
PMA (162 nM)	2.28 ± 0.12[c]	3.82 ± 0.23[c]	2.24 ± 0.16[c]	3.86 ± 0.28[c]	1.86 ± 0.15	1.86 ± 0.11
	(37.3 ± 2.0%)	(62.6 ± 3.8%)	(36.7 ± 2.6%)	(63.3 ± 4.6%)	(52.8 ± 4.3%)	(47.2 ± 3.1%)
Exp. II: Hippocampus						
Control	7.89 ± 0.15	3.63 ± 0.09	7.56 ± 0.27	3.47 ± 0.09	7.23 ± 0.16	3.36 ± 0.08
	(68.5 ± 1.3%)	(31.5 ± 0.8%)	(68.5 ± 2.4%)	(31.5 ± 0.8%)	(68.9 ± 1.5%)	(31.1 ± 0.8%)
PMA (162 nM)	3.59 ± 0.14[d]	7.49 ± 0.07[d]	3.38 ± 0.16[d]	7.50 ± 0.14[d]	2.88 ± 0.20[d]	7.45 ± 0.16[d]
	(32.4 ± 1.3%)	(67.6 ± 0.6%)	(31.1 ± 1.5%)	(68.9 ± 1.3%)	(27.9 ± 1.9%)	(72.1 ± 1.5%)

[a]Cortical and hippocampal brain slices from animals of differing ages were incubated for 20.5 min in K-R (control) or for 20.5 min in PMA. The tissue slices were collected and homogenized and cytosolic and membrane-bound PKC activity determined. Each value represents the mean ±SEM of values obtained from six to eight animals.

[b]$p < 0.001$ as compared with 6-month-old animals.

[c]$p < 0.01$ as compared with respective control group.

[d]$p < 0.001$ as compared with respective control group.

aging process, including direct cofactors for this reaction, e.g., local Ca^{2+} concentrations, availability of phosphatidylserine and DAG, as well as other considerations, including membrane fluidity and content, phosphatase activity, and the concentration of arachidonic acid, its metabolites, or sphingolipids.

The present results were obtained under conditions that optimize PKC activity, at least with regard to Ca^{2+}, phosphotidylserine, and DAG (PMA), and therefore may not reflect physiological changes caused by changes in these factors. Furthermore, the lack of apparent correlation between changes in release and enzymatic activity may point to age-related changes in protein substrates, such as those involved in neurotransmitter release or its regulation. These aspects of the phenomenon are currently under investigation in our laboratory.

ACKNOWLEDGMENT. This study was supported by grant AG07700-01 from the National Institute on Aging.

REFERENCES

Berridge, M. J., 1984, Inositol triphosphate and diacylglycerol as second messengers, *J. Biochem.* **220**:345–360.

Brennan, M., Dallob, A., and Friedman, E., 1981, Involvement of hippocampal serotonergic activity in age-related changes in exploratory behavior, *Neurobiol. Aging* **2**:199–204.

Castagna, M., Takai, Y., Kaibuchi, K., Sano, K., Kikkawa, U., and Nishizuka, Y., 1982, Direct activation of Ca^{2+}-activated phospholipid-dependent protein kinase by tumer-promoting phorbol esters, *J. Biol. Chem.* **257**:7847–7851.

Cooper, J. R., and Meyer, E. M., 1984, Possible mechanisms involved in the release and modulation of release of neuroactive agents, *Neurochem. Int.* **6**:419–433.

Friedman, E., Cooper, T., and Yocca, F., 1986, The effect of imipramine treatment on brain serotonin receptors and beta-adrenoceptors and on pineal beta-adrenergic function in adult and aged rats, *Eur. J. Pharmocol.* **123**:351–356.

Friedman, E., and Wang, H-Y., 1988, Effect of chronic lithium treatment on 5-hydroxytryptamine autoreceptors and release of 5-[³H]-hydroxytryptamine from rat brain cortical, hippocampal, and hypothalamic slices, *J. Neurochem.* **50**:195–201.

Friedman, E., and Wang, H-Y., 1989, The effect of age on brain cortical protein kinase C and its mediation of serotonin release, *J. Neurochem.* **52**:187–192.

Inoue, M., Kishimoto, A., Takai, Y., and Nishizuka, Y., 1977, Studies on a cyclic nucleotide-independent protein kinase and its apoenzyme in mammalian tissues. II. Proenzyme and its activation by calcium-dependent proteins from rat brain, *J. Biol. Chem.* **252**:7610–7616.

Kawamoto, S., and Hidaka, H., 1984, 1-(5-Isoquinolinesulfonyl)-2-methylpiperazine (H-7) is a selective inhibitor of protein kinase C in rabbit platelets, *Biochem. Biophys. Res. Commun.* **125**:258–267.

Kikkawa, U., Go, M., Koumoto, J., and Nishizuka, Y., 1986, Calcium-activated, phospholipid-dependent protein kinase from rat brain, *Biochem. Biophys. Res. Commun.* **135**:636–643.

Kishimoto, A., Takai, Y., Mori, T., Kikkawa, U., and Nishizuka, Y., 1980, Activation of calcium and phospholipid-dependent protein kinase by diacylglycerol, its possible relation to phosphoinositol turnover, *J. Biol. Chem.* **255**:2273–2276.

Kraft, A. S., and Anderson, W. B., 1983, Phorbol esters increase the amount of calcium, phospholipid-dependent protein kinase associated with plasma membrane, *Nature (Lond.)* **301**:621–623.

Lowry, O. H., Rosebrough, N. J., Farr, A. L., and Randall, R. J., 1951, Protein measurement with the Folin phenol reagent, *J. Biol. Chem.* **249**:265–275.

Nichols, R. A., Haycock, J. W., Wang, J. K. T., and Greengard, P., 1987, Phorbol ester enhancement of neurotransmitter release from rat brain synaptosomes, *J. Neurochem.* **48**:615–621.

Nishizuka, Y., 1984, The role of protein kinase C in cell surface signal transduction and tumor promotion, *Nature (Lond.)* **308**:693–696.

Rasmussen, H., Zawalich, W., and Kojima, I., 1985, Ca^{2+} and cAMP in the regulation of cell function, *Calcium and Cell Physiology* (D. Marme, ed.), Springer-Verlag, New York, pp. 1–17.

Wakade, A. R., Malhotra, R. K., and Wakade, T. D., 1985, Phorbol ester, an activator of protein kinase C, enhances calcium-dependent release of sympathetic neurotransmitter, *Naunyn Schmiedebergs Arch. Pharmacol.* **133**:122–127.

Wang, H-Y., and Friedman, E., 1987, Protein kinase C: Regulation of serotonin release from rat brain cortical slices, *Eur. J. Pharmacol.* **141**:15–21.

Wolf, M., Cuatrecasas, P., and Sahyoun, N., 1985, Interaction of protein kinase C with membranes is regulated by Ca^{2+}, phorbol esters and ATP, *J. Biol. Chem.* **260**:15718–15722.

Wood, J. G., Girard, P. R., Mazzei, G. J., and Kuo, J. F., 1986, Immunocytochemical localization of protein kinase C in identified neuronal compartments of rat brain, *J. Neurosci.* **6**:2571–2580.

Worley, P. F., Baraban, J. M., Snyder, S. H., 1986, Heterogeneous localization of protein kinase C in rat brain: Autoradiographic analysis of phorbol ester receptor binding, *J. Neurosci.* **6**:199–207.

Wu, W. C., Walaas, S. I., Nairn, A. C., and Greengard, P., 1982, Calcium/phospholipid regulates phosphorylation of a M "87k" substrate protein in brain synaptosomes, *Proc. Natl. Acad. Sci. USA* **79**:5249–5253.

Zatz, M., Mahan, L. C., and Reisine, T., 1987, Translocation of protein kinase C in anterior pituitary tumor cells, *J. Neurochem.* **48**(1):106–110.

Zurgil, N., and Zisapel, N., 1985, Phorbol ester and calcium act synergistically to enhance neurotransmitters release by brain neurons in culture, *FEBS Lett.* **185**:257–262.

46

Increased Blood Flow Augments CNS Axon Regeneration

J. C. de la TORRE and H. S. GOLDSMITH

1. INTRODUCTION

Aging is known to increase the potential for progressive central nervous system (CNS) deterioration. Often, age-related loss of motor and cognitive function can be linked to reduced CNS blood flow (Grubb *et al.*, 1977; Mann *et al.*, 1986; Ravens, 1978; Sokoloff, 1966). This problem is compounded by the likelihood that extraction of cerebral circulating nutrients such as glucose and oxygen from the microcirculation decreases with aging (Kety, 1956; Grubb *et al.*, 1977; Foster *et al.*, 1983). If such is the case, a cause/effect relationship between cerebrovascular pathology and progressive degeneration of CNS tissue in dementia may exist (Hardy *et al.*, 1986). Support for a blood flow–neural activity interaction is well accepted in head trauma, ischemia, or mass-producing brain lesions (Bowen *et al.*, 1976; Youmans and Albrand, 1973). It would appear, moreover, that a strong correlation exists between the development of dementia-like behavior disorders following reduction of blood flow to the brain brought about by cerebral atherosclerosis (Butler, 1966; Worm-Petersen and Pakkenberg, 1968). The question that has not been answered yet is: If reducing flow is bad for neural activity, can increasing blood flow be good for neural reconstruction? Stated another way, if CNS regeneration can be promoted through increased blood flow, neural impairment resulting from aging-related disorders may be arrested or reversed. To test this premise, two surgical techniques were combined because of the ability of each to support either experimental axon outgrowth through a collagen bridge (de la Torre *et al.*, 1984) or to increase CNS blood flow using a transposed pedicled omentum (Goldsmith *et al.*, 1983, 1984, 1985).

The present experimental design depended on establishing two assumptions: (1) Can an intact pedicled omentum surgically transposed to blanket a spinal cord collagen bridge increase local tissue blood flow? (2) If local tissue blood flow is increased, will the density or rate of spinal fibers regenerating across the bridge matrix be enhanced? Cat spinal cord rather

J. C. de la TORRE • Division of Neurosurgery, University of Ottawa Health Sciences, Ottawa, Ontario K1H 8M5, Canada.   H. S. GOLDSMITH • Department of Surgery, Boston University School of Medicine, Boston, Massachusetts 02118.

than brain was chosen because of the relative reliability in testing neurophysiological and morphological end points of ascending and descending spinal tracts following transection.

2. METHODS

Fourteen female cats were intubated and anesthetized with penthrane–oxygen. A sterile laminectomy was done to expose T7–11. The spinal cord was irrigated for 10 min with ice-cold 15% polyvinyl alcohol and 4 mM chlorpromazine (PVA–CPZ) solution, to cool the tissue and reduce axoplasmic extrusion generally seen after peripheral nerve or spinal transection (de Medinaceli and Church, 1984; de la Torre et al., 1988). The dura was opened around the transection site, and the cord was cleanly divided at T9 with a very fine-edged blade. A gap of 6 mm was consistently obtained following cord transection. The cord stumps were bathed with PVA–CPZ for 15 min. Minimal to no axoplasmic extrusion from the cord stumps was observed after transection. The stumps were irrigated with ice-cold saline until bleeding and cerebrospinal fluid (CSF) leakage had ceased; the gap area was then dried with cotton wicks. Animals were randomly separated into three groups and the gap between cord stumps was filled with (1) collagen matrix (COL), (2) collagen matrix + pedicled omentum (COM), or (3) Gelfoam (GEF). Fluid collagen (type I, 35 mg/ml, obtained from Collagen Corp. Palo Alto, California) was dispensed sterile from a syringe at a temperature of 4°C and required about 60 min at body temperature to harden into a gel. This material has been shown to be biocompatible, bioabsorbable, and capable of creating a tight junction with host CNS tissue (de la Torre et al., 1984; Gelderd, 1987). In the COM group, a small laparotomy incision was made below the left costal margin in order to gently pull the omentum out of the abdominal cavity. The omentum was then surgically lengthened into a pedicle, keeping its vascular supply intact, and then tunneled subcutaneously to the dorsal cord region where it was placed on top of the collagen bridge (de la Torre and Goldsmith, 1987). All incisions were closed in layers. The animals were allowed to recover and received postoperative care for 90 days.

Ninety days after transection, six serial spinal cord blood flows (SCBF) were measured at 10- or 20-min intervals in all groups using the hydrogen clearance technique (Fig. 1). SCBF was determined by the initial slope method (Ingvar and Lassen, 1962). A reference Ag/AgCl electrode was inserted into a subcutaneous pouch. Teflon-insulated platinum/iridium microelectrodes (de la Torre et al., 1984) were inserted midpoint in the collagen matrix of the COM and COL groups and in the tissue growth between the transected stumps of GEF animals. Microelectrodes were also inserted 6 mm below the transection site in the distal cord gray matter and 12 mm above the lesion in the proximal cord. When all blood flows had been obtained, the distal cord microelectrodes were left in place in the COM group, and the pedicled omentum was ligated near its junction with the collagen bridge. Blood flow measurements were repeated until fluctuating values had stabilized (Fig. 1).

Animals underwent left cardiac ventricular perfusion with fixatives, the cord tissue was removed, blocked, and sectioned longitudinally in a cryostat. After incubation with the appropriate antibody, sections were processed for tyrosine hydroxylase immunofluorescence (TH-IF) or immunoreactive (TH-IR) fibers using the peroxidase–antiperoxidase method (Sternberger, 1986). Alternate sections were taken for Palmgren's silver axon and Nissl stains. Using an ocular grid, counts of TH-IR axons/dry high-power field (HPF) were averaged within the collagen bridge and in the distal cord tissue at 1-mm intervals along the cord axis. Blood vessels measuring 20–190 μm were also counted and averaged within the CM bridge in the COL and COM groups (Fig. 2b,d).

FIGURE 1. Spinal cord blood flows recorded 6 mm distal to collagen bridge in COM- and COL-treated groups or center of transection (GEF group) 90 days after total cord transection. Note initially high mean spinal blood flow (68 ml/100 g tissue per min) of COM-treated group as compared with COL- (24 ml) and GEF- (12 ml) treated animals. When pedicled omentum was ligated (arrow) to interrupt anastomotic blood flow from omentum to cord tissue, a rapid, linear decline in the spinal cord blood flow rate resulted that stabilized eventually at about 28 ml after 1 hr. Analysis of variance: ($\square$) $p < 0.0001$; ($\blacksquare$) $p < 0.001$.

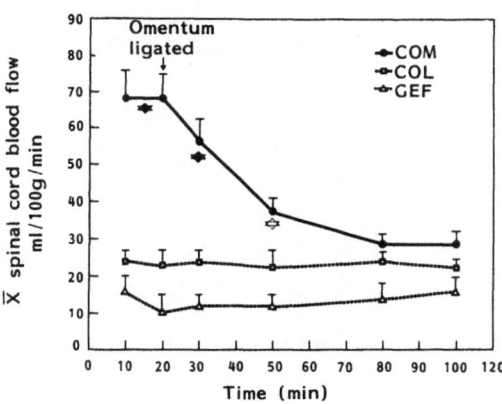

3. RESULTS

The hemodynamic findings showed that blood flows recorded 12 mm above the lesion site in the proximal cord were not significantly different among the three groups, with values ranging from 54 to 62 ml/100 g per min. Blood flow in the midcollagen bridge region (COL, COM) or center of tissue growth (GEF) averaged 38 ml in COM, 18 ml in COL, and 7 ml in GEF groups (Table I). Distal cord blood flows averaged 68 ml in COM, 24 ml in COL, and

TABLE I. 90 Days after Cord Transection[a]

Group	x̄ SCBF[b]	x̄ TH-IR axon counts[c]	x̄ axon travel distance[d] (mm)	x̄ blood vessel density[e]
COM	68 (±12)	23 (±3.38)	9.6 (1.82)	+++
COL	24 (±6)	2 (±0.79)	5.6 (1.24)	+
GEF	12 (±7)	0	0	--

[a]Mean values of spinal cord blood flow (SCBF), axonal and blood vessel density comparing CMO with COL and GEF groups of treated cats 90 days after total transection of the spinal cord. Morphologic longitudinal sections of tyrosine hydroxylase immunoreactive axons (TH-IR). Analysis of variance with ±SEM in parentheses.

[b]ml/100 g tissue per min, recorded 6 mm distal to collagen bridge. Average of six blood flows/cat: SEM ($p < 0.0001$).

[c]TH-IR axons/dry high-power field in collagen bridge; analysis of variance (±SE). Peroxidase antiperoxidase (PAP) method. Sample counts from 1 mm intervals using long spinal cord axis ($p < 0.001$).

[d]TH-IR immunofluorescent axons measured (in mm) from proximal site of cord transection through collagen bridge and below it.

[e]Mean number of blood vessels/dry high-power field (HPF) within CM bridge of COM, COL groups (GEF not determined). Scale: + = 0–2/HPF; ++ = 3–6/HPF; +++ = 7–10/HPF; ++++ = 10/HPF. -- = too low to average.

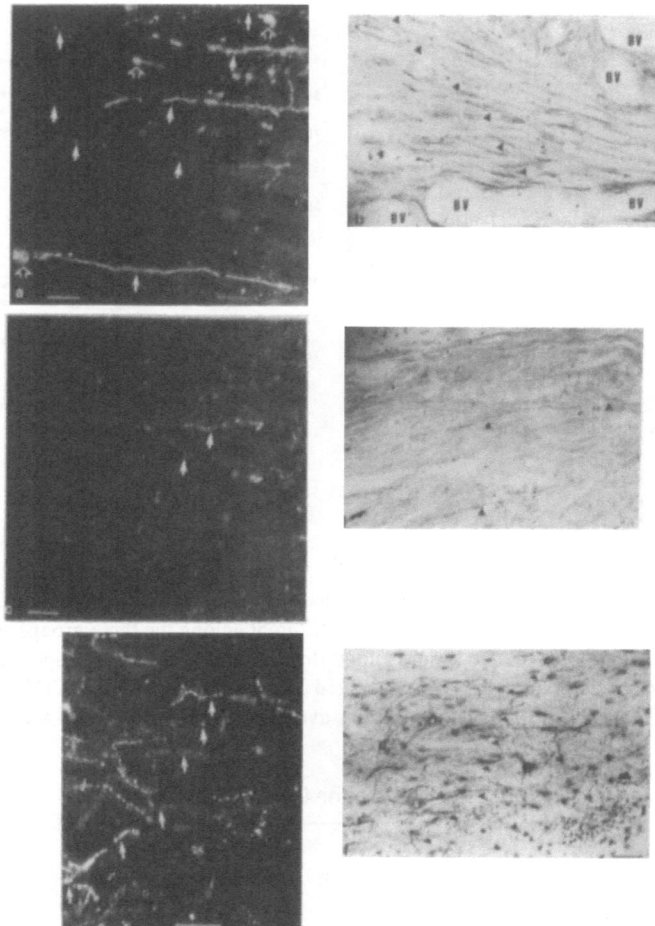

FIGURE 2. Tyrosine hydroxylase immunofluorescent (TH-IF) and immunoreactive (TH-IR) fibers of COM- (a,b), COL- (c,d) treated animals 90 days after total spinal cord transection. Intact gray matter control TH-IF and TH-IR fibers at T_9 is shown for comparison (e, f). Note higher density of TH-IF fibers entering collagen bridge from proximal cord tissue in COM- (↑ ,a) as compared with COL- (↑ ,c) treated group. Midpoint in the collagen bridge, density of TH-IR fibers is in a ratio of 10 : 1 for COM (▲,b) compared with COL (▲,d) treatment. Numerous blood vessels (BV,a) can be seen in the COM-treated animals surrounded by a robust outgrowth of TH-IR fibers. Bar = 25 μm.

12 ml in GEF group (Fig. 1). Midcollagen and distal SCBF differences between COM and COL or GEF were statistically significant using analysis of variance (Table I).

Within a few minutes following ligation of the pedicled omentum in the COM group, a rapid linear fall in blood flow was observed which leveled off around 28 ml within 1 hr postocclusion (see Fig. 1). This drop in blood flow was assumed to be the vascular contribution by the omentum to the collagen bridge and distal cord tissue, which represented an average of 65% difference compared with COL group blood flows in the same general region. Moreover, blood vessel density counts within the collagen matrix showed a 3 : 1 higher ratio for COM as compared with COL-treated animals (Table I).

Ocular grid counts of TH-IR fibers within the collagen matrix bridge showed approximately a 10-fold increase in COM over COL treatments (Table I). Figure 2a,c shows typical TH-IF axon density in COM- and COL-treated animals, respectively, as they enter the collagen bridge area adjoining the proximal cord. Robust outgrowth of TH-IR fibers in the midcollagen bridge region is seen in COM group (Fig. 2b) in contrast to COL-treated animals (Fig. 2c). TH-IR immunofluorescent axons were observed extending 3.5 mm caudal to the collagen bridge–distal cord transection site in COM-treated animals. Maximal distance traveled by regenerated TH-IR fibers was 9.6 mm in COM-treated and 5.6 mm in COL-treated animals during the 12-week recovery period. Many blood vessels (BV) are seen surrounded by TH-IR axons in COM (Fig. 2b) and considerably fewer in COL-treated group (Fig. 2d). Normal control TH-IF and TH-IR fibers in gray matter are shown for comparison (Fig. 2c,f). No TH-IR axons were seen exiting the collagen bridge at its distal junction in the COL-treated group after 90 days. There were no TH-IR axons between the proximal stump and distal cord below the transection site in the GEF group. This finding suggests that TH-IR axons found in COM distal cord did not originate from peripheral nerve sources, since if they had, such axons would also have been routinely observed in COL or GEF groups.

4. DISCUSSION

It is known that tyrosine hydroxylase is the biosynthetic enzyme for catecholamines (CA), and its descending CA tracts in spinal cord originate from neurons located in the brain (Commissiong and Toffano, 1986; Pearson et al., 1983; de la Torre, 1972; Hökfelt et al., 1973). The presence of TH-IR fibers below the level of transection in this model is therefore an indication that these axons regenerated from adrenergic supraspinal tracts. It appears that neuritic outgrowth from segmental spinal neurons also occurred in the COL and COM groups, since Palmgren sections (a general axon stain) revealed considerably more silver-impregnated than did TH-IR fibers near the collagen bridge region in the histologic preparations.

Additional support for "segmental" and "supraspinal" tract regeneration in this model was obtained from a previous experiment in which cats were treated with COM or COL but kept only 45 days after transection. When HRP was injected after 45 days, the label was transported retrogradely across the collagen bridge in the COM but not the COL group. Longitudinal sections revealed HRP-labeled neurons in the COM animals clustered around Rexed lamina VI and VII of the proximal cord (de la Torre and Goldsmith, 1987). Somatosensory evoked potentials were also present after 45 days in COM- but not in COL-treated cats (de la Torre and Goldsmith, 1987).

The results of this study indicate that a substantial increase in the regenerative rate and density of catecholaminergic-derived axons can be achieved by omental transposition to the collagen bridge. The evidence that such increased regeneration results from improved spinal cord blood flow (SCBF) to the transected region is suggested from three findings observed in the present study: (1) increased SCBF measured in omental-treated group; (2) cancellation of SCBF increase by occlusion of omental pedicle; and (3) greater density of blood vessels in collagen bridge of omental than non-omental-treated cats.

Since the omentum has also been shown to harbor neurotrophic material (Goldsmith et al., 1987b), neurotransmitters (Goldsmith et al., 1987a), and a lipid factor that induces rapid angiogenesis in tissue (Goldsmith *et al.*, 1984), it is conceivable that a chemical or chemical–vascular phenomenon may be responsible for the morphologic differences seen between the COM and COL groups.

The concept of adequate vascularization as a basic requirement for CNS regeneration in mammals is not well understood, mainly because in the past, it has not been possible to increase blood flow to the affected brain or cord region in a sustained fashion (Youmans and Albrand, 1973). On the other hand, it has been possible to study the relationship of axonal regeneration and blood flow by the inverse relationship. For example, chemically induced diabetes in rats results in reduced peripheral nerve blood flow and vascular density (Monafo *et al.*, 1988; Tuck and Low, 1984), a condition reported to retard axonal regeneration following nerve transection (Powell *et al.*, 1986). Moreover, sensorimotor transmission impairment can follow a variety of spinal cord ischemic conditions (Darwish *et al.*, 1979; De Girolami and Zivin, 1982; Doppman *et al.*, 1979; Schneider and Dralle, 1973).

The notion that an ''adequate'' vascular supply to traumatized CNS tissue is critical to the outgrowth potential of severed axons is widely accepted by investigators. As Kiernan (1978) has pointed out, growing CNS axonal tips may require proteins released from blood plasma for successful regeneration. However, blood flow or possible derivatives from it are seldom measured or discussed in mammalian CNS regeneration studies (Kiernan, 1979). It is still unclear what ''adequate flow'' or ''minimum flow'' requirements are needed for robust central axonal regrowth. What is known is that when cerebral blood flow (CBF) falls to 20 ml/100 g per min, significant membrane–ionic imbalance associated with reduced neuroelectric brain activity results (Branston *et al.*, 1977). If CBF is furthered lowered to 12–15 ml, neuroelectric activity is abolished (Sharbrough *et al.*, 1973). A CBF drop below 12 ml may generally lead to severe cerebral cell changes and eventual neuronal death (Tamura *et al.*, 1980). We have shown in rodents (de la Torre, 1981, 1984a; de la Torre *et al.*, 1984), and now in cats, that transected cord develops a considerably lower blood flow near the lesion site after 6–12 weeks. It should be pointed out that the ''increased'' blood flow observed in the distal cord area of cats treated with the omentum pedicle is within the range of normal gray matter cord blood flow (Sakurada *et al.*, 1978; de la Torre, 1984b).

5. CONCLUSION

Although the ''minimal'' blood flow rate necessary for significant promotion of CNS axon regeneration remains unknown, the present findings suggest that a proportionately greater number of axons can regenerate and travel faster when blood flow to the transection area is returned to near-normal limits and *sustained* at that level. This concept, if confirmed, could form the basis for potentially useful therapy in aging disorders where neural impairment may follow a reduction of local blood flow.

ACKNOWLEDGMENTS. This work was supported by the Ottawa General Hospital Foundation. The excellent technical assistance of Teresa Fortin and Earl Steward is acknowledged.

REFERENCES

Bowen, D. M., Smith, C., White, P., and Davison, A., 1976, Neurotransmitter-related enzymes and indices of hypoxia in senile dementia and other abiotrophies, *Brain* **99**:459–496.

Branston, N. M., Strong, A., and Symon, L., 1977, Extracellular potassium activity, evoked potentials and tissue flow. Relationship during progressive ischemia in baboon cerebral cortex, *J. Neurol. Sci* **32:**305–321.

Butler, R. N., 1966, Psychiatric aspects of cerebrovascular diseases in the aged, *Res. Publ. Assoc.* **41:**255–266.

Commissiong, J. W., and Toffano, G., 1986, The effect of GM$_1$ ganglioside on coerulospinal, noradrenergic, adult neurons and on fetal monoaminergic neurons transplanted into the transected spinal cord of the adult rat, *Brain Res.* **380:**205–215.

Darwish, H., Archer, C., and Modin, J., 1979, The anterior spinal artery collateral in coarctation of the aorta. A clinical–angiographic correlation, *Arch. Neurol.* **36:**240–243.

De Girolami, U., and Zivin, J., 1982, Neuropathology of spinal cord ischemia in the rabbit, *J. Neuropathol. Exp. Neurol.* **41:**129–149.

de la Torre, J. C., 1972, *Dynamics of Brain Monoamines,* Plenum, New York.

de la Torre, J. C., 1981, Spinal cord injury: Review of basic and applied research, *Spine* **6:**315–335.

de la Torre, J. C., 1984a, Catecholamine fiber regeneration across a collagen bioimplant after spinal cord transection, *Brain Res. Bull.* **9:**545–552.

de la Torre, J. C., 1984b, Spinal cord injury models, *Prog. Neurobiol.* **22:**289–344.

de la Torre, J. C., Hill, P. K., Gonzalez, M., and Parker, J., 1984, Evaluation of transected spinal cord regeneration in the rat, *Exp. Neruol.* **84:**186–206.

de la Torre, J. C., and Goldsmith, H. S., 1987, Collagen-omentum repair after experimental spinal cord transection, *Ann Neurol.* **22:**141–142.

de la Torre, J. C., and Goldsmith, H. S., Fortin, T., Stewart, E., Richard, M., 1988, Transected spinal cord axons cross a 6 mm gap, *Neurology (NY)* **38**(Suppl. 1):232.

de Medinaceli, L., and Church, A., 1984, Peripheral nerve reconnection: inhibition of early degenerative processes through the use of a novel fluid medium, *Exp. Neurol.* **84:**396–408.

Doppman, J. L., Girton, M., and Popovsky, M., 1979, Acute occlusion of the spinal vein. Experimental study in monkeys, *J. Neurosurg.* **51:**201–204.

Foster, N. L., Chase, T., Fedio, P., Patronas, N., Brooks, R., and di Chiro, G., 1983, Alzheimer's disease: focal changes shown by positron emission tomography, *Neurology (NY)* **33:**961–965.

Gelderd, J. B., 1987, Growth of blood vessels and neurites into a collagen matrix placed between the cut ends of transected spinal cord, *Soc. Neurosci. Abs.* **13:**395.

Goldsmith, H. S., Steward, E., Chen, F., and Ducket, S., 1983, Application of intact omentum to the normal and traumatized spinal cord, in: *Spinal Cord Reconstruction* (C. Kao, R. Bunge, and P. Reier,eds.), Raven, New York, pp. 235–242.

Goldsmith, H. S., Griffith, A., Kupferman, A., and Catsimpoolas, N., 1984, Lipid angiogenic factor from omentum, *JAMA* **252:**2034–2036.

Goldsmith, H. S., Steward, E., and Ducket, S., 1985, Early application of pedicled omentum to the acutely traumatized spinal cord, *Paraplegia* **23:**100–112.

Goldsmith, H. S., Marquis, J., and Siek, G., 1987a, Choline acetyltransferase activity in omental tissue, *Br. J. Neruosurg.* **1:**457–460.

Goldsmith, H. S., McIntosh, R., Vezine, and Colton, T., 1987b, Vasoactive neurochemicals identified in omentum, *Br. J. Neurosurg.* **1:**359–364.

Grubb, R. L., Raichle, M., Gado, M., Eichling, J., and Hughes, C., 1977, Cerebral blood flow, oxygen utilization and blood volume in dementia, *Neurology* **27:**905–910.

Hardy, J. A., Mann, D. M., Wester, P., and Winblad, B., 1986, An integrative hypothesis concerning the pathogenesis and progression of Alzeimer's disease, *Neurobiol. Aging* **7:**489–502.

Hökfelt, T., Fuxe, K., and Goldstein, M., 1973, Immunohistochemical studies on monoamine containing cell systems, *Brain Res.* **62:**461–469.

Ingvar, D. H., and Lassen, N. A., 1962, Regional blood flow of the cerebral cortex determined by krypton, *Acta Physiol. Scand.* **54:**325–338.

Kety, S. S., 1956, Human cerebral blood flow and oxygen consumption as related to ageing, *J. Chronic Dis.* **3:**459–477.

Kiernan, J. A., 1978, An explanation of axonal regeneration in peripheral nerves and its failure in the central nervous system, *Med. Hypoth.* **4**:15–26.

Kiernan, J. A., 1979, Hypotheses concerned with axonal regeneration in the mammalian nervous system, *Biol. Rev.* **54**:155–197.

Mann, D. M., Eaves, N., Marcyniuk, B., and Yates, P., 1986, Quantitative changes in cerebral cortical microvasculature in ageing and dementia, *Neurobiol. Aging* **7**:321–330.

Monafo, W. W., Eliason, S., Shimazaki, S., and Sugimoto, H., 1988, Regional blood flow in resting and stimulated sciatic nerve of diabetic rats, *Exp. Neurol.* **99**:607–614.

Pearson, J., Goldstein, M., Markey, K., and Brandeis, L., 1983, Human brainstem catecholamine neuronal anatomy as indicated by immunocytochemistry with antibodies to tyrosine hydroxylase, *Neuroscience* **8**:3–32.

Powell, H. C., Longo, F., LeBeau, J., Myers, R., 1986, Abnormal nerve regeneration in galactose neuropathy, *J. Neuropathol. Exp. Neurol.* **45**:151–160.

Ravens, J. R., 1978, Vascular changes in the human senile brain, in: *Pathology of Cerebrospinal Microcirculation* (J. Cervos-Navarro, ed.), Raven, New York, pp. 487–501.

Sakurada, O., Kennedy, C., Jehle, J., Brown, J., Carbin, G., and Sokoloff, L., 1978, Measurement of local cerebral blood flow with iodo (14-C) antipyrine, *Am. J. Physiol.* **234**:H59–H66.

Schneider, H., and Dralle, J., 1973, Ultrastructural changes in the rat spinal cord after temporary occlusion of the thoracic aorta, Acta Neuropath. **26**:301–306.

Sharbrough, F. W., Messick, J., and Sundt, T., 1973, Correlation of cortical electroencephalograms with cerebral blood flow measurements during carotid endarterectomy, *Stroke* **4**:674–693.

Sokoloff, L., 1966, Cerebral circulatory and metabolic changes associated with aging, in: *Cerebrovascular Disease* (C. Milikan, ed.), Williams & Wilkins, Baltimore, pp. 237–251.

Sternberger, L. A., 1986, *Immunoctyochemistry,* Wiley, New York.

Tamura, A., Asano, T., and Sano, K., 1980, Correlation between CBF and histologic changes following temporary middle cerebral artery occlusion, *Stroke* **11**:487–493.

Tuck, R. R., and Low, P. A., 1984, Endoneurial blood flow and oxygen tension in the sciatic nerves of rats with experimental diabetic neuropathy, *Brain* **107**:935–950.

Worm-Petersen, J., and Pakkenberg, H., 1968, Atherosclerosis of cerebral arteries, pathological and clinical correlates, *J. Gerontol.* **23**:445–449.

Youmans, J. R., and Albrand, O. W., 1973, Cerebral blood flow in clinical problems, in: *Neurological Surgery* (J. R. Youmans, ed.), W. B. Saunders, Philadelphia, pp. 651–697.

47

Free and Bound Polyamines in Normal and Alzheimer Temporal Cortex

PETER J. ANDERSON

1. INTRODUCTION

The polyamines putrescine, spermidine, and spermine are low-molecular-weight polycations that are abundant constituents of all eukaryotic cells, including those of the central nervous system (CNS) (Scalabrino *et al.*, 1985; Shaw, 1979). Although they are present in highly regulated concentrations approaching millimolar, and changes in levels are associated with growth, neoplasia, and differentiation (Hougaard *et al.*, 1986), the biological function of polyamines is unknown. A role in cell secretory processes has been suggested (Hougaard *et al.*, 1986; Thams *et al.*, 1986), possibly through effects on enzymes which regulate intracellular phosphorylation (Ahmed *et al.*, 1986), or through interaction with proteins of the cytoskeleton involved in motile properties (Anderson *et al.*, 1985; Oriol-Audit, 1979).

Of possible value in determining the role of polyamines in the CNS is the examination of the levels of the molecules in normal tissue and in tissue from persons with functional impediments associated with structurally altered tissue. The temporal cortex of patients diagnosed as having had Alzheimer's disease differs structurally from the temporal cortex of persons who have not had the disease (Perry, 1986). Loss of neuronal cells and the formation of abundant characteristic abnormal structures involving insoluble protein, known as senile plaques and neurofibrillary tangles, are associated with decreased levels of certain neurotransmitters in individuals with dementia. Staining with specific antibodies has implicated the cytoskeleton as part of the protein component of such structures (Wischik and Crowther, 1986).

The abnormal protein structures observed in Alzheimer's disease are believed to result from aberrant postsynthetic modification of precursor proteins (Anderton, 1987). Such structures could arise from, or be further altered by, chemical modification with polyamines. Polyamines are substrates for transglutaminases that catalyze the formation of amide bonds between the primary amino groups of polyamines and glutaminyl residues of proteins (Folk *et al.*, 1980). It has been shown that liver, kidney, and testes of rat (Beninati *et al.*, 1985) as

PETER J. ANDERSON • Department of Biochemistry, University of Ottawa, Ottawa, Ontario K1H 8M5, Canada.

well as mouse epidermal cells (Piacentini *et al.*, 1988) contain protein bound polyamines. During the early development of mice, microtubules, a component of the cytoskeleton, are substrates for transglutaminase-catalyzed modifications by polyamines leading to high-molecular-weight material (Maccioni and Arechaga, 1986). Since polyamines contain more than one free amino group, proteins can potentially be crosslinked by transglutaminases using polyamines as substrates. It has been proposed that reactions of this type may lead to the insoluble protein complexes associated with Alzheimer's disease (Selkoe *et al.*, 1982).

Free polyamines levels have been determined for normal human cerebral cortex and compared with levels in tumors of the nervous system (Harik and Sutton, 1979), and it has been found that elevated putrescine levels correlate with the degree of malignancy of astrocytomas. Whether the levels of free or bound polyamines are altered in a disease involving atrophy and abnormal proteins has not been determined. Accordingly, in the present study, free and bound polyamines were determined in postmortem temporal cortex samples from individuals with Alzheimer's disease and from controls.

2. ISOLATION, SEPARATION, AND DETERMINATION OF POLYAMINES

Slices of human temporal cortex taken at 9–20 hr postmortem and stored at −70°C before use were obtained through Dr. M. Ball, Department of Pathology, University of Western Ontario, and Dr. V. Montpetit, Department of Pathology, University of Ottawa. Samples from the Canadian Brain Tissue Bank, Toronto, Ontario, were supplied by Dr. D. Clapin, Department of Pathology, University of Ottawa. Alzheimer samples were identified as such by the University of Western Ontario Senile Dementia Study Group and by the Canadian Brain Tissue Bank.

Weighed amounts of tissue samples (0.5–1.5 g) were placed in a 10-fold excess of cold 10% (w/v) trichloroacetic acid (TCA). After the addition of 200 nmoles 3,3'-iminobispropylamine as internal standard, samples were homogenized for 30 sec using a Brinkman Polytron at one half maximum speed. The pellets obtained by centrifugation at 10,000g for 10 min were rehomogenized with an additional 5 vol 10% TCA. The supernatants were combined and designated as TCA-soluble fractions. After extraction with a 10-fold excess of diethyl ether three times, the aqueous fractions were dried on a Savant Speed Vac. Aliquots were taken for analysis after reconstitution in known volumes of 0.01 N HCl.

The TCA insoluble material was freed of acid by homogenization in 20 vol acetone. The acetone insoluble material was pelleted by centrifugation at 10,000g for 10 min. After decantation of the acetone, the pellets were allowed to air dry. The air-dried pellets were homogenized in 20 vol 8 M urea for 30 sec using the Brinkman Polytron. Insoluble material was pelleted by centrifugation at 10,000g for 20 min and subsequently homogenized in 20 vol distilled water and pelleted by centrifugation twice and finally homogenized in 20 vol acetone, pelleted, and allowed to air dry. In some cases, further extraction of pellets was carried out by homogenization in 5% sodium dodecyl sulfate (SDS) with subsequent washings with water and acetone.

Dried insoluble material was weighed (5–50 mg) and, after addition of agmatine, a polyamine not found in mammalian tissue, as internal standard, hydrolyzed in 6 N HCl for 20 hr at 106°C in sealed evacuated tubes. After removal of HCl using the Speed Vac, and reconstitution in known volumes of 0.01 N HCl, samples were taken for analysis.

Polyamine analysis was carried out on a Varian Vista 5000 Liquid Chromatograph using a Vista 401 for data analysis and a Dionex sulfonated polystyrene column, 2 mm × 40 mm for separation by gradient elution. Buffer A consisted of 0.1 M sodium citrate, pH 7.4. Buffer B contained 0.39 M sodium citrate and 1.98 M KCl, pH 5.8. After elution with buffer A for 25 min at 90°C and a flow rate of 0.2 ml/min, a gradient to 100% buffer B in 10 min was used and the temperature was increased to 98°C. After 45 min, the flow rate was increased to 0.3 ml/min and elution was carried out for an additional 30 min. Detection of polyamines was carried out by monitoring absorbance at 570 nm after postcolumn reaction of eluate with Pierce Nin Sol Reagent (Kamekura *et al.*, 1986). Under the conditions used putrescine was eluted at 62.6 min, spermidine at 84.7 min, and spermine at 116.9 min. The internal standard 3,3'-iminobispropylamine eluted at 78.9 min and agmatine at 95.0 min. Standards were prepared using polyamines purchased from Sigma Chemical Company and used to determine color constants. Under the conditions used, no other ninhydrin peaks greater than 10% that of the putrescine peak other than at the elution times given above were detected. Total primary amines were measured on an Aminco Bowman Spectrophotofluoro-meter from the 450-nm fluorescence upon excitation at 340 nm after reaction with *o*-pht-haldehyde reagent obtained from Pierce Chemical Company. The method was carried out as described (Peterson, 1983) using Pierce Amino Acid Standard and hydrolyzed bovine serum albumin (BSA) for calibration.

3. FREE POLYAMINE LEVELS

Table I shows the free polyamine content of samples from the temporal cortex of four control and four Alzheimer patients. The total amount of polyamine soluble in 10% TCA and the relative amounts of each of the three major polyamines is very similar in both the control and Alzheimer brain. In one of the controls, an elevated putrescine level was detected. This was a tissue sample from a 41-year-old man who died of an abdominal stab wound. Some brain edema was noted on autopsy. The total soluble primary amines also proved very similar in both normal and Alzheimer samples. From fluorescence measurements after reaction with *o*-phthaldelhyde relative to that of the Pierce Chemical Company Amino Acid Standard mixture, normal brain samples contained 14.6 ± 2.2 μmoles of primary amine per gram of tissue. Alzheimer samples contained 16.5 ± 1.4 μmoles of primary amine per gram of tissue. There is no statistically significant difference between samples of control brains and Alz-

TABLE I. Polyamine Content of Human Temporal Cortex Soluble in 10% Trichloroacetic Acid[a]

Subject	Total polyamine (nmoles/g tissue)	Percentage of each polyamine		
		Putrescine	Spermidine	Spermine
Normal	698.3 ± 91	10 ± 7	67 ± 4	23 ± 5
Alzheimer's disease	682.0 ± 123	5 ± 2	67 ± 4	28 ± 3

[a]Samples from four normal males (age 41, 61, 81, and 83 years) and from four Alzheimer males (aged 61, 70, 71, and 78 years) were processed in duplicate. Results are expressed as means ±SD.

heimer brains in soluble polyamine content or composition or in total soluble amine (Student's *t*-test).

4. BOUND POLYAMINE LEVELS

In all samples examined, the TCA-insoluble material still contained polyamines after extraction of the pellets with urea. Exogenous internal standard, 3,3'-iminobispropylamine, added to the samples before homogenization with TCA was not detected in the insoluble material after urea extraction. Bound polyamines were released only under conditions that result in the hydrolysis of peptide bonds. None was detected when protein samples were treated with 6 N HCl for 20 hr at room temperature. Table II summarizes the data obtained for polyamine content of hydrolysates of urea extracted TCA-insoluble material. No statistically significant difference between samples prepared from normal brain and samples from the brains of Alzheimer patients was apparent when calculated as bound polyamine per gram tissue or as bound polyamine per milligram of urea-insoluble protein. Bound polyamines represent about 2% of the total polyamine in brain and the relative proportions of bound spermidine and spermine are similar to the proportions of these polyamines in soluble form. No bound putrescine was detected by the analysis conditions used. Extraction with 5% SDS in addition to urea resulted in the solubilization of additional protein. However, the bound polyamine content of the remaining insoluble material was the same per milligram protein as urea extracted material and there was no difference between material obtained from control brains and from Alzheimer brains.

5. CONCLUSIONS

The total amount of free polyamine in human temporal cortex determined in the present study is similar to reported levels (611 nmoles/g tissue) for normal human cerebral cortex (Harik and Sutton, 1979) although the relative amount of spermidine compared with spermine is somewhat higher than that previously reported. This may be due to the advanced ages of the individuals in the present study. It has been reported that in rats, the proportion of

TABLE II. Polyamine Content of Material from Human Temporal Cortex
Insoluble in 10% Trichloroacetic Acid and 8 M Urea[a]

	Total polyamine		Percentage of each polyamine	
	nmoles/g tissue	nmoles/mg insoluble protein	Spermidine	Spermine
Normal	16.9 ± 8.1	0.86 ± 0.40	63 ± 8	37 ± 9
Alzheimer's disease	14.4 ± 2.4	0.59 ± 0.12	69 ± 1	31 ± 1

[a]Insoluble material from the samples described in Table I was hydrolyzed in 6 N HCl and polyamines released were determined. Results are expressed as means ±SD.

spermidine increases with age (Janne *et al.*, 1964), although recent studies indicate a relatively high spermine content of rat brain (Pashen *et al.*, 1987).

The finding that a fraction of polyamine remains associated with protein and can only be released by hydrolysis in 6 N HCl extends observations made on rat tissues (Beninati *et al.*, 1985). Human brain, like rat liver, kidney, and testis, contains significant amounts of spermidine and spermine bound to protein released by conditions that hydrolyze peptide bonds. The physiological significance of this is uncertain. The amount detected was, as for the free polyamines, similar in normal and Alzheimer samples of temporal cortex of human brain. The ages used in the present study ranged from 41 to 83 years. No differences were apparent when samples were examined for free and bound polyamine content as a function of age. Polyamine levels therefore appear to be highly regulated in human brain suggesting an important role in function. However, the present study does not provide any evidence that effects on proteins due to interactions with altered levels of polyamines are changed with age or accompany structural alterations found in Alzheimer's disease. The role of protein bound polyamine detected in the present study might be clarified by studies examining whether specific proteins are involved in the interactions.

REFERENCES

Ahmed, K., Goueli, S., and Willimans-Ashman, H., 1986, Mechanisms and significance of polyamine stimulation of various protein kinase reactions, *Adv. Enzyme Regul.* **25**:401–421.

Anderson, P. J., Bardocz, S., Campos, R., and Brown, D-L., 1985, The effect of polyamines on tubulin assembly, *Biochem. Biophys. Res. Commun.* **132**:147–154.

Anderton, B. H., 1987, Tangled genes and proteins, *Nature (Lond.)* **329**:106–107.

Beninati, S., Piacentini, M., Argento-Ceriv, M. P., Russo-Caia, S., and Autuori, F., 1985, Presence of di- and polyamines covalently bound to protein in rat liver, *Biochim. Biophys. Acta* **841**:120–126.

Folk, J. E., Park, M. H., Chung, S. I., Schrode, J., Lester, E. F., and Cooper, H. L., 1980, Polyamines as physiological substrates for transglutaminases, *J. Biol. Chem.* **255**:3695–3700.

Harik, S., and Sutton, C., 1979, Putrescine as a marker of malignant brain tumors, *Cancer Res.* **39**:5010–5015.

Hougaard, D., Nielsen, J., and Larsson, L-L., 1986, Polyamines in insulin producing cells, *Biochem. J.* **238**:43–47.

Janne, J., Raina, A., and Simes, M., 1964, Spermidine and spermine in rat tissues at different ages, *Acta Physiol. Scand.* **62**:352–358.

Kamekura, M., Bardocz, S., Anderson, P. J., Wallace, R., and Kushner, D. J., 1986, Polyamines in moderately and extremely halophilic bacteria, *Biochim. Biophys. Act* **880**:204–209.

Maccioni, R. B., and Arechaga, J., 1986, Transglutaminase (TG) involvement in early embryogenesis, *Exp. Cell Res.* **167**:266–270.

Oriol-Audit, C., 1979, Polyamine-induced actin polymerization, *Eur. J. Biochem.* **87**:371–376.

Pashen, W., Schmidt-Kastner, R., Djuricic, B., Meese, C., Linn, F., and Hossman, K-A., 1987, Polyamine changes in reversible cerebral ischemia, *J. Neurochem.* **49**:35–37.

Piacentini, M., Martinet, N., Beninati, S., and Folk, J. E., 1988, Free and protein-conjugated polyamines in mouse epidermal cells, *J. Biol. Chem.* **263**:3790–3794.

Perry, R. H., 1986, Recent advances in neuropathology, *Br. Med. Bull.* **42**:34–41.

Peterson, G. L., 1983, Determination of total protein, *Methods Enzymol.* **91**:95–119.

Scalabrino, G., Ferioli, M. E., and Luccarelli, G., 1985, Polyamine biosynthesis in primary tumors of human central nervous system: Review of current knowledge, *Prog. Neurobiol.* **25**:289–295.

Selkoe, D. J., Abraham, C., and Ihara, Y., 1982, Brain transglutaminase: In vitro crosslinking of human neurofilaments proteins into insoluble polymers, *Proc. Natl. Acad. Sci. USA* **79**:6070–6074.

Shaw, G. G., 1979, The polyamines in the central nervous system, *Biochem. Pharmacol.* **28**:1–6.

Thams, P., Capito, K., and Hedeskov, C., 1986, An inhibitory role for polyamines in protein kinase C activation and insulin secretion in mouse pancreatic cells, *Biochem. J.* **237**:131–138.

Wischik, C. M., and Crowther, R. A., 1986, Subunit structure of the Alzheimer tangle, *Br. Med. Bull.* **42**:51–56.

48

Neurochemical and Behavioral Effects of Bilateral Nucleus Basalis Lesions in the Aged Rat

EDWIN M. MEYER, WILLIAM J. MILLARD,
JENNIFER J. POULAKOS, and GARY W. ARENDASH

1. ALZHEIMER'S DISEASE: EARLY NEUROCHEMICAL CHANGES

Alzheimer's disease is characterized by a progressive, irreversible decline in cognition and memory (Coyle *et al.*, 1983; Whitehouse *et al.*, 1982). Its precise cause remains unknown, with aging and family background the most likely predisposing factors. Although many brain neuronal pathways are eventually rendered hypofunctional by Alzheimer's disease, only a few are consistently affected at its earliest stages. These pathways include the ascending cholinergic projections from the nucleus basalis to the cerebral cortex and from the septum to the hippocampus; the ascending noradrenergic pathway from the locus ceruleus; and cerebral cortical neurons possessing somatostatin, corticotropin-releasing factor (CRF), and neuropeptide Y (Beal *et al.*, 1986; Coyle *et al.*, 1983; Davies, 1986; and DeSouza *et al.*, 1986). One unanswered question central to understanding the etiology and potential treatment of this disease is whether reductions in the activity of these pathways cause, over a period of months or years, transsynaptic neuronal losses and neurochemical changes. We are investigating this question by studying the long-term transsynaptic effects of cholinergic hypofunction in one of the brain regions most sensitive to Alzheimer's disease: the cerebral cortex.

EDWIN M. MEYER and JENNIFER J. POULAKOS • Department of Pharmacology and Therapeutics, College of Medicine, University of Florida, Gainesville, Florida 32610.   WILLIAM J. MILLARD • Department of Pharmacodynamics, College of Pharmacy, University of Florida, Gainesville, Florida 32610.   GARY W. ARENDASH • Department of Biology, University of South Florida, Tampa, Florida 33620.

2. ANIMAL MODELS FOR CEREBRAL CORTICAL CHOLINERGIC HYPOFUNCTION

Several lines of evidence suggest that the cholinergic neurons projecting from the nucleus basalis to the cerebral cortex are particularly involved in the memory-related dysfunctions observed in Alzheimer's disease. Lesioning of this projection or infusion of a long-term cholinergic antagonist AF64A similarly interferes with passive avoidance and other memory-related behaviors in rodents (Arendash *et al.*, 1987; Bartus *et al.*, 1985, 1986; Mouton *et al.*, 1987). Treatment with the cholinergic agonist physostigmine can counteract the memory-related deficits associated with the nucleus basalis lesions, while cholinergic antagonists can mimic these deficits (Murray and Fibiger, 1985; Bartus *et al.*, 1982).

Considerable effort has been expended on developing models for cortical cholinergic hypofunction in order to ascertain both how this hypofunction affects various behavioral processes *in vivo*, as well as how these cholinergic neurons are selectively affected by Alzheimer's disease. Our laboratories have individually or together developed or further characterized several such models, including excitotoxic lesioning of neurons in the nucleus basalis (Arendash *et al.*, 1987); direct infusion into the cerebral cortex of AF64A, an irreversible acetylcholine (ACh)-synthesis inhibitor and potential cholinergic neurotoxin (Mouton *et al.*, 1987); aging itself, which we find to interfere with the calcium-triggered release of ACh (Meyer *et al.*, 1984, 1986); membrane peroxidation, which we find to mimic the effect of aging on ACh release (Meyer *et al.*, submitted); and administration of certain phospholipids such as dipalmitoylphosphatidylcholine that interfere with transmitter synthesis and release (Bottiglieri and Meyer, 1987). Each of these models has caveats and can be used only to answer selected questions that may be relevant to the etiology or treatment of age-related cholinergically associated dementias. With respect to studying transsynaptic changes following cortical cholinergic hypofunction, the only foregoing model conducive to the requisite long-term studies was the nucleus basalis-lesioned rat, since (1) AF64A-treated animals eventually recover their cortical cholinergic activity (Mouton *et al.*, 1987); (2) aged animals (particularly the rats we have been using) often do not live for extended intervals; and (3) the other treatments have so far only been characterized *in vitro*.

3. LONG-TERM EFFECTS OF NUCLEUS BASALIS LESIONS IN THE RAT

In 1987, we demonstrated several transsynaptic changes 10 months after infusing ibotenic acid bilaterally into the nucleus basalis (Arendash *et al.*, 1987). Some of the cerebral cortical changes induced by these lesions were expected of a model for Alzheimer's disease: choline acetyltransferase activity reduced by up to 40%, norepinephrine levels decreased by 18%, and Nissl-stained perikarya reduced by about 15–31%. Thus, long-term cholinergic hypofunction appeared sufficient to cause transsynaptic cell loss over extended intervals.

Yet other transsynaptic, cellular changes did not fit into a simple model for Alzheimer's disease. Levels of neuropeptide transmitters (or modulators) known to be reduced in the disease—somatostatin, neuropeptide Y, and CRF—were tremendously elevated 10 months after bilateral lesions of the nucleus basalis. More recently, we found that unilateral lesions of the nucleus basalis were not sufficient to induce these neuropeptide elevations over similar time intervals (Arendash *et al.*, submitted). Silver-staining plaquelike structures were occasionally observed in the lesioned animals but not in controls; however, unlike the well-known plaques in Alzheimer's disease, these structures had no amyloid core and were seen only rarely. Finally, silver staining of neurofibrillary structures was elevated in the cortices of lesioned animals, but there was no evidence for neurofibrillary tangles characteristic of Alzheimer's disease (Whitehouse et al., 1982).

The increased levels of neuropeptides were of particular importance to us because they were the first evidence of transsynaptic neuronal plasticity following nucleus basalis lesions that could account for the reported recovery of certain memory-related behaviors over similar 6- to 8-month extended intervals following such bilateral lesions (Bartus et al., 1985, 1986). People with Alzheimer's disease never recover memory-related behaviors and consistently present with lower cortical levels of these neuropeptides. We can only speculate at present whether the rat can compensate for cholinergic hypofunction by increasing the levels of other cortical transmitters in a manner that humans cannot. But several points should be noted: (1) the animals used in these lesion studies were young (2 months old) when lesioned, while Alzheimer's disease patients are not, and it is possible that different results may be obtained from lesioning older animals; (2) other neuronal pathways involved in Alzheimer's disease may also affect neuropeptide levels in the cerebral cortex (e.g., noradrenergic neurons); and (3) Alzheimer's disease may directly affect cortical peptidergic neurons and peptide levels in a manner that nucleus basalis lesions do not. Because of the importance of this question for understanding Alzheimer's disease, we began to investigate the first of these possibilities by measuring neuropeptide Y levels and messenger RNA (mRNA) encoding for the peptide in older animals receiving bilateral lesions of the nucleus basalis.

4. EFFECTS OF NUCLEUS BASALIS LESIONS IN OLDER RATS

Senescent rats are deficient with respect to cerebral cortical cholinergic transmission as well as memory-related behaviors associated with this transmission (Bartus et al., 1982). This age-related cholinergic deficit is at least in part due to a reduction in the release of ACh in response to depolarization-induced calcium influx. For example, we found calcium ions to be less potent in senescent nerve terminals with respect to triggering release (Meyer et al., 1986), while others demonstrated that fewer calcium ions enter the neuron during depolarization, in 24-month-old rats compared with 3- to 6-month-old animals (Peterson and Gibson, 1983). Whether these age-related changes in cholinergic transmission have transsynaptic effects on other systems that were interactive with nucleus basalis lesions is unknown. We therefore measured the effects of bilateral nucleus basalis lesions on frontal parietal neuropeptide Y levels as well as mRNA encoding this peptide in 23.5-month-old rats that had received their lesions 2.5 months previously.

4.1. Methods for Nucleus Basalis Lesion Study

Sprague-Dawley albino male rats were anesthetized with 50 mg/kg of sodium pentobarbital (IP) and then infused with two boluses of 1 μl each of 5 μg ibotenic acid in PBS, pH 7.4, into the nucleus basalis as described previously (Arendash et al., 1987). The second infusion was 0.8 mm dorsal to the first. Control rats were sham operated but received no infusions into the nucleus basalis. Following surgery, animals were returned to their individual home cages and fed semisolid mash made from Purina Rat Chow for several days. These ibotenic acid infusions effectively destroyed 85–90% of the acetylcholinesterase (AChE)-staining perikarya in the rostral nucleus basalis (Arendash et al., 1987).

In order to demonstrate that the nucleus basalis lesions affected the ascending cholinergic pathway associated with memory-related behavior, passive-avoidance behavior was measured 2.5 months postlesioning as described previously (Arendash *et al.*, 1987). The maximal latency interval allowed in this model was 300 sec.

Animals were sacrificed by decapitation after passive avoidance testing and assayed for frontal cortical choline acetyltransferase activity (Roskoski, 1973), frontal parietal cortex neuropeptide Y levels (Beal *et al.*, 1986) and mRNA for neuropeptide Y. For measurements of mRNA encoding neuropeptide Y, total cellular RNA was isolated by guanidium–isothiocyanate/phenol extraction. RNA yields were quantitated spectrophotometrically by absorption at 260 nm and the purity assessed by A260–A280 ratios; only ratios over 1.9 were used for analysis. Northern blot analyses used 5–50 μg of RNA electrophoresed on agarose/formaldehyde gels, followed by transferral to nitrocellulose (MSI 2000) and hybridization with labeled complementary (cDNA) probe generously provided by Dr. Janet Allen. This probe was generated from purified plasmid (pGEM, Promega); the 550-basepair (bp) insert was digested from the plasmid with the restriction endonuclease *Eco*RI, purified by agarose/gel electrophoresis and labeled by primer extension with labeled 32-PdCTP. This probe represented a 550-bp sequence that included the 5' untranslated region, the translated region, and the 3' untranslated region. Blots were prehybridized with 50% formamide, 5× SSC, 0.1% SDS, 5× Denhardts solution and 150 μg/ml salmon sperm DNA at 42°C for a minimum of 3 hr. Hybridization was carried out with the same stringent conditions and temperature, with a minimum of 1 million cpm of labeled neuropeptide Y probe per ml of hybridization buffer. Blots were washed with 2× SSC, 0.1% sodium dodecyl sulfate (SDS) for 30 min at room temperature and for 30 min at 60°C, and then with two changes of 0.2× SSC, 0.1% SDS for another hour. Blots were exposed to Kodak XAR-5 X-ray film for 1–5 days with Cronex lighting plus intensifying screens at −70°C. The intensity of the hybridizing siginals was quantitated by scanning laser densitometry.

4.2. Results and Discussion

Passive-avoidance behavior was compromised in lesioned animals as compared with controls 24 hr (sham latency intervals = 300 ± 0 sec, mean ± SEM; lesioned values = 79 ± 38 sec) but not 48 hr after initial training (sham latency values = 300 ± 0 sec; lesioned values = 226 ± 48 sec). These results are similar to those observed in young adult rats, except that there may be more recovery by 48 hr in the older lesioned animals than in the younger ones (not shown).

Nucleus basalis lesions reduced choline acetyltransferase activity to 61 ± 6% of sham-operated control values, demonstrating that the nucleus basalis lesions reduced ascending cholinergic activity. As seen with young adult rats, bilateral nucleus basalis lesions had no effect on neuropeptide Y levels 2.5 months postlesioning in aged rats (sham: 401 ± 90 pg/mg wet weight versus lesioned: 423 ± 61 pg/mg wet weight), suggesting at least that aging did not accentuate the elevation in peptide levels. However, preliminary analysis of four rats indicated that mRNA encoding neuropeptide Y was decreased by about 25% in the lesioned parietal cortices compared to controls. It therefore appears that mRNA levels may decrease prior to elevations in the peptide itself. Further studies at more protracted intervals postlesioning are clearly needed in these animals, and these are being conducted currently.

How might changes in cholinergic activity affect mRNA synthesis encoding neuropeptide Y and to what extent could this phenomenon account for lesion-induced elevations in somatostatin and CRF reported previously? The synthesis of mRNA encoding for both neuropeptide Y and somatostatin has been found to be stimulated by cyclic AMP or drugs (e.g., forskolin) that elevate the levels of this cyclic nucleotide (Higuchi and Sabol, 1987; Montminy and Bilezikjian, 1987). Since cholinergic muscarinic receptors coupled to adenylate cyclase in the cerebral cortex are generally inhibitory (Olianas *et al.*, 1983), a reduction in ascending cholinergic activity would be likely to elevate adenylate cyclase activity over time. This elevation in adenylate cyclase activity could, over extended intervals, allow for sufficient activation of mRNA synthesis that the levels of the peptides would gradually accumulate. Alternatively, other second messengers such as PI-turnover may account for the reduction in mRNA encoding for neuropeptide$_y$ observed at earlier, 1-month intervals. This model is testable and is currently under investigation in our laboratories.

REFERENCES

Arendash, G. W., Millard, W. J., Dunn, A. J., and Meyer, E. M., 1987, Long term neuropathological and chemical changes after lesions of the rat nucleus basalis magnocellularis, *Science* **238**:952–956.

Arendash, G. W., Millard, W. J., Dawson, R., Dunn, A. J., and Meyer, E. M., Different long term neurochemical effects of unilateral and bilateral lesions of the rat nucleus basalis, *Neurochem. Res.* (in press).

Bartus, R. T., Dean, R. L., Beer, B., and Lippa, A. S., 1982, The cholinergic hypothesis of geriatric memory dysfunction, *Science* **217**:408–417.

Bartus, R. T., Flicker, C., Dean, R. L., Pontecorvo, M., Figueiredo, J. C., and Fisher, S. K., 1985, Selective memory loss following nucleus basalis lesions: Long term behavioral recovery despite persistent cholinergic deficiencies, *Pharmacol. Biochem. Behav.* **23**:125–135.

Bartus, R. T., Pontecorvo, M. J., Flicker, C., Dean, R. L., and Figueiedo, J. C., 1986, Behavioral recovery following bilateral lesions of the nucleus basalis does not occur spontaneously, *Pharmacol. Biochem. Behav.* **24**:1287–1292.

Beal, M. F., Mazurek, M. F., Chattha, G. K., Svendsen, C. V., Bird, E. D., and Martin, J. B., 1986, Neuropeptide Y immunoreactivity is reduced in cerebral cortex in Alzheimer's disease, *Ann. Neurol.* **20**:282–289.

Bottiglieri, D. F., and Meyer, E. M., Dipalmitoylphosphatidylcholine liposomes inhibit calcium dependent acetylcholine release, *Neurochem. Res.* **12**:739–744.

Coyle, J. T., Price, D. L., and Delong, M. R., 1983, Alzheimer's disease: A disorder of cortical cholinergic innervation, *Science* **219**:1184–1190.

Davies, P., 1986, Cholinergic and somatostatin deficits in Alzheimer's disease, in: *Treatment Development Strategies for Alzheimer's Disease* (T. Crook, R. Bartus, S. Ferris, and S. Gershon, eds.), Mark Powley Associates, Madison, Connecticut, pp. 385–420.

DeSouza, E. B., Whitehouse, P. J., Kuhar, M. J., Price, D. L., and Vale, W. W., 1986, Reciprocal changes in corticotropin releasing factor (CRF)-like immunoreactivity and CRF receptors in cerebral cortex of Alzheimer's disease, *Nature (Lond.)* **319**:593–595.

Higuchi, H., and Sabol, S. L., 1987, Rat neuropeptide Y precursor mRNA: Characterization, tissue distribution, and regulation by glucocorticoids, cyclic AMP, calcium and NGF, in: *Seventeenth Annual Society for Neurosciences*, abst. 357.12, vol. 13, p. 1286.

Meyer, E. M., and Judkins, J. J., in press, Effects of membrane peroxidation on the release of acetylcholine from rat cerebral cortical synaptosomes, *J. Neuro Chem. Res.*

Meyer, E. M., St. Onge, E., and Crews, F. T., 1984, Effects of aging on rat cortical presynaptic cholinergic processes, *Neurobiol. Aging* **5**:315–317.

Meyer, E. M., Crews, F. T., Otero, D. H., and Larsen, K., 1986, Aging decreases the sensitivity of rat cortical synaptosomes to calcium ionophore-induced acetylcholine release, *J. Neurochem.* **47**:1244–1246.

Montminy, M. R., and Bilezikjian, L. M., 1987, Binding of a nuclear protein to the cyclic AMP response element of the somatostatin gene, *Nature(Lond.)* **328:**175–178.

Mouton, P. R., Meyer, E. M., Dunn, A. J., Millard, W. J., and Arendash, G. W., 1987, Induction of cortical cholinergic hypofunction and memory retention deficits through intracortical AF64A infusions, *Brain Res.* **444:**104–118.

Murray, C. L., and Fibiger, H. C., 1985, Learning and memory deficits after lesions of the nucleus basalis magnocellularis: Reversal by physostigmine, *Neuroscience* **14:**1025–1032.

Olianas, M. C., Onali, P., Neff, N. H., and Costa, E., 1983, Adenylate cyclase activity of synaptic membranes from rat striatum: Inhibition by muscarinic agonists, *Mol. Pharmacol.* **23:**393–398.

Peterson, C., and Gibson, G. E., 1983, Aging and 3,4-diaminopyridine alter synaptosomal calcium uptake, *J. Biol. Chem.* **258:**11482–11486.

Roskoski, R., 1973, Choline acetyltransferase. Evidence for an acetylenzyme reaction intermediate, *Biochemistry* **12:**3709–3713.

Whitehouse, P. J., Price, D. L., Struble, R. G., Clark, A. W., Coyle, J. T., and Delong, M. R., 1982, Alzheimer's disease and senile dementia: Loss of neurons in the basal forebrain, *Science* **215:** 1237–1239.

49

Dopaminergic Neurons in the Substantia Nigra in Normal Aging and MPTP-Lesioned Mice

MADI GUPTA and BHUPENDRA KISHORE GUPTA

1. INTRODUCTION

Parkinson's disease is a slowly progressive neurodegenerative disorder that seldom occurs in patients below the age of 60. Its incidence increases with age, but the cause remains unknown. Typically, the disease is characterized by decreased dopamine levels in the striatum and a loss of pigmented dopamine nerve cells in the substantia nigra pars compacta. 1-Methyl-4-phenyl-1,2,3,6-tetrahydropyridine (MPTP) is a commercially available compound that has been illicitly used as a new type of heroin (Langston *et al.*, 1983). Many users developed a Parkinson-like disorder with bradykinesia, rigidity, tremor, flexed posture, loss of postural reflexes, mutism, and drooling following intravenous (IV) administration of MPTP (Davis *et al.*, 1979; Langston *et al.*, 1983; Langston and Ballard, 1985). Since then, MPTP has been shown to produce parkinsonian symptoms and neuropathology of the nigrostriatal dopamine system in nonhuman primates as well as in mice (Burns *et al.*, 1983; Langston *et al.*, 1985; Heikkila *et al.*, 1984; Gupta *et al.*, 1984–1986).

In humans, dopamine levels in the striatum decrease with age (Carlsson and Winblad, 1976). McGeer *et al.* (1977) showed that neurons of the substantia nigra diminish in number with age. Our previous studies have shown that young adult male Swiss–Webster mice treated with MPTP have a reduced number of fluorescent neurons in the substantia nigra pars compacta and a reduced intensity of fluorescence in the remaining dopaminergic cell bodies (Gupta *et al.*, 1984). Furthermore, when aged male C57BL/6 mice were treated with MPTP, these animals showed marked motor dysfunction characterized by a striking paucity of movements, stiffness of hind limbs, and an initial resting tremor of the whole body. MPTP administration to the young adult mice in a similar manner produced transient slowing of motor activity that quickly recovered.

MADI GUPTA and BHUPENDRA KISHORE GUPTA • Department of Anatomical Sciences and Neurobiology, University of Louisville School of Medicine, Louisville, Kentucky 40292.

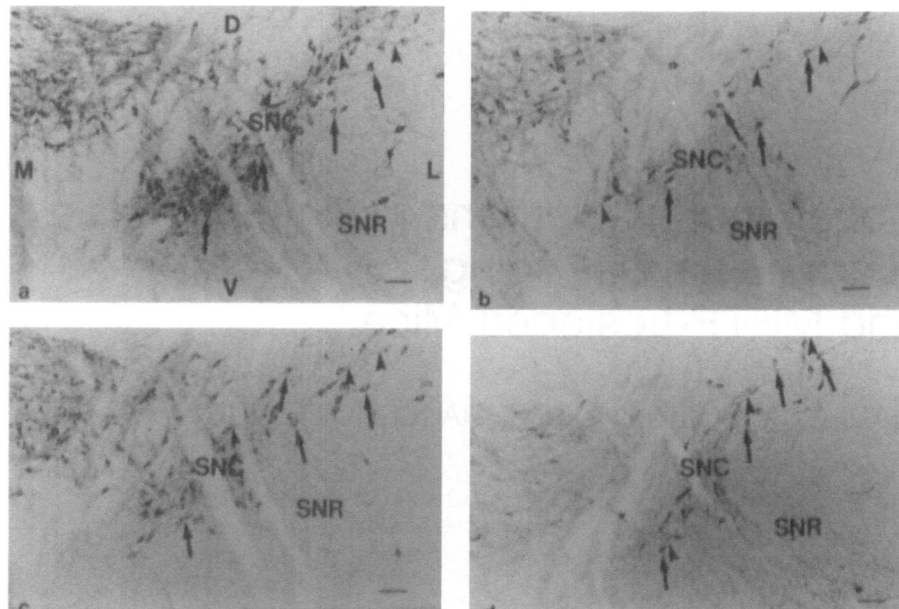

FIGURE 1. Bright-field composite of sections through the substantia nigra stained immunocytochemically for tyrosine hydroxylase (TH). Note the presence of TH-immunoreactive neurons (arrows) and processes (arrowheads). (a) Section from a control young adult mouse. (b) Section from MPTP-treated young adult mouse. (c) Control 21-month-old mouse. (d) MPTP-treated 21-month-old mouse. Note the presence of a reduced number of TH-positive cell bodies in the MPTP-treated young adult (b) and 21-month-old (d) mice compared with their age-matched controls. SNC, substantia nigra pars compacta; SNR, substantia nigra pars reticulata; M, medial; L, lateral; D, dorsal; V, ventral. Bars = 1 mm.

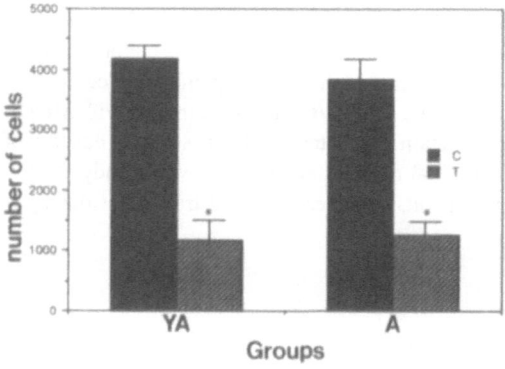

FIGURE 2. Histogram showing the mean number (mean ± SE) of TH-immunoreactive cells in control (C) and MPTP-treated (T) young adult (YA) and aged (A) mice. Asterisk (*) designates statistically significant difference ($p < 0.01$) from controls.

Neuroanatomical studies using fluorescence histochemistry revealed a decreased number of fluorescent cell bodies in the substantia nigra pars compacta in both young adults and aged MPTP-treated mice (Gupta *et al.*, 1986). In aged mice, yellow autofluorescent pigment was present in cells of the substantia nigra pars compacta in both the control and MPTP-treated mice. The present studies were undertaken to investigate whether these severe physical symptoms seen in the aged mice with MPTP treatment were due to a more severe damage to the nigrostriatal system as compared with young adults.

Male C57BL/6 mice at approximately 3 months and 21 months of age were treated with MPTP three times a day 4 hr apart, 16 hr recovery, followed by three more injections 4 hr apart. Control animals received vehicle alone. Treated and control mice at both age groups were sacrificed 3 days after the last injection. Animals were anesthetized with chloropent and perfused intracardially with saline followed by 4% paraformaldehyde and 1.5% sucrose in phosphate buffer (pH 7.4). Brains were dissected out, after which frozen 40-μm-thick serial sections were cut through the substantia nigra. Alternate sections were stained immunocytochemically for tyrosine hydroxylase (TH) using modified Sternberger method (Gupta *et al.*, 1987). The number of TH-immunoreactive neurons was determined in all four groups of animals.

Our results demonstrate a statistically significant decrease ($p < 0.01$) in the number of tyrosine hydroxylase-positive neurons in the substantia nigra in the MPTP-treated young adult and aged mice (Fig. 1). Quantitative analysis of TH-immunoreactive cell counts did not reveal any significant decrease in the number of cells between the young and aged control mice. Furthermore, the number of TH-positive neurons in the substantia nigra was affected equally in both young adult and aged mice (Fig. 2).

These studies demonstrate that MPTP affects the dopamine neurons in both young adult and aged mice. Although the MPTP-treated aged mice displayed more severe behavioral symptoms than did the young adults, the nigrostriatal dopamine system seems to be affected equally in both treated groups. This could be because additional monoaminergic systems are affected in MPTP-treated aged mice (Gupta *et al.*, 1986). This is in agreement with the study of MPTP effects on dopamine turnover and transport function in the striatum of aged mice (Sershan *et al.*, 1985) and more severe effects of MPTP on monoaminergic systems in aged monkeys compared with young adult monkeys (Forno *et al.*, 1986). The effects on these additional monoaminergic systems in aged mice treated with MPTP might lead to more severe behavioral deficits. The reason for the more severe damage in the aged mice could be due to an increased conversion of MPTP to MPP+ through MAO-B. It was reported previously that aged animals have increased MAO activity in the brain (Benedetti and Keane, 1980) and decreased catecholamines in the brain (Knoll *et al.*, 1981). When MPTP treatment is superimposed on the normal age-related decline in catecholamines, the MPTP effects become much more severe because of a large depletion of dopamine. It has already been reported that, in humans, there is an approximately 80% decline of dopamine in the brain before physical symptoms become evident in patients with idiopathic Parkinson's disease. Further studies are in progress to investigate these possibilities.

ACKNOWLEDGMENTS. This work was supported by grants RO3 MH41435 and R29 NS24291 (to M.G.) by the U. S. Public Health Service. The authors thank Rebecca Brown for technical assistance.

REFERENCES

Benedetti, M. S., and Keane, P. E., 1980, Differential changes in monoamine oxidase A and B activity in the aging rat brain, *J. Neurochem.* **35:**1026–1032.

Burns, R. S., Chiueh, C. C., Markey, S. P., Ebert, M. H., Jacobowitz, D. M., and Kopin, I. J., 1983, A primate model of Parkinsonism—Selective destruction of dopaminergic neurons in the pars compacta of the substantia nigra by MPTP, *Proc. Natl. Acad. Sci. USA* **80:**4546–4550.

Carlsson, A., and Winblad, B., 1976, Influence of age and time interval between death and autopsy on dopamine and 3-methoxytyramine levels in human basal ganglia, *J. Neural Transm.* **38:**271–276.

Davis, G. C., Williams, A. C., Markey, S. P., Ebert, M. H., Caine, E. D., Reichert, C. M., and Kopin, I. J., 1979, Chronic Parkinsonism secondary to intravenous injection of meperidine analogues, *Psychiatry Res.* **1:**249–254.

Finch, C. E., 1973, Catecholamine metabolism in the brains of aging male mice, *Brain Res.* **52:**261–276.

Gupta, M., Felten, D. L., and Gash, D. M., 1984, MPTP alters central catecholamine neurons in addition to the nigrostriatal system, *Brain Res. Bull.* **13:**737–742.

Gupta, M., Felten, D. L., and Felten, S. Y., 1985, MPTP alters monoamine levels in systems other than the nigrostriatal dopaminergic system in mice, in: *MPTP—A Neurotoxin Producing a Parkinsonian Syndrome* (S. P. Markey, N. Castagnoli, Jr., A. J. Trevor, and I. J. Kopin, eds.), Academic, Orlando, Florida, pp. 399–402.

Gupta, M., Gupta, B. K., Thomas, R., Bruemmer, V., Sladek, J. R., Jr., and Felten, D. L., 1986, Aged mice are more sensitive to MPTP treatment than young adults, *Neurosci. Lett.* **70:**326–331.

Gupta, M., Felten, D. L., and Ghetti, B., 1987, Selective loss of monoaminergic neurons in weaver mutant mice—An immunocytochemical study, *Brain Res.* **402:**379–382.

Heikkila, R. E., Hess, A., and Duvoisin, R. C., 1984, Dopaminergic neurotoxicity of MPTP in mice, *Science* **224:**1451–1453.

Langston, J. W., and Ballard, P., 1985, Parkinsonism induced by MPTP: Implications for treatment and the pathogenesis of Parkinson's disease, *Can. J. Neurol. Sci.* **11:**160–165.

Langston, J. W., Ballard, P., Tetrud, J., and Irwin, I., 1983, Chronic Parkinsonism in humans due to a product of meperidine analog synthesis, *Science* **219:**979–980.

Langston, J. W., Langston, E. B., and Irwin, I., 1985, MPTP induced Parkinsonism in human and non-human primates—Clinical and experimental aspects, *Acta Neurol. Scand.* **70**(suppl. 100):49–54.

McGeer, P. L., McGeer, E. G., and Suzuki, J. A., 1977, Aging and extrapyramidal function, *Arch. Neurol.* **34:**33–35.

Synaptic Plasticity and Aging

CARL W. COTMAN and CHRISTINE PETERSON

1. INTRODUCTION

Why do certain individuals age successfully? Some elderly subjects perform within the range for normal adult subjects (e.g., age successfully), while others show dramatic losses on various tests of cognitive performance. These deviations may be precipitated by illness or environmental factors rather than by the aging process. In addition to variations in heredity, different life-styles can either enhance or compromise vitality. Heterogeneity within the aged population increases in nearly all aging studies. Until recently, individual variability with respect to physiological or behavioral measures has been ignored. Thus, heterogeneity within the elderly population may be an inherent characteristic that needs to be addressed.

Recent neurochemical studies with animal models, and even humans, suggest that many functions are preserved with aging. This contradicts the prediction that aging is associated with a progressive loss of function until death. Some aged individuals show fewer deficits. Thus, these individuals may possess better adaptive mechanisms to compensate for any losses and thereby preserve key functions.

A new and exciting area of basic research is the identification and modification of the molecular and cellular events that underlie successful aging. Studies are needed to determine more precisely the mechanisms by which the brain normally maintains and repairs itself. Some of the same events that participate in normal brain maintenance and plasticity also operate in age-related neurodegenerative disease, such as Alzheimer's disease.

2. SYNAPSE REPLACEMENT FOLLOWING NEURONAL LOSS

When neurons are lost, the surviving neurons can replace old synapses with new synapses. It is becoming increasingly clear that neuronal loss in the aged brain is less severe than previously thought (see Chapter 42, *this volume*). Nonetheless, neuronal loss can and does occur in the healthy aged brain and in the course of age-related neurodegenerative diseases.

CARL W. COTMAN • Departments of Psychobiology, Neurology, and Psychiatry, University of California–Irvine, Irvine, California 92717.   CHRISTINE PETERSON • Department of Psychobiology, University of California–Irvine, Irvine, California 92717.

For years, it was believed that the adult central nervous system (CNS) was incapable of growth or repair. However, during the past several years, it has become clear that this is no longer true. With the proper stimulus, the brain can rewire its damaged circuitry (e.g., synaptic plasticity). The stimulus may be an injury (e.g., trauma) or a metabolic insult (e.g., low oxygen), or a subtle modification in behavior (e.g., learning a new task), or it may be physical (e.g., graft of neural tissue) or chemical (e.g., neurotrophic factor) (for review, see Cotman *et al.*, 1987). Synapse turnover (e.g., reactive synaptogenesis) is a stimulus-induced loss and replacement of synapses that is not part of the normal developmental process. In several brain regions, sprouting and concurrent synapse turnover appear to be ongoing processes that occur in the absence of injury. Axon sprouting refers to regrowth of un-damaged neurons, whereas regeneration refers to growth of damaged axons and their normal targets.

When some of the input to a neuron or group of neurons is lost, the nerve fibers from undamaged neurons often sprout and form new connections to replace lost ones (Fig. 1). This phenomenon, known as *axon sprouting,* was first described during the 1950s. When pe-ripheral nerve fibers are cut, the remaining ones sprout new branches that connect to the muscle and form new synapses to replace those that are lost (Edds, 1953; Hoffman, 1950). Such synaptic regrowth and replacement is widespread and occurs in both the peripheral and central nervous systems (for review, see Cotman *et al.*, 1981). Understanding the mecha-nisms that underlie neural regeneration in animal models will help us to develop strategies for treating the changes that occur in the aged human CNS.

The phenomenon of sprouting and its robustness can be illustrated by damage to an area of the rodent cerebral cortex (e.g., the entorhinal cortex). The entorhinal cortex provides the major input to the dentate gyrus and terminates in the outer two thirds of the dentate molecular layer. Unilateral ablation of the entorhinal cortex reduces the number of synapses by 80% in the outer molecular layer of the hippocampus. This loss is transient, however, and, over a period of a few weeks, the synapses are replaced (for review, see Cotman and Nieto-Sampedro, 1984; Nieto-Sampedro and Cotman, 1985). After damage, synapse replacement in the mature brain can be virtually complete in the mature brain (Hoff *et al.*, 1982).

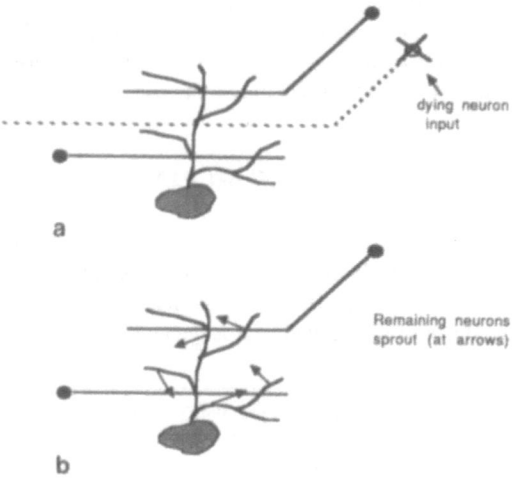

FIGURE 1. Axonal sprouting and re-active synaptogenesis. (a) When neu-rons degenerate (———), the remaining neurons sprout (arrows) to make new connections to replace the lost ones. (b) Time course for the replacement of new synapses in the rodent brain after an entorhinal lesion. (Data from Hoff *et al.*, 1982.)

3. REPLACEMENT OF DAMAGED SYNAPSES IN AGED BRAIN

The aged brain can replace damaged synapses. Reactive synaptogenesis may play an important role during aging, in which the consequences of neuronal death accumulate over a life span, and neurodegenerative diseases are more common. The aged rodent brain demonstrates a remarkable capacity for sprouting and synaptogenesis (for review, see Cotman and Anderson, 1988). Although reinnervation is delayed in aged compared with young animals, eventually the process is as complete. The slower rate of synapse replacement in the aged brain may be due to an inability to remove degenerative debris from the neuropil as rapidly as the young brain. Recent evidence indicates that microglia may play a role in clearing debris (Vijayan and Cotman, 1987). Microglia are inhibited by elevated levels of circulating hormones that are characteristic of aging (Sapolsky et al., 1985) and may play a role in the slower regeneration. Alternatively, the growth-promoting mechanisms may also be reduced.

4. REPLACEMENT OF DAMAGED SYNAPSES IN DISEASED BRAIN

The brain can also replace its synapses during neurodegenerative diseases. Does the brain of a patient with Alzheimer's disease grow new fibers and form new connections? Animal models have helped predict the changes that occur in the human CNS following injury. Experimental evidence derived from research on regenerative growth led to the demonstration of such growth in the Alzheimer's disease brain (for review, see Cotman and Anderson, 1988).

A consistent feature of Alzheimer's disease is the degeneration of selected areas of the limbic system. Alzheimer's disease is accompanied by a loss of large neurons in specific regions of the cerebral cortex (e.g., layer II stellate cells in the entorhinal cortex) and of the pyramidal cells of the hippocampus (Hyman et al., 1984). These findings suggest that Alzheimer's disease is characterized by a selective loss of the major source of input to the hippocampus, a critical brain area for memory processing.

The cholinergic input to the hippocampus appears to facilitate function. Does the cholinergic input to the human hippocampus regenerate after loss of entorhinal neurons in Alzheimer's disease? In some Alzheimer's patients, acetylcholinesterase (AChE)-positive fibers sprout in the hippocampus, even though the cholinergic input to the hippocampus is relatively intact (Geddes et al., 1985). Sprouting generally occurs in areas (e.g., outer molecular layer of the dentate gyrus) in which the cortical input is lost. Similar to the rodent brain, AChE intensification is also seen in the outer molecular layer of the dentate gyrus, corresponding to the zone of perforant path deafferentation. Sprouting may eventually contribute to senile plaque formation, since numerous cholinergic senile plaques are usually seen in areas in which sprouting occurs. The commissural–associational fibers also appear to sprout in the Alzheimer brain, as evidenced by expansion of kainic acid receptor binding (Geddes et al., 1985). Thus, sprouting in the Alzheimer brain may be a natural compensatory mechanism that eventually leads to pathology.

Generally, disease-induced neuronal loss in the entorhinal cortex stimulates regeneration similar to that of an entorhinal lesion in the rat brain. The selective loss of entorhinal neurons removes the perforant path input to the hippocampus and induces a compensatory response from adjacent (e.g., commissural–associational system and septal) inputs. The observed

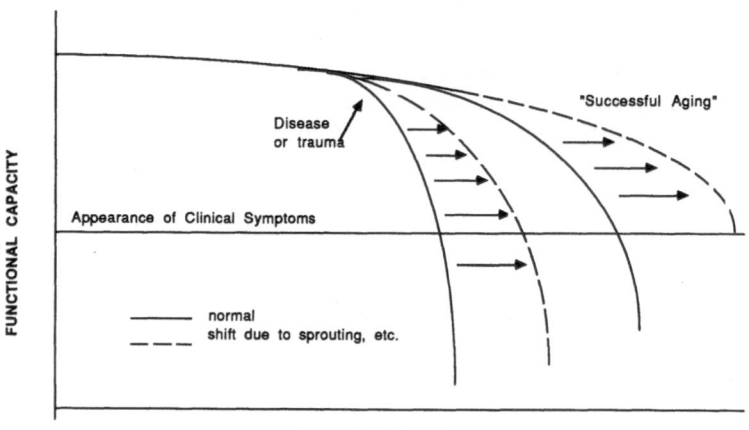

FIGURE 2. Role of synaptic plasticity in normal aging and after injury. As individuals age, their functional capacity (e.g., behavioral, neurochemical) begins to decline slowly, until it reaches a point where deficits can become apparent. The aged brain, however, still makes minor repairs that delay the appearance of functional deficits. Elderly individuals who retain this repair capacity age successfully. Certain diseases or trauma lead to an early decline in function; even so, the aged brain can still repair itself, although eventually even this is ineffective.

expansion of the kainic acid receptor field and the increased AChE activity contrasts with the numerous deficits in transmitter-related parameters in Alzheimer's disease.

Reactive growth can maintain function if a portion of the relay remains intact. Cholinergic input facilitates hippocampal function by inhibition of a calcium-dependent potassium current that increases excitability of hippocampal neurons (Nicoll, 1985; Brown, 1988). As cells are lost, new connections are made by the remaining healthy neurons that assume similar functions of the fibers from the same or converging pathways and may even amplify weakened signals (see Cotman and Anderson, 1988). Thus, following entorhinal damage, the increased cholinergic input may improve hippocampal function. Commisural–associational fibers form a recurrent loop to dentate granule cells; thus, sprouting in this region may amplify signals passing through this relay. Thus, the threshold at which functions appear impaired may be delayed. This maintains functional stability despite cell loss (Fig. 2). As the system continues to compensate, however, it may become progressively more unreliable and unstable.

5. NEUROTROPHIC FACTORS AND NATURAL GROWTH PROCESSES OF BRAIN

Growth factors (neurotrophic factors) are involved in the natural growth processes of the brain. In the developing, mature, and aged nervous system, the trophic support of neurons depends on a special class of chemicals, termed neurotrophic factors. These proteins are essential for the maintenance, survival, and growth of neurons. Some neurotrophic factors are specific to the nervous system but others may interact with non-neural tissues. Elimination of neurotrophic factor-synthesizing target cells, even during development, may deprive neurons of their trophic support, which may lead to a reduction and eventual degeneration of the remaining cells.

Injury induces neurotrophic factor production in the CNS (Nieto-Sampedro *et al.*, 1982, 1983; Cotman and Nieto-Sampedro, 1984) (Fig. 3). These factors may promote sprouting and help repair damaged neurons. After sustaining trauma in the developing, mature, or aged rodent brain, both tissue extracts and fluid around the injury site show increased amounts of neurotrophic factor activity. Maximal levels of trophic activity were found in the neonate; the adult and aged animals contained decreasing amounts. These injury-induced factors probably participate in axon promoting, dendritic sprouting, and even repairing degenerating neurons (for review, see Nieto-Sampedro and Cotman, 1985).

Recent evidence demonstrates that the administration of purified growth factors can retard degeneration. When cholinergic neurons that project to the hippocampus are cut, these neurons atrophy and die over a period of 1–2 weeks. Administration of nerve growth factor (Williams *et al.*, 1986) or of fibroblast growth factor (Anderson *et al.*, 1988), however, retards this degeneration. Fibroblast growth factor administered several hours postinjury still

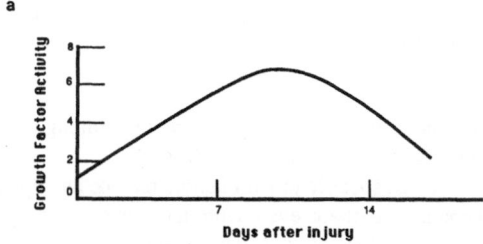

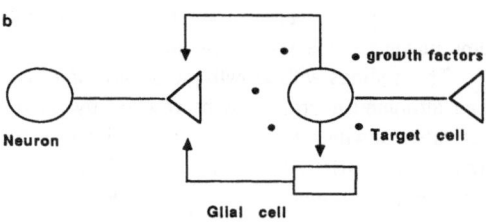

FIGURE 3. Injury-induced growth factor production. (a) After injury, the activity of specific neurotrophic factors increases over the first several days, until it reaches a peak 1–2 weeks later. (b) Growth factors produced by target neurons (or possibly glia) are transported to the cell body, where they provide trophic support. (c) After injury, growth factor production by target cells is increased.

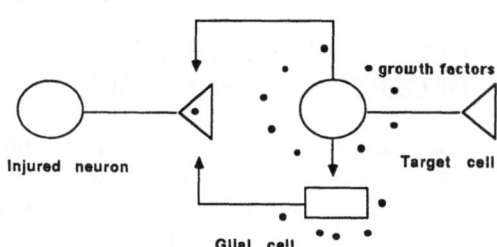

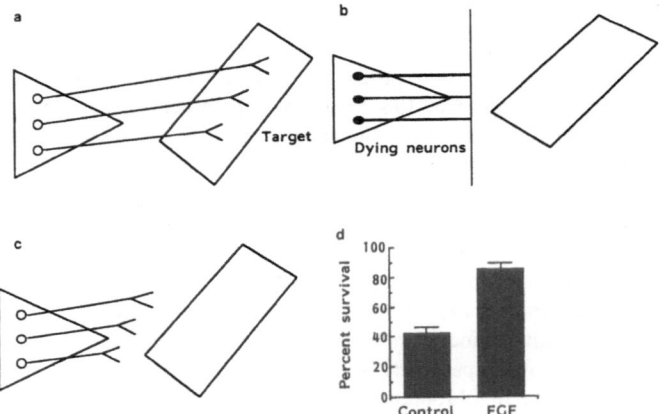

FIGURE 4. Fibroblast growth factor prevents neuronal degeneration. (a) Target cells produce trophic factors. (b) Immediately after injury, trophic support declines and neurons begin to degenerate. (c) Administration of trophic substances, such as fibroblast growth factor, diminishes neuronal degeneration. (d) Neuronal survival after fibroblast growth factor treatment in fimbria fornix-lesioned rats.

prevents neuronal loss and/or atrophy, although its effectiveness after injury diminishes with time (Anderson *et al.*, 1988) (Fig. 4).

Thus, specific growth factors may be an appropriate therapy to minimize injury-induced damage or perhaps even neuronal atrophy with age. Since this injury-induced trophic factor production does not develop immediately, supplying factors earlier may improve their therapeutic effectiveness. Recent data suggest that continuous infusion of nerve growth factor into the brains of aged memory-impaired rats improves behavioral function on a spatial memory task (Fischer *et al.*, 1987). Furthermore, cholinergic neurons in nerve growth factor-treated rats were shown to be larger than in untreated controls. It appears that by acting on the septal cholinergic system, nerve growth factor may improve septohippocampal function in much the same manner as a septal transplant.

The findings with growth factors are significant because they illustrate that damaged or even atrophied neurons can be rescued by pharmacological intervention. Although these factors work within the brain, they are large molecules that are unable to cross the blood–brain barrier (BBB). Thus, they cannot be administered orally or intravenously. Techniques (e.g., drugs or other stimuli) are needed to increase the endogenous production of neurotrophic factors.

6. ROLE OF NEUROTRANSMITTER (*N*-METHYL-D-ASPARTATE) RECEPTORS IN PLASTICITY VERSUS PATHOLOGY

The functional state of the aged brain probably reflects a balance between age-related loss and compensatory mechanisms. It has become increasingly clear that the *N*-methyl-D-aspartate (NMDA) receptor at excitatory pathways plays a pivotal role in maintaining this balance. During development, NMDA receptors participate in directing growth, so that the most active pathways form the most synapses. In the adult or aged brain, NMDA receptors appear to encode particular stimulus patterns at highly adaptive pathways. For example, high-frequency stimulation of NMDA receptors produces a long-lasting increase or potentiation (e.g., long-term potentiation) of synaptic transmission. Ironically, however, their overactivation (such as in seizures, stroke, or vascular insult) can also lead to neuronal injury. NMDA receptor activation increases intracellular calcium (MacDermott *et al.*, 1986), and elevated calcium concentrations can be toxic to neurons. Thus, there is a fine balance between the activation of NMDA receptors for highly integrated functions and that which produces cell damage.

Curiously, in the aged brain, glutamate binding to NMDA receptors decreases, particularly in several specific and highly adaptive brain regions. This would reduce their integrative and storage capacity but would help minimize the damage due to toxicity in those same areas. Many aspects of Alzheimer's disease appear to be related to accelerated aging. In Alzheimer's disease, NMDA receptors appear to be preserved (Geddes *et al.*, 1986), which suggests that there may be a disease-related compensation relative to the accelerated aging. This would in principle help function but would also make the Alzheimer brain more vulnerable to excitotoxic injury associated with excessive receptor activation.

7. BEHAVIORAL FUNCTION IN THE ELDERLY

At a behavioral level, function in the elderly is either adequate, inadequate, or even improved, depending on the task and the individual. Proper integration of brain chemistry is ultimately expressed as behavior. A detailed discussion can be found elsewhere (see Rowe and Kahn, 1987); however, some general points need to be emphasized. Elderly people perform well on tasks that rely on well-established skills and knowledge. Word-finding difficulties are seldom observed in normal aging and, in fact, elderly subjects often perform better than young subjects on certain tasks using verbal abilities. However, on timed tests of cognition and behavior, elderly subjects do not score as well as young individuals, but given further time to respond, aged subjects perform as well as young subjects. With training, there is substantial and retained improvement among individuals who were previously scored as cognitively impaired. As in most studies, there is variability within groups, since some elderly subjects demonstrate no or minimal cognitive losses compared with younger counterparts.

Heterogeneity in learning ability has also been observed in aged rodents. For example, aged (21–23 months) rats were tested for their ability to find a hidden underwater platform in a circular tank placed in a room filled with extra-maze cues (e.g., windows, lamps). Out of a group of 75 aged rats, only 24 rats had impaired performance in the Morris water maze, whereas the others did not (Gage *et al.*, 1986). In studies of behavior during aging, it is essential that deficits in the animal's motivation, motor abilities, and sensory capacity not be misinterpreted as deficits in learning and memory. For example, visual or olfactory impairments may be misinterpreted as learning difficulties in a task that requires searching for objects or food.

8. NON-INJURY FACTORS THAT REMODEL BRAIN CIRCUITRY

Training and/or experience can enrich neuron structure in the mature brain. The brain is capable of growth and remodeling after injury or due to aging. Many studies demonstrate that early developmental experiences can also influence neuronal structure (for review, see Greenough, 1984; Cotman and Lynch, 1987). It is now clear that subtle but significant effects can also be demonstrated in adults. Similar to handedness in humans, rats appear to have a paw preference. The large neurons in the motor cortex on the side of the brain that controls the preferred paw have more elaborate dendrites than do those on the nonpreferred side. However, when mature rats are trained to reach for food with their nonpreferred paw (Greenough *et al.*, 1984), the dendritic branching increases on the side controlling the newly trained paw. Experience and/or learning thus appears capable of building circuitry in the mature brain. Similar experiments on the aged brain have not yet been reported, although the increase in dendrites in the aged human brain (Coleman and Flood, 1986) may reflect in part a lifetime of experience, as well as compensatory mechanisms to counteract cell loss.

9. CONCLUSION AND OUTLOOK FOR THE FUTURE

The nervous system can compensate for some losses due to aging. With age there is an increased incidence of abnormal neurochemical changes and an accumulation of errors over a lifetime. For example, the neuropathological changes that occur in Alzheimer's disease differ quantitatively but not qualitatively from those that occur as part of the natural aging process. It is reasonable to assume that some subtle neurochemical deficits will ultimately lead to distinct pathology. Whether individuals that age successfully escape pathology remains to be determined. When disease and mechanisms of plasticity are considered, few age-related functional changes occur in some individuals (see Fig. 2). While the brain compensates, at least partially, for some minor losses, less than perfect corrections may eventually lead to computational errors and predispose the system to further deficits.

10. SUMMARY

Many aspects of brain structure, metabolism, and function are well maintained despite advancing age. Those age-related changes that occur can be compensated for by various mechanisms. For example, healthy neurons grow new neuronal connections to replace defective ones. This mechanism, known as synaptic plasticity, which was first identified in animal models, also occurs in the human age-related neurodegenerative diseases. Thus, the aged brain appears to have the capacity, and probably even the blueprints, to repair its own connections. Eventually, however, compensatory mechanisms may become ineffective and may even predispose the aged brain to less stable circuit functions, increasing susceptibility to pathology and disease. Various molecules, such as growth factors (e.g., neurotrophic factors), appear to play a role in maintaining neurons, stimulating their growth, and protecting them against various metabolic insults. The mechanisms that underlie these compensatory or plastic processes are now amenable to detailed molecular analysis, which will ultimately lead to the development of effective therapeutic interventions. This will help us to understand why some individuals successfully age as well as provide the basis for improving function in the impaired aged brain.

ACKNOWLEDGMENTS. This work was supported in part by grants AG00538 (C.W.C.) and AG07855 (C.P.) from the National Institute on Aging, by grant 19691 (C.W.C.) from the

National Institute of Mental Health, and by grants from the Alzheimer's Disease and Related Disorders Association and the John D. French Foundation (C.P.).

REFERENCES

Anderson, K. J., Dam, D., Lee, S., and Cotman, C. W., 1988, Basic fibroblast growth factor prevents death of cholinergic neurons *in vivo*, *Nature (Lond.)* **332:**360–361.

Brown, D., 1988, M currents: An update, *Trends Neurosci.* **11:**294–298.

Coleman, P. D., and Flood, D. G., 1986, Dendritic proliferation in the aging brain as a compensatory repair mechanism, *Progr. Brain Res.* **70:**227–236.

Cotman, C. W., and Anderson, K. J., 1988, Synaptic plasticity and functional stabilization in the hippocampal formation: Possible role in Alzheimer's disease, in: *Physiologic Basis for Functional Recovery in Neurological Disease* (S. Waxman, ed.), Raven, New York, pp. 313–336.

Cotman, C. W., and Lynch, G., 1989, The neurobiology of learning and memory, *Cognition* **33:** (in press).

Cotman, C. W., and Nieto-Sampedro, M., 1984, Cell biology of synaptic plasticity, *Science* **255:**1287–1294.

Cotman, C. W., and Peterson, C., 1988, Aging, in: *Basic Neurochemistry* (G. Siegel, W. Albers, B. Agranoff, and R. Katzman, eds.), Raven, New York, pp. 523–540.

Cotman, C. W., Nieto-Sampedro, M., and Harris, E., 1981, Synapse replacement in the nervous system of adult vertebrates, *Physiol. Rev.* **61:**684–784.

Cotman, C. W., Nieto-Sampedro, M., and Geddes, J. W., 1987, Plasticity of brain after injury, in: *The Neuro-Immuno-Endocrine Connection* (C. W. Cotman, R. E. Brinton, A. Galaburda, B. McEwen, and D. M. Schneider, eds.), Raven, New York, pp. 93–116.

Edds, M. V., 1953, Collateral nerve regeneration, *Q. Rev. Biol.* **28:**260–276.

Fischer, W., Wictorin, K., Bjorklund, A., Williams, L. R., Varon, S., and Gage, F. H., 1987, Amelioration of cholinergic neuron atrophy and spatial memory impairment in aged rats by nerve growth factor, *Nature (Lond.)* **329:**65–68.

Gage, F. H., and Bjorklund, A., 1986, Cholinergic septal grafts into the hippocampal formation improve spatial learning and memory in the aged rats by an atropine sensitive mechanism, *J. Neurosci.* **6:**2837–2847.

Gage, F. H., Wictorin, K., Fisher, W., Williams, L. R., Varon, S., and Bjorklund, A., 1986, Chronic intracerebral infusion of nerve growth factor improves memory performance in cognitively impaired rats, *Neurosci. Abs.* **215:**426.5.

Geddes, J. W., Monaghan, D. T., Cotman, C. W., Lott, I. T., Kim, R. C., and Chui, H. C., 1985, Plasticity of hippocampal circuitry in Alzheimer's disease, *Science* **230:**1179–1181.

Geddes, J. W., Chang-Chui, H., Cooper, S. M., Lott, I. T., and Cotman, C. W., 1986, Density and distribution of NMDA receptors in the human hippocampus in Alzheimer's disease, *Brain Res.* **399:**156–161.

Greenough, W. T., 1984, Structural correlates of information storage in the mammalian brain: A review and hypothesis, *Trends Neurosci.* **7:**229–233.

Greenough, W. T., Larson, J. R., and Withers, G. S., 1985, Effects of unilateral and bilateral training in a reaching task on dendritic branching of neurons in the rat motor-sensory forelimb cortex, *Behav. Neural Biol.* **44:**301–314.

Hoff, S. F., Scheff, S. W., Benardo, L. S., and Cotman, C. W., 1982, Lesion-induced synaptogenesis in the dentate gyrus of aged rats. I. Loss and reacquisition of normal synaptic density, *J. Comp. Neurol.* **205:**246–252.

Hoffman, H., 1950, Local reinnervation in partially denervated muscle: A histophysiological study, *Aust. J. Exp. Biol. Med. Sci.* **28:**383–397.

Hyman, B. T., Van Hoesen, G. W., Damasio, A. R., and Barnes, C. L., 1984, Alzheimer's disease: Cell-specific pathology isolates the hippocampal formation, *Science* **225:**1168–1170.

MacDermott, A. B., Mayer, M. L., Westbrook, G. L., Smith, S. J., and Barker, J. L., 1986, NMDA-receptor activation increases cytoplasmic calcium concentration in cultured spinal cord neurons, *Nature (Lond.)* **321:**519–522.

Nicoll, R. A., 1985, The septo-hippocampal projection: A model cholinergic pathway, *Trends Neurosci.* **8:**533.

Nieto-Sampedro, M., and Cotman, C. W., 1985, Growth factor induction and temporal order in CNS repair, in: *Synaptic Plasticity* (C. W. Cotman, ed.), Guilford, New York, pp. 405–455.

Nieto-Sampedro, M., Lewis, E. R., Cotman, C. W., Manthorpe, M., Skaper, S. D., Barbin, G., Longo, F. M., and Varon, S., 1982, Brain injury causes a time-dependent increase in neurotrophic activity at the lesion site, *Science* **217:**860–861.

Nieto-Sampedro, M., Manthorpe, M., Barbin, G., Varon, S., and Cotman, C. W., 1983, Injury-induced neurotrophic activity in adult rat brain: Correlation with survival of delayed implants in the wound cavity, *J. Neurosci.* **3:**2219–2229.

Rowe, J. W., and Kahn, R. L., 1987, Human aging: Usual and successful, *Science* **237:**143–149.

Sapolsky, R. M., Krey, L. C., and McEwen, B. S., 1985, Prolonged glucocorticoid exposure reduces hippocampal number: Implication in aging, *J. Neurosci.* **5:**1222–1227.

Vijayan, V., and Cotman, C. W., 1987, Hydrocortisone administration alters glial reaction to entorhinal lesions in the rat dentate gyrus, *Exp. Neurol.* **96:**197–200.

Williams, L. R., Varon, S., Peterson, G. M., Wictorin, K., Fischer, W., Bjorklund, A., and Gage, F. H., 1986, Continuous infusion of nerve growth factor prevents basal forebrain neuronal death after fimbria fornix transection, *Proc. Natl. Acad. Sci. USA* **83:**9231–9235.

Immunological, Endocrine, and Pharmacological Approaches to Treatment of Diseases of Aging

Influenza and Aging

Immunological Methods of Enhancing Influenza Vaccine Response in Elderly People

WILLIAM B. ERSHLER

1. INTRODUCTION

Despite the marked reduction in mortality from infectious diseases during the twentieth century, infections remain a major cause of morbidity and mortality in the elderly. Pneumonia, for example, is the second leading cause of death in octogenarians (Kohn, 1982). Influenza occurs more frequently in the elderly and is often an antecedent of bacterial pneumonia and death (Alling *et al.*, 1981). Although other factors are certainly involved, such as the presence of underlying disease or the use of immunosuppressive medicines, it is reasonable to assert that age-related immune deficiency contributes to the predisposition to certain infections, such as influenza, in the elderly. This chapter reviews current influenza vaccination recommendations for the elderly and presents indications of the shortcomings or successes of such vaccines. Because age-related changes in immune functions may well account for the diminished antibody response to vaccine, selected research strategies designed to augment vaccine response are also discussed.

2. INFLUENZA: A BRIEF CLINICAL REVIEW

Influenza viruses are orthomyxoviruses that comprise three types; A, B, and C. Influenza A and B, the major pathogens in humans, are composed of four major structural proteins with RNA replicase and transcriptase activity. There are also eight single strands of RNA. A host-derived envelope is rimmed interiorly by repeating sequences of a membrane (M) protein. Traversing the enveloping and projecting outward are approximately 400 spikes of glycoproteins. These glycoproteins are of two types, either hemagglutinin or neuraminidase. These surface glycoproteins are the antigens to which host immune forces are directed

WILLIAM B. ERSHLER • Section of Geriatrics and Gerontology, Department of Medicine, University of Wisconsin–Madison, and William S. Middleton VA Hospital, Madison, Wisconsin 53706.

Hemagglutinin and neuraminidase molecules are susceptible to frequent genetic alteration, and such changes have clinical significance. Small changes in hemagglutinin, for example, may be sufficient to permit escape from immunity established by exposure to parenteral strains. Such change is termed antigenic drift. A large change, such as one that results in major alteration in the hemagglutinin molecule is termed Antigenic Shift, and frequently portends pandemic (for a comprehensive review, see Makinodan, 1980).

Usually influenza is a self-limited upper respiratory tract infection characterized by headache, fever, and tracheobronchitis. Generally more severe than the common cold, it should be considered the most likely cause of these symptoms during the midwinter weeks, especially when influenza has already been isolated in the community.

Although vaccines are available, for reasons discussed below, infection remains a common cause of morbidity and mortality in elderly people. Approximately 10,000 deaths per year occur in the over-65 age group (Kilbourne, 1987). Estimated annual costs for medical treatment for influenza and influenza-related illness in this age group ranges from $3 to $11 billion (Lui and Kendal, 1987).

3. IMMUNE SENESCENCE AND INFLUENZA

It is currently understood that a decline in immune function begins at the time of sexual maturation in all mammalian species and progresses throughout the life span (for a comprehensive review, see Fedson, 1987). In humans, this decline is most notable in the thymus-dependent (or T-cell) component of the immune response. *In vitro* parameters such as the proliferative response to mitogens (Pisciotta *et al.*, 1967), antigens, or alloantigens (i.e., the mixed-lymphocyte culture) (Gerbase-DeLima *et al.*, 1975) show a consistent gradual decline throughout adult years. The production of lymphokines also decreases with age. Relevant to this discussion is the rather marked decline in the lymphokine interleukin-2 (IL-2) (Thoman and Weigle, 1981, 1982; Gillis *et al.*, 1981; Chang *et al.*, 1983; Ershler *et al.*, 1985a). IL-2 is 15-kDa product of T-helper cells that has been shown to augment a variety of immune functions, including the antibody response to certain types of antigens (Gillis, 1983). Despite the observation that T-cell numbers (including T-helper and T-suppressor cells) are not consistently altered in number with age (Fedson, 1987), current evidence indicates that the reduction in IL-2 production reflects an age-associated decline in IL-2-producing precursor cells (Miller and Stutman, 1982). Whether the decline in IL-2 production reflects a quantitative or qualitative defect, there is reason to believe that the consequence of reduced IL-2 activity renders a substantial impairment of the magnitude of immune function. Strategies have been developed, therefore, that are designed to augment T-cell function with the hopeful expectation of rejuvenating IL-2 production.

Within the context of vaccine response, it is of some interest to note that B-cell function is not affected significantly by aging, yet antibody responses are frequently reduced (Callard *et al.*, 1977). In explanation of this apparent paradox it should be recalled that antibody responses to large or complex antigens, such as proteins, require an intricate network of cellular interactions that prominently include non-B-cells, such as antigen-presenting cells and T-helper cells (Wilcox, 1975; Virelizier *et al.*, 1974). Accordingly, antibody responses to these complex antigens are reduced in states of T-cell deficiency, such as that seen with aging (Kishumoto *et al.*, 1980; Ershler *et al.*, 1982, 1984), whereas antibody responses to simple antigens, such as those polysaccharides that comprise the pneumococcal vaccine, are not strikingly affected (Landesman and Schiffman, 1981; Ershler *et al.*, 1985b). This basic observation could explain the clinically observed greater efficacy of certain vaccines such as Pneumovax in the elderly as compared with others, for example, influenza or tetanus toxoid. Similarly, it is for that reason that immunoadjuvants are currently being developed to augment T-cell function in a setting that has classically been considered "humoral" immunity, i.e., vaccine responses.

4. THE INFLUENZA VACCINE

Each year the Immunization Practices Advisory Committee publishes recommendations for annual influenza vaccination (Centers for Disease Control, 1986). Current vaccines are designed in response to epidemiologic predictions of prevailing strains, and recommendations are based on the desire to prevent disease in at-risk populations (Table I).

The virus is particularly evasive because the outer membrane proteins, i.e., those exposed to immune-mediated clearance mechanisms, are constantly changing. The changes can be minor or substantial and have become known as antigenic drift and antigenic shift. Within any influenza subtype, the appearance of a one or two amino acid change in outer surface proteins (reflective of a point mutation within the RNA genome of the virus) is termed antigenic drift and may signal the appearance of a new strain, and potentially the episodic influenza epidemics that seem to occur every 3 years or so. By contrast, antigenic shift refers to a genetic rearrangement or reassortment on a larger scale that results in a new influenza subtype. Its occurrence may herald the development of an influenza pandemic, as occurred in 1918 or in 1957. Epidemiologic surveillance is essential to detect these changes and alter vaccine composition accordingly. Nevertheless, the occurrence of new subtypes is impossible to predict; therefore, the selection of appropriate vaccine constituents is oftentimes fortuitous.

Of the three genera of influenza viruses, type A produces the most severe disease in the elderly. Current vaccines are designed to produce antibody to surface proteins. The most important outer surface protein is hemagglutinin (HA), which is the site of attachment of the virus to the target cell (Laver and Valentine, 1969). In humans, there are five HA types (H0,

TABLE I. Candidates for Influenza Vaccination[a]

Highest risk
    Those with cardiovascular or pulmonary disorders severe enough
        to have caused hospitalization within past year
    Residents of nursing homes

Moderate risk
    Healthy, over 65 years of age
    Adults/children with metabolic disease (e.g., diabetes) or kidney
        failure, or requiring immunosuppressive therapy

Not at increased risk but capable of nosocomial transmission
    Physicians, nurses, and other health care providers
    Family caregivers

---

[a]Based on U.S. Public Health Service (Centers for Disease Control, 1986).

H1, H2, H3, SW), each of which defines a subtype of influenza A; antibody to that particular HA is believed to be the best candidate for effective elimination of infection by virus of that subtype. Another membrane protein is neuraminidase (NA), of which there are two types (N1, N2). NA probably render a virus more invasive by enzymatically degrading host cell neuraminic acid (a constituent of mucin) (Compans *et al.*, 1986). Each subtype of influenza A can therefore be characterized by its HA and NA, (e.g., H3N2).

Current commercially available vaccines are made from purified protein (HA) fractions from egg-grown viruses that are chemically treated (split-virus) and thereby inactivated. The recommended vaccine contains antigen from three virus strains (two type A, one type B) that are considered most likely to be the cause of clinical disease in the next year. The dose of HA in the vaccine was selected because it has been shown to produce "protective" levels of antibody in young healthy recipients, and it is associated with minimal local and systemic morbidity (Centers for Disease Control, 1986). The measured antibody response in older persons has been considerably less, and perhaps as many as one half those vaccinated will not achieve the conventional fourfold titer change indicative of "response" (Ershler *et al.*, 1984a; Howells *et al.*, 1975; Brandiss *et al.*, 1981; Gravenstein *et al.*, 1987). Nevertheless, the evidence supports the contention that the vaccine may be effective in preventing lower respiratory tract disease, even if it is not absolutely protective in most cases. It is also worthy of note that the antibody response to vaccine even under the best of circumstances, is transient. In addition, in the elderly there may be a delay in achieving the peak titer after vaccine (Levine *et al.*, 1987), yet there is evidence that titers have fallen to baseline by 6 months (Arden *et al.*, 1986a). These findings indicate that the timing of vaccination is clinically significant. Because of the rather limited period of detectable antibody, vaccines should be administered in late fall (mid-October through mid-December), to render optimal protection during the peak influenza months of January and February.

5. EVIDENCE OF INFLUENZA VACCINE EFFICACY AND PROPOSED EXPLANATIONS FOR FAILURE

Although influenza vaccine is not uniformly protective, occasional reports cite reduced incidence of infections (Howells *et al.*, 1975; Stuart *et al.*, 1969) or decreased susceptibility to pneumonia (Van Der Veen *et al.*, 1977; Barker and Mullooly, 1980; Strassburg *et al.*, 1986; Arroyo *et al.*, 1984; Ruben, 1982) and to death (Barker and Mullooly, 1980; Ruben, 1982) among vaccinated people, as compared with nonvaccinated people. Some investigators, however, have reported a lack of vaccine-induced protection (D'Alessio *et al.*, 1969; Ruben *et al.*, 1974), but most do believe that if the epidemiologic surveillance predicts the infectious strain correctly, the vaccine is at least partially effective (LaForce, 1987). Nevertheless, despite the fact that millions of elderly people receive the influenza vaccine, influenza epidemics continue to occur with some degree of regularity, and there continues to be substantial morbidity and mortality associated with infection, even in vaccinated individuals.

Several factors may contribute to failure of the vaccine to have eliminated influenza in the elderly:

1. *A change in the prevalent infectious influenza agent, such as that produced by antigenic drift or antigenic shift:* Thus, the vaccine may well have provided immunity to certain strains, yet the person remains relatively or completely unprotected

against the prevalent strain. Despite intense surveillance efforts, this type of failure occasionally occurs (Barker and Mullooly, 1980; Ruben, 1982).

2. *Failure of the vaccine to induce an immune response:* Although young healthy immune competent people produce excellent antibody responses to influenza vaccine, the responses are considerably lower in the elderly, especially those who have underlying medical conditions, such as malignancy or cardiovascular disease (Ershler *et al.*, 1984a; Laver and Valentine, 1969; Phair *et al.*, 1978). Failure to produce antibody could well explain the clinical observation of influenza infection in individuals who had been vaccinated with a vaccine that accurately predicted the infectious influenza strain. An estimated 25–50% of elderly individuals do not achieve the fourfold titer change that has, by convention, become the definition of vaccine response—and, presumably, protection.

3. *Short vaccine response:* Often the vaccine response is short (less than 6 months) (Gravenstein *et al.*, 1987), and early vaccine, even in immunocompetent individuals, may render that individual susceptible to infection late in the flu season (such as March/April in people vaccinated in September or early October).

4. *Failure of susceptible individuals to receive vaccine:* For a variety of reasons, many elderly people refuse to receive the annual vaccine despite recommendations and underwritten costs (Setia *et al.*, 1985; Kendal *et al.*, 1985). Many of these refusals are based on previous experience with less purified or whole virus preparations (Cromwell *et al.*, 1969) or on the reports of serious neurologic sequelae associated with the swine flu vaccine of 1976 (Centers for Disease Control, 1977). There are new strategies to increase vaccination accrual, particularly in nursing homes, and it is predicted that such efforts will result in reduced morbidity and mortality in future epidemics (Stuart *et al.*, 1969; Kendal *et al.*, 1985).

6. GENERAL RESEARCH STRATEGIES TO AUGMENT VACCINE EFFICACY

To date there has been no proven method of increasing vaccine efficacy, although there are certain leads that sound promising. For example, for certain HA it is clear that increasing the dose of the antigen in the vaccine is associated with no toxicity and with greater antibody production (and presumably protection) (Arden *et al.*, 1986b; Gross *et al.*, 1988). This observation may eventually lead to the administration of higher dose vaccines to at-risk populations. However, this may occur only after further confirmation, particularly with other HA. Additional approaches involve the oral administration of RU4170, a glycoprotein from *Klebsiella pneumoniae*, in conjunction with the influenza vaccine (Profeta *et al.*, 1987), or the covalent coupling of diphtheria toxoid to influenza HA (C. S. Brown, personal communication, 1987). In a preliminary trial, both approaches have been shown to augment specific antibody response to the vaccine component. For example, in recent trials from our laboratory, we have shown that the hemagglutinin–diphtheria conjugate (HA–D) vaccine was well tolerated by elderly volunteer recipients; there was also a dose-related enhanced antibody response as compared with the standard subunit vaccine (Miller *et al.*, 1987; Gravenstein *et al.*, 1988). More definitive analyses are needed to confirm the enhanced antibody response and to establish the lack of toxicity. It remains to be seen whether the higher level of antibody achieved is sufficient to result in improved protection during an influenza outbreak.

7. THYMIC HORMONE AND INFLUENZA VACCINE

Such precautionary remarks could also be made regarding vaccine adjuvant studies from our laboratory. In earlier work we had shown that antibody production to influenza vaccine antigens could be enhanced *in vitro* by the addition of thymic hormone to the lymphocyte culture media (Ershler *et al.*, 1984a). Previously, we had also demonstrated this to be true for tetanus toxoid antibody production (Ershler *et al.*, 1984b). These observations seemed logical because of the known requirement of T-cell help for antibody production to these antigens and the known T-cell deficiency associated with the age-related involution of thymic gland. We have expanded our *in vitro* observations to a clinical trial of thymosin α_1 ($T\alpha_1$) in the elderly (Gravenstein *et al.*, 1987). This 28-amino acid peptide is one of several purified components of an earlier described calf thymic hormone preparation (thymosin fraction 5) (Low and Goldstein, 1984; Goldstein, 1984). $T\alpha_1$ has been investigated in a variety of immune-deficient states and is generally thought to be nontoxic but only marginally effective in those with profound immune deficiency. Nevertheless, in those with more mild immune deficiency, such as that associated with certain malignancies (Schulof *et al.*, 1985) and with advanced age (Ershler *et al.*, 1984a; D'Agastaro *et al.*, 1980; Frasca *et al.*, 1982, 1986), it has been shown to have potentially clinically important immunoreconstitutive properties. In a recently completed clinical trial, we showed that elderly men given $T\alpha_1$ twice weekly for 4 weeks, with the first dose immediately after influenza vaccine, had a significantly greater vaccine response rate than placebo-treated controls (Gravenstein *et al.*, manuscript submitted). Certainly, the confirmation of such a finding may lead to a new approach to augmenting vaccine response in elderly people by transiently bolstering T-cell immunity by thymic hormone.

8. SUMMARY

Despite large vaccination programs, influenza remains a major cause of morbidity and mortality in the elderly. Several factors could account for this, including poor vaccine compliance, changing influenza strains, and ineffective response to vaccine antigens. Current research strategies are being developed to improve vaccine response, some directed at augmenting antigenicity of the vaccine (such as by conjugation of hemagglutinin with diphtheria toxoid), and others aimed at reconstituting the antibody response by enhancing age-reduced T-cell function (such as with thymic hormone). Currently all people over 65 years of age, especially those who are frail, with cardiorespiratory disease or malignancy, or who are living in nursing homes, should receive annual influenza vaccination. Furthermore, physicians, nurses, and other personnel, who administer care to high-risk populations should also receive the vaccine.

REFERENCES

Alling, D. W., Blackwelder, W. C., and Stuart-Harris, C. H., 1981, A study of excess mortality during influenza epidemics in the United States, 1968–1976, *Am. J. Epidemiol.* **113**:30–43.

Arden, N. H., Patriarca, P. A., and Kendal, A. P., 1986a, Experiences in the use and efficacy of inactivated influenza vaccine in nursing home, in: *Options for the Control of Influenza* (A. P. Kendal and P. A. Patriarca, eds.), Liss, New York, pp. 155–168.

Arden, N. H., Patriarca, P. A., Lui, K-J., Harmon, M. W., Brandon, F., and Kendal, A. P., 1986b, Safety and immunogenicity of a 45 mg supplemental dose of inactivated split-virus influenza B vaccine in the elderly, *J. Infect. Dis.* **153**:805–806.

Arroyo, J. C., Postic, B., Brown, A., Harrison, K., Birgenheier, R., and Dowda, H., 1984, Influenza A/Philippines/2/82 outbreak in a nursing home: Limitation of influenza vaccination in the aged, *Am. J. Infect. Control* **12**:329–334.

Barker, W. H., and Mullooly, J. P., 1980, Influenza vaccination of elderly persons: Reduction in pneumonia and influenza hospitalizations and deaths, *JAMA* **244**:2547–2549.

Brandriss, M. W., Betts, R. F., Mathur, U., and Douglas, R. G., 1981, Responses of elderly subjects to monovalent A/USSR/77/(HINI) and trivalent A/USSR/77(HINI)-A Texas/77 (H3N2)™ B/Hong Kong/72 vaccines, *Am. Rev. Respir. Dis.* **124**:681–684.

Callard, R. E., Basten, A., and Waters, L. K., 1977, Immune function in aged mice. II. B-cell function, *Cell. Immunol.* **31**:26–36.

Centers for Disease Control, 1977, Influenza vaccine: Recommendations of the Public Health Service Committee on immunization practices, *Ann. Intern. Med.* **87**:316–318.

Centers for Disease Control, 1986, Recommendations for prevention and control of influenza: Recommendations of the Immunization Practices Advisory Committee, *Ann. Intern. Med.* **105**:399–104.

Chang, M. P., Makinodan, T., Peterson, W. J., and Strehler, B. L., 1983, Role of T-cells and adherent cells in age-related decline in murine interleukin-2 production, *J. Immunol.* **129**:2426–2430.

Compans, R. W., Jones, L. U., and Melsen, L. R., 1986, Organization and assembly of influenza virus proteins, in: *Options for the Control of Influenza* (A. P. Kendal and P. A. Patriarca, eds.), Liss, New York, pp. 23–38.

Cromwell, H. A., Brandon, F. B., McLean, I. W., and Sadusk, J. F., 1969, Influenza immunization: A new vaccine, *JAMA* **210**:1438–1442.

D'Agastaro, G., Frasca, D., Garovini, M., and Doria, G., 1980, Immunorestoration of old mice by injection of thymus extract. Enhancement of t-cell–t-cell cooperation in the *in vitro* antibody response, *Cell. Immunol.* **53**:207–213.

D'Alessio, D. J., Cox, P. M., and Dick, E. C., 1969, Failure of inactivated influenza vaccine to protect an aged population, *JAMA* **210**:485–489.

Ershler, W. B., Moore, A. L., and Hacker, M. P., 1982, Specific *in vivo* and *in vitro* antibody response to tetanus toxoid immunization, *Clin. Exp. Immunol.* **49**:552–558.

Ershler, W. B., Moore, A. L., and Socinski, M. A., 1984a, Influenza and aging: Age-related changes and the effects of thymosin on the antibody response to influenza vaccine, *J. Clin. Immunol.* **4**:445–454.

Ershler, W. B., Moore, A. L., Hacker, M. P., Nimomiya, J., Naylor, P., and Goldstein, A. L., 1984b, Specific antibody synthesis *in vitro*. II. Age-associated thymosin enhancement of antitetanus antibody synthesis, *Immunopharmacology* **8**:69–77.

Ershler, W. B., Moore, A. L., Roessner, K., and Ranges, G. E., 1985a, Interleukin-2 and aging: Decreased IL-2 production in healthy older people does not correlate with reduced helper cell numbers or antibody response to influenza vaccine and is not corrected *in vitro* by Thymosin Alpha One, *Immunopharmacology* **10**:11–17.

Ershler, W. B., Hebert, J. C., Blow, A. J., Granter, S. R., and Lynch, J., 1985b, Effect of thymosin alpha one on specific antibody response and susceptibility to infection in young and aged mice, *Int. J. Immunopharmacol.* **7**:465–471.

Fedson, D. S., 1987, Influenza and pneumococcal immunization strategies for physicians, *Chest* **91**:436–443.

Frasca, D., Garavini, M., and Doria, G., 1982, Recovery of t-cell functions in aged mice injected with synthetic thymosin alpha one, *Cell. Immunol.* **72**:384–391.

Frasca, D., Adorini, L., Mancini, C., and Doria, G., 1986, Reconstitution of t-cell functions in aging mice by thymosin alpha one, *Immunopharmacology* **11**:155–163.

Gerbase-DeLima, M., Meredith, P., and Walford, R. L., 1975, Age-related changes, including synergy and suppression in the mixed lymphocytes reaction in long-lived mice, *Fed. Proc.* **34**:159–161.

Gillis, S., 1983, Interleukin 2: Biology and biochemistry, *J. Clin. Immunol.* **3**:1–13.

Gillis, S., Kozak, R., Durante, M., and Weksler, M. E., 1981, Immunologic studies of aging: Decreased production and response to T-cell growth factor by lymphocytes from aged humans, *J. Clin. Invest.* **67**:937–942.

Goldstein, A. L. (ed.), 1984, *Thymic Hormones and Lymphokines. Basic Chemistry and Clinical Applications*, Plenum, New York.

Gravenstein, S., Miller, B. A., Duthie, P., Drinka, P. J., Prathipatti, K., Odiet, F. M., Schicker, J. M., Siewert, M. E., and Ershler, W. B., 1987, Enhancement of anti-influenza antibody response in elderly men by thymosin alpha one, *Clin. Res.* **35**:346a.

Gravenstein, S., Miller, B. A., and Ershler, W. B., 1988, Immunogenicity of an influenza virus hemagglutinin-diphtheria toxoid conjugate vaccine in elderly outpatients: A placebo controlled dose response study, *Clin. Res.* **36**:338a.

Gravenstein, S., Duthie, E. H., Miller, B. A., Roecker, E., Drinka, P., Prathipati, K., and Ershler, W. B., 1989, Augmentation of influenza antibody response in elderly men by thymosin alpha one, *J. Am. Geriatrics Soc.* **37**:1–8.

Gross, P. A., Quinnan, G. V., Weksler, M. E., Gaerlan, P. F., and Denning, C. R., 1988, Immunization of elderly people with high doses of influenza vaccine, *J. Am. Geriatr. Soc.* **36**:209–212.

Howells, C. H. L., Vesselinova-Jenkins, C. K., Evans, A. D., and James, J., 1975, Influenza vaccination and mortality from bronchopneumonia in the elderly, *Lancet* **1**:381–383.

Kendal, A. P., Patriarca, P. A., and Arden, N. H., 1985, Policies and outcomes for control of influenza among the elderly in the USA, *Vaccine* **3**:274–276.

Kilbourne, E. D., 1987, *Influenza*, Plenum, New York.

Kishumoto, S., Tomino, S., Mitsuya, H., Fujiwara, H., and Tsuda, H., 1980, Age-related decline in the *in vitro* and *in vivo* synthesis of anti-tetanus antibody in humans, *J. Immunol.* **125**:2347–2352.

Kohn, R. R., 1982, Causes of death in very old people, *JAMA* **247**:2793–2797.

LaForce, F. M., 1987, Immunization, immunoprophylaxis and chemoprophylaxis to prevent selected infections: A report of the U.S. preventive service task force, *JAMA* **257**:2464–2470.

Landesman, S. H., and Schiffman, G., 1981, Assessment of antibody response to pneumococcal vaccine in high risk population, *Rev. Infect. Dis.* **3**:184–197.

Laver, W. G., and Valentine, R. C., 1969, Morphology of the isolated hemagglutinin and neuraminidase subunits of influenza virus, *Virology* **38**:105–119.

Levine, M., Beattie, B. L., McLean, D. M., and Corman, D., 1987, Characterization of the immune response to trivalent influenza vaccine in elderly men, *J. Am. Geriatr. Soc.* **35**:609–615.

Low, T. L. K., and Goldstein, A. L., 1984, Thymosin, peptidic moieties and related agents, in: *Immune Modulation Agents and Their Mechanisms* (R. L. Fenichel and M. A. Chingos, eds.), Dekker, New York, pp. 135–162.

Lui, K. J., and Kendal, A. P., 1987, Impact of influenza epidemics on mortality in the United States from October 1972 to May 1985, *Am. J. Public Health* **77**:712–716.

Makinodan, T., and Kay, M. M. B., 1980, Age influence on the immune system, *Adv. Immunol.* **29**:287–329.

Miller, R. A., and Stutman, O., 1982, Enumeration of IL-2 secretory helper T-cells by limiting dilution analysis and demonstration of unexpectedly high levels of IL-2 production per responding cell, *J. Immunol.* **128**:2258–2264.

Miller, B. A., Gravenstein, S., Carlson, J., and Ershler, W. B., 1987, Influenza-diphtheria conjugate vaccine study in the elderly, *Gerontologist* **27**:86a.

Phair, J., Kauffman, C. A., Bjornson, A., Adams, L., and Linnemann, C., 1978, Failure to respond to influenza vaccine in the aged: Correlation with B-cell number and function, *J. Lab. Clin. Med.* **92**:822–828.

Pisciotta, A. V., Westring, D. W., DePrey, C., and Walsh, B., 1967, Mitogenic effect of phytohemagglutinin at different ages, *Nature (Lond.)* **215**:193–194.

Profeta, M. L., Guidi, G., Meroni, P. L., Palmieri, R., Palladino, G., Cantone, V., and Zanussi, C., 1987, Influenza vaccination with adjuvant RU41740 in the elderly, *Lancet* **1**:973.

Ruben, F. L., 1982, Prevention of influenza in the elderly, *J. Am. Geriatr. Soc.* **30:**577–580.

Ruben, F. L., Johnston, F., and Streiff, E. J., 1974, Influenza in a partially immunized aged population: Effectiveness of killed Hong Kong vaccine against infection with the England strain, *JAMA* **230:**863–866.

Setia, U., Serventi, I., and Lorenz, P., 1985, Factors affecting the use of influenza vaccine in the institutionalized elderly, *J. Am. Geriatr. Soc.* **33:**856–858.

Shulof, R. S., Lloyd, M. J., Cleary, P. A., Palaszynski, S. R., Mai, D. A., Cox, J. W., Alabaster, O., and Goldstein, A. L., 1985, A randomized trial to evaluate the immunorestorative properties of synthetic thymosin alpha one with lung cancer, *J. Biol. Respir. Modif.* **4:**147–158.

Strassburg, M. A., Greenland, S., Sorvillo, F. J., Lieb, L. E., and Habel, L. A., 1986, Influenza in the elderly: Report of an outbreak and a review of vaccine effectiveness reports, *Vaccine* **4:**38–44.

Stuart, W. H., Dull, B., Newton, L. H., McQueen, J. L., and Schiff, E. R., 1969, Evaluation of monovalent influenza vaccine in a retirement community during the epidemic of 1965–1966, *JAMA* **209:**232–238.

Thoman, M., and Weigle, W. O., 1981, Lymphokines and aging: Interleukin 2 production and activity in aged animals, *J. Immunol.* **127:**2102–2106.

Thoman, M., and Weigle, W. O., 1982, Cell mediated immunity in aged mice: An underlying lesion in IL-2 synthesis, *J. Immunol.* **128:**2358–2361.

Van Der Veen, J., Van Der Werf, P. A. M., Masurel, N., and Polak, M. F., 1977, Influenza in a partially vaccinated community of elderly persons, *Ned. T. Geneesk.* **121:**1259–1262.

Virelizier, J-L., Postlethwaite, R., Schild, G. C., and Allison, D. C., 1974, Antibody response to antigenic determinants of influenza virus hemagglutinin. I. Thymus dependence of antibody formation and thymus independence of immunological memory, *J. Exp. Med.* **140:**1559–1570.

Wilcox, H. N. A., 1975, Thymus dependence of the antibody response to tetanus toxoid in mice, *Clin. Exp. Immunol.* **22:**341–347.

52

Age-Dependent Enhancement of Influenza Vaccine Responses by Thymosin in Chronic Hemodialysis Patients

STEVE Y. SHEN, QUINTINA B. CORTEZA,
JOHN JOSSELSON, STEFAN GRAVENSTEIN,
WILLIAM B. ERSHLER, JOHN H. SADLER, and
PAUL B. CHRETIEN

1. INTRODUCTION

Vaccination against influenza has been recommended for chronic hemodialysis patients (Centers for Disease Control, 1984). Several studies have reported conflicting results of this vaccination in patients with chronic renal disease and in patients who are on chronic hemodialysis (Jordan *et al.*, 1973; Pabico *et al.*, 1974; Ortbals *et al.*, 1978; Osanloo *et al.*, 1978; Cappel *et al.*, 1983). Since previous studies of the immunologic competence in uremic patients have shown that they are suppressed in both cellular and humoral immunity (Wilson *et al.*, 1965; Newberry and Sanford, 1971; Slavin and Fitch, 1971; Birkeland, 1976), we postulated that an immunomodulator capable of enhancing antibody production in immunocompromised patients would improve antibody response to influenza vaccine in hemodialysis patients.

Thymosin α_1 is a 28-amino acid peptide isolated from the parent preparation thymic hormone fraction 5. The major biological properties of this hormone include enhancement of T-cell-dependent specific antibody production, helper T-cell activity, and secondary T-cell

STEVE Y. SHEN, QUINTINA B. CORTEZA, JOHN JOSSELSON, and JOHN H. SADLER • Division of Nephrology, University of Maryland Hospital, Baltimore, Maryland 21201. *Present address for S.Y.S.*: Division of Nephrology, Maryland General Hospital, Baltimore, Maryland 21201. STEFAN GRAVENSTEIN • Division of Hematology, Department of Medicine, University of Wisconsin–Madison, Madison, Wisconsin 53706. WILLIAM B. ERSHLER • Section of Geriatrics and Gerontology, Department of Medicine, University of Wisconsin–Madison, and William S. Middleton VA Hospital, Madison, Wisconsin 53706. PAUL B. CHRETIEN • Department of Surgery, University of Maryland Hospital, Baltimore, Maryland 21201.

dependent IgG, IgM, and IgA antibody responses (Low and Goldstein, 1982, 1984). We undertook this randomized double-blind placebo-controlled study to evaluate the effect of thymosin α_1 on antibody production after influenza vaccination in chronic hemodialysis patients. The effects of age and duration of end-stage renal disease (ESRD) prior to vaccination were also evaluated in this study.

2. METHODS AND MATERIALS

2.1. Subjects

A total of 97 hemodialysis patients with end-stage renal disease participated in this study after giving informed consent that was reviewed and approved by the Human Volunteers Research Committee, University of Maryland, at Baltimore. Each of these patients received 5–6 hr of hemodialysis with Gambro parallel plate dialyzers twice weekly at either our self-care dialysis unit or our chronic staff-assisted dialysis unit. None was allergic to eggs or egg products or was known to have acute illness, liver disease, or neoplastic disease at the time of vaccination. None of the subjects was on any immunosuppressive therapy.

2.2. Study Groups

After matching in age, 48 patients were randomized to group A and 49 to group B. Group A patients received vaccine and thymosin α_1, group B patients received vaccine and placebo injections.

2.3. Influenza Vaccination

Vaccination was performed with a 0.5-ml intradeltoid injection to each patient of the licensed 1986 monovalent influenza vaccine containing A/Taiwan/1/86 (H1N1) antigen.

2.4. Thymosin α_1 and Placebo Injections

Both thymosin α_1 and placebo were manufactured by Hoffman-LaRoche, Inc. (Nutley, New Jersey), and provided to us by Alpha-One Biomedicals, Inc. (Washington, D. C.). Each patient in group A received a subcutaneous injection of thymosin α_1 at a dose of 0.45 ml/m^2 (900 μg/m^2) of body surface area twice weekly for 4 weeks with the first dose given coincident with the vaccine.

Placebo consisted of lyophilized mannitol, U.S.P., ~17 mg in each 5-ml vial of thymosin diluent (sodium bicarbonate), which simulated the appearance of thymosin α_1. Each patient in group B was given a subcutaneous (SC) injection of placebo at a dose of 0.45 ml/m^2 of body surface area at the same schedule as those of thymosin α_1.

2.5. Evaluation of Subjects

Clinical and laboratory evaluations of each participating patient included an initial medical history and a physical examination before vaccination and study drug injections, a brief interview and examination twice weekly during the study period, and routine monthly serum chemistries, liver enzymes, and hepatitis B surface antigen (HB$_s$Ag) screening. Each patient's age and duration of ESRD prior to vaccination were recorded and analyzed for correlation with anti-influenza antibody response to vaccination.

2.6. Anti-Influenza Antibody Determination

In addition to routine monthly chemistries, sera for specific antibody determination were collected before vaccination, and at 4 weeks and 8 weeks thereafter. Antibody analysis was done by enzyme-linked immunosorbent assay (ELISA) in triplicate and compared with a control standard (by S. Gravenstein and W. Ershler in University of Wisconsin, Madison). A positive response to vaccination was defined as an increase in specific anti-influenza antibody level four times greater than the prevaccination level at 4 weeks or later postvaccination.

2.7. Statistical Analysis

The differences in the positive response rates to vaccination between groups A and B were evaluated by chi-square analysis. Student's t-test was used to determine the significance of the differences in age and duration of ESRD prior to vaccination.

3. RESULTS

Except for minor pain at the injection site, there were no side effects or complications related to influenza vaccination or to thymosin α_1 or placebo administration. No patients withdrew from the study. All 97 patients survived to the study's conclusion for analysis.

3.1. Anti-Influenza Antibody Response Rates

At 4 weeks postvaccination, patients in group A (thymosin group) responded to influenza vaccination 71% (34 responders/48 patients at risk), while only 43% (21/49) ($p <$ 0.002) of those in group B (placebo-treated group) responded. At 8 weeks postvaccination, the response rates were 65% (31/48) in group A and 24% (12/49) in group B, respectively ($p < 0.001$). In addition, there were 17 patients in group A but only 2 patients in group B ($p <$ 0.00005) who were able to sustain an increase in specific antibody more than eight times greater than the prevaccination level both at 4 weeks and 8 weeks postvaccination.

3.2. Effect of Duration of ESRD

The duration of ESRD prior to vaccination was not different between groups A and B: group A 1–161 months, mean 79.6 ± 24.4 (SD); group B 1–191 months, mean 81.6 ± 27.6 ($p =$ NS). There were no differences in duration of ESRD between responders and nonresponders in either group A or B, at 4 or 8 weeks postvaccination.

3.3. Effect of Age

The ages of the two groups were similar: group A 22–82 years, mean 50.5 ± 14.8 (SD); group B 22–70 years, mean 49.3 ± 13.5 ($p =$ NS). At 4 weeks postvaccination the mean age of the responders was lower than that of nonresponders, but not significantly, both in group A

TABLE I. Effects of Age and Thymosin α_1
on Response Rates[a] to Influenza
Vaccination in Hemodialysis Patients

	Treatment group			
	Thymosin		Placebo	
Age[b]	N[c]	%	N[c]	%
20–29	5/5	100	5/5	100
30–39	6/6	100	3/7	43
40–49	6/10	60	4/10	40
50–59	8/13	62	5/14	36
60–69	6/9	67	3/9	33
70–79	3/4	75	1/4	25
80–89	0/1		0/0	

[a]At 4 weeks postvaccination.
[b]Age in years.
[c]Responders/patients at risk.

(responders 48.2 ± 15.1 years versus nonresponders 56.2 ± 12.2, p = NS) and in group B (responders 47.5 ± 13.0 years versus nonresponders 52.8 ± 9.8, p = NS). When patients from two groups were combined, the mean age of the responders at 4 weeks postvaccination was significantly lower than that of nonresponders (47.9 ± 14.3 versus 53.9 ± 10.8, $p <$ 0.046). Furthermore, as response rates at 4 weeks postvaccination were stratified by age and compared between group A and group B, the likelihood of responding to influenza vaccination in hemodialysis patients decreased with age in the placebo-treated group but not in the thymosin-treated group (Table I).

4. DISCUSSION

Although influenza vaccine has been available for several years and the efficacy has been satisfactory in a young, healthy population, conflicting results have been reported concerning the antibody responses in patients with ESRD. Data regarding the integrity and the defect of humoral immunity in chronic renal failure patients are not entirely consistent. A number of studies have reported no differences between uremic patients and normal controls in humoral antibody responses to immunization with diphtheria toxoid (Stoloff *et al.*, 1958), tetanus toxoid (Balch, 1955), and blood group substances (Dammin *et al.*, 1957). However, poor antibody responses following typhoid vaccination (Wilson *et al.*, 1965) and keyhole limpet hemocyanin (Boulton-Jones *et al.*, 1973) have been documented in patients with chronic renal failure. The evidence for impairment of cell-mediated immunity in hemodialysis patients is more convincing and seems well established (Dammin *et al.*, 1957; Lawrence, 1965; Wilson *et al.*, 1965; Newberry and Sanford, 1971; Sanders *et al.*, 1971). Several studies have reported that poor antibody response after hepatitis B vaccination in hemodialysis patients (Stevens *et al.*, 1980; Crosnier *et al.*, 1981; Grob *et al.*, 1983; Stevens *et al.*, 1984) is due to incompetency in T-cell-mediated immune responses (Bramwell *et al.*,

1985; Revie *et al.*, 1985). Since antibody response to influenza vaccination is also T-cell dependent (Virelizier *et al.*, 1974; Ershler *et al.*, 1984), the efficacy of this vaccine in hemodialysis patients is questionable.

Similar problems have been evaluated in elderly volunteers. The immune deficiency associated with aging has been found to be directly related to the gradual involution of the thymus gland and subsequent T-cell insufficiency (Weksler *et al.*, 1978; Makinodan and Kay, 1980; Weksler, 1983). The capacity of the antibody response following antigen stimulation is reduced with aging (Makinodan and Peterson, 1962; Kishimoto *et al.*, 1980; Ershler *et al.*, 1985). Therefore, we also directed our attention to the effect of aging on antibody production after influenza vaccination in hemodialysis patients.

It has been demonstrated that specific anti-influenza antibody production could be enhanced by the *in vitro* addition of thymosin α_1 to the culture media (Ershler *et al.*, 1984). In the United States, thymosin α_1 has been studied extensively in many clinical trials on patients with cancer, congenital immune deficiency, and rheumatoid arthritis (Wara and Ammann, 1978; Costani *et al.*, 1979; Goldstein *et al.*, 1982), and the safety of administering this agent to patients has been established. However, no clinical trial of this preparation on hemodialysis patients has ever been conducted. Since thymosin deficiency is one of the putative mechanisms of immune deficiency in patients with end-stage renal failure (Harris *et al.*, 1975), we decided to evaluate the effect of this immunomodulator on enhancing antibody production following influenza A/Taiwan/86 vaccination in hemodialysis patients.

In this study, we have shown that antibody response to influenza A/Taiwan/86 vaccination was poor in hemodialysis patients receiving placebo injections. The response rates declined with increasing age in this group of patients. However, antibody response was significantly better in patients receiving thymosin α_1 injections, and the response rates did not decrease with increasing age in this group. The ages of the two groups were similar, and there was no difference in duration of ESRD between these two groups. The difference in responsiveness to vaccination between these two groups could not be correlated with the serum creatinine level because it was maintained at a similar level by chronic hemodialysis. These results strongly suggest that thymosin α_1 is a useful adjuvant to influenza A/Taiwan/86 vaccination for chronic hemodialysis patients, particularly for patients above 40–50 years of age.

We believe this to be the first randomized double-blind placebo-controlled clinical trial using thymosin α_1 to augment antibody production following vaccination in chronic hemodialysis patients. The precise immune mechanism(s) responsible for this enhancement of response to influenza A/Taiwan/86 vaccine by thymosin α_1 are unknown. The injection schedule and dosage of thymosin used in this study were derived from experiments in laboratory animals and earlier clinical trials on nondialysis patients. Further studies are needed to elaborate the mechanism(s) of the enhancing effect and to determine the best thymosin regimen for improving immune responses to various vaccines and other antigen challenges in hemodialysis patients.

5. SUMMARY

Conflicting results have been reported about antibody responses to influenza vaccine in hemodialysis patients. In this randomized double-blind placebo-controlled study, we evaluated the effects of aging and thymosin α_1 on antibody production after influenza vaccination in 97 hemodialysis patients. Patients were matched for age and randomized into one of two groups, A and B. Each patient received an injection of 1986 monovalent Taiwan influenza A vaccine in the deltoid muscle. Group A (48 patients) also received thymosin α_1 subcutaneous injections at a dose of 0.45 ml/m² (900 µg/m²) of body surface area twice weekly for 4 weeks after vaccination; group B (49 patients) received placebo (thymosin diluent) at a dose of 0.45 ml/m² of body surface area at the same schedule. Sera for specific anti-influenza antibody determinations by enzyme-linked immunosorbent assay were collected from all patients before vaccination and, at 4 and 8 weeks afterward. Response to vaccination was defined as an increase in specific antibody level four times greater than the prevaccination level at 4 weeks or later postvaccination. Response rates at 4 weeks after vaccination were 71% in group A and 43% in group B ($p < 0.002$, chi-square), and at 8 weeks, 65% versus 24% ($p < 0.001$). Seventeen patients in group A versus 2 patients in group B were able to sustain an eight-fold rise in antibody at 8 weeks. Response rates decreased with age in group B, but not in group A. These results suggest that response to influenza vaccination is poor and is age dependent in hemodialysis patients. However, twice-weekly injections of thymosin α_1 for 4 weeks following vaccination can augment antibody production in this patient population, particularly for older patients.

ACKNOWLEDGMENTS. This study was supported in part by a research grant from Alpha-One Biomedical, Inc., Washington, D. C. We are grateful to all nurses and technicians in our dialysis units for their enthusiastic assistance to this study. We want to thank Ms. Donna DeLuca for her excellent preparation of this manuscript.

REFERENCES

Balch, H. H., 1955, The effect of severe battle injury and of post-traumatic renal failure on resistance to infection, *Ann. Surg.* **142:**145–163.

Birkeland, S. A., 1976, Uremia as a state of immune deficiency, *Scand. J. Immunol.* **5:**107–115.

Boulton-Jones, J. M., Vick, R., and Cameron, J. S., 1973, Immune responses in uremia, *Clin. Nephrol.* **1:**351–360.

Bramwell, S. P., Tsakiris, D. J., Briggs, J. D., Follett, E. A., Stewart, J., McWhinnie, D. L., Watson, M. A., Hamilton, D. N., and Junor, B. J., 1985, Dinitrochlorobenzene skin testing predicts response to hepatitis B vaccine in dialysis patients, *Lancet* **2:**1412–1415.

Cappel, R., Van Beers, D., Liesnard, C., and Dratwa, M., 1983, Impaired humoral and cell-mediated immune responses in dialyzed patients after influenza vaccination, *Nephron* **33:**21–25.

Centers for Disease Control, 1984, Prevention and control of influenza: Recommendation of the immunization practices advisory committee, *Ann. Intern. Med.* **101:**218–222.

Costani, J., Daniels, J., Thurman, G., Goldstein, A., and Hokanson, J., 1979, Clinical trials with thymosin, *Ann. NY Acad Sci.* **322:**148–159.

Crosnier, J., Jungers, P., Courouce, A. M., Laplanche, A., Benhamou, E., Pegos, F., Lacour, B., Prunet, P., Cerisier, Y., and Guesry, P., 1981, Randomized placebo-controlled trial of hepatitis-B surface antigen vaccine in French hemodialysis units. II, *Lancet* **1:**797–800.

Dammin, G. J., Couch, N. P., and Murray, J. E., 1957, Prolonged survival of skin homografts in uremic patients, *Ann. NY Acad. Sci.* **64:**967–976.

Ershler, W. B., Moore, A. L., and Socinski, M. A., 1984, Influenza and aging: Age-related changes and the effects of thymosin on the antibody response to influenza vaccine, *J. Clin. Immunol.* **4:**445–454.

Ershler, W. B., Hebert, J. L., Blow, A. J., Granter, S. F., and Lynch, J., 1985, Effects of thymosin alpha one on specific antibody response and susceptibility to infection in young and aged mice, *Int. J. Immunopharmacol.* **7**:465–471.

Goldstein, A., Low, T., Thurman, G., Zatz, M., Hall, N. R., McClure, J. E., Hu, S. K., and Schulof, R. S., 1982, Thymosins and other hormone-like factors in the thymus gland, in: *Immunological Approaches to Cancer Therapeutics* (J. Michich, ed.), Wiley, New York, pp. 137–190.

Grob, P. J., Binswanger, U., Zaruba, K., Joller-Jemelka, H. I., Schmid, M., Hacki, W., Blumberg, A., Abplanalp, A., Herwig, W., Iselin, H., and Pescoeudres, C., 1983, Immunogenicity of a hepatitis B subunit vaccine in hemodialysis and in renal transplant recipients, *Antiviral Res.* **3**:43–52.

Harris, J., Sengar, D., Rashid, A., Hyslop, D., Green, L., and Goldstein, A., 1975, Immunodeficiency in chronic uremia: Preliminary evidence for thymosin deficiency, *Transplantation* **20**:176–178.

Jordan, M. C., Rousseau, W. E., Tegtmeier, G. E., Noble, G. R., Muth, R. G., and Chin, T., 1973, Immunogenicity of inactivated influenza virus vaccine in chronic renal failure, *Ann. Intern. Med.* **79**:790–794.

Kishimoto, S., Tomino, S., Mitsuya, H., Fujiwara, H., and Tsuda, H., 1980, Age-related decline in the *in vitro* and *in vivo* synthesis of anti-tetanus antibody in humans, *J. Immunol.* **125**:2347–2352.

Lawrence, H. S., 1965, Uremia-nature's immunosuppressive device (Editorial), *Ann. Intern. Med.* **62**:166–170.

Low, T., and Goldstein, A., 1982, Role of the thymosins as immunomodulating agents and maturation factors, in: *Maturation Factors and Cancer* (M. A. Moore, ed.), Raven, New York, pp. 129–152.

Low, T., and Goldstein, A., 1984, Thymosin, peptide moieties, and related agents, in: *Immune Modulation Agents and Their Mechanisms* (R. L. Fenichel and M. A. Chirigus, eds.), Dekker, New York, pp. 135–162.

Makinodan, T., and Kay, M., 1980, Age influence on the immune system, in: *Advances in Immunology* (H. G. Kunkel and F. J. Dixon, eds.), Academic, Orlando, Florida, pp. 287–330.

Makinoden, T., and Peterson, W., 1962, Relative antibody-forming capacity of spleen cells as a function of age, *Proc. Natl. Acad. Sci. USA* **48**:234–238.

Newberry, W., and Sanford, J., 1971, Defective cellular immunity in renal failure: Depression of reactivity of lymphocytes to phytohemagglutinin by renal failure serum, *J. Clin. Invest.* **50**:1262–1271.

Ortbals, D., Marks, E., and Liebhaber, H., 1978, Influenza immunization in patients with chronic renal disease, *JAMA* **239**:2562–2565.

Osanloo, E., Berlin, B., Popli, S., Ing, T., Cumings, J., Gies, W., and Hano, J., 1978, Antibody responses to influenza vaccination in patients with chronic renal failure, *Kidney Int.* **14**:614–618.

Pabico, R., Douglas, R., Betts, R., McKenna, B., and Freeman, R., 1974, Influenza vaccination of patients with glomerular diseases, *Ann. Intern. Med.* **81**:171–177.

Revie, D., Shen, S. Y., Ordonez, J., Welik, R., Litkowski, L., Dagher, F., Sadler, J. H., and Chretien, P. B., 1985, T-cell subsets and status of hepatitis-B surface antigen and antibody in end-stage renal disease patients, *Kidney Int.* **27**:150 (abst.).

Sanders, C. V., Jr., Luby, J. P., Sanford, J. P., and Hull, A. R., 1971, Suppression of interferon response in lymphocytes from patients with uremia, *J. Lab. Clin. Med.* **77**:768–776.

Slavin, R. G., and Fitch, C. D., 1971, Inhibition of lymphocyte transformation by guanidinosuccinic acid, a surplus metabolite in uremia, *Experientia* **27**:1340–1341.

Stevens, C. E., Szmuness, W., Goodman, A., Weseley, S., and Fotino, M., 1980, Hepatitis-B vaccine: Immune responses in hemodialysis patients, *Lancet* **2**:1211–1213.

Stevens, C. E., Alter, H., Taylor, P. E., Zang, E. A., Harley, E., and Szmuness, W., 1984, Hepatitis-B vaccine in patients receiving hemodialysis, *N. Engl. J. Med.* **311**:496–501.

Stoloff, I. L., Stout, R., Myerson, R. M., and Havens, W. P., Jr., 1958, Production of antibody in patients with uremia, *N. Engl. J. Med.* **259**:320–323.

Virelizier, J. L., Postelwaite, R., Schild, G. C., and Allison, A. C., 1974, Antibody responses to antigenic determinants of influenza virus hemagglutinin I: Thymus dependence of antibody formation and thymus independence of immunologic memory, *J. Exp. Med.* **140**:1559–1570.

Wara, D. W., and Ammann, A. T., 1978, Thymosin treatment of children with primary immunodefi-
    ciency disease, *Transplant. Proc.* **10**:203–209.
Weksler, M. E., Innes, J. B., and Goldstein, G., 1978, Immunologic studies of aging. IV. The
    contribution of thymic involution to immune deficiencies of aging mice and reversal with thymopro-
    tein, *J. Exp. Med.* **148**:996–1006.
Weksler, M. E., 1983, The thymus gland and aging, *Ann. Intern. Med.* **98**:105–107.
Wilson, W. E., Kirkpatrick, C. R., and Talmage, D. W., 1965, Suppression of immunologic respon-
    siveness in uremia, *Ann. Intern. Med.* **62**:1–14.

53

Lipid and Lipoprotein Changes Due to Estrogen Replacement Therapies and Their Association with Prevention of Cardiovascular Disease in Postmenopausal Women

VALERY T. MILLER, JOHN C. LAROSA, and
RICHARD A. MUESING

1. INTRODUCTION

Postmenopausal estrogen replacement is prescribed for nearly 2.3 million women in the United States for the relief of symptoms and more recently for the prevention of osteoporosis (Kennedy *et al.*, 1985; Peck *et al.*, 1984). Numerous cohort and case-control studies, however, suggest that estrogen replacement therapy (ERT) may have a more important indication (Ross *et al.*, 1987). These studies show that ERT decreases the risk of coronary artery disease (CAD) in women by as much as one half to two thirds. More than 250,000 women die each year of CAD, and it is the number one cause of death in women. ERT could therefore have a major role in the prevention of heart disease in women.

Estrogen given over long periods of time, however, appears to increase the risk of endometrial cancer (Ziel *et al.*, 1975). Because the addition of a progestogen has been shown to protect the endometrium, the current recommended regimen for ERT is the cyclical use of estrogen and a progestogen (Whitehead *et al.*, 1979; Gambrell, 1982). Concerns have been raised, however, about the potential long-term negative effects of progestogens in CAD prevention in women. It is well established that ERT decreases circulating low-density lipoprotein cholesterol (LDL-C) and increases high-density lipoprotein cholesterol (HDL-C), lipoprotein changes that are antiatherogenic (Bush *et al.*, 1985; Castelli, 1986). It is believed that these changes at least in part account for the significant reduction in risk provided by estrogen in ERT. By contrast, progestogens have the opposite effect on LDL-C and HDL-C; that is, they increase LDL-C and decrease HDL-C (Wahl *et al.*, 1983).

VALERY T. MILLER, JOHN C. LAROSA, and RICHARD A. MUESING • Lipid Research Clinic, George Washington University School of Medicine and Health Sciences, Washington, D. C. 20037.

These two hormones then have opposing effects on lipoproteins. The net effect on LDL-C and HDL-C of a combination regimen is related to the kind of estrogen and progestogen used, the doses administered, and the method of administration. Research is being directed toward identification of a combination of estrogen and progestogen that will protect the endometrium but will also allow the fullest expression of the positive effects of the estrogen on lipoproteins.

2. ESTROGEN EFFECTS ON LIPIDS AND LIPOPROTEINS

Estrogens can be divided into natural (conjugated and micronized) and synthetic. In general, synthetic estrogens have greater lipoprotein effects than do natural estrogens. This is probably related more to dose than to chemical structures. Table I shows the percentage changes in lipids and lipoproteins from several oral preparations of estrogen. LDL-C levels are decreased by estrogen and HDL-C and triglyceride levels are increased. HDL_2-C, the subfraction of HDL-C thought to be most closely associated with decreased risk of CAD (Miller et al., 1988) is increased substantially by estrogen in all reported studies (Cauley et al., 1983; Blumenfeld et al., 1983; Miller et al., 1988; Tikkanen et al., 1982; Krauss et al., 1979).

The route of administration of estrogen has important effects on lipid and lipoprotein levels. Estrogens have been administered in the menopause orally, vaginally, intramuscularly, transdermally, and subcutaneously in the form of pellets. Most commonly, however, it is given by mouth. This route of administration has the greatest effect on lipoproteins (Bush et al., 1987). The explanation for this is believed to be related to the high concentrations of estrogen reaching the liver via the portal system, the so-called first pass phenomena (Geola et al., 1980). Each method of administration is, however, capable of producing lipoprotein changes if high enough doses of estrogen are used. Neither vaginal nor transdermal estrogen administration as prescribed in the United States has been shown to have beneficial effects on lipoproteins (Mandel et al., 1983; Chetkowski et al., 1986). Thus, at this time it appears that only oral estrogen affords cardiovascular protection by beneficial alterations in lipoproteins.

TABLE I. Adjusted[a] Percentage Change in Lipids and Lipoproteins
Due to Various Estrogen Preparations

Estrogen	Dose (mg)	% change			
		LDL-C	HDL-C	HDL_2-C	Triglycerides
Conjugated equine estrogen	0.625	−4	+10	+20	+11
	1.25	−8	+14	—	+17
Estradiol valerate	2	−16	+15	+20	+4
Estradiol succinate	1	0.0	+12	—	+2
Ethinyl estradiol	0.05	−21	+26	+29	+50

[a]Adjusted for sample size and duration of study.

3. ESTROGEN /PROGESTOGEN EFFECTS ON LIPIDS AND LIPOPROTEINS

Three progestogens are commonly used worldwide in ERT: norethindrone and its acetate, norgestrel, and medroxyprogesterone acetate (MPA). Norethindrone and norgestrel are derived from 19-nortestosterone. By weight they are far more androgenic than is MPA, which is derived from 17 α-hydroxyprogesterone (Whitehead et al., 1987). Hirvonen et al. (1981) demonstrated that the more androgenic compounds, norethindrone and norgestrel, reduced HDL-C far below baseline in the presence of 2 mg of estradiol valerate. The doses of norgestrel and norethindrone used in that study were high (500 mg and 10 mg, respectively) compared with those currently in use. At these doses, the 19-nortesterone-derived progestogens were less desirable from the standpoint of lipoprotein changes than was MPA. However, MPA at 10 mg also reduces HDL-C below baseline levels. Recent research has therefore been directed toward using lower doses of both MPA as well as norgestrel and norethindrone.

The lipoprotein effects of various estrogen/progestogen regimens are presented in Table II. Remarkable consistency is shown in LDL-C change among studies using cyclical 0.625 mg conjugated equine estrogen (CE) and 10 mg MPA. LDL-C is lowered by about 12% with this regimen. Furthermore, in the continuous regimen, doses of norethindrone acetate and norgestrel (1 mg and 150 μg, respectively) are identified that are similar in LDL-C effects to those of 10 mg MPA. Regimens of continuous estrogen and progestogen, using smaller daily doses of progestogens, also reduce LDL-C in four of five studies (Weinstein, 1987; Miller et al., 1988; Prough et al., 1987; Luciano et al., 1988; Farish et al., 1983; Jensen et al., 1987).

There is less consistency in HDL-C change among the studies than LDL-C change. However, most studies support a dose relationship; that is, HDL-C levels are higher in the presence of less progestogen. Table III presents the percentage change in HDL-C levels with increasing monthly doses of MPA. The dose of estrogen is the same except in one study. The dose of MPA per month is calculated by multiplying the amount taken per day by the number of days taken. The regimens were cyclical or continuous daily doses of MPA. From their presentation, the concept of progestogen load emerges. With lower monthly doses of MPA (65–75 mg), the estrogen effects of increasing the HDL-C are seen. As the progestogen load is increased, however, HDL-C levels decline. Prough et al. (1987) reported higher HDL-C levels than did other studies for the similar progestogen loads. These higher values may be attributable to the fact that their study is the only study of 9 months' duration. Indeed, Prough et al. report that they measured lipoproteins at 3 months in the continuous-regimen group and found changes to be negligible.

Only two studies state the times of sampling when a cyclical regimen was administered (Miller et al., 1988; Prough et al., 1987). This is an important consideration, since sampling at different points in the month would likely show different results from those where sampling occurs during progestogen loading.

The data of Luciano et al. (1988) are difficult to interpret because these authors combined the results from one group of subjects given 0.625 mg CE and another group given 1.25 mg CE. Thus, in spite of a progestogen load of 130 mg, the influence of a comparatively higher dose of estrogen may be reflected in the 8% increase in HDL-C. The data presented in Table III indicate that, irrespective of the regimen (cyclical or continuous), the monthly progestogen dose determines the overall effect on lipoprotein levels. Each of these studies reported on small groups of women and, while a trend has been identified, the ideal combina-

TABLE II. Effects of Estrogen/Progestogen Regimens on Lipoproteins[a]

Study	N	Duration (months)	Estrogen	Dose (mg)	Progestogen	Dose (mg)	LDL-C	HDL-C	HDL$_2$-C
Cyclical regimens									
Weinstein (1987)	12	3	CE	0.625	MPA	5	−18	+11	—
Miller et al. (1988)	7	3	CE	0.625	MPA	10	−11.6	−6	—
Prough et al. (1987)	10	9	CE	0.625	MPA	10	−11.6	+25	—
Luciano et al. (1988)	10	3	CE	0.625–1.25	NE	10	−12	+8	—
Miller et al. (1988)	10	3	CE	0.625	NG	1	−10	−10	—
Miller et al. (1988)	10	3	CE	0.625	NG	150 µg	−6	−2	−19.3
Farish et al. (1987)	21	6	CE	0.625	NG	150 µg	−13	−5	−10
Continuous regimens									
Weinstein (1987)	12	3	CE	0.625	MPA	2.5	−21	+3.7	—
Prough et al. (1987)	16	9	CE	0.625	MPA	2.5	+2	+12	—
Weinstein (1987)	12	3	CE	0.625	MPA	5	−19	+3.5	—
Luciano et al. (1988)	10	3	CE	0.625–1.25	MPA	10	−11	−16	—
Jensen et al. (1987)	21	12	CE	0.625	NE	1	−20	−5	—

[a]CE, conjugated equine estrogen; MPA, medroxyprogesterone acetate; NE, norethindrone; NG, norgestrel.

TABLE III. Effects of Various Doses of MPA on HDL-C Change

Study	N	Duration (months)		Conjugated estrogen dose (mg)	MPA dose (mg)	Monthly dose (mg)	Change HDL-C (%)
Weinstein (1987)	12	3	Cyclical[a]	0.625	5	65	+11
Prough et al. (1987)	16	9	Daily	0.625	2.5	75	+12
Weinstein (1987)	12	3	Daily[b]	0.625	2.5	75	+4
Weinstein (1987)	12	3	Daily	0.625	5.0	150	+4
Luciano et al. (1988)	10	3	Cyclical	0.625–1.25	10	130	+8
Miller et al. (1987)	7	3	Cyclical	0.625	10	130	−6
Prough et al. (1987)	10	9	Cyclical	0.625	10	130	+25
Luciano et al. (1988)	10	3	Daily	0.625–1.25	10	300	−16

[a]Cyclical administration of MPA 10–13 days per month.
[b]Daily or continuous administration of MPA.

tion of an estrogen and progestogen has not. More investigations are needed on large numbers of women to examine both the qualitative as well as quantitative changes in lipoproteins.

Continuous administration of MPA at the doses listed in Table III has been reported to provide adequate protection for the uterus (Weinstein et al., 1987; Prough et al., 1987); a 10-mg dose of MPA administered cyclically ensures adequate protection in most women (Whitehead et al., 1981). Low doses of norethindrone and norgestrel (1 mg and 150 µg, respectively) have also been demonstrated to protect the endometrium (Whitehead et al., 1987).

4. SUMMARY

Because heart disease is the number one cause of death in women, the finding that postmenopausal replacement with estrogen substantially reduces cardiovascular risk in women is very important. The effects of estrogen on lipids and lipoproteins are antiatherogenic. Current practice, however, is to add a progestogen to the replacement regimen because protestogens protect the uterus from endometrial cancer. The opposite effect (i.e., atherogenic) of progestogens on lipoproteins is cause for concern. Recent data indicate that low doses of progestogens preserve some LDL-C lowering in all studied regimens but that HDL-C levels are more sensitive to the progestogen load. Monthly doses of 65–75 mg of medroxyprogesterone acetate, whether administered cyclically or continuously, appear to have the most beneficial lipoprotein effects. More studies are needed to identify more precisely the best regimens of estrogen and progestogen.

ACKNOWLEDGMENT. We wish to thank Mary-Alice Goodridge for her secretarial assistance in the preparation of this manuscript.

REFERENCES

Blumenfeld, Z., Aviram, M., and Brook, G. J., 1983, Changes in lipoprotein and subfractions following oophorectomy and estrogen replacement in perimenopausal women, Maturitas 5:77–83.

Bush, T. L., and Barrett-Conner, E., 1985, Noncontraceptive estrogen use and cardiovascular disease, *Epidemiol. Rev.* **7**:80–104.

Bush, T. L., and Miller, V. T., 1987, Effects of pharmocologic agents used during the menopause, in: *Menopause: Physiology and Pharmacology* (D. R. Mishell, Jr., ed.), Year Book, Chicago, pp. 187–208.

Castelli, W. P., 1984, Epidemiology of coronary heart disease: The Framingham Study, *Am. J. Med.* **76**(suppl. 2A):4–12.

Cauley, J. A., LaPorte, R. E., Kuller, L. H., Bates, M., and Sandler, R. B., 1983, Menopausal estrogen use, high density lipoprotein cholesterol subfractions and liver function, *Atherosclerosis* **49**:31–39.

Chetkowski, R. J., Meldrum, D. R., Steingold, K. A., Randle, D., Lu, J. K., Eggena, P., Hershman, J. M., Alkjaersig, N. K., Fletcher, A. P., and Judd, H. L., 1986, Biologic effects of transdermal estradiol, *N. Engl. J. Med.* **314**:1615–1620.

Farish, E., Fletcher, C. D., Hart, D. M., Teo, H. T., Alazzawi, F., and Howie, C., 1986, The effects of conjugated equine estrogens with and without a cylical progestogen on lipoproteins, and HDL subfractions in postmenopausal women, *Acta Endocrinol. (Copenh.)* **113**:123–127.

Gambrell, R. D., Jr., 1982, Clinical use of progestins in the menopausal patient, dosage and duration, *J. Reprod. Med.* **27**:531–538.

Geola, F. L., Frumar, A. M., Tataryn, I. V., Lu, K. H., Hershman, J. M., Eggena, P., Sambhi, M. P., and Judd, H. L., 1980, Biological effects of various doses of conjugated equine estrogens in postmenopausal women, *J. Clin. Endocrinol. Metab.* **51**:620–625.

Hirvonen, E., Malkonen, M., and Manninen, V., 1981, Effects of different progestogens on lipoproteins during postmenopausal replacement therapy, *N. Engl. J. Med.* **304**:560–563.

Jensen, J., Riis, B. J., Strom, V., and Christiansen, C., 1987, Continuous estrogen–progestogen treatment and serum lipoproteins in postmenopausal women, *Br. J. Obstet. Gynaecol.* **94**:130–135.

Kennedy, D. L., Baum, C., and Forbes, M. B., 1985, Noncontraceptive estrogens and progestins: Use patterns overtime, *Obstet. Gynecol.* **65**:441–446.

Luciano, A. A., Turksoy, N., Carleo, J., and Hendrix, J. W., 1988, Clinical and metabolic responses of menopausal women to sequential versus continuous estrogen and progestin replacement therapy, *Obstet. Gynecol.* **71**:39–43.

Mandel, F. P., Geola, F. L., Meldrum, D. R., Lu, J. H. K., Eggena, P., Sambhi, M. P., Hershman, J. M., and Judd, H. L., 1983, Biological effects of various doses of vaginally administered conjugated equine estrogens in postmenopausal women, *J. Clin. Endocrinol. Metab.* **57**:133–139.

Miller, V. T., Muesing, R. A., and LaRosa, J. C., 1989, Lipoprotein and apoprotein effects of conjugated estrogen and three progestogens, submitted for publication.

Peck, W. A., Barrett-Conner, E., and Buckwater, J., 1984, Consensus development conference on osteoporosis, *JAMA* **252**:799–802.

Prough, S. G., Aksel, S., Wiebe, H., and Shepard, J., 1987, Continuous estrogen/progestin therapy in menopause, *Am. J. Obstet. Gynecol.* **157**:1449–1453.

Ross, R. K., Paganini-Hill, A., Mack, T. M., and Henderson, B. E., 1987, Estrogen use and cardiovascular disease, in: *Menopause: Physiology and Pharmacology* (D. R. Mishell, Jr., ed.), Year Book, Chicago, pp. 209–223.

Wahl, P., Walden, C., Knopp, R., Hoover, J., Wallace, R., Heiss, G., and Rifkind, B., 1983, Effect of estrogen/progestin potency on lipid/lipoprotein cholesterol, *N. Engl. J. Med.* **308**:862–867.

Weinstein, L., 1987, Efficacy of a continuous estrogen–progestin regimen in the menopausal patient, *Obstet. Gynecol.* **69**:929–932.

Whitehead, M. I., Townsend, P. T., Pryse-Davies, J., Ryder, T. A., and King, R. J. B., 1981, Effect of estrogens and progestins on the biochemistry and morphology of the postmenopausal endometrium, *N. Engl. J. Med.* **305**:1599–1605.

Whitehead, M. I., Siddle, N., Lane, G., Padwick, M., Ryder, T. A., Pryse-Davies, J., and King, R. J. B., 1987, The pharmacology of progestogens, in: *Menopause: Physiology and Pharmacology* (D. R. Mishell, Jr., ed.), Year Book, Chicago, pp. 317–334.

Ziel, H. K., and Finkle, W. D., 1975, Increased risk of endometrial carcinoma among users of conjugated estrogens, *N. Engl. J. Med.* **293**:1167–1170.

54

Immunopotentiating Activity of Thymopentin Treatment in Elderly Subjects

PIER LUIGI MERONI, WILMA BARCELLINI,
MARIA ORIETTA BORGHI, DANIELA FRASCA,
ALESSANDRO VISMARA, PAOLO BAMBERGA,
GIANNI FERRARO, GINO DORIA,
and CARLO ZANUSSI

1. INTRODUCTION

The involution of the thymus gland and subsequent decline of thymic hormone serum levels is involved, to a considerable extent, in the development of age-associated immune deficiency (Weksler and Siskind, 1984). Thymus grafting or substitutive therapy with thymic hormones was reported to improve and/or restore age-associated immune defects in experimental animals (Doria *et al.*, 1986).

Thymopentin (TP-5), a synthetic pentapeptide displaying the same biological activities as natural thymopoietin (Goldstein *et al.*, 1979), administered in immunocompromised elderly subjects, was shown to enhance interleukin-2 (IL-2) production, which could account for the concomitant improvement of delayed-type hypersensitivity (DTH) to recall antigens and blastogenesis to lectins (Meroni *et al.*, 1987).

The aim of this study was to investigate further in immunocompromised elderly subjects the immunopharmacological activity of TP-5. The results confirm the enhanced IL-2 production and show increased IL-2 receptor expression after treatment, further stressing that IL-2/IL-2R binding may be the crucial mechanism of the immunopotentiating activity of TP-5 in aging humans. Estimation of phytohemagglutinin (PHA)-responding precursors by

PIER LUIGI MERONI, WILMA BARCELLINI, MARIA ORIETTA BORGHI, ALESSANDRO VISMARA, PAOLO BAMBERGA, GIANNI FERRARO, and CARLO ZANUSSI • Institute of Internal Medicine, Infectious Disease, and Immunopathology, University of Milan, Padiglione Granelli Polyclinic Hospital, 20122 Milan, Italy.   DANIELA FRASCA and GINO DORIA • Laboratory of Pathology, C.R.E. ENEA, Casaccia, Rome, Italy.

limiting dilution analysis (LDA) and studies with TP-5 in vitro were also carried out in order
to investigate additional immunopotentiating mechanisms.

2. MATERIALS AND METHODS

2.1. Subjects

Eighteen institutionalized elderly subjects (14 women and 4 men, mean age ±SD 75.4
± 5.2 years) were studied before (T0) and after (T1) TP-5 treatment, 50 mg subcutaneously
(SC) three times/week for 4 weeks. Dose and schedule of TP-5 administration were chosen
according to previous report in the literature (Duchateau et al., 1983). The subjects were
selected from a group of institutionalized elderly patients on the basis of their skin hypoergy
or anergy to recall antigens. None of the selected subjects was affected by neoplastic,
infectious, or autoimmune disease, nor did they receive any drug influencing immune functions at the time of the study.

The control group consisted of 54 healthy adults (35 women and 19 men, mean age
±SD 34.8 ± 7 years, range 23–39) tested during a period of 6 months, corresponding to the
time of recruitment and follow-up of the elderly subjects into the study.

2.2. Delayed-Type Hypersensitivity

Delayed-type hypersensitivity was evaluated by using a multipuncture instrument (Multitest, Institut Mérieux, Lyon, France) that assesses the response to seven recall antigens
simultaneously (tetanus, diphtheria, Streptococcus, tuberculin, Candida, Tricophyton, and
Proteus) (Frazer et al., 1985): the size of the induration was measured at 48 hr in two
diameters; reactions of <2 mm were scored as negative. The subjects were defined anergic
when unresponsive to all the antigens and hypoergic when responsive only to one antigen.

2.3. Lymphocyte Isolation and Culture Conditions

Peripheral blood mononuclear cells (PBM) were obtained from fresh heparinized venous
blood by Ficoll-Isopaque (Lymphoprep, Neygaard Co., Norway) density-gradient centrifugation, according to Boyum (1968). PBM were cultured in RPMI 1640 (Gibco, Grand Island,
New York), supplemented with 10% Foetal Calf Serum (FCS—Flow Labs., Irvine,
Scotland, U.K.), Penicillin 100 U/ml, streptomycin 100 μg/ml (Eurobio, Paris, France), and
L-glutamine 1% (Flow Laboratories, Irvine, Scotland). The mitogenic stimulus was provided
by (1) phytohemagglutinin (PHA) (Gibco, Grand Island, New York) at the final concentra-
tions of 5, 1.2, and 0.3%; (2) Concanavalin A (Con A) (Sigma Chemicals Co., St. Louis,
Missouri), at the final concentration of 75, 18, and 4.5 μg/ml, and pokeweed mitogen
(PWM) at the final concentration of 0.8%.

Standard cultures were performed in 5% humidified incubator for 72 hr. The PBM
proliferative response was assessed by [3H]thymidine uptake as previously described (Meroni
et al., 1982). In vitro PWM-induced immunoglobulin (IgG and IgM) synthesis was evaluated
as described (Meroni et al., 1984).

Interleukin-2 production was induced by stimulating PBM (2×10^6 cells in 1 ml of
complete medium) in 12×75 mm round-bottomed glass tubes fitted with Morton closures

(Sterilin Ltd., Teddington, Middlesex) with 5% PHA (final concentration) for 48 hr in 5% CO_2 humidified incubator. Culture supernatants were collected by centrifugation (10 min at 1500 rpm) filtered through 0.2 μm Millex filters (Millipore, Molsheim, France) and stored at −80°C until use.

2.4. IL-2 Titration

The assay was based on the method of Gillis *et al.* (1978) but involved statistical validation of titration data according to the principles of the biological assay by parallel lines as applied to probit analysis of quantitative responses, as previously described (Sette *et al.*, 1986). Briefly, supernatants were twofold serially diluted in medium from $\frac{1}{2}$ to $\frac{1}{256}$, and 100-μl samples of each dilution were added to triplicate microwells containing 100 μl of IL-2-dependent CTLL cell suspension (1×10^4 cells/well). After 20-hr incubation at 37°C, all cultures received 0.5 μCi of [^{3}H]thymidine (specific activity 2Ci/mmoles, Amersham International plc, Amersham); 4 hr later, cells were harvested by an automated cell harvester (Titertek cell harvester, Flow Labs., Irvine, Scotland), and radioactivity was measured in a liquid scintillation counter (Packard, Downers Grove, Illinois).

2.5. Effect of Exogenous IL-2 on PHA-Blast Proliferation

In the first-step culture, 1×10^6 PBM was cultured in 12×75-mm tubes in a final volume of 1 ml of complete medium without or with mitogenic (1.2%) and submitogenic (0.3%) doses of PHA, at 37°C in a humidified atmosphere of 5% CO_2 and air for 48 hr. In the second-step culture, blasts were washed at 37°C twice with phosphate-buffered saline (PBS) and twice with Hank's balanced salt solution (HBSS) (Flow Laboratories, Irvine, Scotland) and adjusted to the concentration of 10^5 cells/ml in complete medium. Then, 100 μl of this suspension was further cultured for 24 hr in a 5% CO_2 incubator in the presence of 100 μl of twofold dilutions (from $\frac{1}{4}$ to $\frac{1}{256}$) of exogenous IL-2 from EL-4 line, obtained as described below. Briefly, 1×10^6 EL-4 thymoma cells were cultured in RPMI 1640 added with FCS 2%, penicillin 100 U/ml, streptomycin 100 μg/ml, L-glutamine 1%, 2-mercaptoethanol 2×10^{-5} M (Merck, Darmstadt, West Germany) and stimulated by phorbol-12-myristate-13-acetate (PMA) (Sigma Chemicals Co., St. Louis) 10 ng/ml for 48 hr at 37°C in humidified atmosphere of 5% CO_2. PMA-stimulated EL-4 supernatants were collected by centrifugation (10 min at 1500 rpm) and filtered through 0.22-μm Millex filters. They were defined to contain 10 U/ml of IL-2, as described above. At the end of the second-step culture, cells were pulsed with 1 μCi of [^{3}H]thymidine (specific activity 2 Ci/mmoles, Amersham International plc, Amersham); 8 hr later, cells were harvested, and radioactivity was measured in a liquid scintillation counter (Packard, Downers Grove, Illinois).

2.6. Evaluation of Tac-Positive Lymphocytes

In evaluating Tac-positive lymphocytes, 1×10^6 PBM were cultured in 12×75-mm tubes in a final volume of 1 ml with 1.2% PHA or medium alone in a 5% CO_2 incubator for 48 hr. At the end of the culture period, blasts were washed twice with PBS and twice with HBSS; the percentage of Tac-positive lymphocytes was evaluated by indirect immunofluorescence using anti-Tac monoclonal antibody (Becton & Dickinson, Mountain View, California) (Uchiyama *et al.*, 1981), as described (Meroni *et al.*, 1984).

2.7. Limiting Dilution Assay

Cultures were set up in round-bottomed 96-well microtiter plates; each well contained varying numbers of PBM (from 100 to 25) as responders, 10^5 irradiated (5000 rad) autologous PBM as feeders and 0.3% PHA in a final volume of 0.2 ml of RPMI 1640, supplemented with 10% fetal calf serum (FCS), 2% IL-2 (from PMA-stimulated EL-4 line), 2×10^{-5} M 2-mercaptoethanol, 100 U/ml penicillin, 100 μg/ml streptomycin, and 1% L-glutamine; 32 replicates were set up for each cell concentration or for feeders alone. Plates were cultured in a 5% CO_2 humidified incubator for 10 days and pulsed with 1 μCi of [³H]thymidine (specific activity 2 Ci/mmoles) during the last 18 hr of culture. Positive cultures were defined as those in which proliferation exceeded by 3 SD the mean from 32 control wells containing feeders alone. The log fraction of nonresponding cultures was plotted as a function of the number of cells added to culture, and a straight line was forced through the origin by the least-squares method (Steel and Torrie, 1960) for graphic representation of the data. Statistical analysis was performed by the method of maximum likelihood (Fazekas de St. Groth, 1982), which gives the most likely mitogen-responsive T-cell precursor frequency in a cell population and an error factor by which the frequency should be multiplied or divided to obtain the variations due to 1 SE. Validity of the estimate was assessed by the chi-square criterion to test the goodness of fit of the data to a Poisson distribution, as previously described (Frasca *et al.*, 1987).

2.8. Peripheral Blood Subpopulations

Lymphocyte subsets were detected by indirect immunofluorescence with monoclonal antibodies against CD3, CD4, CD8, CD11 and CD10 antigens as previously described (Meroni *et al.*, 1984).

2.9. *In Vitro* Immunoglobulin Synthesis

For the evaluation of *in vitro* immunoglobulin synthesis, 1×10^6 PBM were cultured for 8 days in 12×75 round-bottomed tubes (Sterilin) in the presence or absence of PWM 1% final concentrations. The amounts of IgG and IgM in the culture supernatants were determined as previously described (Meroni *et al.*, 1984).

2.10. *In Vitro* Effects of TP-5

Thymopentin-acetate powder (lot No. 855039, kindly provided by Italfarmaco Laboratories, Milan) was dissolved in sterile distilled water at 100 mg/ml and stored at $-80°C$ until use. PBM (2×10^6) were incubated in 12×75-mm tubes for 30 min at 37°C in serum-free HBSS (to avoid inactivation of the drug by serum proteases) without or with different TP-5 concentrations (0.1–10,000 ng/ml). Cells were washed and further cultured with the same concentrations of TP-5 in FCS 10% complete medium. The cultures, either unstimulated or stimulated with PHA 0.3%, were performed in 96 microwell plates for 72 hr in a 5% CO_2 incubator; 1 μCi of [³H]thymidine/well was added 18 hr before harvesting.

2.11. Statistical Analysis

Statistical analysis was carried out using Student's *t*-test for paired and unpaired data; correlations were calculated by linear regression.

3. RESULTS

3.1. Impaired Immune Response in Elderly Subjects

All subjects entering the study displayed impaired DTH to recall antigens (13 anergic and 5 hypoergic) and significantly depressed baseline proliferative responses to PHA, Con A, and PWM, compared with healthy adult controls (data not shown).

As shown in Fig. 1, PHA-induced IL-2 production by elderly PBM before treatment (T0) was not significantly reduced with respect to adult values. By contrast, baseline values of IL-2R expression, as identified by the percentage of PHA-induced Tac-positive blasts, were decreased compared with adult controls ($p < 0.001$) (Fig. 2a).

The response to all concentrations of exogenous IL-2 by elderly PHA blasts was significantly impaired, after either PHA 1.2% ($p < 0.001$) or PHA 0.3% ($p < 0.005$) activation, compared with adult controls. Figure 2b shows the T0 values using preactivation with PHA 1.2% and serial dilution of IL-2.

3.2. Effect of TP-5 Treatment on the Different Immune Parameters Investigated

TP-5 was able to restore the DTH in 11 subjects (from anergic or hypoergic to normoergic) and to improve the DTH in 7 subjects (from anergic to hypoergic). The overall mean ±SD diameters of induration was 1.6 ± 1.3 mm at T0 versus 4.9 ± 1.7 mm at T1 ($p <$

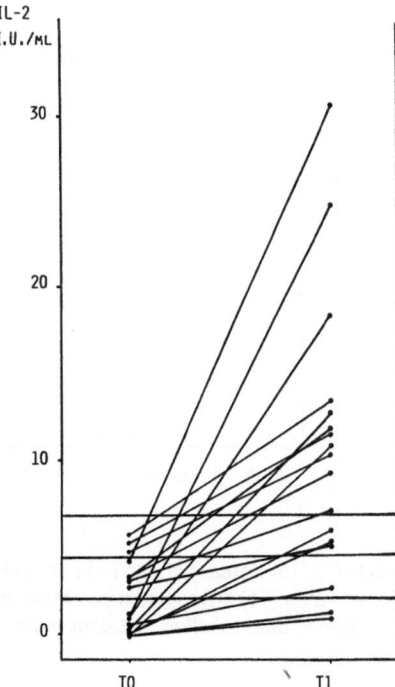

Figure 1. IL-2 activity (Units/ml) of PHA-stimulated cultures from elderly subjects, before (T0) and after (T1) thymopentin treatment. Horizontal lines represent the mean ±SD of 21 adult controls.

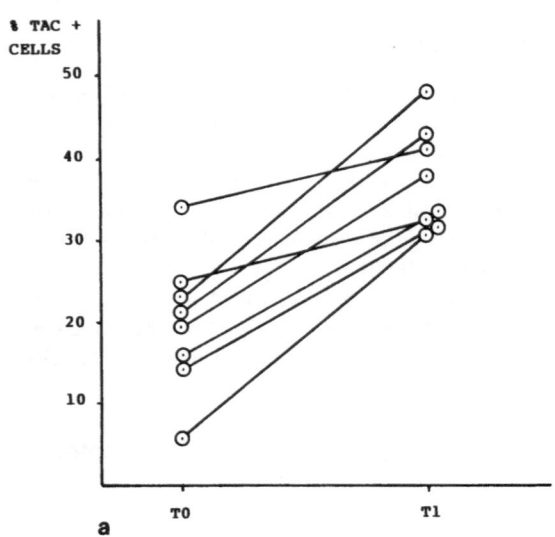

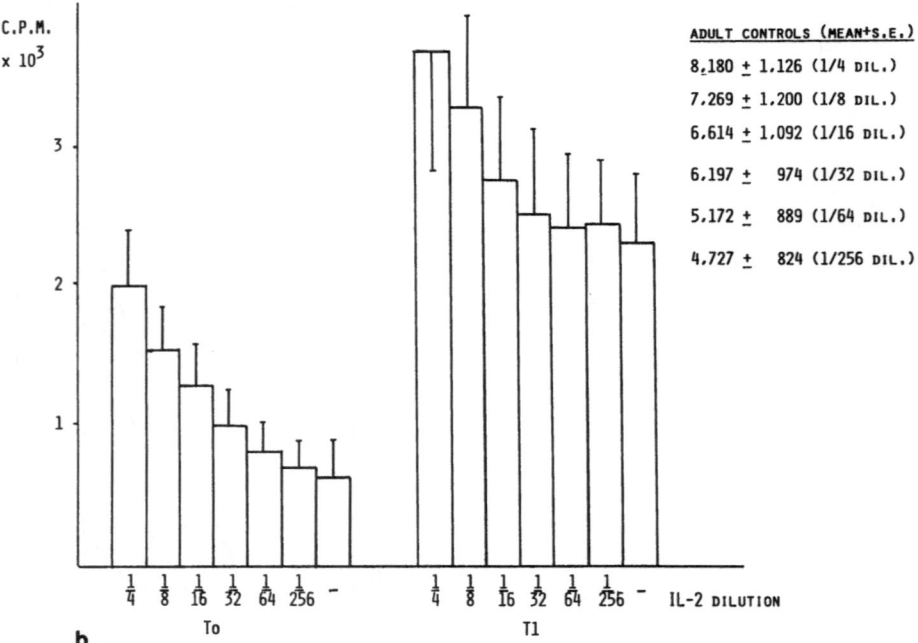

FIGURE 2. (a) Percent of Tac (+) cells in PHA-stimulated cultures from elderly subjects before (T0) and after (T1) thymopentin treatment. (b) Proliferative responses (mean ±SE) of PHA 1.2%-preactivated cells to different IL-2 dilutions, before (T0) and after (T1) thymopentin treatment.

0.01). At the same time, impaired PHA (Fig. 3), Con-A (Fig. 4), and PWM-induced proliferation of PBM from elderly subjects were significantly improved up to levels displayed by adult controls (horizontal lines: mean ±SD of 21 subjects) after treatment.

In the elderly subjects investigated, the PWM-induced IgG and IgM synthesis was significantly impaired ($p < 0.005$) as compared with that in normal adults; no changes were found after treatment (data not shown).

We confirmed increased IL-2 production after TP-5 treatment ($p < 0.025$, T1 versus T0) (see Fig. 1). Also, the percentage of Tac-positive blasts in PHA-stimulated cultures was significantly augmented ($p < 0.0005$) after TP-5 administration (Fig. 2a). It should be pointed out that baseline values of IL-2 production and Tac-positive cells in unstimulated cultures were comparable between elderly and adult controls and were not affected by TP-5 treatment (data not shown).

As shown in Fig. 2b, the response to different concentrations of exogenous IL-2 by PHA 1.2%-pulsed PBM was significantly increased, even if not restored to normal values ($p < 0.01$, T1 versus adult controls), after TP-5 administration. TP-5 treatment had a weak effect on the response to exogenous IL-2 by PHA 0.3%-activated lymphocytes (data not reported). It should be noted that PBM control cultures preincubated in medium without PHA (first-step culture) displayed negligible proliferation upon addition of exogenous IL-2 in the second-step culture. TP-5 treatment had no effect on this parameter.

Six of 18 treated subjects were also tested 3 (T2) and 6 (T3) months after the end of TP-5

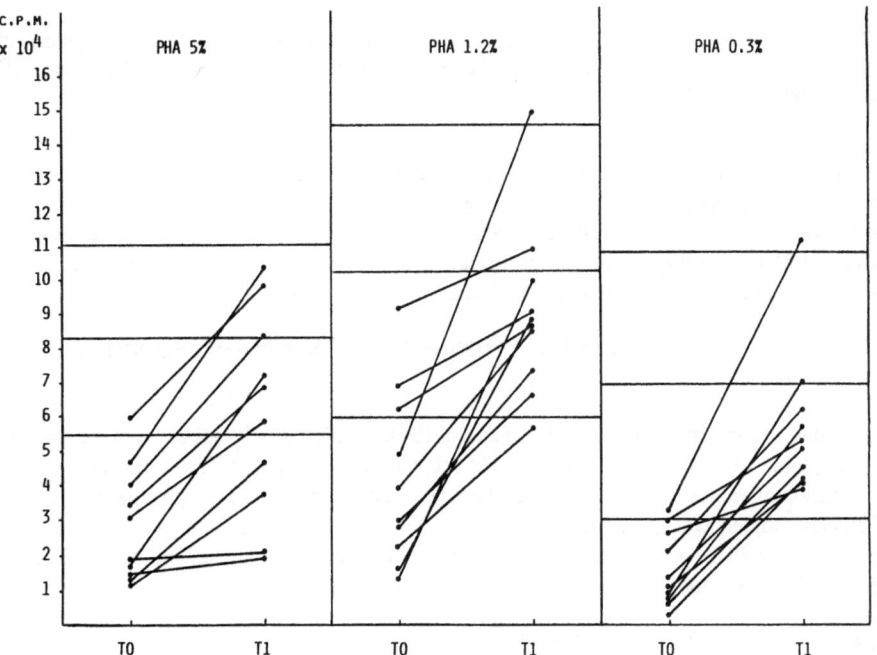

FIGURE 3. Proliferative responses of PBM from elderly subjects to different concentrations of PHA before (T0) and after (T1) thymopentin treatment. Horizontal lines represent the mean ±SD from 21 adult controls.

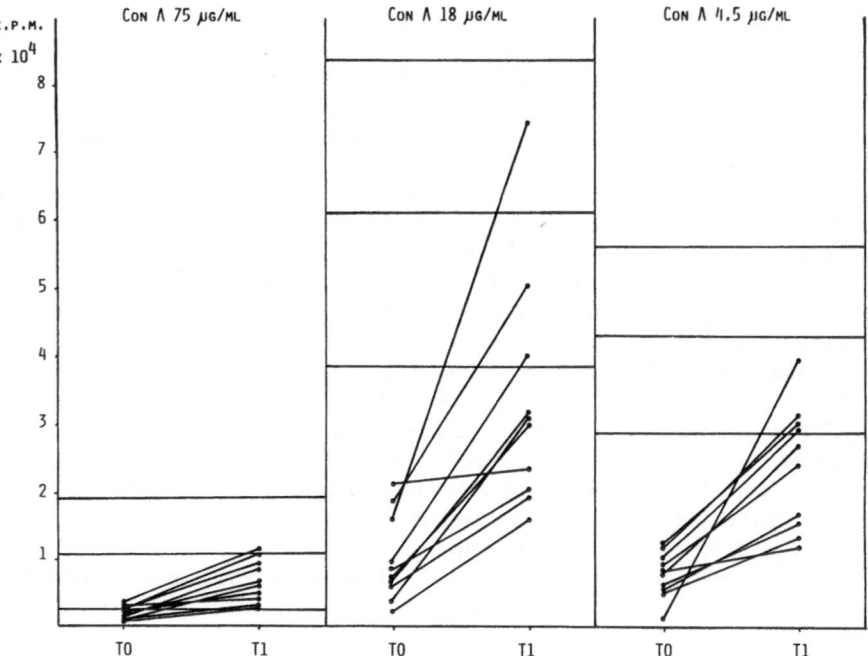

FIGURE 4. Proliferative responses of PBM from elderly subjects to different concentrations of ConA before (T0) and after (T1) thymopentin treatment. Horizontal lines represent the mean ±SD from 21 adult controls.

treatment. PHA-induced proliferation (Fig. 5) and PHA-induced IL-2 production (Fig. 6) still persisted at augmented levels at T2 and decreased at T3. A control group of six untreated institutionalized elderly subjects, comparable to the treated group concerning the baseline values of *in vitro* mitogen-induced proliferation and immunoglobulin synthesis, was tested twice over a period of 6 months and did not show significant variations.

3.3. Estimation of Precursor Frequencies for PHA-Responding Cells

Table I shows the precursor frequencies of PHA-proliferating lymphocytes as responsive cell/10^4 input cells in culture from 6 elderly subjects before and after TP-5 treatment. A wide distribution of values was observed in all cultures, and the mean baseline precursor frequency of elderly subjects was not significantly reduced compared with adult controls. The precursor frequencies of PHA-proliferating cells after TP-5 treatment were unchanged in 3 of 6 cases, decreased in one, and increased in two of six subjects tested.

3.4. Lymphocyte Subpopulations

In the subjects investigated, the lymphocyte subsets did not show differences with the control groups, either before or after treatment. The only exception was a slight increase in CD11-positive cells (not statistically significant) (Fig. 7).

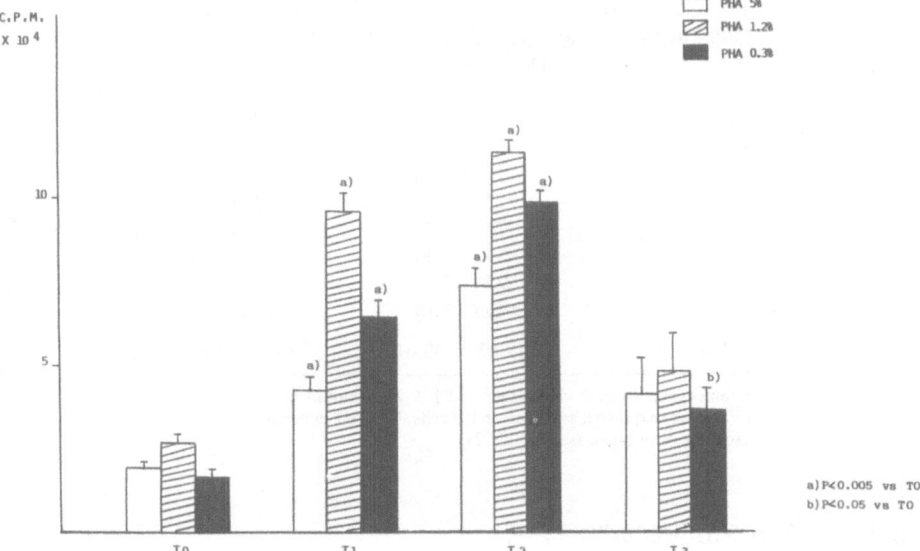

FIGURE 5. Proliferative responses by PBM from six elderly subjects to different concentrations of PHA before (T0), 4 weeks (T1), 3 (T2), and 6 months (T3) after thymopentin therapy.

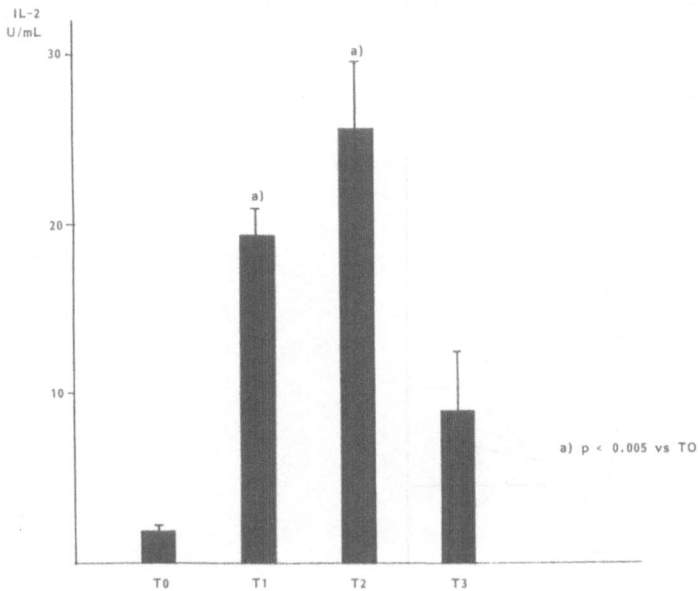

FIGURE 6. PHA-induced IL-2 production by PBM from six elderly subjects before (T0), 4 weeks (T1), 3 (T2), and 6 months (T3) after thymopentin therapy.

TABLE I. Precursor Frequencies of PHA-Proliferating
Cells from Elderly Subjects before (T0) and after (T1)
TP-5 Treatment[a]

Subject	T0	T1
1	28 (1.156)[b]	25 (1.161)
2	277 (1.148)	62 (1.131)
3	77 (1.147)	75 (1.148)
4	59 (1.158)	59 (1.157)
5	25 (1.217)	52 (1.165)
6	13 (1.310)	132 (1.136)
Mean $\pm$SE	79.83 $\pm$ 40.61	67.5 $\pm$ 14.56

[a]Values from 10 adult controls are 112.1 $\pm$ 25.29 (mean $\pm$SE).
[b]Values are expressed as precursor/10^4 cells. Numbers in parentheses represent the error factor (see Section 2).

3.5. *In Vitro* Studies with TP-5

Lymphocytes obtained from elderly subjects before treatment and cultured *in vitro* with TP-5 as described under Materials and Methods (Section 2) showed a dose-dependent increase of PHA-induced blastogenesis (Fig. 8). This enhancement was statistically significant for TP-5 doses of 100 ng/ml ($p < 0.01$), 1000 ng/ml ($p < 0.001$), and 10,000 ng/ml ($p < 0.01$). By contrast, no variations of PHA-induced blastogenetic response of adult lymphocytes were observed in the presence of TP-5. The *in vitro* effect of TP-5 was also explored in

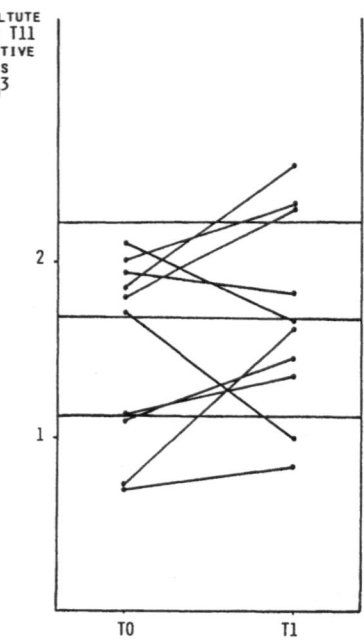

ABSOLTUTE
N OF T11
POSITIVE
CELLS
x 10^3

2

1

T0   T1

FIGURE 7. Absolute number/ml of CD11 (+) lymphocytes in elderly subjects, before (T0) and after (T1) thymopentin treatment. Horizontal lines represent the mean $\pm$SD from 21 adult controls.

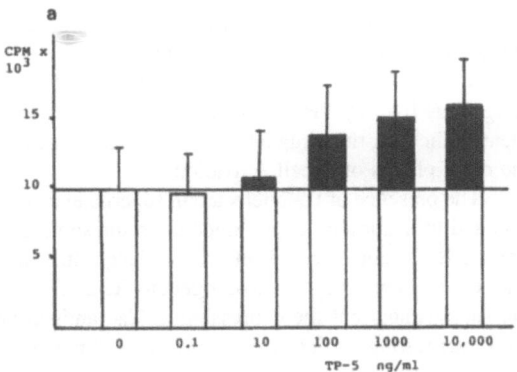

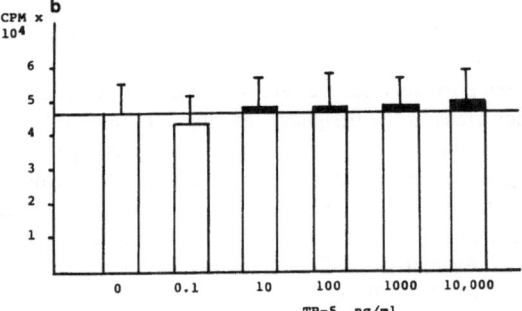

FIGURE 8. *In vitro* effect of TP-5 on PHA-induced blastogenesis. Values are expressed as c.p.m. ±SE of 7 aged subjects and 10 adult controls.

unstimulated lymphocytes. Both elderly and adult spontaneous proliferation was unaffected by the different doses of TP-5 tested (data not shown).

An attempt was made to correlate the *in vitro* effect of TP-5 with the *in vivo* response after treatment. We were unable to find any correlation between the degree of *in vitro* enhancement of PHA-induced blastogenesis and the *in vivo* increase of IL-2 production, percentage of Tac-positive blasts, and response to exogenous IL-2 after treatment.

4. DISCUSSION

The results in this chapter show that TP-5 treatment is able to correct to a great extent the impaired T-cell functions in the elderly. In a previous report (Meroni *et al.*, 1987), we demonstrated that TP-5 administration increased [^{3}H]thymidine incorporation into DNA after lectin activation as well as IL-2 production by PHA-stimulated lymphocytes. The improved IL-2 production might account for the immunopotentiating activity of the drug as suggested also by the comparable behavior of the proliferation and IL-2 values during the follow-up study.

Further experiments to investigate the IL-2R expression after TP-5 treatment were planned: (1) the evaluation of Tac expression in PHA-activated cells, which identifies both high- and low-affinity IL-2R (Robb *et al.*, 1984); and (2) the response to exogenous IL-2 by PHA-activated cells. Since proliferation is strictly dependent on the expression of high-affinity IL-2R (Robb *et al.*, 1981), the latter procedure gives more direct information on the expression of high-affinity IL-2-binding sites.

Results show that either the percentage of Tac-positive lymphocytes or the response to exogenous IL-2 by PHA 1.2% activated blasts are significantly enhanced after TP-5 treatment, indicating that drug administration can effectively upregulate IL-2R expression during the early phases of T-cell activation.

The presence of IL-2 detected in supernatants represents only a balance between production and utilization by cells. Since the same subjects display reduced IL-2R expression, the normal IL-2 content could reflect a reduced utilization of the lymphokine by cells, in line with the impaired response to exogenous IL-2. TP-5 administration increased IL-2 content in the supernatants but the expression of Tac antigen and the response to exogenous IL-2 as well, suggesting an increased utilization of the lymphokine by the cells. Altogether, our findings support that the improvement of both IL-2 synthesis and IL-2R expression may be instrumental in promoting T-cell functions after TP-5 treatment.

More controversial are the mechanism(s) by which TP-5 exerts its immunopotentiating activity. The induction of T-cell maturation and differentiation markers in the thymus gland is well documented (Scheid *et al.*, 1975; Ranges *et al.*, 1982). This maturative effect has also been postulated for the relatively immature extrathymic T cells undergoing the final maturation steps in the periphery (Stutman, 1978; Scollary *et al.*, 1984).

Since lectin responsiveness is displayed by well-differentiated T lymphocytes, we investigated the precursor frequencies of PHA-responding cells by LDA both before and after TP-5 treatment. We did not find a clear effect of the treatment on LDA-estimated precursor frequencies: in fact, an increased precursor frequency was demonstrated only in two subjects.

By contrast, a direct immunomodulating activity of thymic hormones on human mature peripheral T cells has also been reported (Zatz and Goldstein, 1985; Sztein *et al.*, 1986). *In vitro* experiments show that TP-5 increases PHA-induced proliferative response by peripheral lymphocytes. This finding suggests that the drug could directly modulate responses of peripheral T cells, although the immunoregulatory activity is evident only in elderly hyporesponsive lymphocytes. In line with our results, Sztein *et al.* (1986) demonstrated that the *in vitro* thymosin fraction 5-induced increase of IL-2 production and IL-2R expression were more evident in cells exhibiting suboptimal responses to PHA alone.

Of note, TP-5 displays a potentiating activity only on activated lymphocytes, since it has no effect on unstimulated cell functions in both *in vitro* and *in vivo* studies.

5. CONCLUSION

We confirm that TP-5 *in vivo* improves IL-2 production; we also demonstrate that the increased expression of IL-2R is a clear effect of the drug. The enhanced T-cell responses after TP-5 treatment may reflect an enhanced IL-2/IL-2R efficiency, but an increase in the size of the responsive T-cell pool cannot be excluded, at least in some subjects, as suggested in animal studies (Frasca *et al.*, 1987). Studies are now in progress in our laboratory to investigate whether TP-5 might affect also the non-T-lymphocyte cells, as suggested by the increase of CD11- but not CD3-positive cells after treatment.

6. SUMMARY

The *in vivo* immunopharmacological activity of thymopentin was investigated using age-associated immune deficiency as a model. Subcutaneous administration of thymopentin was able to increase IL-2 production and IL-2 receptor expression, evaluated as percentage of Tac-positive cells and response to exogenous IL-2 of PHA-activated lymphocytes. Using limiting dilution analysis, increased precursor frequency of PHA-responding lymphocytes was observed in two of six subjects tested after treatment. *In vitro* experiments show that thymopentin was able to enhance directly the PHA or anti-CD3-induced proliferation of elderly lymphocytes but not of adult cells.

Increased IL-2 synthesis/IL-2 receptor expression seems to be the key mechanism of the immunopotentiating activity of the drug in the age-associated immune defect. It is difficult to state whether this activity is mediated by a simple increase in intrinsic T-cell responsiveness or by an increase in the size of the responsive T-cell pool, at least in some subjects.

REFERENCES

Boyum, A., 1968, Isolation of mononuclear cells and granulocytes from human blood, *Scand. J. Clin. Lab. Invest.* **21**(suppl. 97):77–81.

Doria, G., Adorini, L., and Frasca, D., 1986, Immunoregulation of antibody responses in aging mice, in: *Aging and the Immune Response* (E. Goidl, eds.), Dekker, New York, pp. 143–176.

Duchateau, J., Delespesse, G., and Bolla, K., 1983, Phase variation in the modulation of the human immune response, *Immunol. Today* **4**:213–214.

Frasca, D., Adorini, L., and Doria, G., 1987, Enhanced frequency of mitogen-responsive T cell precursor in old mice injected with thymosin alpha-1, *Eur. J. Immunol.* **17**:727–734.

Frazer, I. H., Collins, E. J., Fox, J. S., Jones, B., Oliphant, R. C., and Hackey, I. R., 1985, Assessment of delayed-type hypersensitivity in man: A comparison of the "Multitest" and conventional intradermal injection of six antigens, *Clin. Immunol. Immunopathol.* **35**:182–190.

Gillis, S., Ferm, M. M., Ou, W., and Smith, K. A., 1978, T cell growth factor: Parameters of production and a quantitative microassay for activity, *J. Immunol.* **120**:2027–2031.

Goldstein, G., Scheid, M. P., Boyse, E. A., Schlesinger, D. H., and Van Wauwe, J., 1979, A synthetic pentapeptide with biological activity characteristic of the thymic hormone thymopoietin, *Science* **204**:1309–1310.

Meroni, P. L., Barcellini, W., Messina, C., DeBartolo, G., Capsoni, F., and Invernizzi, F., 1982, Defective suppressor cell activity in essential mixed cryoglobulinemia, *J. Clin. Lab. Immunol.* **8**:177–182.

Meroni, P. L., Barcellini, W., De Bartolo, G., Invernizzi, F., and Zanussi, C., 1984, Abnormalities of *in vitro* immunoglobulin synthesis by peripheral blood lymphocytes from patients with essential mixed cryoglobulinemia, *Clin. Immunol. Immunopathol.* **33**:245–257.

Meroni, P. L., Barcellini, W., Frasca, D., Sguotti, C., Borghi, M. O., De Bartolo, G., Doria, G., and Zanussi, C., 1987, *In vivo* immunopotentiating activity of thymopentin in aging humans, *Clin. Immunol. Immunopathol.* **42**:151–159.

Ranges, G. E., Scheid, M. P., Goldstein, G., and Boyse, E. A., 1982, T cell development in normal and tymopentin-treated nude mice, *J. Exp. Med.* **156**:1057–1064.

Robb, R. J., Munck, A., and Smith, K. A., 1981, T cell growth factor receptors: Quantitation, specificity and biological relevance, *J. Exp. Med.* **154**:1455–1461.

Robb, R. J., Greene, W. C., and Rusk, C., 1984, Low and high affinity cellular receptors for interleukin 2. Implications for the level of Tac antigen, *J. Exp. Med.* **160**:1126–1146.

Scheid, M. P., Goldstein, G., and Boyse, E. A., 1975, Differentiation of T cells in nude mice, *Science* **190**:1211–1214.

Sette, A., Adorini, L., Marubini, E., and Doria, G., 1986, A microcomputer program for probit analysis of interleukin 2 titration data, *J. Immunol. Methods* **86**:265–277.

Steel, R. G. D., and Torrie, J. H. (eds.), 1960, *Principles and procedures of Statistics*, McGraw-Hill, New York.

Fazekas de St. Groth, S., 1982, The evaluation of limiting dilution assay, *J. Immunol. Methods* **49.**

Stutman, O., 1978, Intrathymic and extrathymic T cell maturation, *Immunol. Rev.* **42**:139.

Sztein, M. B., Serrate, S. A., and Goldstein, A. L., 1986, Modulation of interleukin 2 receptor expression by thymic hormones, *Proc. Natl. Acad. Sci. USA* **83**:6107–6111.

Uchiyama, T., Broder, S., and Waldmann, T. A., 1981, A monoclonal antibody (anti-Tac) reactive with activated and functionally mature human T cells. I. Production of anti-Tac monoclonal antibody and distribution of Tac(+) cells, *J. Immunol.* **126**:1393–1401.

Weksler, M. E., and Siskind, G. W., 1984, The cellular basis of immune senescence, *Monog. Dev. Biol.* **17**:110–121.

Zatz, M. M., and Goldstein, A. L., 1985, Thymosin increases production of T cell growth factor by normal human peripheral blood lymphocytes, *Proc. Natl. Acad. Sci. USA* **81**:2082–2085.

55

Thymopentin Therapy in Elderly Patients with Chronic Bronchitis

A Clinical and Cellular Study

ALBERTO DEGRASSI, ERMINIA MARIANI,
PATRIZIA RODA, MARCO SINOPPI, DONATO ZOCCHI,
ADRIANA RITA MARIANI, and ANDREA FACCHINI

1. INTRODUCTION

Aging has been reported to be the most common immune deficiency syndrome (Kay and Makinodan, 1981), since major pathological events and diseases are associated with advancing age. The decline in immune responsiveness affects both the T- and B-cell compartment, although T-cell functions seem to be the most impaired (Facchini *et al.*, 1986, 1987). In particular, a reduced number of T-cell subsets (Abo *et al.*, 1981) has been reported during human aging together with a depleted production of lymphokines as interleukin-2 (IL-2) and its receptor (IL-2R) (Gillis *et al.*, 1981; Facchini *et al.*, 1983).

These immunological findings, together with the recent demonstration of an increased incidence of chronic bronchitis (Carratu', 1986) particularly evident in the aged, led to a clinical and immunological study on the effectiveness of thymic hormone therapy in such pathology.

The clinical improvement observed in treated patients suggests the possible application of thymopentin in therapy for chronic bronchitis. Furthermore, the enhancement of CD4+ T-cell subset together with an increased lymphocyte proliferative response to mitogens could account for the cellular mechanism of action of this molecule.

ALBERTO DEGRASSI, ERMINIA MARIANI, PATRIZIA RODA, and ANDREA FACCHINI • Institute of Clinical Medicine and Gastroenterology, St. Orsola University Hospital, 40138 Bologna, Italy.   MARCO SINOPPI and DONATO ZOCCHI • Institute of Recovery and Cure of Giovanni XXIII, 40133 Bologna, Italy.   ADRIANA RITA MARIANI • Institute of Normal Human Anatomy, University of Bologna, 40138 Bologna, Italy.

2. MATERIALS AND METHODS

2.1. Subjects

Patients with chronic bronchitis were selected from residents in an old age home (Istituto Giovanni XXIII, Bologna). Two groups of 15 elderly patients were studied; the first group had a mean age of ±SE: 81 ± 1.5 years; the second group had a mean age of ±SE: 80 ± 1.9 years. Patients who were not self-sufficient or who had severe chronic, autoimmune, or neoplastic diseases were excluded, as were patients receiving steroids, immunomodulating drugs, or antibiotics. The two groups of patients under study were randomized for age, sex, and severity of pulmonary disease. The diagnosis of chronic bronchitis was made on the basis of the presence of excessive tracheobronchial mucus production sufficient to cause a cough with expectoration for at least 3 months of the year for more than 2 consecutive years (American Thoracic Society, 1962).

2.2. Treatment

The first group of patients was treated with thymopentin 32–36 (TIMUNOX–CILAG) by 50 mg subcutaneous (SC) injection three times a week for 6 weeks. Treatment was administered in March–April 1987, and clinical observations from March–July 1987 were compared with those collected during the same period of the previous year (March–July 1986).

The second group of patients acted as controls; no immunomodulatory treatment was carried out during the study. The acute events of patients from both groups were treated with antibiotics, mucolytics, and bronchodilators.

2.3. Clinical Parameters

The number of acute events and the number of days of illness were examined in the period of treatment. Data were compared for statistical analysis with the data from the same period of the previous year. A clinical score was used to define each acute event. The score provided three steps of severity, each with an increasing numerical value: low = 1, medium = 2, and high = 3. Severity of acute events was assessed on the basis of clinical parameters such as fever, day of therapy, hospitalization, quality and quantity of bronchial expectorate, and oxygen administration. Total value of each acute event was the clinical score; the score from the year of the study was compared with that of the same period in the previous year. To exclude the influence of seasonal or external factors that could interfere with the clinical course of the treated group, clinical results from the control group were examined by comparing data from the period of the study with data from the same period of the previous year.

2.4. Laboratory Findings

Laboratory and immunological findings were performed before therapy (time 0), at the end of treatment (time 1), and 6 weeks later (time 2). The following hematological findings were examined: white blood cells (WBC), red blood cells (RBC), platelets, percentage and absolute number of lymphocytes, polymorphonuclear cells, and monocytes. Serum glucose levels and blood urea nitrogen (BUN) were also tested together with serum levels of three immunoglobulins: IgG, IgA, and IgM.

2.5. Cell Preparation

Blood was collected in Heparin (Liquemin, Roche, Switzerland) and peripheral blood lymphocytes (PBL) were collected after density-gradient centrifugation (Ficoll–Hypaque) according to Boyum (1968).

2.6. Monoclonal Antibodies

The following monoclonal antibodies (MoAb) (Becton-Dickinson Monoclonal Center, Mountain View, California) were used: anti-Leu 1 (CD5) (reacting with a common T-cell antigen), anti-Leu 2a (CD8) (cytotoxic/suppressor T cells), anti-Leu 3a (CD4) (helper/inducer T cells), and anti-Leu 11a (CD16) directed against the Fc receptor present in human large granular lymphocytes. Staining of lymphocytes with MoAb was performed as reported by Mariani *et al.* (1987a). The reactivity of PBL with MoAb was determined by counting cells under a fluorescent microscope.

2.7. Lymphocyte Proliferative Response

Mononuclear cells were stimulated with two different mitogens: phytohemagglutinin (PHA) (Gibco, Basel, Switzerland), and Concanavalin A (Con A) (Pharmacia, Upsala, Sweden). Mitogens were used at different concentrations: PHA from 1 : 6 to 1 : 400 dilution and Con A from 3.1 μg/ml to 50 μg/ml. Cells were cultured in triplicate in round-bottomed plates at a concentration of 1×10^5 cells in 200 μl of RPMI 1640, buffered with 25 mM Hepes, and supplemented with 10% inactivated fetal calf serum (FCS). Control cultures were performed incubating cells in mitogen-free medium. The proliferative response was measured by [^{3}H]thymidine uptake (0.4 μCi/well) (specific activity 25 Ci/mmoles, Amersham, Buckinghamshire, England), added after 3 days of culture; cells were harvested on filters (Skatron, Norway) 18 hr later, and radioactivity was measured in a Beta-counter.

2.8. Statistics

Student's *t*-test and Wilcoxon analysis were used to compare experimental data.

3. RESULTS

3.1. Clinical Parameters

Subcutaneous thymopentin injection had no local or systemic side effects. The clinical course of both groups was similar during the period March–July 1986, when no treatment was administered. Analysis of clinical data from the control group in the year of the study and in the previous year also failed to show any difference.

After thymopentin therapy, within the above-mentioned period of study, a significant decrease ($p < 0.005$) in acute events was observed in the treated group with respect to the previous year (Fig. 1). Furthermore, the treated group showed a significant ($p < 0.005$) decrease in total days of illness when data from the period of the study were compared with data from the previous year (Fig. 2).

Evaluation of the seriousness of each acute event by means of a clinical score is reported

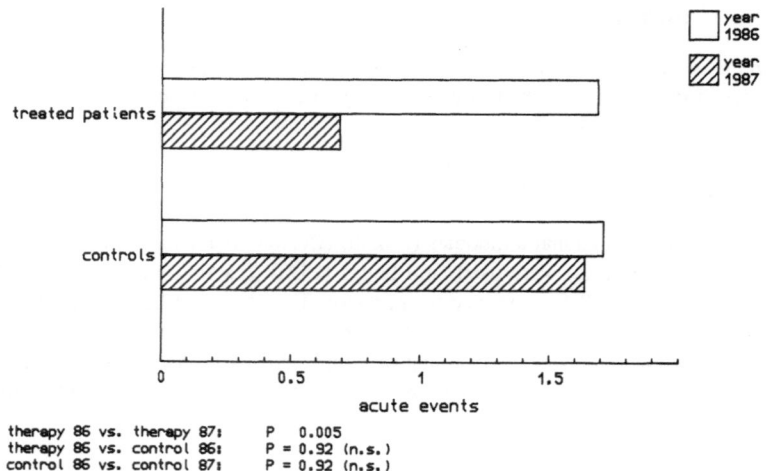

FIGURE 1. Number of acute events in treated patients and controls evaluated in the year of the study and in the previous one.

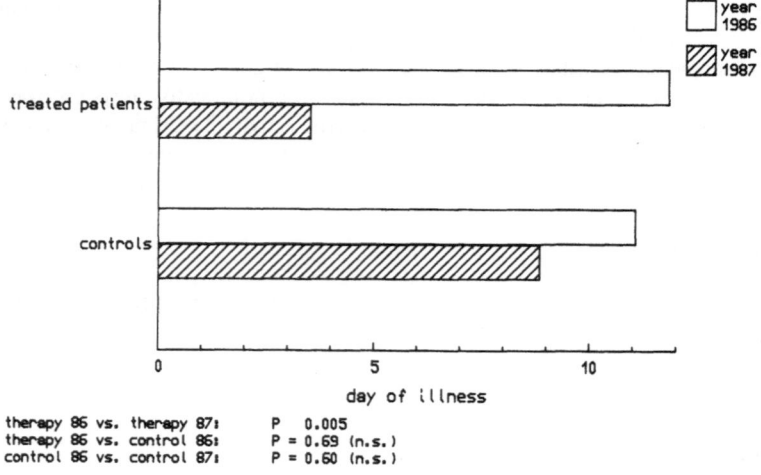

FIGURE 2. Total day of illness in treated patients and controls evaluated in the year of the study and in the previous one.

in Fig. 3. After thymopentin therapy, a significant decrease in the clinical score was observed in the treated group with respect to the previous year.

3.2. Laboratory Findings

Data from laboratory findings before therapy (time 0), at the end (time 1), and after 6 weeks (time 2) are summarized in Table I. At the end of therapy, there was an increase in

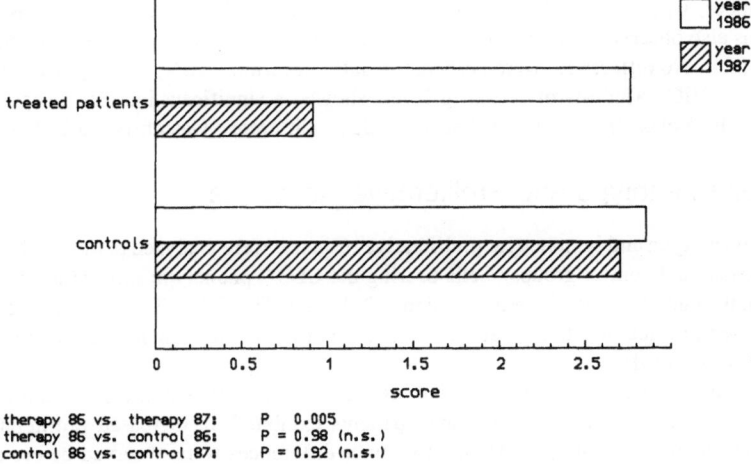

therapy 86 vs. therapy 87: P 0.005
therapy 86 vs. control 86: P = 0.98 (n.s.)
control 86 vs. control 87: P = 0.92 (n.s.)

FIGURE 3. Clinical score of treated patients evaluated in the year of the study and in the previous one. Three steps of severity were considered: low = 1, medium = 2, high = 3.

TABLE I. Laboratory and Immunological Findings
Evaluated at Different Times in Treated Patients

Parameters	Units	Time 0	Time 1	Time 2
RBC	/μl (× 10³)	4620	4520	4500
WBC	/μl	5653	6177	5546
Platelets	/μl (× 10³)	259	250	255
Lymphocytes	%	36[a]	42[a]	36
	/μl	1572[b]	2747	2094
Neutrophils	%	62	55	61
	/μl	2907	3268	3315
Monocytes	%	1	2	1
	/μl	46	69	63
Eosinophils	%	2	2	3
	/μl	125	148	153
BUN	mg/dl	17	18	17
Glucose	mg/dl	93	93	93
IgG	mg/dl	1492[c]	1582	1569
IgA	mg/dl	319	319	341
IgM	mg/dl	118	133[a]	146

[a] $p \leq 0.05$.
[b] $p \leq 0.005$.
[c] $p \leq 0.001$.

WBC number, which returned to previous values within time 2. A significant increase ($p <$ 0.005) was also observed in lymphocyte number at time 1, while values from time 0 and time 2 were similar. No differences were observed in data concerning BUN, serum glucose levels, platelets, or RBC. Analysis of serum Ig levels showed a significant increase in IgG ($p <$ 0.001) and IgM class ($p < 0.05$) at time 1, while no difference was observed in IgA class.

3.3. Cell Phenotype and Proliferative Response

Cell phenotype and lymphocyte proliferative response were analyzed at time 0, 1, and 2, both in treated and control groups. Cells bearing the CD3 + phenotype showed a significant increase at the end of therapy in treated patients (Table II). The CD4/CD8 ratio was increased after treatment, attributable to a greater enhancement of CD4 + subpopulation with respect to CD8 + cells (Table II).

Data from the lymphocyte proliferative response after stimulation of cells with mitogens are shown in Table III. PBL from treated patients exhibited an increased proliferation 6 weeks after the end of treatment, while only minor differences were observed before and at the end of treatment.

4. DISCUSSION

Thymopentin is a synthetic pentapeptide corresponding to the active part of the thymic hormone thymopoietin. Studies on mice have shown that the synthetic pentapeptide has an effect similar to that of the purified hormone, inducing a selective differentiation of T lymphocytes (Schlesinger *et al.*, 1975). It has also been demonstrated that cyclic adenosine monophosphate (cAMP) is the second signal used by thymopentin to induce effects (Goldstein *et al.*, 1977; Nash *et al.*, 1981).

These results were confirmed by other studies on humans, and thymopentin has been used with good clinical results in many different pathologies: autoimmune disease (Veys, 1982), allergic (Kooper *et al.*, 1983; Genova *et al.*, 1983), neoplastic (Berengo *et al.*, 1987), and dermatologic (Djawari *et al.*, 1982; Thivolet *et al.*, 1983) disorders.

Thymopentin was recently used to treat children's recurrent bronchopulmonary infections with positive clinical results (De Martino *et al.*, 1984; Agosti *et al.*, 1986). In these patients, many immunological alterations have been demonstrated that could be related to chronic bronchitis disease (Lepore *et al.*, 1982, 1984).

During aging, a general functional impairment of the immune system has been demonstrated. In particular, a reduced proliferative response to mitogen stimulation and a reduced production of lymphokines (Mariani *et al.*, 1986, 1987b) have been demonstrated together with an increased number of circulating natural killer (NK) cells (Mariani *et al.*, 1987c,d) not accompanied by enhanced functional activity (Facchini *et al.*, 1987; Pazzaglia *et al.*, 1987). This experimental evidence allowed the clinical application of thymopentin in elderly patients with chronic bronchitis.

In this study, we report a significant clinical improvement of patients treated with thymopentin. Thymopentin-treated patients showed a significant decrease in infective acute events associated with a lower severity of each event and with an improvement in clinical score with respect to the same period of the previous year. Since these data are paralleled by an increase in lymphocyte number, the effects of thymopentin could be mediated by a numerical rise in the circulating lymphocyte compartment. This seems to be confirmed by the

TABLE II. Phenotype of Circulating Lymphocytes Evaluated at Different Times in Treated Patients[a,b]

Phenotype	Time					
	0		1		2	
	%	Absolute No. (μl)	%	Absolute No. (μl)	%	Absolute No. (μl)
CD3[+c]	66.40 ± 4.95	888 ± 150	62.30 ± 3.05	1722 ± 127	59.31 ± 2.87	1201 ± 164
CD4[+d]	44.69 ± 2.89	668 ± 82	44.38 ± 2.19	1249 ± 83	42.77 ± 2.08	891 ± 141
CD8[+e]	24.00 ± 2.81	319 ± 59	19.15 ± 1.49	546 ± 67	19.23 ± 2.38	342 ± 35
CD4/CD8 ratio	2.08 ± 0.19		2.55 ± 0.30		2.72 ± 0.38	

[a]Results are expressed as mean ±SE.
[b]Statistical analysis: Student's t-test.
[c]Absolute No. time 0 vs. time 1: $p \leq 0.01$; absolute No. time 1 vs. time 2: $p \leq 0.05$.
[d]Absolute No. time 0 vs. time 1: $p \leq 0.005$.
[e]Absolute No. time 0 vs. time 1: $p \leq 0.05$; absolute No. time 1 vs. time 2: $p \leq 0.01$.

TABLE III. Lymphocyte Proliferative Response after Stimulation
of Cells from Treated Patients with Different Mitogens[a,b]

Mitogen	Time		
	0	1	2
PHA	100.36 ± 9.32	115.82 ± 15.97	189.25 ± 36.13
ConA	53.92 ± 8.33	51.08 ± 7.97	59.23 ± 14.20

[a]Results are expressed as mean stimulation index $\pm$ SE.
[b]Statistical analysis: Student's t-test. Stimulation index time 1 vs. time 2: $p \leq 0.05$.

demonstration of an increased proliferative response to mitogens, although it was more evident 6 weeks after the end of therapy. The greater enhancement of the CD4+ compartment in treated patients suggests that these cells could be involved in the clinical improvement of elderly patients with chronic bronchitis. An *in vitro* thymopentin-mediated modulation of IL-2R expression on the surface of PBL from normal has recently been demonstrated (Szein *et al.*, 1986). The expansion of the CD4+ compartment could be related to the IL-2R modulation by thymopentin and the subsequent proliferation and differentiation of T-helper cells may be involved in the delayed clinical and proliferation response. Other soluble factors could be involved in this mechanism and further studies are necessary for a fuller understanding of the overall mechanism of action of thymopentin.

REFERENCES

Abo, T., Morimoto, C., Toguchi, T., Kiyotachi, M., and Homma, M., 1981, Evidence of aberration of T cell subsets in aged individuals, *Scand. J. Immunol.* **13**:151.

Agosti, E., and Panizon, F., 1986, Trattamento con timomodulina per os delle infezioni ricorrenti delle vie respiratorie in età pediatrica, in: *Atti del Simp. Int. Inquadramento della Timomodulina negli Immunomodulanti Biologici, St. Vincent, dicembre 12–13*, pp. 51–60.

American Thoracic Society (Statement by Committee on Diagnostic Standards for Nontubercolous Respiratory Diseases), 1962, Definitions and classification of chronic bronchitis, asthma and pulmonary emphysema, *Am. Rev. Respir. Dis.* **85**:762.

Berengo, M. G., Fra, P., Lisa, F., Meregalli, M., and Zina, G., 1983, Thymostimulin therapy in melanoma patients: Correlation of immunologic effects with clinical course, *Clin. Immunol. Immunopathol.* **28**:311.

Boyum, A., 1968, Isolation of mononuclear cells and granulocytes from human blood, *Scand. J. Clin. Lab. Invest.* **97**:77.

Carratu', L., 1986, Generalità sui meccanismi di difesa dell' apparato respiratorio, in: *Atti del Simp. Int. Inquadramento della Timomodulina negli Immunomodulanti Biologici, St. Vincent, dicembre 12–13*, pp. 97–101.

De Martino, M., Rossi, M. E., Muccioli, A. T., and Vierucci, A., 1984, T lymphocytes in children with recurrent respiratory infections: Effect of the use of thymostimulin on the alterations of T-cell subset, *Int. Tissue React.* **6**:223.

Djawari, D., Hornstein, O. P., and Hancke, E., 1982, Immunomodulation therapy of pyostomatitis vegetans in *Arch. Dermatol. Res.* **273**:174.

Facchini, A., Papa, S., Mariani, A. R., Mariani, E., Pazzaglia, M. G., and Manzoli, F. A., 1984, Expression of early activation antigens on lymphocytes from aged subjects, in: *Lymphoid Cell*

Function in Ageing, Vol. 3, *Topics in Ageing Research in Europe* (A. L. De Weck, ed.), pp. 149–153.

Facchini, A., Mariani, E., and Pazzaglia, M., 1986, Immunological changes during ageing, *IRCS Med. Sci.* **14**:859.

Facchini, A., Mariani, E., Mariani, A. R., Papa, S., Vitale, M., and Manzoli, F. A., 1987, Increased number of circulating Leu11c⁺ (CD16) large granular lymphocytes and decreased NK activity during human ageing, *Clin. Exp. Immunol.* **68**(2):340.

Genova, R., and Guerra, A., 1983, Un estratto di timo (timomodulina) nella profilassi dell' asma infantile, *Pediatr. Med. Chir.* **5**:395.

Gillis, S., Kozak, R., Durante, M., and Weksler, M. E., 1981, Decrease production of and response to T cell growth factor by lymphocytes from aged humans, *J. Clin. Invest.* **67**:937.

Goldstein, G., Scheid, M., Boise, E. A., Brand, A., and Gilmour, G. D., 1977, Thymopoietin and bursopoietin: Induction signals regulating early lymphocyte differentiation, *Cold Spring Harbor Symp. Quant. Biol.* **41**:32–38.

Kay, M. M. B., and Makimodan, T., 1981, Relationship between aging and the immune system, *Prog. Allergy* **29**:139.

Kooper, K. D., Kang, K., and Hanifin, J. M., 1983, Effects of thymopoietin pentapeptide on in vitro and in vivo IgE production by atopic dermatitis cell subset, *Diagn. Immunol.* **1**:211.

Lepore, L., Longo, F., Presani, G., and Perticari, S., 1982, Difetto della immunità ritardata nelle infezioni respiratorie ricorrenti, *Immunol. Pediatr.* **2**:3.

Lepore, L., Longo, F., Presani, G., and Panizon, F., 1984, Il profilo immunologico nei bambini con infezioni respiratorie ricorrenti, *Riv. Ital. Pediatr.* **10**:138.

Mariani, E., Mariani, A. R., Mingari, M. C., Sinoppi, M., and Facchini, A., 1986, Lymphokine production in normal old subjects, in: *Immunoregulation in Ageing,* Vol. 9 (A. Facchini, J. J. Haaijman, and G. Labò, eds.), *Topics in Ageing Research in Europe,* Eurage Series, The Hague, pp. 101–108.

Mariani, E., Mariani, A. R., Roda, P., Vitale, M., Degrassi, A., and Facchini, A., 1987a, Proliferative capacity of lymphocyte clones from old subjects, in: *Protides of the Biological Fluids,* Vol. 35 (H. Peeters, ed.), Pergamon, Oxford, pp. 209–212.

Mariani, E., Mariani, A. R., Roda, P., Sinoppi, M., and Facchini, A., 1987b, IFN-gamma production in elderly subjects in *Fed. Proc.* **46**:4511.

Mariani, E., Vitale, M., Roda, P., Degrassi, A., Mariani, A. R., and Facchini, A., 1987c, T and NK clones in old individuals in *Fed. Proc.* **46**:4512.

Mariani, E., Roda, P., Mariani, A. R., Vitale, M., Degrassi, A., Papa, S., Manzoli, F. A., and Facchini, A., 1987d, Lymphocyte clones from old subjects: Growing rate and functional activity, *Cytotechnology* **1**:103.

Nash, L., God, R. A., Hatzfeld, A., Goldstein, G., and Incefy, G. F., 1981, In vitro differentiation of two surface markers for immature T-cell by the synthetic pentapeptide thymopoietin 32-36, *J. Immunol.* **126**:150.

Pazzaglia, M., Sinoppi, M., Papa, S., Mariani, E., Mariani, A. R., Degrassi, A., Facchini, A., Savorani, G., and Manzoli, F. A., 1987, Il sistema immunitario durante l'invecchiamento. 1. Analisi fenotipica e funzionale linfocitaria, *Gli Osp. Vita* **14**:57.

Schlesinger, D. H., Goldstein, G., Schein, M. P., and Boise, E. A., 1975, Chemical synthesis of a peptide fragment of thymopoietin II that induces selective T-cell differentiation, *Cell* **5**:367.

Sztein, M. B., Serrate, S. A., and Goldstein, A. L., 1986, Modulation of interleukin 2 receptor expression on normal human lymphocytes by thymic hormones, *Proc. Natl. Acad. Sci. USA* **83**:6107.

Thivolet, J., Faure, M., Nicolas, J. F., Mauduit, G., and Claudy, A., 1983, Therapeutic use of TP-5 (thymopoietin 32-36) in sarcoidosis of the skin, *Clin. Immunol. Immunopatol.* **26**:350.

Veys, E. M., 1982, Clinical response to therapy with thymopoietin pentapeptide (TP-5) in rheumatoid arthritis, *Ann. Rheum. Dis.* **41**:401.

56

Aspirin and Risks of Cardiovascular Disease in the Physicians' Health Study

CHARLES H. HENNEKENS

1. INTRODUCTION

In the United States today, cardiovascular disease is the leading cause of mortality, accounting for approximately one half of the more than two million annual deaths. Fatal myocardial infarction (MI) is the primary cause of cardiovascular death and the single greatest cause of all mortality, accounting for roughly one of every three deaths in the United States. The potential public health impact of a primary prevention measure that could reduce cardiovascular mortality by even 20% is therefore large. Such an intervention could, at least in theory, prevent 160,000 of the 800,000 deaths from MI and more than 28,000 of the 144,000 annual stroke deaths.

Low-dose aspirin is a plausible intervention for primary prevention of cardiovascular disease. The biologic mechanism for the hypothesis relates to its effect on platelet aggregation. The British scientist Sir John Vane (Moncada and Vane, 1979) and others have demonstrated that, in platelets, small amounts of aspirin irreversibly acetylate the active site of cyclo-oxygenase, which is required for the production of thromboxane A_2, a powerful promoter of aggregation. This tendency is so profound that higher doses provide no additional benefit. In fact, it has been speculated that higher doses might even reverse this tendency, due to activation of vessel wall enzymes.

2. ASPIRIN IN SECONDARY PREVENTION

Further evidence suggesting the possibility of a beneficial effect of aspirin comes from epidemiologic research among patients with a history of cardiovascular disease. A large number of trials have tested aspirin among patients with a history of MI, stroke, or angina pectoris. In 1986, investigators conducting trials of antiplatelet therapy among patients with a

CHARLES H. HENNEKENS • Departments of Medicine and Preventive Medicine, Harvard Medical School and Brigham and Women's Hospital, Brookline, Massachusetts 02146.

history of cardiovascular disease began to collaborate in a comprehensive overview, or meta-analysis, of all completed trials involving aspirin or two other antiplatelet agents, dipyridamole and sulfinpyrazone (Anti-Platelet Trialists Collaboration, 1988). We identified a total of 25 completed randomized trials of aspirin, dipyridamole, or sulfinpyrazone, either alone or in combination. These included nearly 29,000 patients with a history of myocardial infarction, stroke, transient ischemic attacks (TIAs), or unstable angina. This overview found a statistically significant 25% reduction from aspirin in risk of developing what we termed an "important vascular event." This term includes nonfatal MI, nonfatal stroke, or vascular death. For nonfatal MI, the reduction in risk, when all available trials were considered, was 32%, while for nonfatal stroke, there was a statistically significant 27% reduction in risk. Finally, with respect to vascular mortality, for all trials combined, there was a statistically significant 15% reduction in risk.

3. ASPIRIN IN EVOLVING MI

The findings on secondary prevention or treatment of cardiovascular disease raised the possibility that aspirin may also be effective in the acute stages of MI. It was to test this hypothesis, as well as to assess the role of intravenous (IV) streptokinase in treating acute MI in a 2 × 2 factorial design, that the Second International Study of Infarct Survival (ISIS-2) was designed. This trial randomized over 17,000 patients from more than 400 hospitals in 16 different countries to taking either 160 mg of aspirin or placebo daily for 30 days, beginning immediately upon hospital admission for evolving myocardial infarction. Patients were also randomized to receiving either a single dose of 1.5 million units of streptokinase or placebo intravenously over 60 min. The data on mortality five weeks after randomization, which represents the period during which patients are at greatest risk of reinfarction or death, indicated a 49% reduction in MI, a 46% reduction in stroke, and a 23% decrease in vascular mortality among those assigned to aspirin (ISIS-2 Collaborative Group, 1988).

The overview of secondary prevention trials indicates a moderate, but clinically important benefit of aspirin among these patient populations. The ISIS-2 results from treatment of acute MI suggest a slightly stronger benefit of aspirin on reinfarction, stroke, and vascular mortality during the critical five-week period following an initial MI. However, none of these trials is able to directly answer the broader question of a possible benefit of aspirin among healthy individuals. In order to address this question, a randomized trial of aspirin for the primary prevention of cardiovascular disease was initiated among 22,071 U.S. physicians (Steering Committee of the Physicians' Health Study Research Group, 1988).

4. ASPIRIN IN PRIMARY PREVENTION

In planning for the U.S. Physicians' Health Study, a chief objective was of course to minimize the risks to participants while maximizing the potential benefit. As regards the risks of aspirin, in the Aspirin Myocardial Infarction Study (Aspirin Myocardial Infarction Study Research Group, 1980), a secondary prevention trial, 23.7% of those receiving 500 mg of aspirin twice daily experienced gastrointestinal side effects, compared with 14.9% of those receiving placebo. Thus, 8.8% experienced some degree of gastric discomfort directly attributable to aspirin. Other trials have suggested a possible small but significant increased risk of gastrointestinal hemorrhage. As regards the relationship between dose of aspirin and risk of side effects, the recently completed UK–TIA trial (UK–TIA Study Group, 1988) tested two different doses of aspirin in addition to placebo, thus allowing for a direct assessment of whether the reported GI side effects are dose related. In this trial, the group receiving 300 mg aspirin experienced only 30% of the side effects experienced in the group taking 1200 mg, strongly indicating that the side effects of aspirin are, indeed, dose dependent. Gastroscopic study data suggested that an alternate-day regimen might reduce side effects even further, by allowing time for the gastric muscosa to heal in between doses. Thus, both lower doses of aspirin and less frequent administration appear to lower the risk of side effects. As regards the benefits of lower doses of aspirin, there were no apparent differences in cardiovascular risk reductions at high and low doses in the secondary prevention trials. We therefore elected to test one commercially available 325-mg tablet on alternate days in the Physicians' Health Study.

To assess further the potential benefits of this regimen, we conducted a small trial of this dose and frequency of administration on platelet aggregation, bleeding time, and thromboxane production (Stampfer *et al.*, 1986). We randomly assigned subjects to 325-mg regular aspirin or placebo on alternate days for two weeks. Measurements were taken at baseline as well as 4 and 24 hr after the first dose to assess acute effects, and at 48 hr after the last dose to test for chronic effects. For each individual on active aspirin, there was virtually complete inhibition of platelet aggregation, prolongation of bleeding time, and complete suppression of platelet thromboxane A_2 production even 48 hours after the last dose. There were no such changes in the placebo group. Thus, a single 325-mg dose of aspirin every other day provides continuous suppression of platelet function, and, even after 48 hr, there is virtually no recovery.

The Physicians' Health Study is a randomized, double-blind, placebo-controlled trial designed to evaluate two primary prevention hypotheses: (1) whether 325 mg of aspirin taken every other day reduces cardiovascular mortality, and (2) whether 50 mg of β-carotene on alternate days decreases cancer incidence. We chose physicians as subjects for several ethical, scientific, and practical reasons. First, as a group, physicians are obviously in the best position to give true informed consent to participation in such a study. Moreover, their training permits them to recognize possible side effects promptly and to report their medical history and health status with a greater degree of completeness and accuracy than most other population groups. Physicians are also far less mobile and easier to trace than the general population, ensuring that we will be able to obtain complete follow-up information from them over an extended period of time. Finally, from a practical point of view, our pilot studies showed that the collaboration of doctors would result in excellent compliance with their assigned regimens as well as the receipt of completed questionnaires, thus allowing us to conduct the trial entirely by mail, at a small fraction of the usual costs for other National Institutes of Health (NIH)-funded trials of primary prevention.

Thus, in 1982, we mailed introductory letters and questionnaires to all 261,248 potentially eligible male physicians in the United States, aged 40–84, who were identified from a tape purchased from the American Medical Association (AMA). Of those to whom we mailed, 112,528 returned the questionnaire, with 59,285 indicating that they were willing to participate in the trial. Willing physicians were excluded if they had a personal history of cancer, MI, TIA, or stroke, current liver or renal disease, peptic ulcer or gout; contraindications to aspirin consumption; current use of aspirin, other platelet-active drugs, or non-steroidal anti-inflammatory drugs (NSAID); or current use of a vitamin A or β-carotene supplement. It is interesting to note that the single chief exclusion criterion among doctors willing to enroll in this trial was regular use of aspirin. The 33,223 initially willing and eligible participants were then enrolled into a run-in phase, where, for approximately 18 weeks, all physicians took their daily pills from calendar packs containing active aspirin and β-carotene placebo. At the end of the 18-week period, we sent the participants question- naires, and individuals who reported side effects or a desire to discontinue participation, as well as those who developed an exclusion criterion or even those who wished to continue but whose compliance we deemed inadequate, were excluded from the trial before randomiza- tion. Thus, a total of 22,071 physicians who were proven good compliers were randomized into the trial.

These 22,071 physicians were randomly assigned first to two groups, one taking aspirin and the other aspirin placebo. Each of these groups was further randomized into two sub- groups taking either β-carotene or β-carotene placebo. Thus an individual participant could be receiving aspirin only, carotene only, both aspirin and carotene, or both placebos. Follow- up questionnaires asking about compliance with the treatment regimens and the development of disease outcomes since the return of the last questionnaire were mailed twice a year for the first 12 months and then annually.

Reported diagnoses are confirmed by an end points committee of physicians, including two internists, one cardiologist, and one neurologist, all blinded to treatment assignment. Diagnoses of nonfatal myocardial infarction are confirmed on the basis of World Health Organization (WHO) criteria. Cardiovascular death is documented by convincing evidence of a cardiovascular mechanism on the basis of all available information, including death certifi- cates, hospital records, and, for deaths outside the hospital, observers' impressions. Nonfatal stroke is defined as a typical neurologic deficit, sudden or rapid in onset, lasting more than 24 hours and attributable to a cerebrovascular event. Strokes are further classified according to severity of residual impairment at hospital discharge as well as whether their etiology is ischemic or hemorrhagic, based on the medical records, which in most cases include a computed tomography (CT) scan, and the judgment of the neurologist.

After an average of 4.8 years of follow-up, 87.6% of randomized subjects were still taking at least one of their two types of pills, and 83.0% were still taking both types of pills regularly. Thus, only 12.4% had stopped taking pills entirely after this extended period of follow-up. These self-reported compliance figures have been confirmed by analysis of blood samples from a sample of participants for levels of thromboxane B_2, the stable degradation product of thromboxane A_2, as well as serum β-carotene. In addition, after 4.8 years of follow-up, 99.7% of participating doctors had provided complete questionnaire data by either mail or telephone. This left 0.3% on whom we obtained only vital status. Thus, to date, not a single participant has been lost to follow-up. Both our compliance and follow-up results are exceptionally high, reflecting very gratifying levels of cooperation among the participating physicians.

An independent Data Monitoring Board has been meeting twice yearly to review the accumulating data and monitor the progress of the trial. A specific charge of the Board is to evaluate the unblinded data for the emergence of extreme treatment effects that might warrant alteration or early termination of one or both arms of the trial. As a general rule, results from a blinded trial are neither known by the investigators nor reported until the scheduled end of the study. However, on December 18, 1987, the Data Monitoring Board took the unusual step of recommending to the Steering Committee that the randomized aspirin component of the trial be terminated early.

Table I presents the data on which this recommendation was based. Overall, there was a 47% reduction in risk of total MI ($RR = 0.53$) that was highly statistically significant and reflects significant benefits of aspirin on both nonfatal and fatal events. For total stroke, RR

TABLE I. Cardiovascular End Points in the Aspirin Arm
of the Physicians' Health Study

End point	Aspirin	Placebo	Relative risk	95% confidence interval	p value
Myocardial infarction					
Fatal	5	18	0.25	0.11–0.56	0.006
Nonfatal	99	171	0.56	0.44–0.71	<0.00001
Total	104	189	0.53	0.42–0.67	<0.00001
Total stroke					
Fatal	6	2	3.00	0.75–11.98	0.16
Nonfatal	74	68	1.09	0.78–1.52	0.61
Total	80	70	1.15	0.84–1.58	0.41
Stroke[a]					
Ischemic					
Mild	50	49	1.02	0.69–1.51	0.92
Moderate, severe, or fatal	13	12	1.08	0.50–2.37	0.84
Unknown	1	0			
Total	64	61	1.05	0.74–1.49	0.79
Hemorrhagic					
Mild	3	4	0.75	0.17–3.30	0.70
Moderate, severe, or fatal	10	2	5.06	1.63–15.70	0.02
Total	13	6	2.19	0.89–5.39	0.11
Unknown	3	3			

[a]Subdivided by etiology and severity.

among those receiving aspirin was 1.15, but this finding was not significant. When strokes were subdivided by whether the event was ischemic or hemorrhagic as well as by the severity of any residual disability, the only significant result was an increased risk of moderate to severe or fatal hemorrhagic strokes among those in the aspirin-treated group, where the p value was 0.02. However, the 95% confidence limits were very wide, reflecting the fact that this finding was based on 10 events in the aspirin-treated group and on two events in placebo-treated subjects.

To help clarify the risk–benefit ratio in a manner analogous to the overview of trials of secondary prevention, we analyzed an end point that included all important vascular events, by combining nonfatal MI and stroke with cardiovascular death. For this combined end point, there was a highly significant 23% reduction in risk among those allocated to the aspirin-treated group.

As regards gastrointestinal (GI) discomfort on this regimen of 325 mg of aspirin on alternate days, such symptoms were reported by 24.2% of the active group and 23.6% of the placebo group, leaving only 0.6% of such symptoms attributable to the aspirin. This very low rate of GI side effects is likely to be due, in part, to the low dose and frequency of administration as well as to the prerandomization run-in, which excluded those unable to

TABLE II. Cardiovascular Deaths according to Treatment Group

Category of CV deaths (ICD codes)	Aspirin	Placebo	Relative risk	95% confidence interval	p value
Acute myocardial infarction (410)	5	18	0.25	0.11–0.56	0.006
Stroke (430, 431, 434, 436)	6	2	3.00	0.75–11.98	0.16
Ischemic heart disease (411–414)	9	8	1.08	0.42–2.79	0.81
Sudden death (798)	13	9	1.49	0.65–3.43	0.40
Other cardiovascular (402, 424, 425, 428, 429, 440, 441)	10	6	1.79	0.67–4.76	0.31
Other cerebrovascular (431, 436)	1	1	1.00	0.06–15.96	1.00
Total cardiovascular deaths	44	44	0.99	0.65–1.50	0.99

tolerate the drug. Furthermore, with respect to fatal GI hemorrhage, in the PHS not a single case has been confirmed, and only one was reported.

With respect to the issue of total cardiovascular mortality, the physicians randomized into this trial have had extraordinarily good cardiovascular health. In fact, while we would have expected to see 733 cardiovascular deaths among a general population of U.S. white males of the same age distribution during the same period of follow-up, we confirmed only 88. As shown in Table II, these deaths were divided equally between the aspirin- and placebo-treated groups. Moreover, there was no significant excess risk among any one of the specific categories that would counterbalance the large deficit of fatal MI among the aspirin-treated group. We are continuing to identify deaths that occurred through January 25, 1988, and at present there is a 13% reduction in the aspirin-treated group. This, of course, is not significant and provides no more evidence of a benefit than the earlier comparison indicating no effect. In fact, the data are simply insufficient for a sound judgment.

Several factors affected the decision of the Data Monitoring Board to recommend terminating the randomized aspirin component of the Physicians' Health Study. The first was the extreme beneficial effect of aspirin on both fatal and nonfatal MI. The second was the inability to accumulate sufficient numbers of cardiovascular deaths to detect any effects of aspirin on this end point until the year 2000 or beyond. Furthermore, although total cardiovascular mortality could not be evaluated, it was predicted that any overall benefit would show up first in fatal MI. In fact, the benefit of aspirin on that end point achieved statistical significance, along with the finding on nonfatal MI. Finally, more than 85% of participants who experienced a nonfatal MI were subsequently prescribed aspirin as therapy.

The only other data on the role of aspirin in the primary prevention of cardiovascular disease derive from a randomized trial of 5139 British doctors that tested 500 mg of aspirin daily using an open design, where the control group was asked to avoid all products containing aspirin rather than to take a placebo (Peto et al., 1988). Doctors were considered ineligible if they reported regular use of aspirin, any contraindication to aspirin, or a history of peptic ulcer, stroke, or MI. Twice yearly, participating doctors were asked to complete a brief questionnaire about their health and their use of aspirin or other antiplatelet agents over the preceding 6 months, as well as about possible MI, strokes, and TIAs. For any reported events, further details were obtained from the participants or their treating physicians. This information was then examined by a cardiologist or neurologist at Oxford who was blinded as to treatment assignment and who classified the reported events as definite, probable, or doubtful. Although information was sought about the likely etiology of strokes, a firm distinction between cerebral infarction and hemorrhage was not usually possible.

With respect to ascertainment of end points, fatal events were identified by replies from relatives to correspondence, records of the General Medical Council, and National Health Service records. Whenever possible, certified causes of death recorded as vascular were supplemented by scrutiny of clinical or other records. At the end of the study, a further questionnaire was sent to ensure that no cardiovascular events had been missed, and this was completed either by mail or by telephone for 99% of all surviving participants.

Overall, there were 169 total MI among the 3429 doctors in the aspirin-treated group and 88 among the 1710 participants in the control group, giving a *RR* of 0.97, with 95% CL from 0.75 to 1.26. This reflects similar findings for both fatal and nonfatal events. For total stroke, *RR* among those receiving aspirin was 1.17, but this finding was not significant, with 95% CL from 0.80 to 1.70. Again, the findings were similar for fatal and nonfatal events. Strokes were then subdivided by whether the event was hemorrhagic, occlusive, or of unknown etiology, as well as by the severity of any residual disability for nonfatal events. The only significant result was an increased risk of disabling strokes among those in the aspirin-treated group. While this finding may reflect more severe strokes among those taking aspirin, some bias may have been introduced by the subjective nature of the assessment of residual impairment, which was done through self-reports, as well as the lack of placebo control. On the other hand, this may also reflect the fact that disabling strokes are more likely to be hemorrhagic, and these may be increased by aspirin use. With respect to mortality, there were no significant differences in either vascular or nonvascular deaths among this population.

In evaluating the evidence from these two primary prevention trials of British and U.S. doctors, it is informative to compare their methodologic features (Table III). First, with respect to dosage and frequency of administration, the British trial tested 500 mg aspirin daily, while the U.S. study tested one 325-mg tablet every other day. The U.K. trial used an open design, with no placebo control, while the U.S. study was double-blind and placebo controlled. Compliance in the two studies also varied: in the British trial, during the first 3 years, average compliance was 70%, while in the U.S. trial, overall compliance at the end of 5 years was 83% and during this interval averaged more than 90%. The most striking difference, however, and the most significant in terms of impact on interpretation of the results, is in sample size, with 5139 subjects randomized in the British trial and 22,071 in the U.S. trial.

Because of this large sample size difference and despite other differences in design

TABLE III. Comparison of Methodologic Features of Aspirin Primary Prevention Trials

	British	United States
Dose	500 mg	325 mg
Frequency of administration	Daily	Alternate-day
Blindness	Open	Double-blind
Placebo control	No	Yes
Compliance	70% average during first 3 years	83% at the end of 5 years
Sample size	5139	22,071

TABLE IV. Summary of Current Knowledge on Role of Aspirin in Prevention
of Cardiovascular Disease

Type of trial	Myocardial infarction	Stroke	Vascular death
Secondary prevention	Conclusive benefit	Conclusive benefit	Conclusive benefit
Treatment of early MI	Conclusive benefit	Conclusive benefit	Conclusive benefit
Primary prevention	Conclusive benefit	Inconclusive	Inconclusive

features, it may be useful to view these two studies in aggregate (Hennekens *et al.*, 1988). For nonfatal MI, the risk reduction in the U.S. trial was 42% and that in the United Kingdom trial 3%. Because the U.S. trial was so much larger, an overview of this finding shows an overall 33% reduction in nonfatal MI that was highly statistically significant.

5. CURRENT STATUS OF KNOWLEDGE REGARDING ASPIRIN

Table IV illustrates the current status of our knowledge concerning the role of aspirin in the prevention of cardiovascular disease. With respect to secondary prevention, the evidence indicates a conclusive benefit of aspirin on MI, stroke, and vascular death. Similarly, for the treatment of evolving MI, a conclusive benefit seems to be present for all three of these end points. For primary prevention, a conclusive benefit has been demonstrated for MI, but the evidence concerning stroke and vascular death remains inconclusive due to inadequate numbers of end points in both the U.S. and British trials as well as the overview.

It is important to view the results of these two primary prevention trials within the context of what we already know about modification of risk factors to prevent cardiovascular disease. Specifically, as regards blood cholesterol, a 10% decrease corresponds to roughly a 20–30% decrease in risk of coronary heart disease (Peto *et al.*, 1985). For blood pressure, a 7–8 mm decrease in diastolic pressure results in a 12% lower risk of coronary heart disease as well as a 40% reduction in risk of stroke (Hebert *et al.*, 1988). Finally, cessation of cigarette smoking yields about an 50% decrease in risk of coronary heart disease even within a matter of months (Hennekens *et al.*, 1984).

It would be tragic if middle-aged or older smokers were to elect to take aspirin instead of quitting, as the benefits from quitting smoking far exceed any protective effect of aspirin on coronary heart disease. Furthermore, a continuing smoker will remain exposed to hazards that render this habit a risk factor for both ischemic and hemorrhagic stroke as well as the leading preventable cause of cancer deaths and total mortality in the United States. Similar arguments hold for management of other risk factors. Thus, it seems most prudent to view aspirin as a possible adjunct, not an alternative, to risk-factor management, which should be prescribed by a physician. Such a decision by a physician should include consideration of the cardiovascular risk profile of the patient, the known side effects of aspirin, as well as the recently demonstrated benefit in reducing the risks of a first myocardial infarction.

REFERENCES

Anti-Platelet Trialists Collaboration, 1988, Secondary prevention of vascular disease by prolonged antiplatelet therapy, *Br. Med. J.* **296**:320–331.

Aspirin Myocardial Infarction Study Research Group, 1980, A randomized, controlled trial of aspirin in persons recovered from myocardial infarction, *JAMA* **243**:661–669.

Hebert, P. R., Fiebach, N. H., Eberlein, K. A., Taylor, J. O., and Hennekens, C. H., 1988, The community-based randomized trials of pharmacologic treatment of mild-to-moderate hypertension, *Am. J. Epidemiol.* **127**:581–590.

Hennekens, C. H., Buring, J. E., and Mayrent, S., 1984, Smoking, aging and coronary heart disease, in: *Smoking and Aging* (R. Bosse and C. Rose, eds.), D. C. Heath, Lexington, Massachusetts, pp. 117–129.

Hennekens, C. H., Peto, R., Hutchison, G. B., and Doll, R., 1988, An overview of the British and American aspirin studies (Letter to the editor), *N. Engl. J. Med.* **318**:923–924.

ISIS-2 Collaborative Group, 1988, Randomised trial of intravenous streptokinase and/or oral aspirin in acute myocardial infarction: ISIS-2, *Lancet* **2**:349–360.

Moncada, S., and Vane, J. R., 1979, Arachidonic acid metabolites and the interactions between platelets and blood-vessel walls, *N. Engl. J. Med.* **300**:1142–1147.

Peto, R., Yusuf, S., and Collins, R., 1985, Cholesterol-lowering trial results in their epidemiologic context, in: *Fifty-eighth Scientific Sessions, American Heart Association, November, 1985* (abst.).

Peto, R., Gray, R., Collins, R., Wheatley, K., Hennekens, C., Jamrozik, K., Warlow, C., Hafner, B., Thompson, E., Norton, S., Gilliland, J., and Doll, R., 1988, A randomised trial of the effects of prophylactic daily aspirin among male British doctors, *Br. Med. J.* **296**:313–316.

Stampfer, M. J., Jakubowski, J. A., Deykin, D., Schafer, A. I., Willett, W. C., and Hennekens, C. H., 1986, Effect of alternate-day regular and enteric-coated aspirin on platelet aggregation, bleeding time, and thromboxane A_2 levels in bleeding-time blood, *Am. J. Med.* **81**:400–404.

Steering Committee of the Physicians' Health Study Research Group, 1988, Preliminary Report: Findings from the aspirin component of the ongoing Physicians' Health Study, *N. Engl. J. Med.* **318**:262–264.

UK–TIA Study Group, 1988, United Kingdom transient ischaemic attack (UK–TIA) aspirin trial interim results, *Br. Med. J.* **296**:316–320.

Participants

L. ABEL • Department of Cell Biology, Weizmann Institute of Science, Rehovot, Israel 76100

CARMELA R. ABRAHAM • Department of Neurobiology, Harvard Medical School, Boston, Massachusetts 02115. *Present address:* Arthritis Center, Boston University School of Medicine, Boston, Massachusetts 02118

G. N. ABRAHAM • Departments of Medicine, and Microbiology and Immunology, and Clinical Immunology Unit, University of Rochester School of Medicine and Dentistry, Rochester, New York 14642

OLAF ADAM • Medical Polyclinic, University of Munich, D-8000 Munich, Federal Republic of Germany

JOSEPH F. ALBRIGHT • Department of Microbiology, George Washington University School of Medicine, Washington, D.C. 20037

JULIA W. ALBRIGHT • Department of Microbiology, George Washington University School of Medicine, Washington, D.C. 20037

CAROLYN M. ALDWIN • Normative Aging Study, Veterans Administration Outpatient Clinic, Boston, Massachusetts 02108

DAVID AMINOFF • Institute of Gerontology, Department of Biological Chemistry, University of Michigan, Ann Arbor, Michigan 48109-2007

PETER J. ANDERSON • Department of Biochemistry, University of Ottawa, Ottawa, Ontario K1H 8M5, Canada

ROBERT J. ANDERSON • Department of Medicine, University of Colorado Health Science Center and VA Hospital, Denver, Colorado 80220

GARY W. ARENDASH • Department of Biology, University of South Florida, Tampa, Florida 33620

PAOLO BAMBERGA • Institute of Internal Medicine, Infectious Disease, and Immunopathology, University of Milan, Padiglione Granelli Polyclinic Hospital, 20122 Milan, Italy

WILMA BARCELLINI • Institute of Internal Medicine, Infectious Disease, and Immunopathology, University of Milan, Padiglione Granelli Polyclinic Hospital, 20122 Milan, Italy

AVI BEN-ABRAHAM • American Cryonics Society, San Francisco, California 94102

D. BEN-MENAHEM • Department of Cell Biology, Weizmann Institute of Science, Rehovot, Israel 76100

RICHARD N. BERGMAN • Department of Physiology and Biophysics, University of Southern California Medical School, Los Angeles, California 90033

CONSTANTIN A. BONA • Department of Microbiology, Mount Sinai School of Medicine, New York, New York 10037

FRANCISCO A. BONILLA • Department of Microbiology, Mount Sinai School of Medicine, New York, New York 10037

MARIA ORIETTA BORGHI • Institute of Internal Medicine, Infectious Disease, and Immunopathology, University of Milan, Padiglione Granelli Polyclinic Hospital, 20122 Milan, Italy

MATTHEWS O. BRADLEY • Department of Safety Assessment, Merck Institute for Therapeutic Research, West Point, Pennsylvania 19486

ELAINE BRESNAHAN • Gerontology Research Center, National Institute on Aging, National Institutes of Health, Baltimore, Maryland 21224

JACOB A. BRODY • School of Public Health, University of Illinois at Chicago, Chicago, Illinois 60680

NIAN-SHENG CAI • Departments of Biological Sciences and Chemistry, Illinois State University, Normal, Illinois 61761

FRANCESCO CAVAZZUTI • Department of Geriatric Medicine, Malpighi Hospital USL 28, 40138 Bologna, Italy

H. TAK CHEUNG • Departments of Biological Sciences and Chemistry, Illinois State University, Normal, Illinois 61761

MARIELLA CHIRICOLO • Department of Experimental Pathology, University of Bologna, 40126 Bologna, Italy

PAUL B. CHRETIEN • Department of Surgery, University of Maryland Hospital, Baltimore, Maryland 21201

GEORGE A. CLARK • Normative Aging Study, Veterans Administration Outpatient Clinic, Boston, Massachusetts 02108

MARIGRAZIA CLERICI • Institute of Internal Medicine, University of Milan, 20122 Milan, Italy

QUINTINA B. CORTEZA • Division of Nephrology, University of Maryland Hospital, Baltimore, Maryland 21201

CARL W. COTMAN • Departments of Psychobiology, Neurology, and Psychiatry, University of California–Irvine, Irvine, California 92717

JOZSEF CSONGOR • First Department of Medicine, University Medical School of Debrecen, 4012 Debrecen, Hungary

BARBARA J. DAVIS • Department of Neurology, University of Rochester School of Medicine and Dentistry, Rochester, New York 14642

ALBERTO DEGRASSI • Institute of Clinical Medicine and Gastroenterology, St. Orsola University Hospital, 40138 Bologna, Italy; Institute Rizzoli, University of Bologna, 40136 Bologna, Italy

MARIAN C. DIAMOND • Department of Integrative Biology, University of California–Berkeley, Berkeley, California 94720

MARK A. DILLINGHAM • Department of Medicine, University of Colorado Health Science Center, and VA Hospital, Denver, Colorado 80220

GINO DORIA • Laboratory of Pathology, C.R.E. ENEA, Casaccia, Rome, Italy

J. M. EDINGTON • Department of Pathology, New York University Medical Center, New York, New York 10016

R. EREN • Department of Cell Biology, Weizmann Institute of Science, Rehovot, Israel 76100

WILLIAM B. ERSHLER • Section of Geriatrics and Gerontology, Department of Medicine, University of Wisconsin–Madison, and William S. Middleton VA Hospital, Madison, Wisconsin 53706

NICOLA FABRIS • Gerontology Research Department, Italian National Research Center on Aging, 60100 Ancona, Italy

ANDREA FACCHINI • Institute of Clinical Medicine and Gastroenterology, St. Orsola University Hospital, 40138 Bologna, Italy; and Institute Rizzoli, University of Bologna, 40136 Bologna, Italy

GIANNI FERRARO • Institute of Internal Medicine, Infectious Disease, and Immunopathology, University of Milan, Padiglione Granelli Polyclinic Hospital, 20122 Milan, Italy

GABRIELLA FORIS • First Department of Medicine, University Medical School of Debrecen, 4012 Debrecen, Hungary

DANIELA FRASCA • Laboratory of Pathology, C.R.E. ENEA, Casaccia, Rome, Italy

E. FRIEDMAN • Division of Neurochemistry, Departments of Psychiatry and Pharmacology, Medical College of Pennsylvania, Philadelphia, Pennsylvania 19129

BARBARA G. FROSCHER • Department of Immunology, Scripps Clinic and Research Foundation, La Jolla, California 92037

TAMÀS FÜLÖP, JR. • First Department of Medicine, University of Medical School of Debrecen, 4012 Debrecen, Hungary

RUTH GABIZON • Department of Neurology, University of California–San Francisco, San Francisco, California 94143-0518

D. CARLETON GAJDUSEK • Laboratory of Central Nervous System Studies, National Institute of Neurological Disorders and Stroke, National Institutes of Health, Bethesda, Maryland 20892

C. JOSEPH GIBBS, JR. • Laboratory of Central Nervous System Studies, National Institute of Neurological Disorders and Stroke, National Institutes of Health, Bethesda, Maryland 20892

GEORGE G. GLENNER • Department of Pathology, University of California–San Diego, School of Medicine, La Jolla, California 92093

A. GLOBERSON • Department of Cell Biology, Weizmann Institute of Science, Rehovot, Israel 76100

A. M. GOATE • Department of Biochemistry and Molecular Genetics, St. Mary's Hospital Medical School, Norfolk Place, London W2 1PG, England

EDMOND A. GOIDL • Department of Microbiology and Immunology, School of Medicine, University of Maryland at Baltimore, Baltimore, Maryland 21021

H. S. GOLDSMITH • Department of Surgery, Boston University School of Medicine, Boston, Massachusetts 02118

ALLAN L. GOLDSTEIN • George Washington University Medical Center, Washington, D.C. 20037

P. D. GOREVIC • Clinical Allergy and Rheumatology Unit, Department of Medicine, State University of New York at Stony Brook, Stony Brook, New York 11794

SUSAN R. S. GOTTESMAN • Department of Pathology, New York University Medical Center, New York, New York 10016

STEFAN GRAVENSTEIN • Division of Hematology, Department of Medicine, University of Wisconsin–Madison, Madison, Wisconsin 53706

MONICA GRAZIOLI • Institute of Internal Medicine, University of Milan, 20122 Milan, Italy

DARLENE GROTH • Department of Neurology, University of California–San Francisco, San Francisco, California 94143-0518

BHUPENDRA KISHORE GUPTA • Department of Anatomical Sciences and Neurobiology, University of Louisville School of Medicine, Louisville, Kentucky 40292

MADI GUPTA • Department of Anatomical Sciences and Neurobiology, University of Louisville School of Medicine, Louisville, Kentucky 40292

NICHOLAS R. HALL • Department of Psychiatry and Behavioral Medicine, and Center of Psychoimmunology, University of South Florida Medical College, Tampa, Florida 33613

ROBERT W. HAMILL • Department of Neurology, University of Rochester School of Medicine and Dentistry, Rochester, New York 14642

J. A. HARDY • Department of Biochemistry and Molecular Genetics, St. Mary's Hospital Medical School, London W2 1PG, England

A. R. HAYNES • Department of Biochemistry and Molecular Genetics, St. Mary's Hospital Medical School, London W2 1PG, England

CHARLES H. HENNEKENS • Departments of Medicine and Preventive Medicine, Harvard Medical School, and Brigham and Women's Hospital, Brookline, Massachusetts 02146

KATSUIKU HIROKAWA • Department of Pathology, Tokyo Metropolitan Institute of Gerontology, 35-2, Sakaecho, Itabashi-ku, Tokyo 173, Japan

DONALD K. INGRAM • Molecular Physiology and Genetics Section, Laboratory of Cellular and Molecular Biology, Gerontology Research Center, National Institute on Aging, National Institutes of Health, Francis Scott Key Medical Center, Baltimore, Maryland 21224

MARIE-PAULE JACOB • Laboratory of the Biochemistry of Connective Tissue, CNRS UA 1174, Faculty of Medicine, University of Paris–Val de Marne, 94010 Créteil, France

L. A. JAMES • Department of Biochemistry and Molecular Genetics, St. Mary's Hospital Medical School, London W2 1PG, England

THOMAS E. JOHNSON • Department of Molecular Biology and Biochemistry, University of California–Irvine, Irvine, California 92717. *Present address:* Institute for Behavioral Genetics, University of Colorado, Boulder, Colorado 80309

G. JONES • Departments of Medicine, and Microbiology and Immunology, and Clinical Immunology Unit, University of Rochester School of Medicine and Dentistry, Rochester, New York 14642

JOHN JOSSELSON • Division of Nephrology, University of Maryland Hospital, Baltimore, Maryland 21201

MICHIYUKI KASAI • Department of Pathology, Tokyo Metropolitan Institute of Gerontology, 35-2, Sakaecho, Itabashi-ku, Tokyo 173, Japan

AZAD KAUSHIK • Department of Microbiology, Mount Sinai School of Medicine, New York, New York 10037

MARGUERITE M. B. KAY • Departments of Medicine, and Medical Biochemistry and Genetics, and Medical Microbiology and Immunology, Texas A&M University, and Teague Veterans Center, Temple, Texas 76504

E. KENEDI • Department of Chemical Pathology, School of Pathology, Medical School, University of the Witwatersrand, and The South African Institute for Medical Research, Johannesburg 2000, Republic of South Africa

YOUNG TAI KIM • Department of Medicine, Cornell University Medical College, New York, New York 10021

NORMAN R. KLINMAN • Department of Immunology, Scripps Clinic and Research Foundation, La Jolla, California 92037

RAJABATHER KRISHNARAJ • Division of Geriatric Medicine, Department of Medicine, College of Medicine, University of Illinois at Chicago, Chicago, Illinois 60612; and Center on Aging/Northwestern University, McGaw Medical Center, Chicago, Illinois 60611

DAVID KRITCHEVSKY • Wistar Institute of Anatomy and Biology, Philadelphia, Pennsylvania 19104

R. A. KYLE • Department of Medicine, Clinical Immunology Unit, Mayo School of Medicine, Mayo Clinic, Rochester, Minnesota 55905

CHRISTOPHER S. LANGE • Department of Radiation Oncology, SUNY Health Science Center at Brooklyn, Brooklyn, New York 11203

JOHN C. LAROSA • Lipid Research Clinic, George Washington University School of Medicine and Health Sciences, Washington, D.C. 20037

ANDRÀS LEOVEY • First Department of Medicine, University Medical School of Debrecen, 4012 Debrecen, Hungary

FEDERICO LICASTRO • Department of Experimental Pathology, University of Bologna, 40126 Bologna, Italy

PHYLLIS-JEAN LINTON • Department of Immunology, Scripps Clinic and Research Foundation, La Jolla, California 92037

SUSAN J. MARTIN McEVOY • Department of Microbiology and Immunology, School of Medicine, University of Maryland at Baltimore, Baltimore, Maryland 21201

MICHAEL P. McKINLEY • Department of Neurology, University of California–San Francisco, San Francisco, California 94143-0518

THOMAS H. McNEILL • Department of Neurology, University of Rochester School of Medicine and Dentistry, Rochester, New York 14642. *Present address:* Andrus Gerontology Center, University of Southern California, Los Angeles, California 90089

CAMILLO MANCINI • Laboratory of Pathology, C.R.E. ENEA, Casaccia, Rome, Italy

FRANCESCO ANTONIO MANZOLI • Institute of Normal Human Anatomy, University of Bologna, 40138 Bologna, Italy

ADRIANA RITA MARIANI • Institute of Normal Human Anatomy, University of Bologna, 40138 Bologna, Italy

ERMINIA MARIANI • Institute Rizzoli, University of Bologna, 40136 Bologna, Italy; and Institute of Clinical Medicine and Gastroenterology, St. Orsola University Hospital, 40138 Bologna, Italy

PETER J. MAYER • Department of Radiation Oncology, SUNY Health Science Center at Brooklyn, Brooklyn, New York 11203

D. MENDELSOHN • Department of Chemical Pathology, School of Pathology, Medical School, University of the Witwatersrand, and The South African Institute for Medical Research, Johannesburg 2000, Republic of South Africa

PIER LUIGI MERONI • Institute of Internal Medicine, Infectious Disease, and Immunopathology, University of Milan, Padiglione Granelli Polyclinic Hospital, 20122 Milan, Italy

EDWIN M. MEYER • Department of Pharmacology and Therapeutics, College of Medicine, University of Florida, Gainesville, Florida 32610

WILLIAM J. MILLARD • Department of Pharmacodynamics, College of Pharmacy, University of Florida, Gainesville, Florida 32610

VALERY T. MILLER • Lipid Research Clinic, George Washington University School of Medicine and Health Sciences, Washington, D.C. 20037

EUGENIO MOCCHEGIANI • Gerontology Research Department, Italian National Research Center on Aging, 60100 Ancona, Italy

RICHARD A. MUESING • Lipid Research Clinic, George Washington University School of Medicine and Health Sciences, Washington, D.C. 20037

M. J. MULLAN • Department of Neurology, St. Mary's Hospital Medical School, London W2 1PG, England

MARIO MUZZIOLI • Gerontology Research Department, Italian National Research Center on Aging, 60100 Ancona, Italy

PIRUZ NAHREINI • Division of Hematology and Oncology, Departments of Medicine, Microbiology and Immunology, Indiana University School of Medicine, Indianapolis, Indiana 46202

WARREN W. NICHOLS • Department of Safety Assessment, Merck Institute for Therapeutic Research, West Point, Pennsylvania 19486

ALEXANDER P. OSMAND • Department of Medicine, University of Tennessee Medical Center, Knoxville, Tennessee 37920

M. J. OWEN • Department of Biochemistry and Molecular Genetics, St. Mary's Hospital Medical School, London W2 1PG, England

MOHAMMAD A. PAHLAVANI • Departments of Biological Sciences and Chemistry, Illinois State University, Normal, Illinois 61761

STEFANO PAPA • Institute of Normal Human Anatomy, University of Bologna, 40138 Bologna, Italy

A. PERL • Departments of Medicine, and Microbiology and Immunology, and Clinical Immunology Unit, University of Rochester School of Medicine and Dentistry, Rochester, New York 14642

CHRISTINE PETERSON • Department of Psychobiology, University of California–Irvine, Irvine, California 92717

HUNTINGTON POTTER • Department of Neurobiology, Harvard Medical School, Boston, Massachusetts 02115

JENNIFER J. POULAKOS • Department of Pharmacology and Therapeutics, College of Medicine, University of Florida, Gainesville, Florida 32610

GORDON D. POWERS • Department of Immunology, Scripps Clinic and Research Foundation, La Jolla, California 92037

MAURO PROVINCIALI • Gerontology Research Department, Italian National Research Center on Aging, 60100 Ancona, Italy

STANLEY B. PRUSINER • Departments of Neurology and Biochemistry and Biophysics, University of California–San Francisco, San Francisco, California 94143-0518

ARLAN RICHARDSON • Departments of Biological Sciences and Chemistry, Illinois State University, Normal, Illinois 61761

SYLVIA C. RILEY • Department of Immunology, Scripps Clinic and Research Foundation, La Jolla, California 92037

LADISLAS ROBERT • Laboratory of the Biochemistry of Connective Tissue, CNRS UA 1174, Faculty of Medicine, University of Paris–Val de Marne, 94010 Créteil, France

PATRIZIA RODA • Institute Rizzoli, University of Bologna, 40136 Bologna, Italy; and

Institute of Clinical Medicine and Gastroenterology, St. Orsola University Hospital, 40138 Bologna, Italy

P. ROQUES • Department of Neurology, St. Mary's Hospital Medical School, London W2 1PG, England

M. N. ROSSOR • Department of Neurology, St. Mary's Hospital Medical School, London W2 1PG, England

GEORGE S. ROTH • Molecular Physiology and Genetics Section, Gerontology Research Center, National Institute on Aging, National Institutes of Health, Francis Scott Key Medical Center, Baltimore, Maryland 21224

JOHN H. SADLER • Division of Nephrology, University of Maryland Hospital, Baltimore, Maryland 21201

AFRO SALSI • Department of Geriatric Medicine, Malpighi Hospital USL 28, 40138 Bologna, Italy

GABRIELE SARTI • Department of Geriatric Medicine, Malpighi Hospital USL 28, 40138 Bologna, Italy

GIANCARLO SAVORANI • Department of Geriatric Medicine, Malpighi Hospital USL 28, 40138 Bologna, Italy

ROBERT M. SCHMIDT • Health Watch Program, Center for Preventive Medicine and Health Research, Pacific Presbyterian Medical Center and San Francisco State University, San Francisco, California 94132-1789

RISE SCHWAB • Department of Medicine, Cornell University Medical College, New York, New York 10021

PAUL E. SEGALL • Trans Time Inc., Oakland, California 94603

STEVE Y. SHEN • Division of Nephrology, University of Maryland Hospital, Baltimore, Maryland 21201. *Present address:* Division of Nephrology, Maryland General Hospital, Baltimore, Maryland 21201

MARCO SINOPPI • Institute of Recovery and Cure of Giovanni XXIII, 40133 Bologna, Italy

GREGORY W. SISKIND • Department of Medicine, Cornell University Medical College, New York, New York 10021

ARUN SRIVASTAVA • Division of Hematology and Oncology, Departments of Medicine, Microbiology and Immunology, Indiana University School of Medicine, Indianapolis, Indiana 46202

PATRIZIA STEFANONI • Institute of Internal Medicine, University of Milan, 20122 Milan, Italy

R. CLAYTON STEINER • George Washington University Medical Center, Washington, D.C. 20037

HAL STERNBERG • Department of Physiology and Anatomy, University of California–Berkeley, Berkeley, California 94720; and Trans Time Inc., Oakland, California 94603

ROBERT C. SWITZER III • Department of Pathology, University of Tennessee Medical Center, Knoxville, Tennessee 37920

SÀNDOR SZUCS • First Department of Medicine, University Medical School of Debrecen, 4012 Debrecen, Hungary

ROBERT D. TERRY • Department of Neurosciences, School of Medicine, University of California–San Diego, La Jolla, California 92093

J. C. de la TORRE • Division of Neurosurgery, University of Ottawa Health Sciences, Ottawa, Ontario K1H 8M5, Canada

GIUSEPPE TUCCI • Department of Geriatric Medicine, Malpighi Hospital USL 28, 40138 Bologna, Italy

MASANORI UTSUYAMA • Department of Pathology, Tokyo Metropolitan Institute of Gerontology, 35-2, Sakaecho, Itabashi-ku, Tokyo 173, Japan

RENÉ VAN DE GRIEND • Radiobiological Institute, TNO, 2280 HV Rijswijk, The Netherlands

ZSUZSA VARGA • First Department of Medicine, University Medical School of Debrecen, 4012 Debrecen, Hungary

CARLO VERGANI • Institute of Internal Medicine, University of Milan, 20122 Milan, Italy

ALESSANDRO VISMARA • Institute of Internal Medicine, Infectious Disease, and Immunopathology, University of Milan, Padiglione Granelli Polyclinic Hospital 20122, Milan, Italy

MARCO VITALE • Institute of Normal Human Anatomy, University of Bologna, 40138 Bologna, Italy

HAROLD WAITZ • Trans Time Inc., Oakland, California 94603

H.-Y. WANG • Division of Neurochemistry, Departments of Psychiatry and Pharmacology, Medical College of Pennsylvania, Philadelphia, Pennsylvania 19129

RICHARD WEINDRUCH • Biomedical Research and Clinical Medicine Program, National Institute on Aging, National Institutes of Health, Bethesda, Maryland 20892

PETER WEISWEILER • Metabolic Research Munich, D-8000 Munich 5, Federal Republic of Germany

MARC E. WEKSLER • Department of Medicine, Cornell University Medical College, New York, New York 10021

GEORGE Z. WILLIAMS • Health Watch Program, Center for Preventive Medicine and Health Research, Pacific Presbyterian Medical Center and San Francisco State University, San Francisco, California 94132-1789

J. M. WILLIAMS • Departments of Medicine, and Microbiology and Immunology, and Clinical Immunology Unit, University of Rochester School of Medicine and Dentistry, Rochester, New York 14642

R. WILLIAMSON • Department of Biochemistry and Molecular Genetics, St. Mary's Hospital Medical School, London W2 1PG, England

PATRICIA D. WILSON • Department of Physiology and Biophysics, UMNJ–Robert Wood Johnson (formerly Rutgers) Medical School, Piscataway, New Jersey 08854

MEIWEN WU • Health Watch Program, Center for Preventive Medicine and Health Research, Pacific Presbyterian Medical Center and San Francisco State University, San Francisco, California 94132-1789

LUCIO ZANICHELLI • Department of Geriatric Medicine, Malpighi Hospital USL 28, 40138 Bologna, Italy

CARLO ZANUSSI • Institute of Internal Medicine, Infectious Disease, and Immunopathology, University of Milan, Padiglione Granelli Polyclinic Hospital, 20122 Milan, Italy

DORITH ZHARHARY • Department of Immunology, Scripps Clinic and Research Foundation, La Jolla, California 92037

DONATO ZOCCHI • Institute of Recovery and Cure of Giovanni XXIII, 40133 Bologna, Italy

Index

A68 protein in Alzheimer's disease, 111
Acetylcholine deficiency in Alzheimer's disease, 110
Adeno-associated virus replication in fibroblasts, 98–105
Adenovirus 2 replication in fibroblasts, 90–98
Adenylate cyclase in renal collecting ducts, response to vasopressin in aging, 291–295
Adrenal tyrosine hydroxylase activity, dietary restriction affecting, 285, 288–289
Adrenergic receptors in parotid glands, activity of, 143, 222
age-1 gene activity, 46–48
Age-dependent conditions, 138, 141
Age-related conditions, 138–141
Agmatine in temporal cortex, in Alzheimer's disease, 487
Alzheimer's disease
  as age-dependent condition, 138
  amyloid gene expression in, 5–6, 40
  amyloid β-protein in, 51–59, 76
  α_1-antichymotrypsin in amyloid deposits, 76–85
    expression in specific brain areas, 78–82
  chromosome 21 in, 40, 41
  and Down's syndrome, 40, 51
  and effects of cerebral cortical cholinergic hypofunction, 491–495
  FAD marker in, 58
  immunochemical markers in, 111
  lactoferrin immunoreactivity in, 109–122
  mitogen response of lymphocytes in, 128, 130
  molecular genetics of, 39–41
  neuritic plaques in, 5–6, 7, 25, 56–57, 76, 110–111
    biochemical properties of, 110
    distribution of, 110
    lactoferrin immunoreactivity with, 114

Alzheimer's disease (*cont.*)
  neurofibrillary tangles in, 110–111
  neuronal populations in, 110, 439
  olfactory tract pathology in, 112, 121
  and polyamines in temporal cortex, 485–489
  proteolytic enzyme defect in, 59
  regional pathology in, 111–112
  subtypes of, 126
  synapse replacement in, 503–504
  thymulin levels in, 127–128, 130
  zinc levels in, 127–128, 130
cAMP
  and action of vasopressin in renal collecting ducts, 293–294
  aging affecting, in cells, 188, 222
Amygdaloid nucleus measurements in aging, 444–445
Amyloid in brain, 3–15
  α_1-antichymotrypsin in, 76–85
  in congophilic angiopathy with hemorrhage, 55, 56, 83
  formation from precursor protein, 4–6, 110
  gene expression in Alzheimer's disease, 5–6, 40
  mineral deposits affecting, 11
  in neuritic plaques in Alzheimer's disease, 5–6, 7, 25, 56–57, 76, 110–111
  in prion disorders, 25
  two forms of, 6–8
Amyloid β-protein
  in Alzheimer's disease, 51–59, 76
  association with α_1-antichymotrypsin, 84–85
  gene localization on chromosome 21, 5, 57–58, 83
  precursor protein, 57–58, 76
  purification and analysis of, 52–55
Amyloidotic polyneuropathy, familial, variant prealbumin in, 57, 84